GLAUCOMA

GLAUCOMA

Associate Editors
PAUL L. KAUFMAN, MD
Professor of Ophthalmology
University of Wisconsin Medical School
Madison, WI

THOMAS W. MITTAG, PhD
Research Professor of Ophthalmology
Mt. Sinai School of Medicine
New York, NY

VOLUME 7

TEXTBOOK OF OPHTHALMOLOGY

EDITED BY
STEVEN M. PODOS, MD, FACS
Professor and Chairman
Department of Ophthalmology
Mt. Sinai School of Medicine
New York, NY

MYRON YANOFF, MD, FACS
Professor and Chairman
Department of Ophthalmology
Hahnemann University
Philadelphia, PA

Mosby
London St. Louis Baltimore Boston Chicago Philadelphia Sydney Toronto

For full details of all Mosby-Year Book Europe Limited titles, please write to Mosby-Year Book Europe Limited, Lynton House, 7–12 Tavistock Square, London, WC1H 9LB, England.

LIBRARY OF CONGRESS CATALOGING-IN-PUBLICATION DATA
(Revised for vol. 7)

Textbook of ophthalmology.

Includes bibliographical references and index.
Contents: v. 1. Optics and refraction / David Miller—
v. 2. The uvea / Narsing A. Rao, David J. Forster, James J. Augsburger—[etc.]—
v. 7. Glaucoma / associate editors, Paul L. Kaufman, Thomas W. Mittag.
1. Ophthalmology. I. Podos, Steven M. II. Yanoff, Myron.
[DNLM: 1. Ophthalmology. WW 100 T355]
RE46.T26 1991 617.7 91-34425
ISBN 1-56375-011-2 (v. 1)

BRITISH LIBRARY CATALOGUING-IN-PUBLICATION DATA:
A catalogue record for this book is available from the British Library.

ISBN Volume 7: 1-56375-098-8
ISBN Set: 0-397-44692-6

10 9 8 7 6 5 4 3 2 1

Project Manager: DIMITRY POPOW
Editor: SHARON RULE
Art Director and Cover Design: KATHRYN GREENSLADE
Interior Design and Layout: JEFFREY S. BROWN, JENNIFER BERGAMINI
Illustrators: WENDY JACKELOW, KIMBERLEY CONNERS
Illustration Director: CAROL KALAFATIC

Originated in Hong Kong by Bright Arts, Ltd.
Produced by Imago Productions, Pte., Ltd.
Printed and bound in Singapore, 1994.

EDITORS' PREFACE

As we approach the twenty-first century it is apparent that the half-life of medical knowledge is continuing to shrink and the amount of current dogma is continuing to expand. Packaging today's relevant ophthalmic knowledge is a difficult chore, yet one that periodically demands doing. Every editor or author desires to accomplish this task in a new and unique fashion. This ten-volume series represents our vision of a *Textbook of Ophthalmology* for the 1990s: one that integrates the basic visual science and clinical information of each subspecialty in a separate volume that is edited or written by noted basic scientists and clinicians; one that is manageable, readable, and affordable for the ophthalmic expert as well as the neophyte; and one that contains original diagrams, figures, and photographs—all in full color—designed to depict the necessary knowledge we hope to impart.

We are grateful to our associate editors and authors for sharing their superb expertise in the compilation of this unique ophthalmic resourse, to our assistants Barbara Zoldessy and Roe Brennan for their unstinting efforts in organizing and coordinating this project, and to our wives Wendy Donn Podos and Karin L. Yanoff for their continued patience and encouragement throughout the many phases of this endeavor.

STEVEN M. PODOS, MD, FACS
DEPARTMENT OF OPHTHALMOLOGY
MT. SINAI SCHOOL OF MEDICINE
NEW YORK, NY

MYRON YANOFF, MD, FACS
DEPARTMENT OF OPHTHALMOLOGY
HAHNEMANN UNIVERSITY
PHILADELPHIA, PA

ASSOCIATE EDITORS' PREFACE

PAUL KAUFMAN, MD
DEPARTMENT OF OPTHALMOLOGY
UNIVERSITY OF WISCONSIN
CLINICAL SCIENCE CENTER
MADISON, WI

THOMAS MITTAG, PHD
DEPARTMENT OF OPTHALMOLOGY
MT. SINAI SCHOOL OF MEDICINE
NEW YORK, NY

Unlike most of the other volumes in this series, *Glaucoma* deals not with a specific ocular tissue, biophysical discipline, or bodily system, but rather with a disease family that necessitates integrating all of these approaches. Nonetheless, in keeping with the overall philosophy of the series, we have sought to encompass and integrate the basic biology and pathobiology of the tissues and physiologic processes with the clinical manifestations, diagnostic technologies, and therapeutic modalities relevant to this disease family. This required the cooperation of 43 authors, all of whom were timely with their contributions and gracious in consenting to our aggressive "mix and match" editing which led to truly joint ventures. We hope that this approach, combined with the publisher's unique, creative, and copious use of illustrative materials, will provide a natural and more easily understandable and assimilable flow of information than other currently available glaucoma texts.

Special thanks go to Bernadette Bull, PLK's unfailingly loyal and efficient secretary, who routinely wrests order from chaos, and to Dimitry Popow, our edtor, who stifled his own reservations to support and facilitate our concept of broad-based, multidisciplinary authorship despite the extra work it created for him.

DEDICATION

To Margaret, who understands why the balcony is *never* closed, and to Bianca, for her great understanding

CONTRIBUTORS

Ted S. Acott, MD
Associate Professor
Department of Ophthalmology
Department of Biochemistry and Molecular Biology
Oregon Health Sciences Center
Portland, Oregon

P. Juhani Airaksinen, MD
Professor and Chairman
Department of Ophthalmology
University of Oulu
Oulu, Finland

Anders Bill, MD
Professor and Chairman
Department of Physiology and Medical Biophysics
University of Uppsala
Uppsala, Sweden

Ivan Bodis-Wollner, MD
Professor
Division of Neurology
Department of Internal Medicine
University of Nebraska Medical Center
Omaha, Nebraska

Scott E. Brodie, MD, PhD
Assistant Professor
Department of Ophthalmology
Mount Sinai School of Medicine
New York, New York

Richard F. Brubaker, MD
Professor
Department of Ophthalmology
Mayo Clinic and Medical School
Rochester, Minnesota

Joseph Caprioli, MD
Professor
Department of Ophthalmology and Visual Science
Yale University School of Medicine
New Haven, Connecticut

Stephen M. Drance, MD
Professor
Department of Ophthalmology
University of British Columbia
Vancouver, BC, Canada

Anders Heijl, MD
Professor and Chairman
Department of Ophthalmology
Malmö General Hospital
Malmö, Sweden

M. Rosario Hernandez, DDS
Assistant Professor
Department of Ophthalmology
Harvard Medical School
Boston, Massachusetts

Jonathan Herschler, MD
Private Practice
Sheridan, Wyoming

John R. Hetherington, Jr., MD
Clinical Professor
Department of Ophthalmology
University of California Medical School
San Francisco, California

Eve Juliet Higginbotham, MD
Associate Professor of Ophthalmology
W.K. Kellogg Eye Center
University of Michigan
Ann Arbor, Michigan

Paul L. Kaufman, MD
Professor of Ophthalmology
University of Wisconsin Medical School
Madison, WI

Theodore Krupin, MD
Professor
Department of Ophthalmology
Northwestern University Medical School
Chicago, Illinois

Jeffrey Liebmann, MD
Clinical Assistant Professor of Ophthalmology
The New York Medical College
New York Eye and Ear Infirmary
New York, New York

Elke Lütjen-Drecoll, MD
Professor and Chairman
Department of Anatomy
University of Erlangen–Nürnberg
Erlangen, Germany

Wayne F. March, MD
Robertson-Poth Professor and Chairman
Department of Ophthalmology
The University of Texas Medical Branch at Galveston
Galveston, Texas

Thomas H. Maren, MD
Graduate Research Professor
Department of Pharmacology and Therapeutics
College of Medicine
University of Florida Health Science Center
Gainesville, Florida

Thomas W. Mittag, PhD
Research Professor
Department of Ophthalmology
Mt. Sinai School of Medicine
New York, NY

Siv F.E. Nilsson, PhD
Assistant Professor
Department of Physiology and Medical Biophysics
University of Uppsala
Uppsala, Sweden

Richard K. Parrish, MD
Associate Professor
Bascom Palmer Eye Institute
University of Miami School of Medicine
Miami, Florida

Todd W. Perkins, MD
Assistant Professor
Department of Ophthalmology
University of Wisconsin Medical School
Madison, Wisconsin

Lutz E. Pillunat, MD
Department of Ophthalmology
University of Ulm
New Ulm, Germany

Ronald L. Radius, MD
Professor
Department of Ophthalmology
Medical College of Wisconsin
Milwaukee, Wisconsin

Robert Ritch, MD, FACP
Professor
Clinical Ophthalmology
The New York Medical College
Chief, Glaucoma Service
New York Eye and Ear Infirmary
New York, New York

Johannes W. Rohen, MD
Professor Emeritus and Former Chairman
Department of Anatomy
University of Erlangen–Nürnberg
Erlangen, Germany

Lisa F. Rosenberg, MD
Assistant Professor
Department of Ophthalmology
Northwestern University Medical School
Chicago, Illinois

Jon M. Ruderman, MD
Associate Professor
Department of Ophthalmology
Northwestern University Medical School
Chicago, Illinois

Michael J. Sakamoto, MD
Private Practice
Sacramento Eye Care and Surgicenter
Sacramento, California

Bernard Schwartz, MD, PhD
Professor of Ophthalmology
Tufts University School of Medicine
Boston, Massachusetts

M. Bruce Shields, MD
Professor
Department of Ophthalmology
Duke University Medical Center
Durham, North Carolina

Gregory L. Skuta, MD
Clinical Associate Professor
Department of Ophthalmology
University of Oklahoma Medical School
The Dean A. McGee Eye Institute
Oklahoma City, Oklahoma

Barbara A. Smythe, MD
Private Practice
Ft. Worth, Texas

Robert L. Stamper, MD
Professor and Chairman
Department of Ophthalmology
Pacific University Medical Center
San Francisco, California

Richard Stodtmeister, MD
Professor
Department of Ophthalmology
University of Ulm
Neu Ulm, Germany

Anja Tuulonen, MD
Department of Ophthalmology
University of Oulu
Oulu, Finland

E. Michael Van Buskirk, MD
Chief and Chairman
Department of Ophthalmology
Legacy Portland Hospitals
Portland, Oregon

Robert N. Weinreb, MD
Professor
Department of Ophthalmology
University of California, San Diego
La Jolla, California

Jacob T. Wilensky, MD
Professor
Department of Ophthalmology
Eye and Ear Infirmary
University of Illinois Hospital and Clinics
Chicago, Illinois

Ruth D. Williams, MD
Private Practice
Wheaton Eye Clinic
Wheaton, Illinois

Martha M. Wright, MD
Department of Ophthalmology
University of Minnesota Medical School
Minneapolis, Minnesota

Alan H. Zalta, MD
Associate Professor
Department of Ophthalmology
University of Cincinnati Medical Center
Cincinnati, Ohio

CONTENTS

1 The Normal Anterior Segment

Section I

Anatomy of Aqueous Humor Formation and Drainage

E. Lütjen-Drecoll
J.W. Rohen

Aqueous humor is formed by the ciliary processes of the ciliary body (Figs. 1.1 and 1.2). It derives primarily from blood circulating in the capillaries of the ciliary processes. After having passed the two-layered ciliary epithelium the fluid enters the posterior chamber and reaches the anterior chamber by way of the pupil. In the chamber angle, aqueous humor modified by exchange with surrounding tissues, leaves the anterior chamber, mainly by

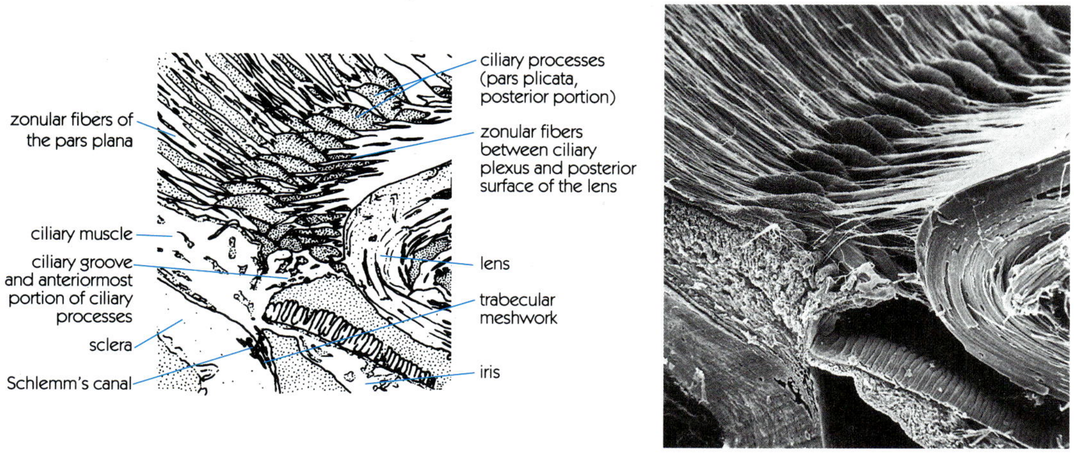

1.1 | Scanning electron micrograph of the ciliary body, zonular apparatus, lens and iris root (sagittal section, cynomolgus monkey, x50.) (After Rohen JW: Scanning electron microscopic studies of the zonular apparatus in human and monkey eyes. *Invest Ophthalmol Vis Sci 1979; 18:133–144.)*

way of Schlemm's canal, after having passed the trabecular meshwork. Schlemm's canal is connected by a number of collector channels to the intra- and episcleral venous network, so that the fluid finally reenters the bloodstream (Fig. 1.3).

MORPHOLOGY OF AQUEOUS INFLOW

The ciliary processes in which aqueous humor is formed are heavily vascularized. Each of the 70 to 80 processes contains a large number of capillaries which are supplied mainly by branches of the major arterial circle of the iris. Aqueous humor formation results from a combination of ultrafiltration in the ciliary process vasculature and the adjacent stromal layer and active, energy-requiring secretory processes within the ciliary epithelial lining. Aqueous secretion is a biological process subject to circadian rhythms.[1] The main site of aqueous secretion appears to be the part of the ciliary process that protrudes into the posterior chamber (see Fig. 1.1). The epithelium and the vasculature of the valleys between the processes, the posterior pars plicata, and the pars plana are so different from those of the protruding major ciliary processes that they probably serve different functions. From the standpoint of functional morphology, there are six different regions of the ciliary body (see Fig. 1.2):

1. The major ciliary processes protruding into the aqueous humor of the posterior chamber.
2. The anteriormost portion of the ciliary processes, formed by the anterior part of the major processes and their interprocess connections.
3. The posterior part of the pars plicata facing the vitreous body.

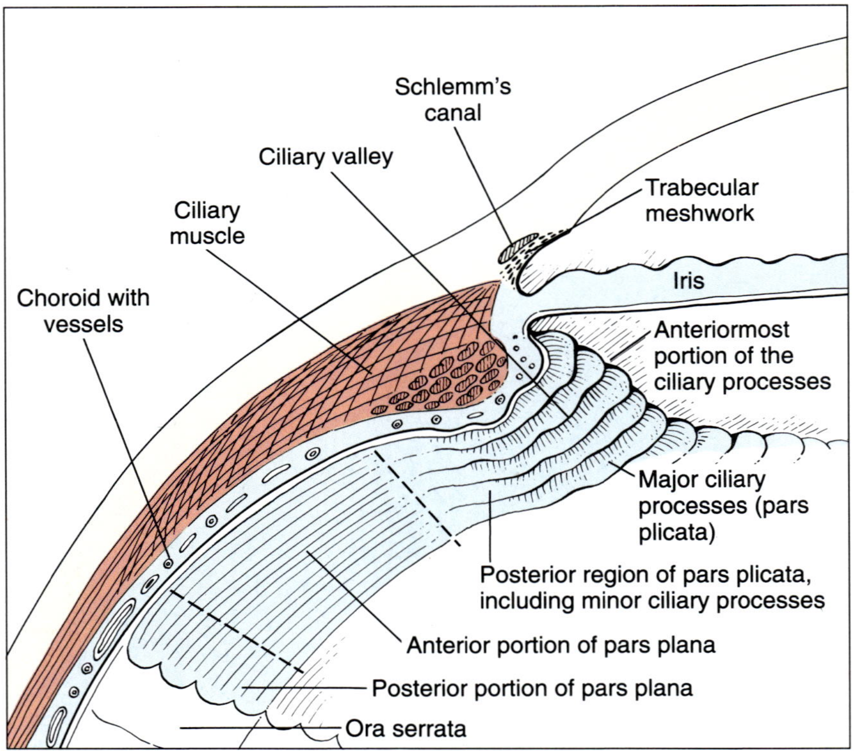

1.2 | Regions of the ciliary body.

4. The valleys between the major processes, in which the ciliary epithelium is covered by zonular fibers.
5. The anterior pars plana leading posteriorly towards the posterior tips of the ciliary muscle.
6. The posterior pars plana which reaches posteriorly nearly to the ora serrata.

CILIARY PROCESSES

THE MAJOR CILIARY PROCESSES (REGION 1)

The capillary network of the major ciliary processes is supplied by arterioles which derive from the major arterial circle of the iris located in the anterior region of the ciliary muscle or in the iris root. This circle is mainly formed by the two long posterior ciliary arteries, which run without branching along the temporal and nasal side of the eye, through choroid and ciliary muscle. In the latter, they divide into two main arteries bending in an equatorial direction.[2-4] Here, the perforating branches of the anterior ciliary arteries may join the circle, but these branches predominantly supply the ciliary muscle rather than the ciliary processes. The arterioles supplying the ciliary processes radiate from the major iris circle and enter the anterior portion of

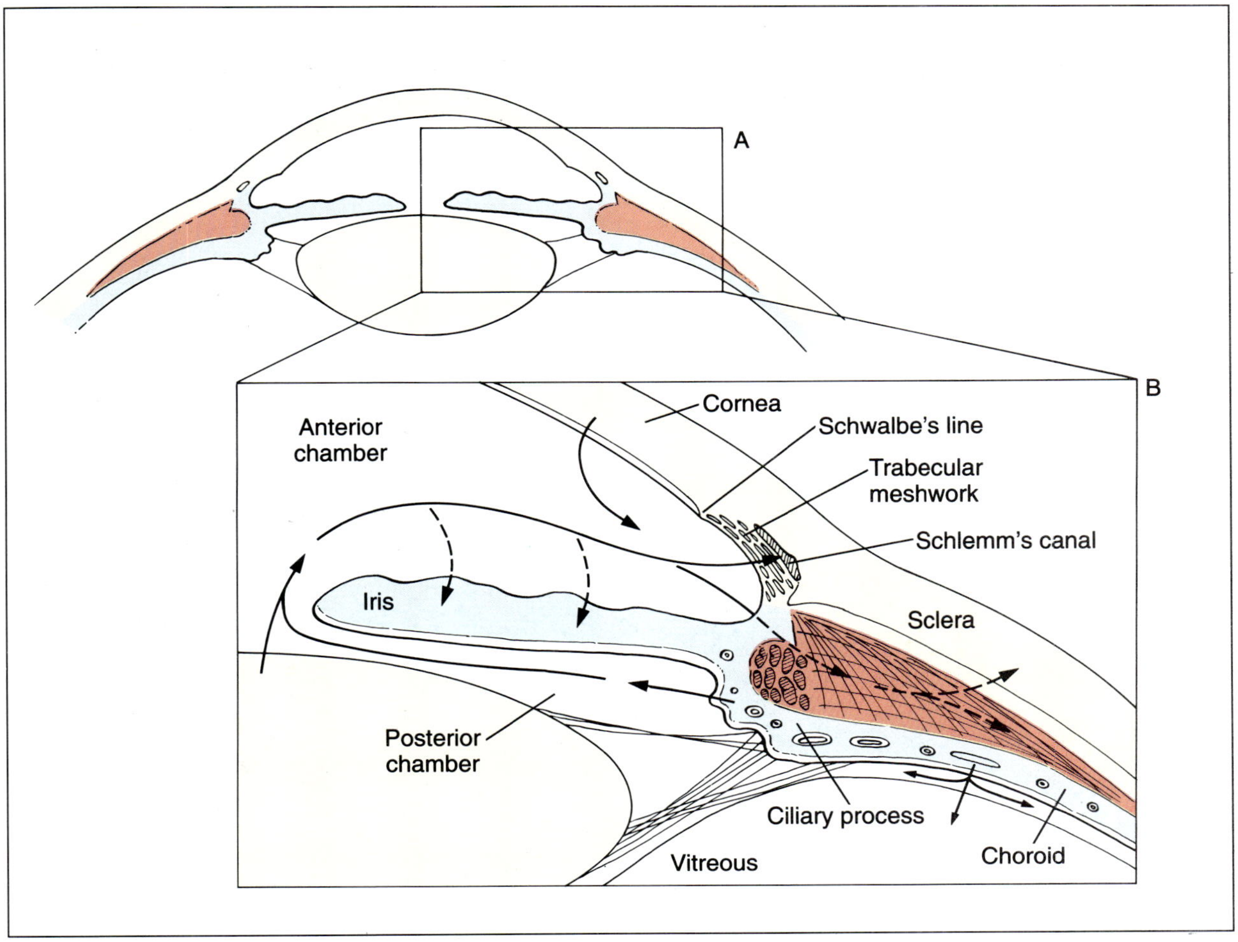

1.3 | *A:* Aqueous circulation system in the anterior eye segment. *B:* Higher magnification of the chamber structures outlined in *A* (the arrows show the direction of aqueous flow).

the processes. Subsequently, they split into tufts and form long capillaries which run in parallel and frequently anastomose with each other (Fig. 1.4). Usually, one larger capillary bends directly towards the margin of the process, where it forms the wide marginal venule that drains most of the ciliary process capillaries into the posterior pars plana veins (see Figs. 1.4 and 1.5). In scanning electron micrographs (SEM), the arterioles supplying the capillary network of the major processes often show localized constrictions, which represent sphincter-like segments of the terminal arterioles. The blood flow in the capillaries may be regulated by these sphincter-like structures.[3]

The marginal venule and the capillaries of the major ciliary processes are fenestrated and are rather highly permeable to protein.[5–7] The fenestrations in the endothelial lining are found mainly in the part of the capillary wall that faces the ciliary epithelium.[8] In primates, the fenestrated endothelium stains histochemically for the enzyme carbonic anhydrase (CA), like the fenestrated endothelium of other mucous membrane vessels.[9] The functional significance of the enzyme in this location is still not clear.

The *ciliary epithelium* consists of two layers. The inner layer is made up of nonpigmented columnar cells (NPE). Their basement membrane, termed the internal limiting membrane, faces the posterior chamber or the vitreous body. Apically, the cells are connected to the second or outer layer of the ciliary epithelium, which consists of pigmented, mainly cuboidal cells (PE), resting on a thin basal lamina and the connective tissue of the ciliary body stroma. During early development of the eye, the inner, nonpigmented cell layer becomes inverted so that the apices of the pigmented and nonpigmented cells are in contact with one another[7] (see Fig. 1.5).

In region 1 an elaborate system of membrane infoldings is developed at the basolateral surfaces of both the nonpigmented and the pigmented epithelium (Fig. 1.5). The enzymes Na,K-ATPase and CA are incorporated into these infoldings. The cytoplasm of the NPE contains a remarkable number of large mitochondria, which almost completely fill the basolateral portions of the PE and NPE cells adjacent to the membrane infoldings (Fig. 1.6). Therefore, these cells possess all the characteristics of cells involved in active, energy-dependent transport processes.

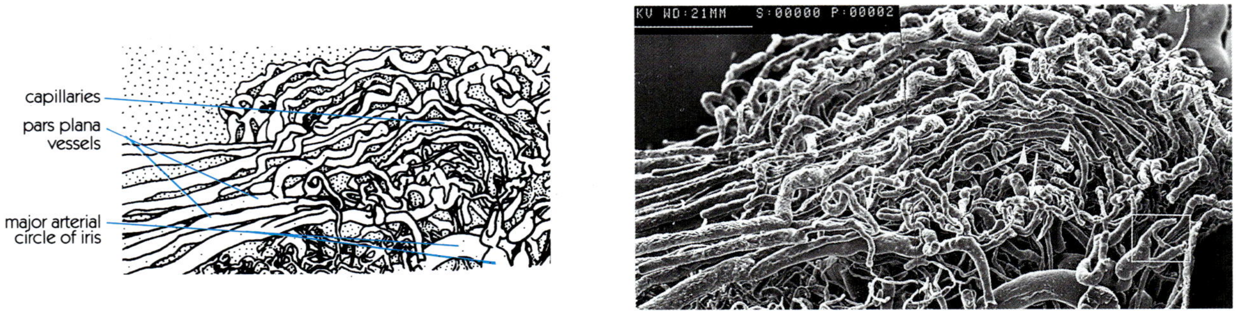

1.4 | Scanning electron micrograph of a resin cast of the ciliary body vasculature in the human eye (bar = 500 μm). The pars plana vessels appear on the left. Note the capillaries arranged in parallel in the major ciliary processes (arrows). Bottom right: major arterial circle of the iris. (From Funk R, Rohen JW: Functional morphology of the vasculature in the anterior eye segment, in Lütjen-Drecoll E, Rohen JW (eds): *Basic Aspects of Glaucoma Research,* Vol II. Stuttgart, New York: Schattauer Verlag, 1990, 179.)

Junctional Complexes and Fluid Transport

For directional fluid transport through the epithelial lining to occur, there must be differences between the apical and basal membranes of the cells, and adjacent cells of one layer must be connected to each other by tight junctions (zonulae occludentes). In the ciliary epithelium, tight junctions are

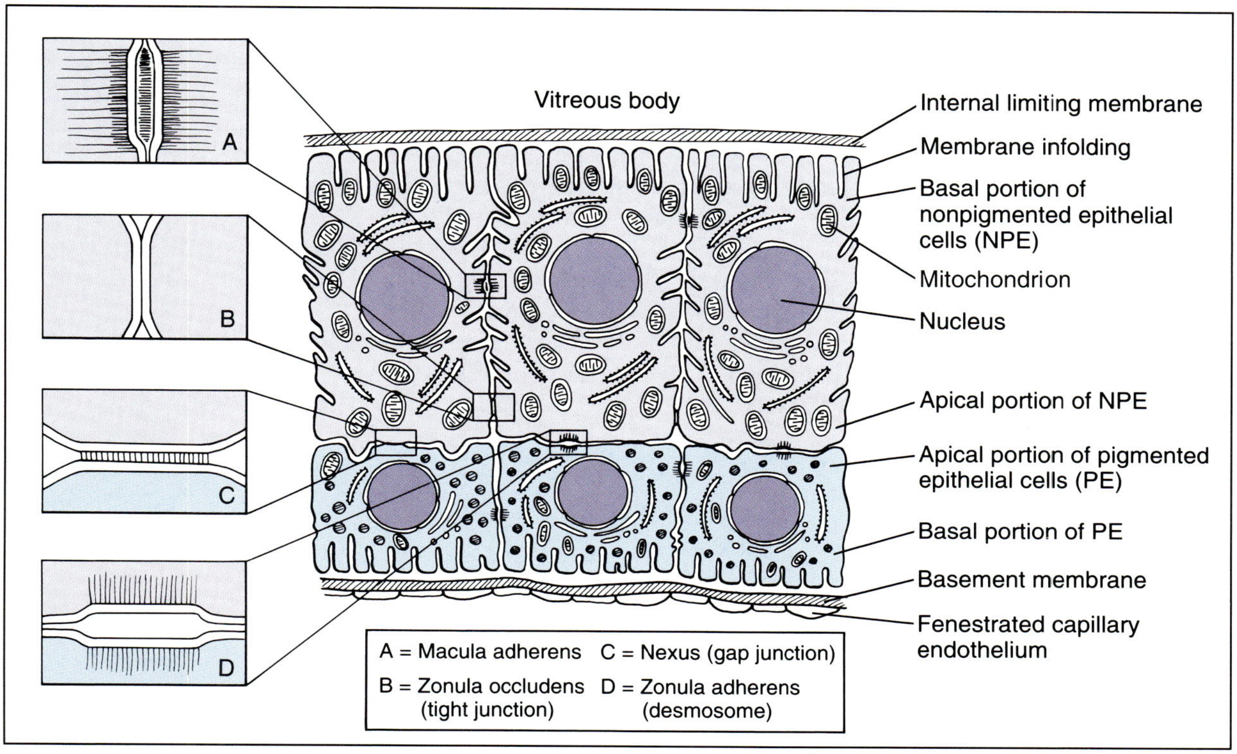

1.5 | Ultrastructure of the ciliary epithelium with different types of junctions.

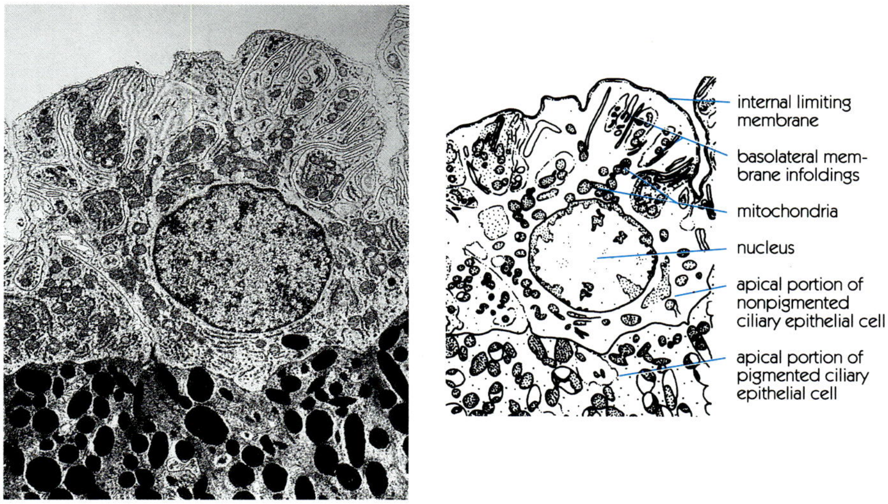

1.6 | Electron micrograph of the ciliary epithelium (x9,500).

located in the apical region of the NPE cells, but not between adjacent PE cells (see Fig. 1.5).

Because experimentally applied tracer substances, such as horseradish peroxidase, penetrate the intercellular spaces only up to the apical region of the NPE, these junctions are considered to be the main site of the blood–aqueous barrier.[10–13]

Sodium and other ions are actively pumped into the intercellular spaces of the NPE, building up an osmotic gradient. Water and small molecules follow this osmotic gradient and flow into the posterior chamber (Fig. 1.7). This flow takes place as long as the NPE cells are pumping sodium or other ions into the apical portion of the intercellular spaces. The internal limiting membrane presents no barrier to aqueous flow.

At the interface between the NPE and PE cell layer are many gap junctions (nexus).[5,6,14] These junctions allow exchange of ions between the coupled cell layers. It is possible that NPE and PE are electrically coupled to ensure coordination of the secretory activity.

Desmosomes, puncta, and maculae adherentes are intercellular junctions that serve mechanical functions. They are evenly distributed between the two cell layers or between the NPE cells in their basal portion (see Fig. 1.5).

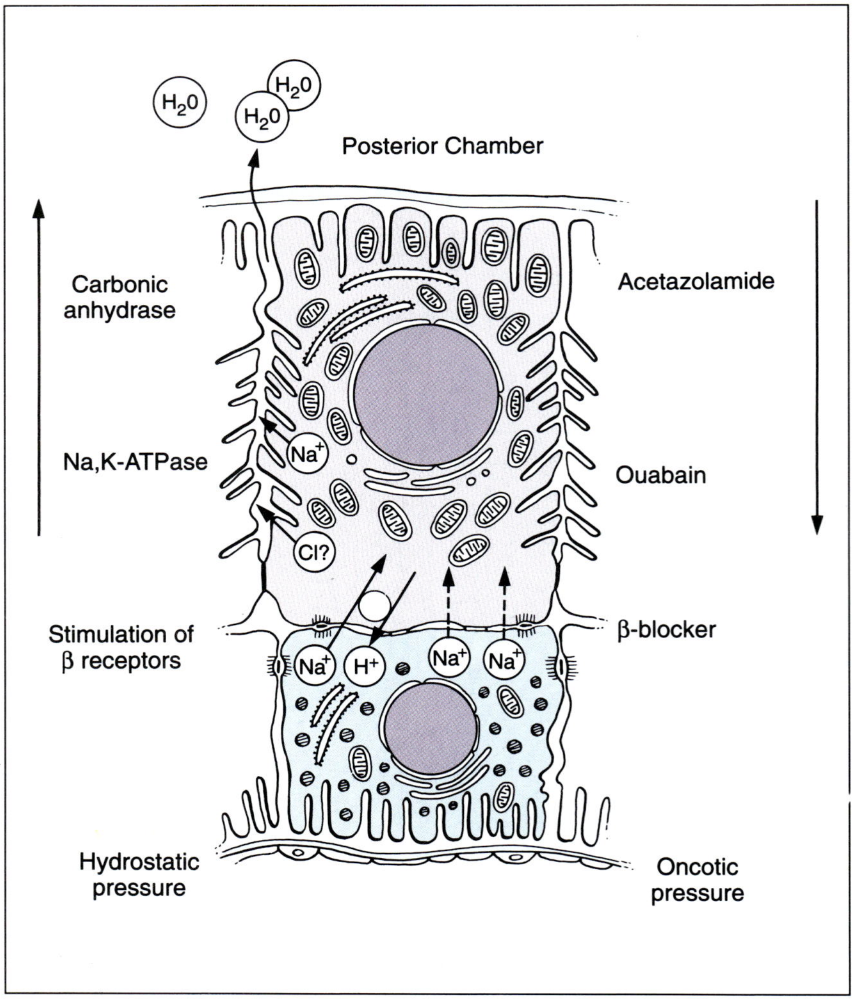

1.7 | Schematic drawing of the two-layered ciliary epithelium. The mechanism of aqueous secretion and some of the factors influencing the secretory processes are shown.

ANTERIORMOST PORTION OF THE CILIARY PROCESSES (REGION 2)

The NPE cells in the anteriormost portion of the pars plicata are similar to those of the major portion of the ciliary processes. The cytoplasm contains many mitochondria and elaborate basolateral membrane infoldings which stain for Na,K-ATPase and CA. SEM studies have shown that the vasculature of the anteriormost portion of the ciliary processes differs from that of the major processes[4] (Fig. 1.8D). It is morphologically and functionally separate

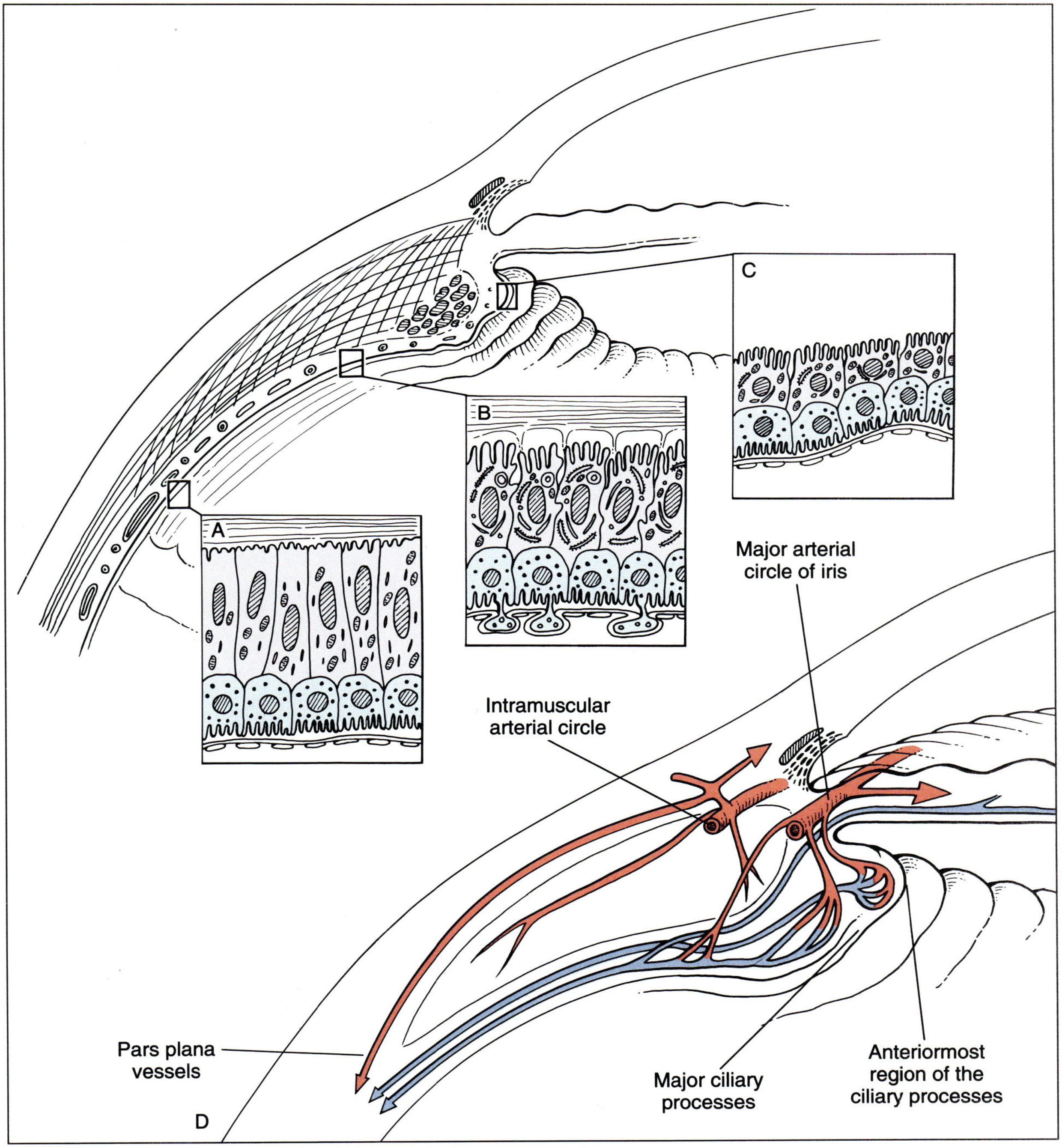

1.8 | Regional differences of the ciliary epithelium and of the ciliary body vasculature in the primate eye. *A:* Posterior pars plana (region 6). *B:* Posterior pars plicata (region 3). *C:* Major ciliary processes (region 1). *D:* Ciliary body vasculature.

and is supplied by separate arterioles that derive from the major iris arterial circle. The vasculature of this region is particularly sensitive to pressure changes in the eye. The vascular reactivity and the structural characteristics of the ciliary epithelial cells of this region resemble to some extent those of the iridial processes in the rabbit. These regions may serve for volume regulation and reabsorption rather than for secretion of aqueous humor, perhaps preventing protein from entering the anterior chamber.

POSTERIOR PART OF THE CILIARY PROCESSES FACING THE VITREOUS BODY (REGION 3)

As one passes from region 1 to the posterior part of the pars plicata, which is also supplied by a separate arteriole from the major iris arterial circle, the number of rough endoplasmic reticulum (rER) profiles increases. Single cells contain fingerprint-like profiles of rER and/or many Golgi vesicles[7] (see Fig. 1.8D). Whether these cells produce peptides, proteins, or proteoglycans to be released into the aqueous or vitreous body is not yet clear.

VALLEYS OF THE PARS PLICATA (REGION 4)

The ciliary epithelium of the valleys is covered by a plexus of zonular fibers, including tension fibers attached to the NPE cells.[6,15] The structure of the ciliary epithelium in the valleys differs from that on the crests of the processes in that fewer basolateral membrane infoldings are present and staining for Na,K-ATPase and CA is lacking.[7,8] The NPE cytoplasm contains few mitochondria, indicating that active, energy-dependent transport is not a predominant function. On the other hand, the basal part of the NPE cells, to which the zonule is attached, exhibits extensions and invaginations. Desmosomes are more numerous between NPE and PE cells than at the crests of the processes,[6] and the stromal layer between the capillaries and the PE is thicker. The capillaries are not fenestrated.

PARS PLANA

ANTERIOR PARS PLANA (REGION 5)

The ciliary epithelium overlying the pars plana vessels is covered by zonular fibers. In contrast to the valleys of the pars plicata, the main portion of the zonule does not adhere directly to the NPE cells but rather is separated from them by a small cleft (Fig. 1.9). Only thin, fine fibers penetrate this space and insert on the lateral surface of the NPE cells.[15] The NPE cells in this region are of the high columnar type and exhibit long basal membrane infoldings. The cytoplasm adjacent to the infoldings contains mitochondria. Quantitatively, both the infoldings and the number of mitochondria are less numerous than in the NPE of the major ciliary processes, but the basolateral membranes also stain for Na,K-ATPase, indicating that these cells, too, are involved in active ion transport (see Fig. 1.8B). It is unclear whether fluid secretion takes place in this area or whether freshly secreted fluid is reabsorbed into the underlying venous capillaries.

POSTERIOR PARS PLANA (REGION 6)

In the posterior pars plana between the posterior tips of the ciliary muscle and the ora serrata, the morphology of the NPE cells changes significantly. The high columnar cells become connected to each other by many desmosomes, located mainly between the basal parts. The cytoplasm is filled with intermediate filaments. Only few mitochondria and a small number of rER profiles are seen here (see Fig. 1.8A). The zonular plate is directly attached to the internal limiting membrane and the basal surface of the NPE cells (see Fig. 1.9). The morphology of these cells suggests a mainly mechanical function.

The venous capillaries in the posterior pars plana differ from the anterior pars plana vessels insofar as they also drain the venous blood from the ciliary muscle. They exhibit only sparse connections with the choroid and instead join the vortex vein tributaries directly.

The long, straight pars plana veins are situated in the stroma between the ciliary muscle and the ciliary epithelium. The elastic network of Bruch's membrane is also located in this layer. The posterior elastic tendons of the ciliary muscle insert into both Bruch's membrane and the basal lamina of the capillary vessel wall.[16] Therefore, ciliary muscle contraction might influence blood flow in this region. Indeed, after long-term treatment with miotics in monkeys,[17] the pars plana veins were significantly dilated, and ciliary epithelium and peripheral retina near the ora showed signs of cystic degeneration.[18]

Interestingly, large nerve endings or varicosities containing various types of synaptic vesicles have been observed within the elastic network of the stromal layer of the pars plana. Their functional significance is not yet known. They may be pain receptors to prevent overshooting contractions of the ciliary muscle system.

Near the ora serrata is a narrow region in which the PE cells reveal an elaborate system of basolateral membrane infoldings, with many mitochondria and membrane-bound Na,K-ATPase. On the other hand, the NPE cell membranes do not stain for ATPase. In addition, ciliary channels are present between the two cell layers. It is possible that this small zone is engaged in outward transport of fluid to prevent retinal detachment.[19]

MORPHOLOGY OF AQUEOUS OUTFLOW

TRABECULAR MESHWORK

Most of the aqueous humor leaves the eye through the trabecular meshwork and Schlemm's canal. This outflow is pressure dependent. In addition, there is a pressure-independent bulk flow through the ciliary body and the choroid, the so-called uveoscleral flow.[20-22] In monkeys with relaxed ciliary muscle, uveoscleral outflow can account for up to 30%–50% of the total outflow; however, in humans its magnitude is probably somewhat less.[23] Some

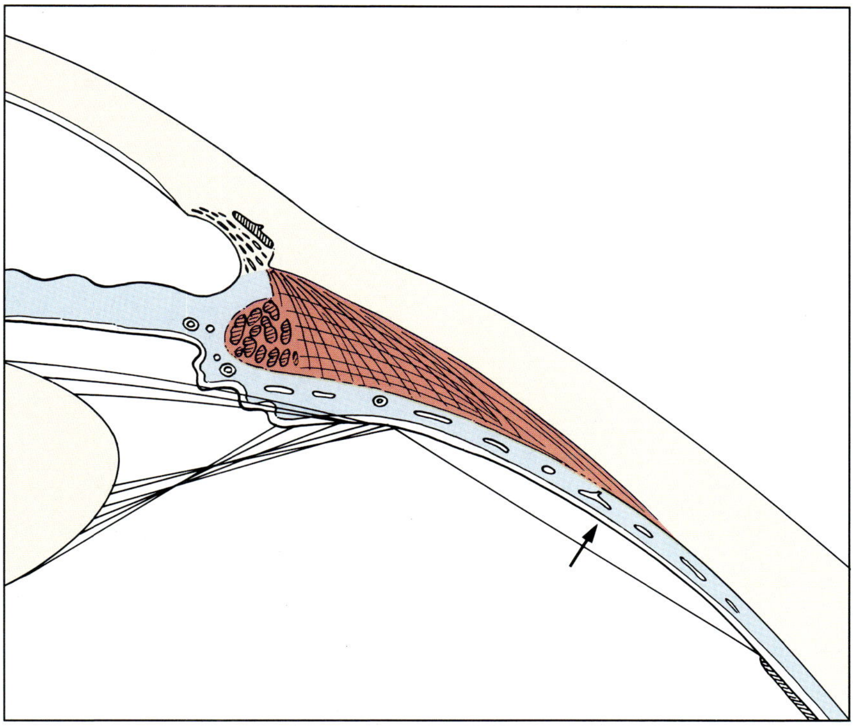

1.9 | Organization of the zonular apparatus in relation to the different regions of the ciliary body. Note that in the anterior pars plana the zonular plate is not fixed to the ciliary epithelium so that a small space filled with aqueous humor is formed (arrow).

fluid may also be absorbed by the iris vessels, but this amount probably is insignificant. Schlemm's canal and the trabecular meshwork lie within the internal scleral groove between the scleral spur and the ring of Schwalbe's line at the termination of Descemet's membrane. Schlemm's canal, measuring 360–500 μm in diameter, does not occupy the entire anterior–posterior length of the groove. In contrast, the trabecular meshwork extends from the level of the scleral spur to Schwalbe's line. Thus, an anterior nonfiltering portion can be distinguished from a posterior filtering portion of the meshwork (Figs. 1.10 and 1.11). The trabecular meshwork itself consists of three functionally and structurally different parts: the iridic and uveal part, which represents the innermost portion of the meshwork; the corneoscleral part, which extends between the scleral spur and the cornea; and the juxtacanalicular part or cribriform layer, which forms the inner wall of Schlemm's canal.

The iridic, uveal, and corneoscleral portions of the trabecular meshwork consist of connective tissue plates or lamellae which are completely covered by endothelial cells resting on a basement membrane.

The iridic and uveal meshwork is posteriorly contiguous with the ciliary body and the iris root. The *iridic portion* (pectinate ligament, trabeculum iridis) consists mainly of intermeshed, radially oriented, more or less round tissue strands which originate in the stroma of the iris root or in the connective tissue in front of the ciliary muscle (seen gonioscopically as the ciliary body band). They become fixed anteriorly in the corneal stroma or the nonfiltering portion of the trabecular meshwork (see Figs. 1.10 and 1.11). Between the radial strands, large spaces or openings (25–75 μm in diameter) can be observed.

In the uveal meshwork, as in the corneoscleral part of the meshwork, the trabecular lamellae form net-like sheets oriented mainly in an equatorial direction. The endothelial cells completely covering these sheets or beams connect the sheets also in the radial, outward–inward direction so that a three-dimensional sponge-like mesh is formed. The intertrabecular spaces and openings are relatively large in the inner parts of the meshwork but become smaller towards the cribriform layer (see Figs. 1.10 and 1.11). Each trabecular lamella has a central core containing ground substance, rich in

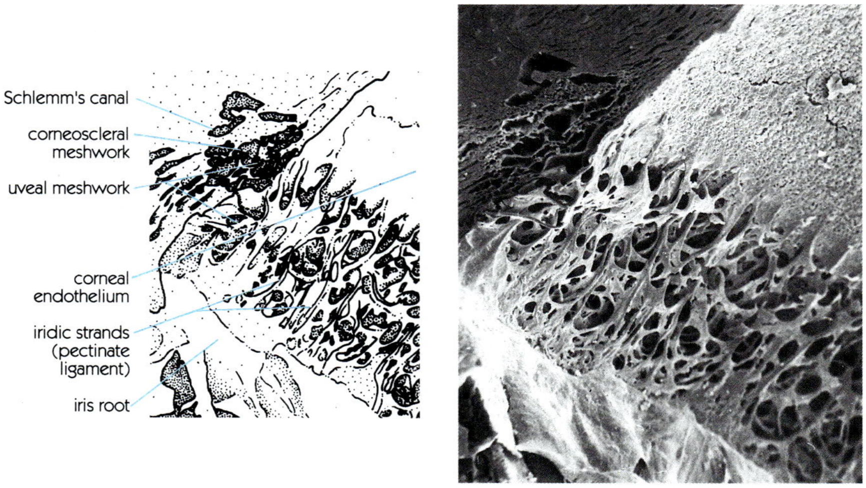

1.10 | Scanning electron micrograph of the trabecular meshwork of a cynomolgus monkey, internal aspect (x300).

glycoproteins and hyaluronic acid, and collagenous and elastic-like fibers. The collagenous and elastic-like fibers form a regular network of interlacing bundles, their main course following an equatorial direction.[24]

The cribriform or *juxtacanalicular layer* comprises the outermost portion of the meshwork and forms part of the inner wall of Schlemm's canal. It contains a number of elongated cells which are arranged in layers and are interspersed within the extracellular material. In contrast to the corneoscleral meshwork, the cribriform layer is not organized into cell-covered lamellae, so that aqueous humor directly penetrates this tissue layer, thereby coming in contact with the extracellular substances and fibrous material. The cribriform layer is supported by an elastic-like fiber network and fine collagen fiber bundles,[25] having the same orientation as the elastic-like network in the central core of the trabecular lamellae. This network is connected to the inner wall endothelium of Schlemm's canal by fine, bent, connecting fibrils.

Schlemm's canal itself possesses a complete endothelial lining which does not rest on a continuous basement membrane. A subendothelial cell layer is oriented predominantly in a radial direction, whereas the endothelial cells of the canal run mostly in an equatorial direction.[26] The two cell layers

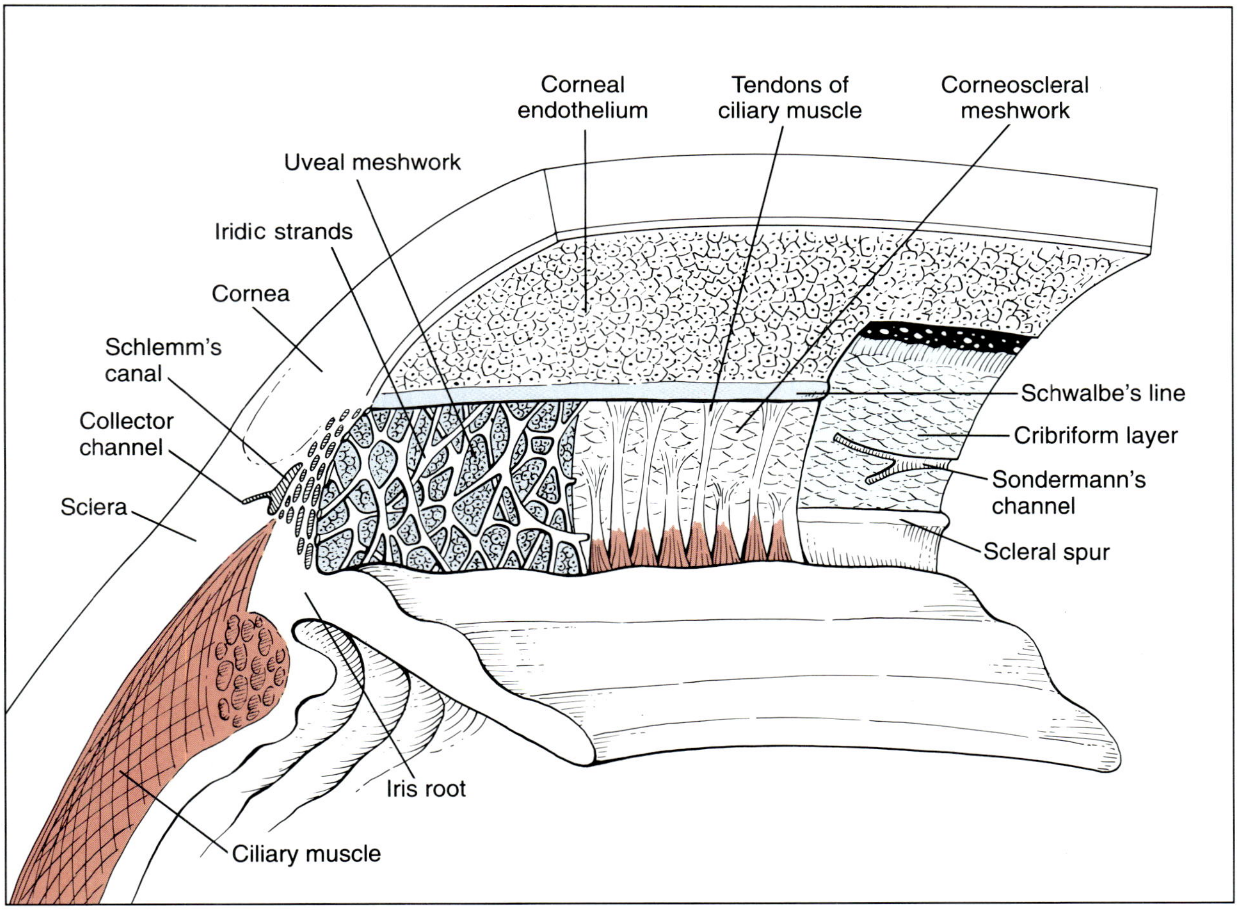

1.11 | Organization of the human trabecular meshwork.

are closely related to each other by interdigitating cell processes. The extracellular material between the cells, rich in glycoproteins and fine collagenous fibrils, might serve for fixation of the two cell layers (Fig. 1.12).

Site of Outflow Resistance

The morphologic structure of the trabecular meshwork, with wide spaces between the trabecular beams or strands in the uveal and corneoscleral layers, suggests that resistance to fluid movement is maximal either in the outermost or cribriform layer or in the endothelial lining of Schlemm's canal. Recent experimental studies in monkeys have indeed shown that nearly 90% of the resistance is located in the inner wall region.[27]

Aqueous humor must pass the endothelial lining of Schlemm's canal in order to reenter the general circulation. The lining endothelium differs from other endothelial monolayers in that it is subject to considerable variation in pressure and flow in the normal physiological environment. Therefore, it is not surprising that this monolayer should have a functional modification that allows rapid fluid transfer, i.e., the ability to form transcellular channels. Many cells in this monolayer contain large so-called "giant vacuoles," the majority of which communicate with the subendothelial space via an opening, whereas a smaller number communicate with the lumen of the canal via a pore (see Fig. 1.12). By serial sectioning it can be shown that some "vacuoles" have openings on the inner *and* outer sides, so that they can be considered as transcellular microchannels.[28,29] When the intraocular pressure is experimentally elevated, the number and the size of these giant vacuoles are increased, whereas vacuolization decreases at lower pressure gradients.[30,31] Because the openings of these microchannels at the adluminal (meshwork) side are often larger than at the luminal side, and because their apical pores are usually located not directly opposite the basal openings, some authors have assumed that these structures provide a valvular function.[32,33]

Recent experimental studies of the transendothelial passage of ferritin particles in monkeys have indicated that ferritin also traverses tortuous paracellular routes that lie between the endothelial cells of Schlemm's canal[34] (Fig. 1.12). At present, no definite statements can be made about the functional significance of these paracellular routes for aqueous outflow.

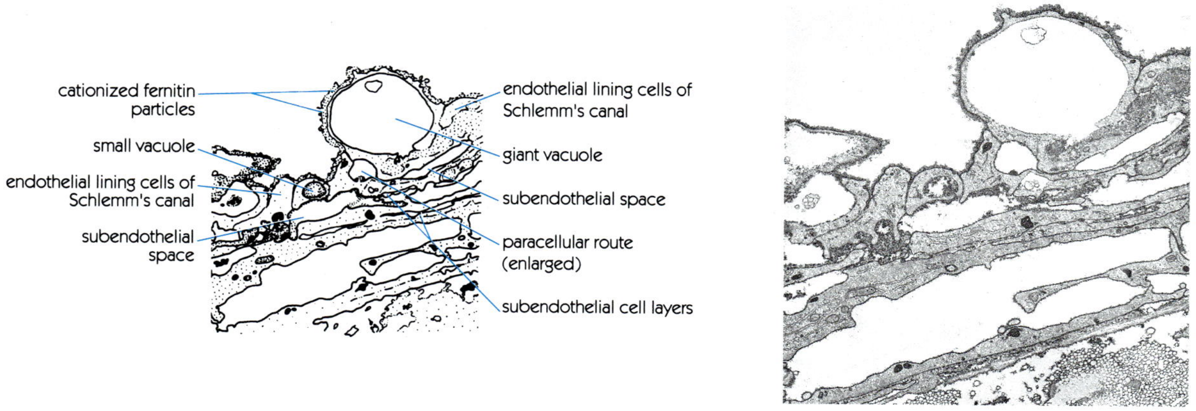

1.12 | Electron micrograph of the inner wall of Schlemm's canal in a cynomolgus monkey after anterior chamber perfusion with cationized ferritin (black) (x21,000). (From Epstein DL, Rohen JW: Morphology of the trabecular meshwork and inner wall endothelium after cationized ferritin perfusion in the monkey eye. *Invest Ophthalmol Vis Sci 1991;32:160–171.)*

According to calculations, the number of pores and openings in the inner wall endothelium of Schlemm's canal is too large to account for most of the outflow resistance. These and other findings lead to the assumption that the main resistance to aqueous outflow is located internal to the endothelial lining, i.e., within the subendothelial or cribriform layer. In fact, a combined physiologic and morphometric study in stumptailed macaques revealed a positive correlation between outflow facility after pilocarpine treatment and the area of the so-called "empty spaces" in the cribriform area.[35] Even if these optically empty spaces are not really empty, they appear to represent "preferential aqueous pathways" for aqueous outflow towards the inner wall endothelium.

Obstruction of these cribriform pathways or a collapse of the cribriform layer as a whole could result in increased outflow resistance and, if compensatory mechanisms fail, increased IOP.

Modulation of Outflow Pathways and Resistance

The outflow resistance can be modulated by ciliary muscle contraction. The ciliary muscle is connected to the trabecular meshwork by three different types of tendons[36] (see Figs. 1.11 and 1.13). One type comprises small elastic tendons that bend into the scleral spur, and a second type comprises tendons

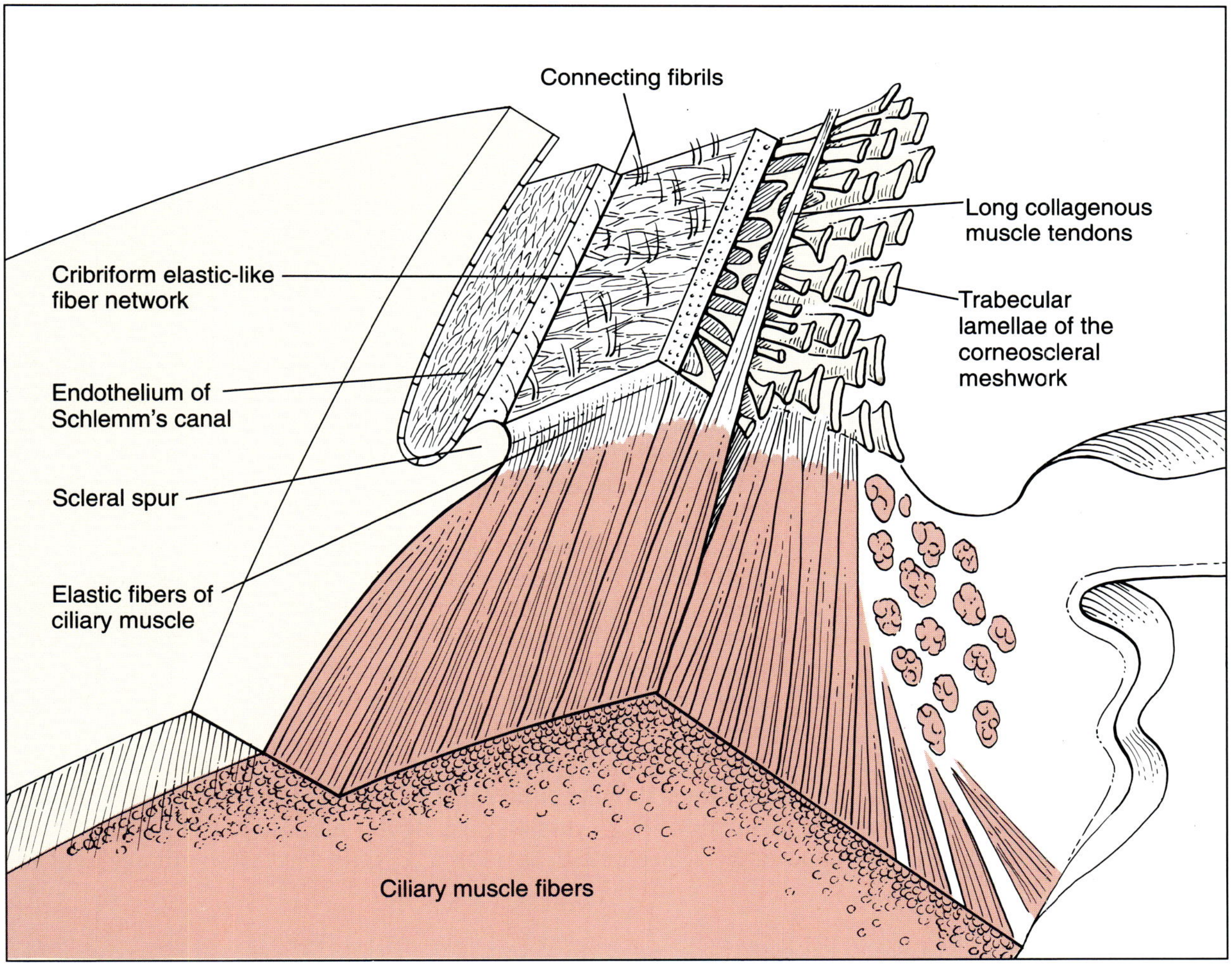

1.13 | Insertion of the anterior ciliary muscle tendons within the trabecular meshwork and corneosclera.

that form broad collagenous bands passing straight through the trabecular meshwork and anchoring in the cornea. The third type of tendon consists of brush-like elastic fibers that bend into the trabecular lamellae and into the cribriform region (see Fig. 1.13).

All of these tendons may be capable of expanding the trabecular lamellae in response to increased ciliary muscle tone. The uveal lamellae are separated from each other by an inward movement of the muscle directly, whereas the corneoscleral lamellae are spread by movements of the scleral spur.[37–39] However, spreading of the lamellae alone cannot explain the increase in outflow facility, if the resistance is located mainly within the cribriform layer.

In fact, ultrastructural tangential sections through the cribriform region reveal that tendons of the third type insert directly into the cribriform plexus of elastic-like fibers. These tendons appear to be especially important for movements of the cribriform layer and the inner wall of Schlemm's canal. If the ciliary muscle pulls the cribriform elastic network inwardly, the connecting fibrils are straightened and the cribriform area, and possibly the aqueous pathways through this region, are enlarged. In addition, if the canal is collapsed, inward movement of the endothelium would reopen the lumen and, thereby, increase the filtration area. Furthermore, widening of the canal lumen and enlargement of the cribriform layer seem to lead to a washout of extracellular material, debris, or cells that otherwise might accumulate in this region. Experimentally induced underperfusion of the meshwork results in an accumulation of extracellular homogeneous material in the subendothelial region.[40]

Functional Significance of the Corneoscleral and Uveal Meshwork

Although the uveal and corneoscleral part of the trabecular meshwork is of minor importance for outflow regulation, it fulfills additional functions that also support the outflow mechanisms. Any debris or exogenous material deposited within the aqueous pathways would certainly disturb normal passage of aqueous fluid. Therefore, it is not surprising that the trabecular meshwork has great phagocytic capability. The cells of the corneoscleral and uveal meshwork are capable of incorporating various kinds of particles: larger and smaller molecules, microspheres, pigment granules, and even red blood cells.[41–43] In addition, macrophages derived from the ciliary body or iris can also be found within the intertrabecular spaces. They appear to move freely through the trabecular meshwork, and they leave the tissue predominantly via Schlemm's canal.

Little is known about the functional significance of the trabecular cells with regard to the biologic properties of the meshwork. Under tissue culture conditions the trabecular cells are capable of synthesizing hyaluronic acid and various types of glycosaminoglycans, probably in the form of proteoglycans.[44] There seems to be a turnover (production and removal) of extracellular material within the meshwork, particularly of collagenous fibers and glycoproteins.

Age-Related Changes

In old eyes the trabecular endothelial cells contain large numbers of pigment granules within their cytoplasm, giving the meshwork as a whole a brown appearance. The number of trabecular cells decreases with age, and the underlying basement membrane thickens.[45] Within the central core of the lamellae, the elastic-like fibers, which consist of only a small amount of elastin embedded in an electron-dense material, become surrounded by a sheath of fine fibrils (elastic microfibrils and type VI collagen) embedded in proteoglycans (Fig. 1.14). The lamellae as a whole become thickened, and in places the sheets come into close contact with each other or even fuse. In the cribriform layer the amount of extracellular material also increases.[46] The sheaths surrounding the elastic-like fibers of the cribriform network thicken

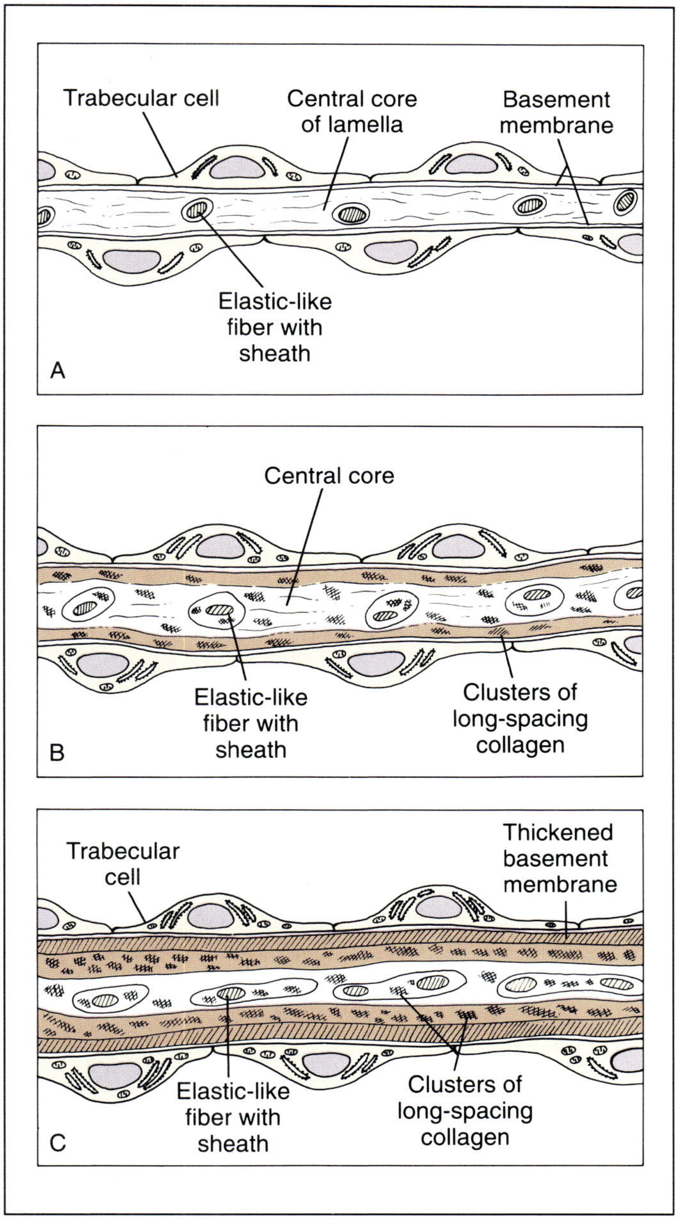

1.14 | Structural changes in the trabecular lamellae with increasing age and in cases of POAG (primary open-angle glaucoma). *A:* Trabecular lamella in young normal eyes. *B:* Trabecular lamella in older eyes. Note the increase in long-spacing fibrils and the thickening of basement membranes. *C:* Trabecular lamella in a glaucomatous eye. Note the thickening of the basement membranes with clusters of long-spacing collagen, and the increase in elastic-like fiber sheaths.

so that the spaces within the network become smaller (Fig. 1.15). Therefore, it appears that the area of the aqueous pathways within the cribriform region is reduced, so that outflow resistance will increase.

In the presbyopic eye the contractility of the ciliary muscle and movement of the scleral spur are also reduced, so that spreading of the trabecular lamellae is minimal. Possibly the washout of extracellular material is therefore reduced and a vicious circle develops. In normal eyes the IOP increases with age, but the increase is not marked because the increase in outflow resistance is partly compensated for by a decrease in aqueous formation. However, if additional material leads to further obstruction of the aqueous pathways through the trabecular meshwork, the equilibrium between outflow and inflow is disturbed and the IOP may rise substantially, producing glaucoma.

ACKNOWLEDGEMENTS

This work was supported by the Academy of Science and Literature, Mainz/Rh., Germany, and by the Deutsche Forschungsgemeinschaft, Bonn-Bad Godesberg (Grant Dre 124/6–1), Germany.

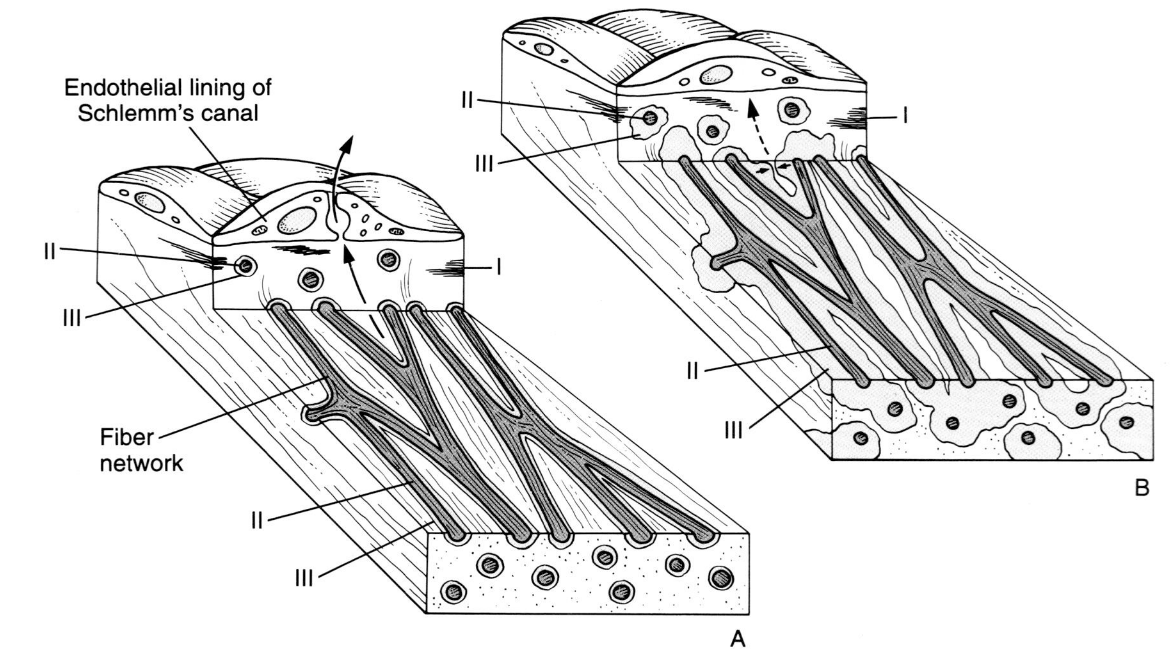

1.15 | Inner wall of Schlemm's canal and the subendothelially located elastic-like fiber network in normal (*A*) and primary open-angle glaucoma (*B*). The thickening of the sheaths by so-called sheath-derived plaques (type III) is shown in *B*. I, II, and III indicate type I, II, or III plaques. The long arrows indicate the direction of aqueous outflow through a giant vacuole. In primary open-angle glaucoma the outflow pathways are narrowed by SD plaque material (small arrows), so that the giant vacuole disappears.

Section II

Physiology and Neurophysiology of Aqueous Humor Inflow and Outflow

Siv F. E. Nilsson
Anders Bill

The aqueous humor is continuously formed by the ciliary processes as a result of active secretion into the posterior chamber. Ions, glucose, amino acids, and ascorbate are transported from the ciliary processes into the posterior chamber, causing a net secretion of fluid. Other substances, e.g., prostaglandins and organic acids, are transported in the other direction, i.e., from the posterior chamber into the ciliary processes (Fig. 1.16).

A small part of the newly formed aqueous humor probably enters the vitreous body, but most of it passes between the anterior surface of the lens and the posterior surface of the iris, entering the anterior chamber via the pupil. The temperature is normally slightly higher in the posterior than in the anterior chamber, which causes a thermal circulation of aqueous humor in the anterior chamber. The aqueous humor entering through the pupil is warmer and moves upward, whereas the aqueous humor closest to the cornea is colder and moves downward (see Fig. 1.16).

The aqueous humor is drained from the anterior chamber at the iridocorneal chamber angle. Some of it is drained via the trabecular meshwork into Schlemm's canal; from there, it enters (via the collector channels) intrascleral and episcleral veins. This outflow is usually referred to as "conventional" or "trabecular" outflow. Aqueous humor can also enter the ciliary muscle, pass through the supraciliary and suprachoroidal spaces and be drained through the sclera. This outflow constitutes the uveoscleral outflow (see Fig. 1.16).

The formation and flow of aqueous humor have two very important functions. First, the aqueous humor supplies nutrients to the lens, cornea, and chamber angle tissues, all of which are metabolically active but nonvascularized. Second, the resistance in the outflow routes for aqueous humor is relatively high, which creates a high pressure in the eye as compared with the interstitial pressure in other tissues. The high intraocular pressure (IOP) keeps the eyeball distended and prevents it from being deformed even during vigorous eye movements. Therefore, the high IOP is a prerequisite for maintaining good optics of the eye under variable conditions.

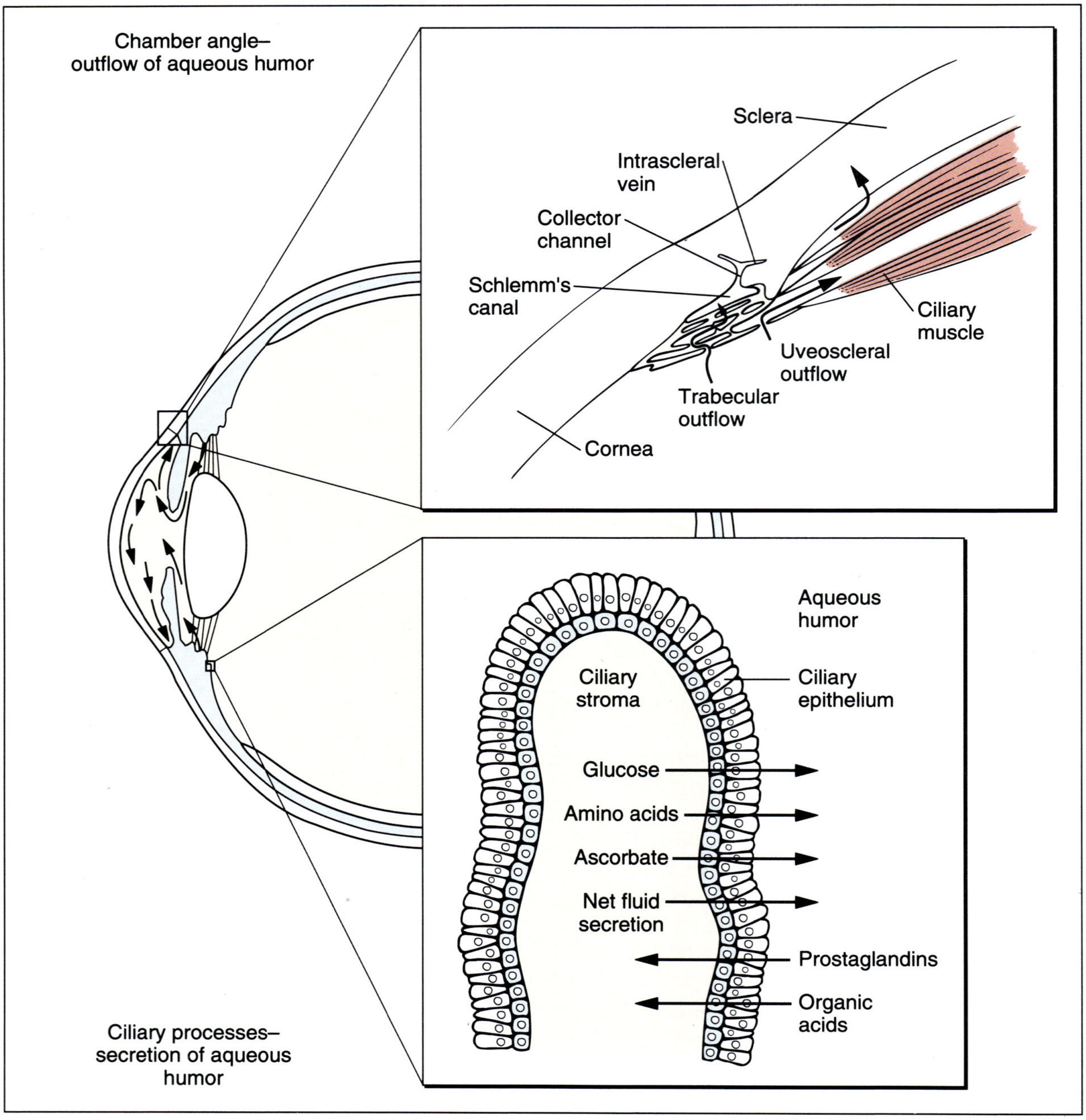

1.16 | Flow of aqueous humor in the eye. Secretion of aqueous humor by the ciliary processes. Thermal circulation in the anterior chamber. Outflow of aqueous humor at the chamber angle via trabecular and uveoscleral pathways.

INTRAOCULAR PRESSURE

FACTORS INFLUENCING THE INTRAOCULAR PRESSURE AND THEIR MEASUREMENT

Although the IOP is normally discussed as a single entity, it is not exactly the same in all parts of the eye. For instance, the pressure in the posterior chamber must be slightly higher than that in the anterior chamber to induce flow from the posterior to the anterior chamber.

Under normal conditions, there are only moderate variations in the IOP. Some small fluctuations are synchronous with the changes in the arterial blood pressure: the intraocular blood volume and IOP increase during systole and decrease during diastole. These fluctuations are 1–2 mm Hg at normal IOP and pulse pressure (systolic minus diastolic pressure), but may increase considerably at high IOP and with increased pulse pressure. The IOP is slightly higher during the day than during the night. This diurnal variation in IOP appears to be secondary to a diurnal variation in aqueous humor formation (see below).

Under steady-state conditions with a stable IOP, the inflow of aqueous humor via the pupil is equal to the total outflow of aqueous humor. Thus,

$$F_{in} = F_{out} = F_{trab} + F_u \qquad \text{(I)}$$

where F_{in} = inflow of aqueous humor to the anterior chamber, F_{out} = total outflow of aqueous humor, F_{trab} = outflow through Schlemm's canal, and F_u = uveoscleral outflow. According to Ohm's law, the flow through a system (Q) is directly proportional to the pressure difference between the inlet and the outlet of the system (ΔP) and inversely proportional to the resistance in the system (R).

$$Q = \Delta P/R \qquad \text{(II)}$$

This equation can also be applied to the fluid dynamics in the eye, but with one important distinction. The outflow through the trabecular meshwork is pressure dependent, whereas the uveoscleral outflow (at least in monkeys) is relatively pressure independent within the normal range of intraocular pressures.[47,48] The driving force for the flow of aqueous humor through the trabecular meshwork is the hydrostatic pressure difference between the anterior chamber and the episcleral veins, into which the aqueous humor drains. Ohm's law applied to the fluid dynamics in the eye can therefore be written as

$$F_{trab} = (F_{in} - F_u) = (IOP - P_v)/R \qquad \text{(III)}$$

or rearranged as

$$IOP = P_v + (F_{in} - F_u)R \qquad \text{(IV)}$$

where P_v = episcleral venous pressure and R = the resistance in the conventional outflow routes. Ocular physiology usually prefers the term "conductance" or "facility" instead of resistance. As the conductance (C) is the reverse of resistance, equation IV can be written as

$$IOP = P_v + (F_{in} - F_u)/C \qquad \text{(V)}$$

Determination of these parameters in normal human eyes has given the following values: IOP = 15-16 mm Hg, P_v = 8–9 mm Hg, F_{in} = 2.5–2.8 µl/min, and C = 0.3–0.4 µl/min/mm Hg. The uveoscleral outflow (F_u) has not been determined in normal human eyes, but theoretical calculation has given a value of ~0.8 μl/min.[49]

The high IOP in high-tension glaucoma is almost exclusively caused by increased outflow resistance. In some rare cases, pathologically elevated IOP can be seen as a result of increased episcleral venous pressure. Treatment of glaucoma is usually intended either to decrease the formation of aqueous humor or to increase the outflow facility. Increasing the uveoscleral outflow by medical or surgical treatment is another possibility that has recently gained interest.

There are several methodological problems with the determination of the different parameters that affect the IOP. First, the method used to measure a parameter may change the parameter under study. Second, measurement of one variable sometimes includes changing one of the other variables. Third, the accuracy of the methods is not always great enough to detect small changes that occur normally. This can be especially difficult in human studies in which noninvasive techniques are used.

In humans, the IOP is commonly measured with applanation tonometry. Although the design of different tonometers varies, the fundamental principle is the same: the force necessary to applanate a certain area of the cornea is measured, and because pressure equals force per area, the pressure can be determined accordingly (see Higginbotham, Chapter 3). In experimental animals under general anesthesia, the IOP can be measured by inserting a cannula, connected to a pressure transducer into the anterior chamber. This procedure gives more accurate measurement of the IOP, but may cause irritation of the eye due to release of prostaglandins and sensory neuropeptides. These substances may cause disruption of the blood–aqueous barrier and, secondary to this, disturbances in the aqueous humor dynamics. Furthermore, the anesthetic agent may in itself affect the IOP.

Episcleral Venous Pressure

The episcleral venous pressure can be determined in experimental animals by direct cannulation of episcleral veins. This technique has problems similar to those of measuring IOP with direct cannulation, e.g., local irritation may affect the results. The episcleral venous pressure can also be measured by different nontraumatic techniques. These techniques, equally effective in humans, follow one common principle. An increasing force is applied to the outside of the vessel and the venous pressure is determined as the pressure required to cause an almost complete collapse of the vein. The episcleral venous pressure is not exactly the same in all parts of the limbus region. The P_v in equation V is, therefore, to be considered as an average value.[50]

Vasoactive substances affect the episcleral venous pressure differently, depending on whether they cause local vasoconstriction/vasodilation only or whether they also increase/decrease the arterial blood pressure. A decrease in the arterial blood pressure resulting from general vasodilation decreases the blood flow through the uvea, anterior sclera, and conjunctiva, and thus the episcleral venous pressure as well. However, local vasodilation in these tissues decreases the vascular resistance and diminishes the pressure drop over these vascular beds, which increases the episcleral venous pressure provided that the arterial blood pressure remains unchanged. Substances that cause local vasodilation in the anterior segment therefore increase the episcleral venous pressure and, hence, also the IOP. Vasoconstrictors have the opposite effects. When their effect is local only, they decrease episcleral venous pressure and IOP; however, they may increase episcleral venous pressure and IOP when there is a rise in the arterial blood pressure. A good illustration of how local vasodilation can affect the intraocular pressure is given by the effects of facial nerve stimulation on IOP and intrascleral venous pressure (ISVP) in cats,[51] as shown by the experiment depicted in Figure 1.17. In this species, the aqueous humor is drained into an intrascleral venous plexus, which can easily be cannulated to measure the ISVP. Facial nerve stimulation causes a marked vasodilation in the uvea, which increases the ISVP and, concomitantly, also the IOP.[51] Initially, the increase in IOP is greater than the increase in ISVP, but after a few minutes the increase in IOP is about equal to the increase in ISVP. The initial overshoot in IOP is most likely due to an increased intraocular blood volume. However, the increased intraocular blood volume will displace an equal volume of aqueous humor from the anterior chamber. Therefore, after a few minutes the IOP falls to a level that corresponds to the increase in ISVP (see Fig. 1.17).

Aqueous Humor Flow

As can be easily understood from the anatomic arrangement of the outflow routes for aqueous humor, the aqueous humor cannot be quantitatively sampled. Therefore, different dilution techniques have been developed for determination of aqueous humor formation. Fluorophotometry is one such commonly used method for determination of the aqueous humor flow in both humans and experimental animals. Briefly, fluorescein is applied topically to the eye, allowed time to enter the anterior chamber, and its rate of disappearance from the anterior chamber is then determined (see Brubaker,

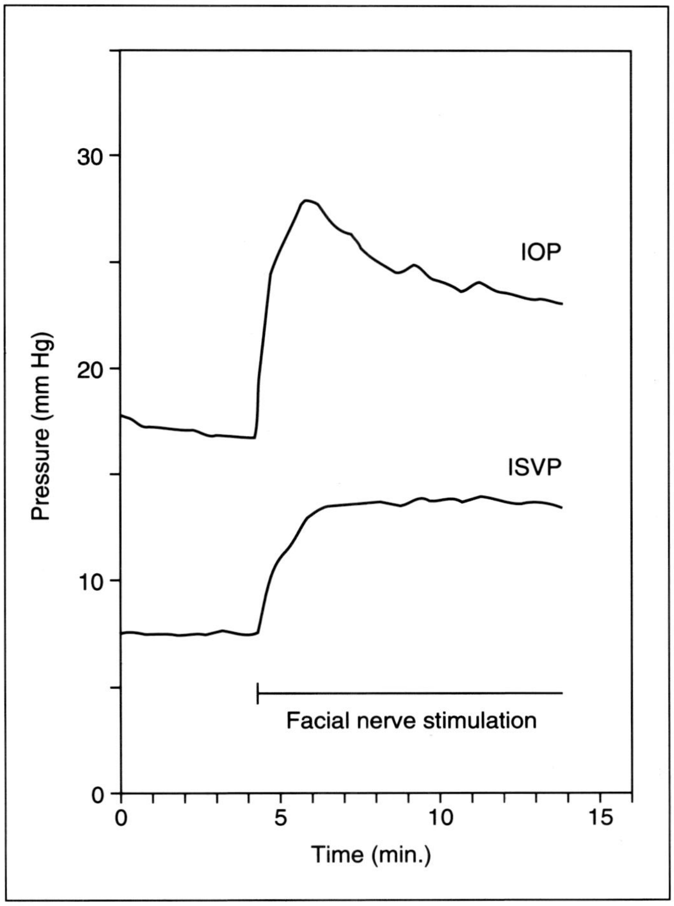

1.17 | Increase in intraocular pressure (IOP) and intrascleral venous pressure (ISVP) caused by vasodilation in the anterior segment during stimulation of the facial nerve in the cat. (Adapted from Nilsson SFE: Studies on ocular blood flow and aqueous humor dynamics. *Acta Univ Ups 1986;43:1–38.*)

Chapter 3). In experimental animals, the anterior chamber can be perfused with a tracer (e.g., radioactively labeled albumin) and its dilution can be continuously recorded. This technique gives better time resolution and provides an opportunity to measure the uveoscleral outflow simultaneously.[52] These dilution techniques measure only the net flow of aqueous humor from the posterior to the anterior chamber, however. The amount of aqueous humor actually secreted by the ciliary epithelium per minute may be higher, some aqueous humor already having been drained behind the iris.

Outflow Facility

The outflow facility can be determined by tonography in humans (see Higginbotham, Chapter 3). In experimental studies, the outflow facility is best measured by Bárány's method. Briefly, the anterior chamber is cannulated by two needles. One is used for IOP measurement and the other is coupled to a reservoir, the weight of which is continuously recorded. First, the IOP is determined with the connection to the reservoir closed. Then the reservoir is raised to a level that causes a slight inflow from the reservoir to the anterior chamber and a slight rise in IOP. A steady state is ensured for a few minutes and the reservoir is raised about 10 cm and a new steady state is established. The facility is calculated as the difference in inflow between the two levels divided by the pressure difference between the two levels. The facility determined in this way is usually referred to as "total" or "gross" facility. However, the aqueous humor formation is slightly depressed by an artificial rise in IOP.[50] As can be seen from equation V, this will cause an overestimate of the total facility. The suppression of aqueous humor formation by an increase in IOP is about 0.02 µl/min/mm Hg and is referred to as the "pseudofacility." Therefore, the true facility equals the gross facility minus the pseudofacility.

Uveoscleral Outflow

The uveoscleral outflow is the parameter of equation V that is most difficult to determine. In experimental animals, the uveoscleral outflow can be determined by perfusing the anterior chamber with mock aqueous humor containing radioactively labeled albumin (or some other labeled substance of high molecular weight) for 1 to 2 hours. The anterior chamber is then rinsed with nonradioactive perfusion fluid, the animal is killed, and the content of radioactive material in the intraocular and periocular tissues determined. Another way to determine the uveoscleral outflow is to measure the aqueous humor flow by the dilution technique with radioactively labeled albumin and to simultaneously determine the plasma radioactivity.[52] Because the labeled albumin that leaves the eye via the uveoscleral outflow route is drained by the lymphatic system outside the eye, it does not appear in plasma until several hours after it has left the eye. Thus, the plasma radioactivity can be used to calculate the conventional outflow, and the uveoscleral outflow is calculated as the difference between the aqueous humor flow and the conventional outflow. With this technique the animal does not need to be killed, an additional advantage.

There is no method for nontraumatic determination of uveoscleral outflow, which makes the available human data very limited. As can be predicted from equation V, the uveoscleral outflow can be calculated if the IOP, episcleral venous pressure, aqueous humor flow, and outflow facility are known. Assuming an episcleral venous pressure of 8 mm Hg, Townsend and Brubaker calculated the uveoscleral outflow to be ~0.8 µl/min in young adult humans. It should be noted that there is some uncertainty in the measurement of each variable and that such calculations may therefore contain considerable errors. By the use of radioactively labeled albumin (the former of the techniques described above), the uveoscleral outflow has been determined in middle- and older-aged humans undergoing surgery for intraocular tumors. These data suggested that the uveoscleral outflow in humans is ~10% of total drainage.[47,49] It may, of course, be higher in normal human eyes, and may also be age dependent.

FORMATION OF AQUEOUS HUMOR

BASIC MECHANISMS IN THE FORMATION OF AQUEOUS HUMOR

The ciliary epithelium consists of two cell layers, one of them pigmented and facing the stroma of the ciliary processes, and the other nonpigmented and facing the posterior chamber (see Lütjen-Drecoll and Rohen, this chapter). The cells in the nonpigmented layer are attached to each other by tight junctions, which prevent free diffusion between the ciliary stroma and the posterior chamber. The capillaries in the ciliary stroma are fenestrated, which allows rapid exchange of solutes between the blood and the ciliary stroma. Even albumin and other large molecules pass out of the ciliary capillaries and can penetrate the intercellular clefts between the pigmented cells, as far as the tight junctions on the nonpigmented cells. The tight junctions between the nonpigmented cells constitute one part of the blood–aqueous barrier. The other component of this barrier is the endothelium of the iridic capillaries, which restricts diffusion of low molecular weight solutes and plasma proteins from the iridic blood vessels into the anterior chamber.[53,54]

Although ultrafiltration was long considered to be the main driving force for the formation of aqueous humor, it is presently acknowledged that active transport across the ciliary epithelium is the most important mechanism.[55] Two facts speak against ultrafiltration as the main mechanism. First, the hydrostatic and oncotic pressure differences across the ciliary epithelium do not favor ultrafiltration. On the contrary, these forces are more likely to cause some reabsorption of newly formed aqueous.[56] Second, the concentrations of different low molecular weight solutes differ considerably between the plasma and the aqueous humor, which would not be the case if the aqueous humor were simply an ultrafiltrate of plasma.

Even if ultrafiltration is of little importance for the normal formation of aqueous humor, it may significantly affect the movement of fluid across the ciliary epithelium when there is damage to the blood–aqueous barrier, caused, for example, by inflammation. Under such conditions the blood–aqueous barrier is likely to be leakier, which will allow even large molecules, such as albumin, to enter the posterior chamber. A leaky barrier also makes the aqueous humor formation more susceptible to changes in the IOP, i.e., the pseudofacility increases.

The double layer of epithelial cells makes it more difficult to study the secretory processes in the ciliary epithelium than in other epithelia. The nonpigmented and the pigmented cells are connected by gap junctions, and an electrical coupling between the two cell layers has been demonstrated.[57,58] There are also gap junctions between the cells within both layers, indicating that the epithelium works as a functional syncytium.

The nonpigmented cells are considered to be the main site for active secretion of aqueous humor. The reasons for this are that the blood–aqueous barrier is located at the tight junctions of the nonpigmented cells and that active secretion requires energy, which is supplied by mitochondria. Mitochondria are more numerous in the nonpigmented than in the pigmented cells, suggesting a higher metabolic activity in the former.[59] Finally, the aqueous humor formation is markedly reduced by Na,K-ATPase inhibitors such as ouabain, suggesting that this enzyme has a key role in the aqueous humor secretion. Although Na,K-ATPase is present in the cell membrane of both cell types, its activity in the nonpigmented epithelium is two- to threefold higher than in the pigmented epithelium.[55]

It is assumed that the active secretion takes place chiefly in the pars plicata region, and more so in the crests of the processes than in the valleys; the mitochondria and gap junctions are more numerous in the pars plicata than in the pars plana, and the nonpigmented cells in the processes have more mitochondria and gap junctions than the cells in the valleys.[59]

Na,K-ATPase and Aqueous Humor Secretion

Histochemically, the Na,K-ATPase has been localized to the basolateral cell membranes of the nonpigmented cells. Its function in the secretion of aqueous humor can be explained by the standing-gradient osmotic flow model,[55] as illustrated in Figure 1.18. The Na,K-ATPase pumps sodium ions out of the nonpigmented cells at the same time as it moves potassium ions from the aqueous humor into the cells. The Na,K pump is electrogenic, i.e., it transports more sodium ions than potassium ions (3 Na^+ are exchanged with 2 K^+). This increases the local Na^+ concentration in the intercellular clefts and in the invaginations of the basal cell membrane, which creates a hyperosmotic environment and subsequent diffusion of water into the clefts and invaginations. As the aqueous humor passes through the clefts towards the posterior chamber, more and more water will be added. When the aqueous humor reaches the posterior chamber, the osmolarity is approximately equal to the posterior chamber osmolarity.

The active transport of Na^+ causes an excess of positive charges in the clefts, which causes the diffusion of negative ions to maintain electroneutrality; bicarbonate and chloride are the most important of these ions (see Maren, this chapter).

An attractive hypothetical model for the transport systems involved in aqueous humor secretion has been presented by Wiederholt et al, based on their studies of human nonpigmented ciliary epithelial cells in tissue culture.[60] These authors found evidence for an electrogenic Na,K pump combined with outward-directed K^+ and Cl^- conductances as indicated in Figure 1.18. This suggests that Na^+ is actively transported out of the nonpigmented cells at the same time as K^+ is pumped into the cells. The K^+ channel allows recirculation of K^+, and Cl^- diffuses passively out of the cells via the Cl^- channels.

Although the importance of the Na,K-ATPase in the formation of aqueous humor is generally acknowledged, there is very little information on how the activity of the Na,K-ATPase is regulated. The Na,K-ATPase enzyme complex consists of two subunits, a catalytic α-subunit and an enzymatic β-subunit. There are three different isoforms of the catalytic α-subunit (α_1, α_2, and α_3), which have different tissue localization. The α_1 and α_3 isoforms are localized to both the pigmented and the nonpigmented ciliary epithelium, whereas the α_2 isoform appears only in the nonpigmented layer.[61] Because the α_2 isoform in adipocytes has been suggested to be hormonally regulated, it is tempting to assume that the α_2 isoform has a key role in aqueous humor secretion.[62]

Active Transport of Other Solutes Across the Ciliary Epithelium

Although the active transport of sodium ions over the ciliary epithelium is the most important transport system as regards fluid secretion, many other transport systems have other important functions in the ciliary epithelium.

Several amino acids are present in higher concentrations in the aqueous humor than in the plasma, indicating that these are actively transported across the ciliary epithelium. At least four different transport systems for amino acids have been demonstrated, one each for basic, neutral, and acidic amino acids, and one for β-amino acids.[63] These transport systems are critically important to the function of the aqueous humor as a nutritional medium for the avascular tissues of the eye. The aqueous humor concentration of some amino acids is lower than the plasma concentration; however, this does not necessarily mean that they are not actively transported. The

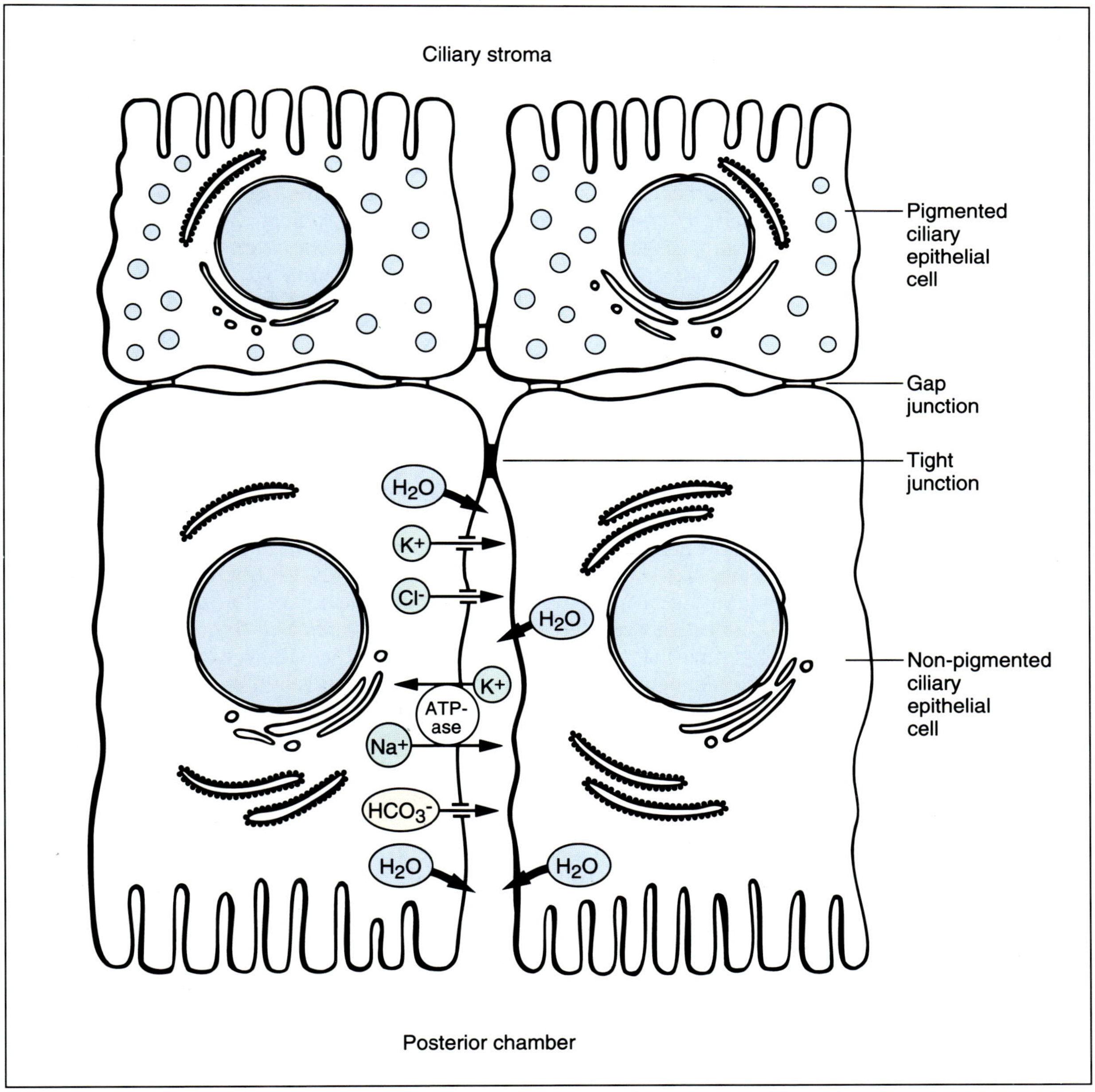

1.18 | Standing gradient, osmotic flow model for secretion of aqueous humor.

steady-state concentration in aqueous humor is not dependent only on the transport into the posterior chamber. Utilization of the amino acids by the intraocular tissues and diffusional loss to surrounding tissues also affects the steady-state concentration. Amino acids and many other compounds can pass freely from the posterior chamber into the vitreous body, whence they are taken up by the retina.

Glucose is another very important substance that must be able to enter the aqueous humor to provide energy to the avascular tissues. However, glucose enters the posterior chamber by facilitated diffusion rather than by active transport.[63]

A phenomenon that has attracted great interest is the high level of ascorbic acid in the aqueous humor, ~20 times higher than the plasma concentration. The high concentration of ascorbic acid is achieved by active transport across the ciliary epithelium. Recently, it was shown in tissue culture that ascorbic acid is transported into the pigmented ciliary epithelial cells by an electrogenic cotransport with sodium (2 Na^+:1 ascorbic acid).[60] The mechanisms by which ascorbic acid passes from the pigmented cells to the posterior chamber remain to be established. The molecule is small enough to pass through the gap junctions, but then has to enter the posterior chamber by some unknown mechanism. It has been suggested that the high concentration of ascorbic acid protects the eye against free radicals formed by ultraviolet radiation.

The ciliary epithelium is not only capable of transporting different solutes into the posterior chamber; transport in the other directions also occurs. It has long been known that substances such as iodide and organic acids, e.g, iodopyracet and *p*-amino-hippurate (PAH), are removed from the posterior chamber by the ciliary processes. Iodopyracet and PAH are removed by a system similar to the hippurate-transporting system in the kidney. There is also a liver-like transport system for organic acids, causing uptake of iodipamide into the ciliary body.[56] Bito and Wallenstein have shown that prostaglandins are actively removed from the aqueous humor by the ciliary processes, suggesting that these may comprise one of the natural substrates for this transport system. The transport of prostaglandins is inhibited by probenecid, indicating that they are removed by the same transport system as PAH.[64]

Carbonic Anhydrase and Aqueous Humor Secretion

Inhibitors of carbonic anhydrase decrease the IOP by decreasing the formation of aqueous humor. Carbonic anhydrase is present in both the pigmented and the nonpigmented ciliary epithelium, where it catalyses the formation of bicarbonate, one of the most important negative ions involved in the secretion of aqueous humor (see Maren, this chapter).

REGULATION OF AQUEOUS HUMOR FORMATION

There is normally little need for variation in the rate of aqueous humor formation, and it is doubtful that a true regulatory mechanism exists. However, there is a diurnal variation in the formation of aqueous humor, with higher flow rates during the day than during the night. The normal flow rate in humans is about 1.5 µl/min during the night, increasing to about 2.5 µl/min during the day.[65,66] The mechanism behind this diurnal variation is not known. It may be caused by a higher activity in the sympathetic nervous system during the day, but other neural and hormonal effects may contribute.

Autonomic Nervous System

The eye is extensively innervated by both the sympathetic and the parasympathetic nervous systems. This fact has focused much research on the possible involvement of the autonomic nervous-system in control of the IOP.[67]

The innervation comprises both the ciliary processes and the outflow apparatus, as well as the uveal blood vessels, which makes the effects of nerve stimulation very complex and difficult to study. Simultaneous effects on aqueous humor formation and outflow may counteract each other, making the resulting effect on the IOP minimal. Marked blood flow changes in the anterior segment may change the episcleral venous pressure and IOP significantly, without having any effect on the inflow or outflow of aqueous humor.

The sympathetic nerve fibers of the eye have their origin in the superior cervical sympathetic ganglion; the innervation is most extensive in the iris dilatator muscle and the uveal blood vessels, but there are also nerve fibers that innervate the ciliary processes and the chamber angle, indicating that the sympathetic nervous system may influence both inflow and outflow of aqueous humor. Although experimental data on the direct effects of sympathetic nerve stimulation on aqueous humor formation are limited, there is an extensive literature on the effects of adrenergic agonists and antagonists.

Epinephrine is one of the most studied substances with regard to its effects on aqueous humor dynamics. Nevertheless, the results obtained by different investigators have been conflicting. There appear to be several reasons for this. Epinephrine is a nonselective adrenergic agonist, and therefore interacts with both α- and β-receptors. In addition, epinephrine affects both inflow and outflow of aqueous humor. Species differences, dosage, and time for measurement play an important role. Finally, some of the effects attributed to epinephrine may actually be secondary to release of prostaglandins.

Selective β-receptor agonists, such as isoproterenol and terbutaline, stimulate aqueous humor flow in monkeys under general anesthesia as well as in humans during sleep.[66,68–70] However, the α_2-receptor agonists clonidine and apraclonidine reduce the formation of aqueous humor.[71,72] Therefore, nonselective adrenergic agonists such as epinephrine may have dual effects on aqueous humor flow: stimulation via β-receptors and inhibition via α_2-receptors.

In awake humans, β-receptor agonists have no effect on aqueous humor flow.[66,69] However, the β-receptor antagonist timolol, which is commonly used in the medical treatment of glaucoma, reduces the formation of aqueous humor during the day but not during sleep.[65] These observations suggest that the aqueous humor formation at night is at a basal, unstimulated level, and that it increases during the day owing to β-receptor activation secondary to increased activity in the sympathetic nervous system and/or to increased levels of circulating catecholamines.

The eyes receive parasympathetic innervation from two sources, oculomotor and facial nerves.[67] Oculomotor-nerve stimulation has marked effects on the outflow of aqueous humor, but it is doubtful that it has any effect on the formation of aqueous humor. The postganglionic nerve fibers in the facial nerve to the eye originate in the pterygopalatine ganglion, and most contain both the classical neurotransmitter acetylcholine and the neuropeptide vasoactive intestinal polypeptide (VIP). Stimulation of the facial nerve increases the IOP in experimental animals, including monkeys, whereas blocking of the pterygopalatine ganglion reduces IOP in glaucoma patients. Lesions to the facial nerve or the pterygopalatine ganglion decrease the IOP in both monkeys and humans. Although the main part of the rise in IOP during facial nerve stimulation appears to be caused by increased episcleral venous pressure secondary to intraocular vasodilation,[51] there are some indications that the facial nerve is involved in regulation of aqueous humor flow.

VIP (or a VIP-like peptide), which is likely to be released in the eye during facial nerve stimulation, stimulates the formation of aqueous humor in the cynomolgus monkey.[51]

Reports on the effects of muscarinic agonists on aqueous humor formation are conflicting; decreased formation rate, no effect, and increased formation rate have been reported.[73] As with the adrenergic receptors, the muscarinic receptors can be divided into different subtypes, which have been designated as M_1 to M_5. The ciliary processes contain predominately the M_3 subtype, but small amounts of the M_2 and M_4 subtypes are also present.[74] Therefore, future studies with selective muscarinic agonists and antagonists may shed light on the conflicting results.

Aqueous Humor Formation and the Adenylate Cyclase System

The membrane-bound adenylate cyclase system, which increases the intracellular formation of cAMP, has long been considered important in aqueous humor formation. In the ciliary epithelium, as in many other epithelia, neurotransmitters and hormones known to influence the secretion rate also affect the intracellular formation of cAMP. There have been conflicting opinions as to how the generation of cAMP is coupled to the aqueous humor formation. Sears has suggested that there is a negative correlation between cAMP and aqueous humor flow, i.e., decreased cAMP formation leads to increased formation of aqueous humor, and vice versa.[75] This hypothesis has been questioned, and present knowledge favors a positive correlation between cAMP formation and aqueous humor formation (Fig. 1.19). Binding of a neurotransmitter or a hormone to a receptor activates a guanine nucleotide-binding protein (G-protein), which subsequently stimulates or inhibits the adenylate cyclase system.

Cell membranes from the ciliary processes contain β-receptors of the β_2 subtype.[76] Activation of these receptors by β-agonists in vitro increases the formation of cAMP in the ciliary body.[76,77] Stimulation of the β-receptor most likely activates a stimulatory G-protein (G_s), which subsequently activates the adenylate cyclase system and hence increases the intracellular formation of cAMP. The α_2-adrenoceptor agonists (e.g., clonidine and apraclonidine) have little or no effect on basal cAMP formation but inhibit β-receptor-mediated stimulation of the adenylate cyclase system in the ciliary epithelium.[78,79] The α_2-receptors are probably coupled to the adenylate cyclase system via an inhibitory G-protein (G_I).

In addition to norepinephrine, the sympathetic nerve fibers to the eye, as to most other tissues, contain neuropeptide Y (NPY). NPY has attracted interest chiefly because of its potent vasoconstrictor effects in various tissues, including the eye.[80] However, it also has effects on nonvascular smooth muscle and on secretory processes. At least some of the effects of NPY are coupled to inhibition of cAMP formation. Because NPY also inhibits β-receptor-mediated cAMP formation in the ciliary body preparation,[81–83] it is tempting to suggest that NPY has an inhibitory effect on the formation of aqueous humor. If so, the effects of the sympathetic nervous system and its transmitters may be even more complex than presently understood.

Specific binding sites for VIP have been identified in isolated cell membranes from the ciliary processes.[84] Neither the effect of VIP on aqueous humor formation in vivo nor the effect on cAMP-formation in vitro are influenced by the β-receptor antagonist timolol.[70] However, VIP-stimulated cAMP formation is reduced by both α_2 agonists and NPY.[81–83,85]

The nonpigmented ciliary epithelium also has muscarinic receptors, which are negatively coupled to the adenylate cyclase system.[86,87] VIP- and β-stimulated cAMP formation is inhibited by the muscarinic agonist carbamylcholine, but the effect is not additative to the effect of an α_2-agonist, which suggests a common site of action.[87]

Therefore, it appears that different stimulatory (β, VIP) and inhibitory (α_2, NPY, muscarinic) receptors in the cell membranes of the nonpigmented cells are coupled to a common adenylate cyclase system (see Fig. 1.19). The β-agonists and VIP stimulate both the formation of cAMP and aqueous humor, whereas α_2-agonists decrease cAMP and aqueous humor formation. Furthermore, the β-receptor antagonist timolol, which reduces the formation of aqueous humor, can inhibit the increase in cAMP caused by β-receptor activation.[76,77] How the changes in intracellular cAMP are coupled to the function of ion channels and/or the active transport of different ions across the ciliary epithelium remains to be elucidated.

Other second-messenger systems, such as formation of cGMP or phosphoinositide metabolism leading to formation of inositol 1,4,5-triphosphate (IP_3) and diacylglycerol (DG) and Ca^{2+} signaling, may also be involved in the secretion of aqueous humor. However, very little is known about how these second-messenger systems are coupled to the formation of aqueous humor or which endogenous substances are their natural agonists. One possible endoge-

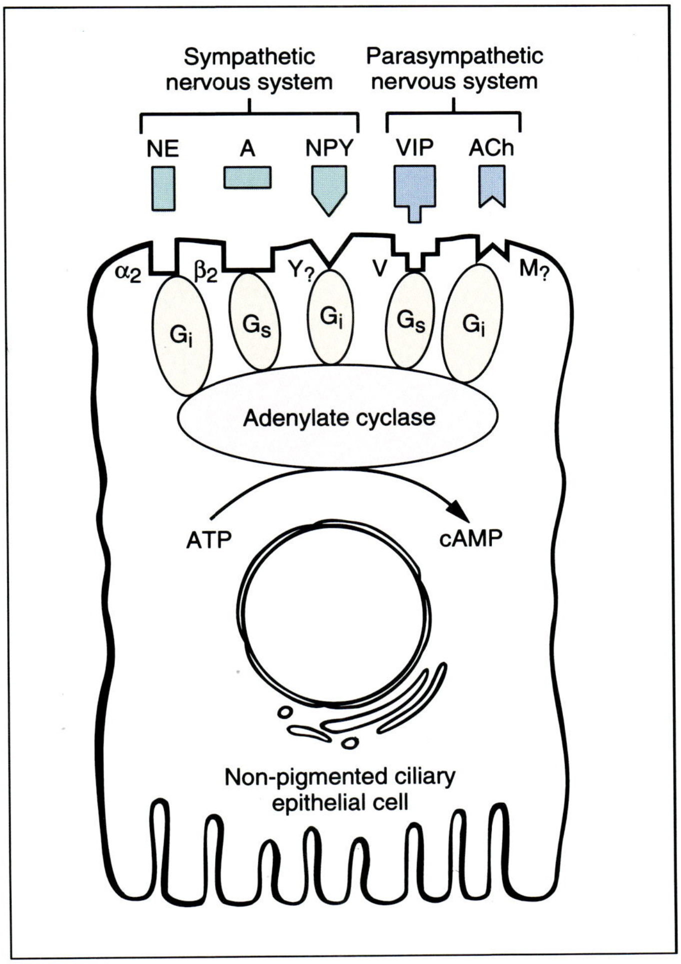

1.19 | Influence of the autonomic nervous system on the formation of cAMP in the ciliary epithelium. Agonists: NE = norepinephrine, E = epinephrine, NPY = neuropeptide Y, VIP = vasoactive intestinal polypeptide, ACh = acetylcholine. Receptors: α_2 and β_2 = adrenergic receptors, $Y_?$ = NPY receptor (subtype unknown), V = VIP receptor, $M_?$ = muscarinic receptor (subtype unknown). G_s = stimulatory guanine nucleotide binding protein, G_I = inhibitory guanine nucleotide binding protein.

nous activator of the guanylate cyclase system is the atrial natriuretic factor (ANF), which stimulates the formation of cGMP in ciliary processes in vitro and increases the aqueous humor flow in cynomolgus monkeys in vivo.[88]

OUTFLOW OF AQUEOUS HUMOR

As discussed above, there is no barrier between the posterior chamber and the vitreous body, which makes it possible for water and low molecular weight substances to enter the vitreous body freely. This exchange between the posterior chamber and the vitreous body changes the composition of the secreted aqueous humor. It seems likely that there is a slight net flow of aqueous humor from the posterior chamber into the vitreous body, but that this flow is probably negligible compared with the flow via the pupil. As the aqueous humor enters the anterior chamber, its composition is further altered by exchange with the surrounding tissues; metabolic substrates are removed, and metabolic endproducts are added. Furthermore, the anterior surface of the iris lacks an epithelial barrier, which allows free exchange between the anterior chamber and the iris stroma. Nevertheless, there seems to be very little net movement of fluid from the anterior chamber to the iridic blood vessels.[54] The net movement of water into the cornea also appears to be minimal. Therefore, the flow of aqueous humor through the pupil is essentially equal to the drainage at the chamber angle, at which location the aqueous humor can be drained either via Schlemm's canal or by the uveoscleral route.

CONVENTIONAL OUTFLOW

The trabecular meshwork consists of three different layers, the uveal meshwork, the corneoscleral meshwork, and the cribriform layer (from inside to outside), through which the aqueous humor must pass before entering Schlemm's canal. The endothelial cells of the inner wall of Schlemm's canal are very thin and are attached to each other by rather "leaky" tight junctions. Some of the aqueous humor is probably drained between the cells, but most of it passes into the canal via transendothelial channels, which are made up of invaginations and pores in the endothelial cells (see Lütjen-Drecoll and Rohen, this chapter). The invaginations and pores appear to be transient structures; they increase in number when the IOP is increased and almost completely disappear when the IOP is lowered.[50] From Schlemm's canal, the aqueous humor enters the collector channels, which are drained into intrascleral and episcleral veins.

As pointed out in the beginning, the flow through the conventional outflow route is pressure-dependent. In the range of normal IOPs, the outflow increases almost linearly with the IOP (Fig. 1.20). At higher IOPs, the slope of the trabecular outflow line diminishes (not shown in figure). This effect is thought to be caused by increased outflow resistance owing to mechanical compression of the meshwork and Schlemm's canal.[89] Reducing the IOP to a level below the normal episcleral venous pressure causes reflux from the collector channels and episcleral veins into Schlemm's canal and the anterior chamber. The invaginations in the endothelial cells in the inner wall of Schlemm's canal collapse when the pressure in the canal is higher than the pressure in the anterior chamber. Thus, the invaginations and pores in the inner wall of Schlemm's canal function as one-way valves that limit the reflux and prevent blood cells from entering the anterior chamber. Furthermore, at very low IOP the inner wall of Schlemm's canal bulges inward (towards the anterior chamber), which causes compression of the juxtacanalicular tissue and further limits the reflux. An abrupt decrease in IOP to extreme levels, as can occur after paracentesis, may cause ruptures in the delicate tissues and reflux of blood into the anterior chamber.[50,54]

Removal of the trabecular meshwork in enucleated human eyes decreases the outflow resistance by 75%, which indicates that the main part of the resistance is located in the trabecular meshwork, most probably within the cribriform layer.[50] Measurements in monkeys of the pressure in the episcleral veins, Schlemm's canal, and the trabecular meshwork, using a micropuncture technique, have further strengthened this suggestion; the main part of the pressure drop occurs between the anterior chamber and Schlemm's canal, whereas there is only a minimal difference in pressure between the canal and the episcleral veins.[48] These authors calculated that about 90% of the resistance was located between the anterior chamber and Schlemm's canal and that more than 50% of it was located near the inner wall of the canal.

The outflow resistance in the conventional outflow route can be altered by three different mechanisms: change in ciliary muscle tone, direct effects on the trabecular meshwork (see below), and washout or change in composition of the ground substance (see Acott, this chapter).

UVEOSCLERAL OUTFLOW

The lack of an epithelial barrier between the anterior chamber and the ciliary body makes it possible for aqueous humor to enter the ciliary body from the chamber angle. The aqueous can pass freely between the muscle bundles and

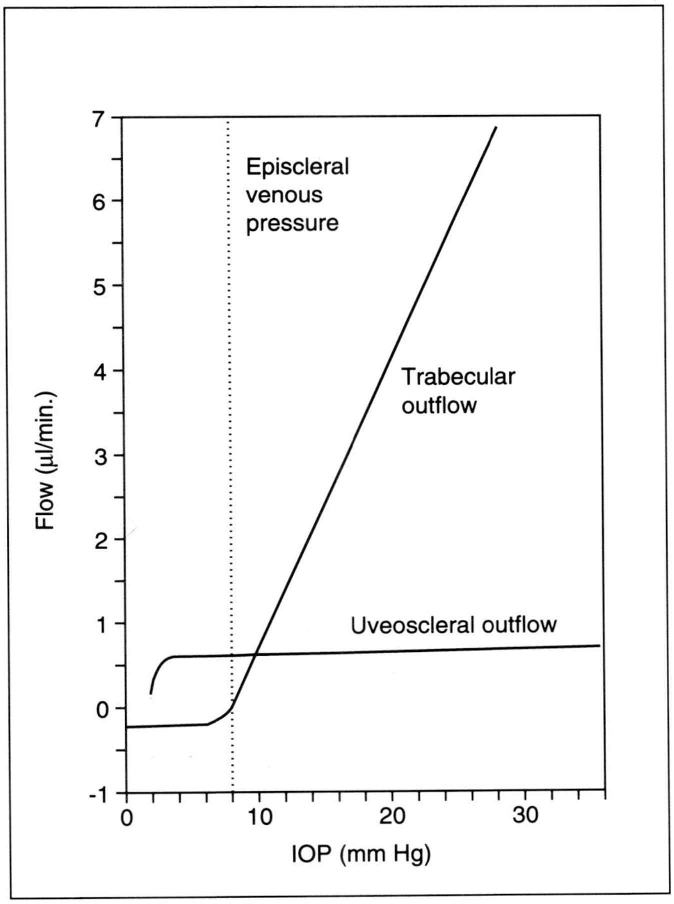

1.20 | Influence of the intraocular pressure (IOP) on outflow via Schlemm's canal (trabecular outflow) and the uveoscleral pathway. (Adapted from Bill A: Uveoscleral drainage of aqueous humor in Bito LZ, Stjernschantz J (eds): *The Ocular Effects of Prostaglandins and Other Eicosanoids.* New York: Alan R Liss, 1989, 417.)

thus enter the supraciliary and suprachoroidal spaces. From there, it can either flow through the sclera or pass through the emissarial channels, where blood vessels and nerves penetrate the sclera. Outside the eye, the fluid becomes part of the orbital tissue and is partly reabsorbed into the orbital blood vessels and partly drained via the lymph vessels of the conjunctiva. Also, posterior drainage may occur via the orbital veins through the orbital fissure.

The uveoscleral outflow is relatively pressure insensitive within the normal range of IOP (see Fig. 1.20). The reason for this is not quite clear, but it is believed that the driving force for the uveoscleral outflow is the difference in pressure between the anterior chamber and the suprachoroidal space. The pressure in the suprachoroidal space has been found to be about 4 mm Hg lower than the IOP in the monkey. At normal IOPs, an increase in the IOP causes an almost equal change in the suprachoroidal pressure, thus making the pressure head for the uveoscleral outflow relatively constant.[90] A contributing factor may be that when the IOP increases the ciliary muscle and supraciliary space become compressed, causing increased resistance to the uveoscleral flow.[49,90]

CILIARY MUSCLE FUNCTION AND OUTFLOW OF AQUEOUS HUMOR

The attachment of the trabecular meshwork to the anterior tips of the ciliary muscle bundles makes it possible for the ciliary muscle to alter the configuration of the meshwork. When the ciliary muscle contracts, the anterior part of the muscle thickens and the meshwork is moved towards the anterior chamber, making the meshwork packing looser (Fig. 1.21). The widening of the spaces between the sheets in the meshwork decreases the resistance in the meshwork. Simultaneously, as the muscle fiber bundles thicken, the spaces between the bundles narrow, which impedes the uveoscleral outflow. Thus, depending on the degree of contraction in the ciliary muscle, aqueous humor can be redistributed via the conventional or the uveoscleral outflow route (see Fig. 1.21).

The ciliary muscle is innervated by both the parasympathetic (oculomotor nerve) and the sympathetic nervous systems, indicating that both divisions of the autonomic nervous system may cause alterations in ciliary muscle tone and, thus, also conventional and uveoscleral outflow of aqueous humor. Oculomotor nerve stimulation causes contraction of the ciliary muscle, whereas sympathetic stimulation relaxes it. However, the parasympathetic effects on outflow of aqueous humor are more pronounced than the sympathetic effects. The outflow facility is increased by both oculomotor nerve stimulation and the muscarinic agonist pilocarpine. After disinsertion of the ciliary muscle from the trabecular meshwork, pilocarpine has no effect on outflow facility, supporting the hypothesis that ciliary muscle contraction is the main cause of the increase in facility.[91] Simultaneously, as pilocarpine increases the outflow facility it stops the uveoscleral outflow almost completely, whereas the muscarinic antagonist atropine increases uveoscleral outflow.[49]

Sympathetic nerve stimulation decreases the outflow facility in monkeys,[92] but there is no effect on uveoscleral outflow.[68] Adrenergic agonists do not mimic the effects of sympathetic nerve stimulation, however, as they also have direct effects on the trabecular meshwork and also affect uveoscleral outflow, perhaps via release of prostaglandins (see below).

HORMONAL AND NEURAL INFLUENCES ON OUTFLOW FACILITY

The trabecular meshwork receives innervation from both the parasympathetic and the sympathetic nervous systems, in addition to sensory innervation. Many different peptidergic (VIP, NPY, CGRP, substance P) nerve fibers are also present,[67] but the significance of the trabecular innervation in relation to the outflow of aqueous humor is still largely unknown.

β-adrenergic agonists increase the outflow facility via activation of β-receptors, although these do not seem to be innervated. It appears that this effect may mask a possible negative effect on outflow facility caused by ciliary muscle relaxation, due to sympathetic stimulation and adrenergic agonists. The increase in outflow facility caused by β-adrenergic agonists is probably mediated by increased formation of cAMP; cAMP and stable analogues of cAMP also increase the outflow facility.[93]

Muscarinic agonists do not appear to have any direct facility-increasing effect on the trabecular meshwork, but the parasympathetic neurotransmitter VIP causes a slight increase in outflow facility in the cynomolgus monkey.[51] Because VIP, like β-agonists, is a potent stimulator of the adenylate

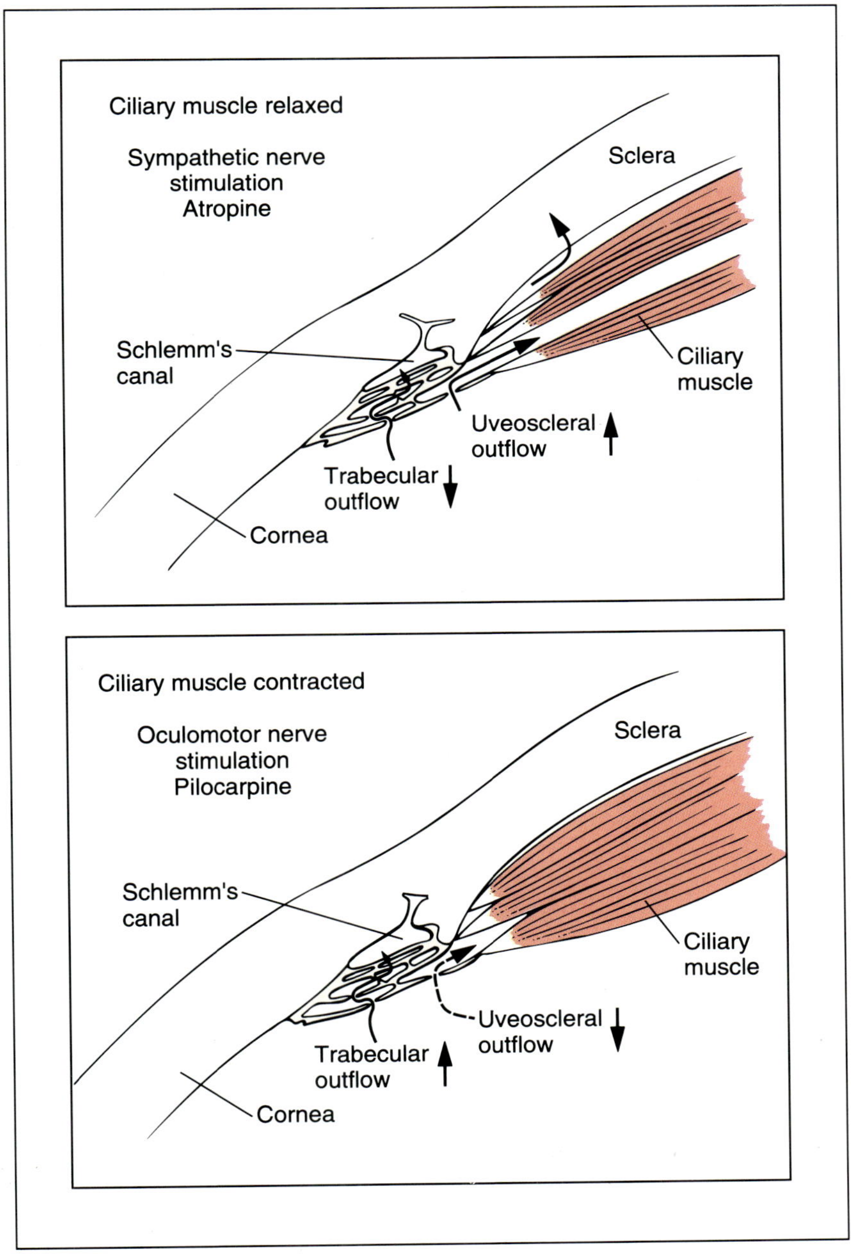

1.21 | Influence of the ciliary muscle tone on the outflow via Schlemm's canal (trabecular outflow) and the uveoscleral outflow. (Adapted from Bill A: Blood circulation and fluid dynamics in the eye. *Physiol Rev 1975;55: 383–417.*)

cyclase system, it seems plausible to assume that VIP also increases the facility via cAMP. That VIP may change the ciliary muscle tone is yet another possibility.

PROSTAGLANDINS AND UVEOSCLERAL OUTFLOW

It has long been known that the uveoscleral outflow can be decreased by ciliary muscle contraction (pilocarpine) and increased by ciliary muscle relaxation (atropine, β-agonists).[49] Uveoscleral outflow can also be increased by cyclodialysis,[94] but there has been no evidence of the existence of a physiologic mechanism for changing the uveoscleral outflow by any means other than changing the tone of the ciliary muscle. Recently, however, it has been shown that the ocular hypotensive effect of prostaglandins is due to their ability to increase uveoscleral outflow.[52,95] This effect may in part be due to relaxation of the ciliary muscle, but structural changes within the muscle may contribute. Lütjen-Drecoll and Tamm have shown that the spaces between the muscle bundles are enlarged during prostaglandin treatment, suggesting a loosening of the connective tissue which may in turn decrease the resistance in the uveoscleral pathway.[96] It also appears that other substances (e.g., epinephrine) may in part exert their hypotensive effect via release of prostaglandins, because the hypotension is reduced by inhibitors of prostaglandin synthesis.[97] It remains to be established whether or not endogenous prostaglandins have a physiologic function in regulating uveoscleral outflow or whether their effect is merely pathophysiologic, which contributes to the hypotension and increase in uveoscleral outflow associated with ocular inflammation.[98]

SECTION III

BIOCHEMISTRY OF AQUEOUS HUMOR INFLOW

Thomas H. Maren

This section will outline the biochemical basis for the formation or flow of aqueous humor. The basic concept is that the 3 µl/min formed from plasma by human ciliary processes has the same Na^+ concentration as plasma, 150 mM. In other words, aqueous humor is isotonic with plasma. This means that 0.45 µmol of Na^+ is transferred each minute from plasma to the posterior aqueous, dissolved in 3 µ1 of the new fluid. How is the sodium moved? First we must account for the Na^+ transport itself, and then we must account for the companion anions in the fluid.

Apart from flow and concentration data, ionic movements cannot be studied in human subjects; indeed, there are still no measurements of ion concentrations in human posterior aqueous. However, studies in rabbit, cat, dog, and monkey all agree in support of the basic principles, so it is likely that these animal data are directly applicable to humans. Studies on teleost and elasmobranch fish also support the idea of Na^+-mediated secretion, coupled to anions in a pattern similar to what we shall describe for mammals. Therefore, aqueous humor secretion according to this pattern is a fundamental element of vertebrate physiology.

The underlying chemistry of aqueous humor secretion is shared with other systems, notably the cerebrospinal fluid, pancreatic juice, and salivary flow.[99] The same chemical or enzymic systems also operate in the kidney, linked not to the formation of new fluid but to the reabsorption of glomerular filtrate.

Figure 1.22 gives the ionic composition of both chambers of aqueous humor in several mammalian species. Note that the Na^+ concentration is nearly the same throughout, whereas the anions, particularly $HC0_3^-$, vary. Particularly striking is the high $HC0_3^-$ in the posterior aqueous of the rabbit, which provided an early clue to the chemistry of the secretion. Unfortunately, at one time it was widely held that the difference in posterior aqueous $HC0_3^-$ between rabbit and dog or primate represented a different mechanism, but this has been disproven. This is discussed, along with a history of the development of the field, in Reference 100.

SODIUM
ACCESSION RATE

The accession rate of Na^+ from plasma to posterior chamber of dog and monkey has been measured by intravenous injection of isotopic sodium as the chloride salt and sampling of the aqueous 1–10 minutes later. Figure 1.23 shows the rate constant obtained in monkey, 0.017 per min.[101] This is agreeably close to the rate constant for fluid formation in this species (flow ÷ volume of chamber), 0.016 min^{-1}. In the dog, k_{in} for sodium is 0.044 min^{-1} and for fluid formation 0.03 per min.[100] This is the basis for the central principle cited above, that sodium and fluid move together, so that the fluid formed is isotonic. The rate constant for fluid formation in human is about 0.04 min^{-1}; that for sodium has not been directly determined but is presumably the same.

Other aspects of Figure 1.23 will be considered below: effect of ouabain on Na^+ accession, effect of acetazolamide on Na^+ accession, and the movement of HCO_3^- and chloride.

Figure 1.22. Ionic Composition of Posterior Aqueous in Several Species (mM)*

	Plasma (All)	Rabbit	Dog	Monkey
Na^+	145	145	150	148
Cl^-	115	100	130	125
HCO_3^-	23	39	25	21

*From various sources.

Figure 1.23. Entry Rates of Ions to the Posterior Chamber of Cynomolgus Monkey: Effect of Carbonic Anhydrase Inhibition

	1 Plasma Concentration (mM)	2 K_{in} (min^{-1})	3 Accession Rate (mM/min) Col. 1 x Col. 2	4 Calc. Conc. in Newly Formed Fluid* (mM)
Na^+				
Control	158	0.017	2.7	162
CAI†		0.009	1.4	168
Cl^-				
Control	103	0.016	1.6	96
CAI†		0.012	1.2	144
HCO_3^-				
Control	20	0.054	1.1	66
CAI†		0.019	0.4	48

$$\text{*Column 3x}\ \frac{\text{vol. posterior chamber (60 µl)}}{\text{aqueous flow (1 µl/min in control; 0.5 µl/min in CAI)}}$$

†Following 50 mg/kg acetazolamide IV 1 hr before isotope injection. See Ref. 101 for details and bibliography.

NA^+,K^+-ADENOSINE TRIPHOSPHATASE (ATPASE)

ATPases are a family of enzymes that can convert chemical work or energy into osmotic work, i.e., movement of electrolytes and associated fluid. In general, the hydrolysis of ATP to adenosine diphosphate (ADP) liberates "energy-rich phosphate," usually designated ~P. One of these enzymes, in the presence of the proper complements of K^+, Mg^{++}, Ca^{++}, and H^+, is activated by Na^+ so that hydrolytic catalysis of ATP increases linearly in the range of 0–100 mM Na^+. This affinity implies a carrier function for sodium which is borne out by anatomic and pharmacologic studies of this enzyme, called Na,K-ATPase.

This protein consists of dimeric cross-linked chain families (alpha, 96 kilodalton; beta, 55 kilodalton) which span the plasma membrane in such a fashion as to facilitate movement of Na^+ (Fig. 1.24).[102] In most tissues thus far studied, this enzyme is contained in the basolateral membrane but not the apical. (An exception is the retinal pigment epithelium.) This has special implications for the ciliary processes; since the two cell layers, pigmented and nonpigmented, face each other at their apical borders, it is the basolateral borders that face both stroma and posterior aqueous (see Section 1, Figs. 1.5–1.7; Section 2, Fig. 1.18; and Fig. 1.29 in this section). Specific staining for Na,K-ATPase shows its presence in both basolateral membranes (including their interdigitations), albeit considerably more in the nonpigmented layer.[103] There are detailed and excellent reviews of the chemistry[104] and physiology of this enzyme in eye[103] and kidney.[105]

The critical and intriguing question about Na,K-ATPase is how its two functions, hydrolytic cleavage to yield ~P and transport of Na^+, are related. In the following paragraph an attempt is made to link them.

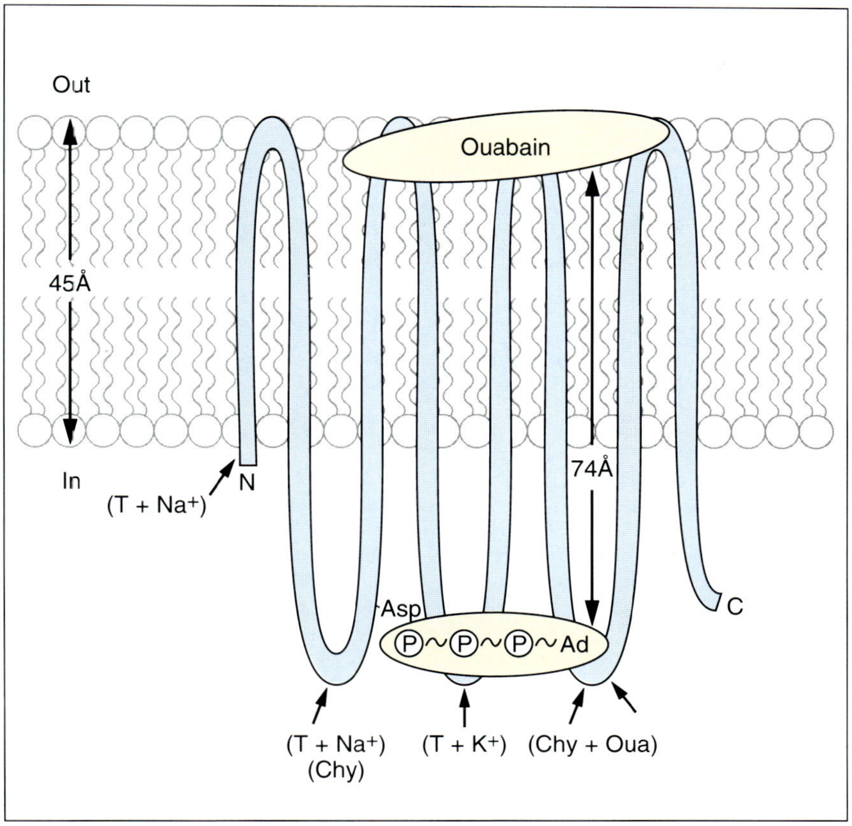

1.24 | Presumed model for the α-subunit of Na,K-ATPase. T (trypsin) and Chy (chymotrypsin) indicate cleavage sites. Ad = adenine; C = carboxy terminal; N = amino terminal; P = phosphate; ASP = active site aspartate residue. (Adapted from Cantley L, Carilli CT, Farley RA, et al: Location of binding sites on the (Na,K)-ATPase for fluorescein-5-isothiocyanate and ouabain. *Ann NY Acad Sci* *1982;402:289–291.*)

The α forms of the enzyme contain the catalytic machinery, including the binding sites for cations and for ouabain. They traverse the membrane in seven to nine loops (Figs. 1.24 and 1.25). The β forms can tentatively be considered as "chaperones" and may face only the outer surface. Let us start with the nonphosphorylated form of the dimer, E_1, always containing Mg^{++}. In the first step, sodium invokes phosphorylation.

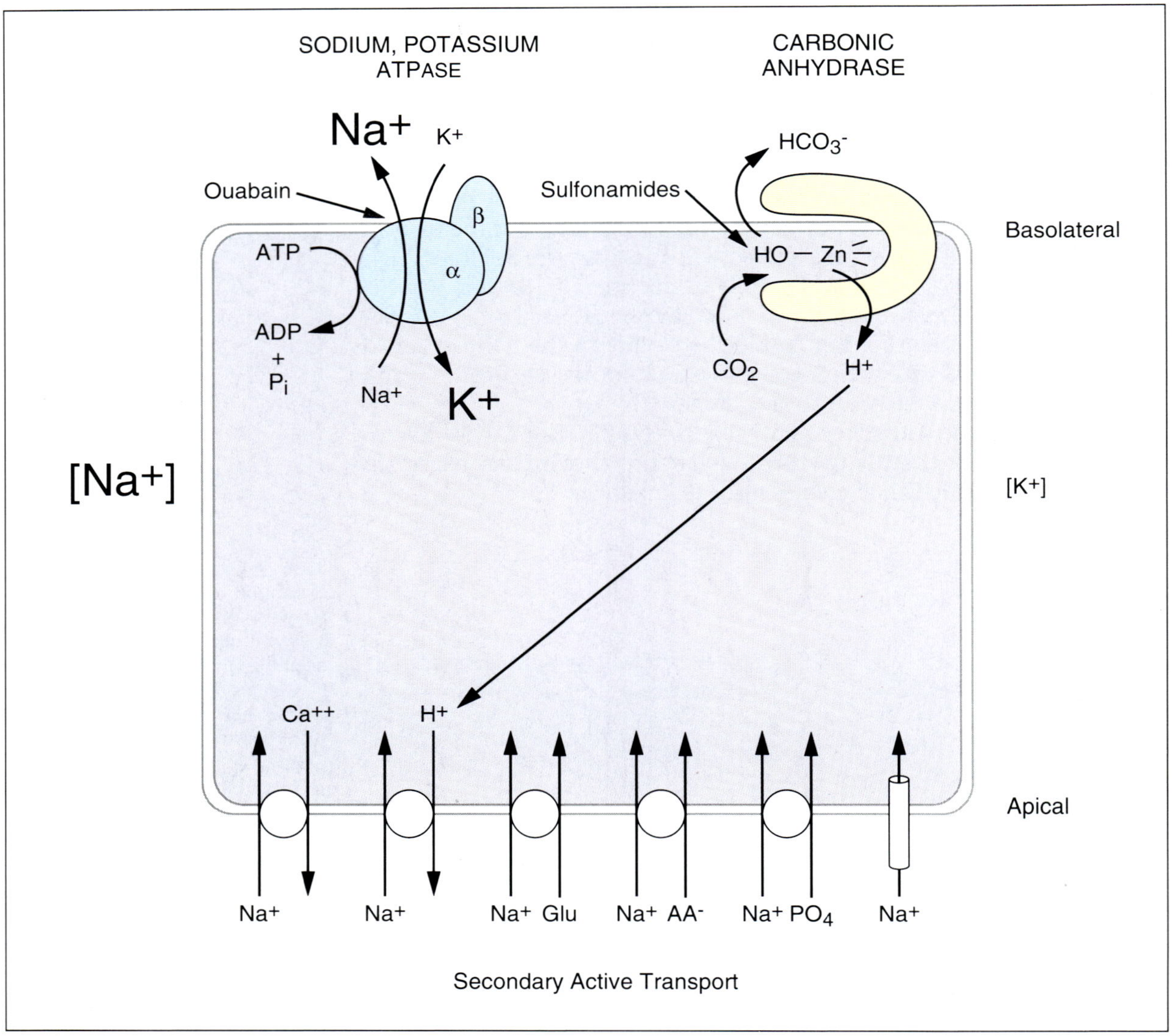

1.25 | Model for Na^+ transport based on ATPase and HCO_3^- formation on carbonic anhydrase. Open circles show Na^+ entering the cell by cotransport or exchange, secondary to action of the ATPase pump on the opposite border. The bar at the right suggests a conductive pathway for Na^+. Carbonic anhydrase is shown in the membrane (isozyme IV). This enzyme is also in cytoplasm (isozyme II), but its role in secretion is most simply relegated to the membrane. (Based on a drawing by Dr. Bruce Kohn.)

$E_1 + 3\ Na + ATP \rightarrow E_1Na_3ATP$ (I)

Hydrolytic cleavage then occurs, on the inner side of the membrane.

$E_1Na_3ATP \rightarrow E_1Na_3P + ADP$ (II)

Now an all-important conformational change in the enzyme ($E_1 \rightarrow E_2$) occurs.

$E_1Na_3\text{-}P \rightarrow E_2Na_3P$ (III)

Here the sodium is in a new state, ready to move out of the membrane into the aqueous as follows.

$E_2Na_3P \rightarrow E_2P + 3\ Na$ (IV)

The next step liberates P and is K^+ dependent. Ouabain acts here in step V to repress dephosphorylation, competing with K^+.

$E_2P + K^+ \rightarrow E_2K + P$ (V)

The K^+ bond formed in step V is relatively strong. In the final steps involving ATP, again there is a conformational change regenerating E_1K, which is a weaker bond with the cation, then freeing E_1 to begin the cycle again, and the K^+ ion.

$E_2K \xrightarrow{ATP} E_1K \rightarrow E_1 + K^+.$ (VI)

The conformational change $E_1 \rightarrow E_2$ is the-key to Na^+ transport, and this depends on phosphorylation and dephosphorylation steps. Therefore, the carrier protein must be an ATPase type; "pump" and enzyme are identical.

Figure 1.25 is a general scheme showing that the pumping of Na^+ out of the cell by the ATPase mechanism, thus keeping its concentration low (about 15 mM), permits the exchange or cotransport of a large number of substances with sodium at the apical border. This is aptly termed "secondary active transport." The dependency on Na,K-ATPase is readily shown, because ouabain or lack of K^+ represses these functions. We will return to this issue below. The part of Figure 1.25 (upper right) that deals with carbonic anhydrase will also be discussed below. As will be shown, this scheme is modified anatomically in the ciliary process, because here Na^+ both enters and leaves basolaterally.

As for all putative relations between enzyme activity and physiologic action, a critical link is the effect of specific enzyme inhibitors on the biologic effect. In the present case, the cardiac glycosides are the closest approach to such drugs. Ouabain, the most widely used, actively inhibits 50% of enzyme in the tissues of most species, including ciliary processes of the rabbit, at about 10^{-6} M. Its mechanism is given above: competition with K^+ at the dephosphorylation step V. Note that this is a considerable distance from the adenosine phosphate site (see Fig. 1.24). As Figure 1.25 shows, ouabain binds at the outer membrane to the alpha chain. Unfortunately, the uses of ouabain are limited by other effects at higher concentrations and by its general toxicity. Nevertheless, by use of judiciously low doses, by application to the vitreous, or by close intra-arterial (lingual) injection, effects on aqueous humor formation, sodium transport, and the blood aqueous potential difference are obtained. Figure 1.26 shows such data.[106] Note that Na^+ and fluid move together precisely; sodium concentration is constant at 150 mM, whereas the ion and fluid transport are reduced 62%. The dose used (0.05 μmol/min x 40 min) is very small, and almost certainly the enzyme was not fully inhibited; yet this very striking effect suggests that virtually all Na^+ transport may be dependent on this mechanism. Inhibition of Na,K-ATPase appears at first glance to be the ideal treatment for glaucoma. However, despite an extensive search, no drugs have been found with low enough toxicity to be clinically useful.

$HC0_3^-$ ACCESSION

The transfer of $HC0_3^-$ from plasma to aqueous is about one third that of sodium (see Fig. 1.23). Similar data to that of Figure 1.23 (monkey) have been obtained in the dog.[101] Most importantly, Figure 1.23 shows that the concentration of $HC0_3^-$ in newly formed (or nascent) fluid (66 mM) is much higher than that in plasma (20 mM), or indeed in the posterior aqueous measured in the steady state (21 mM). Nascent chloride is correspondingly low; as shown above, Na^+ concentration is constant. One might properly ask how the high nascent $HC0_3^-$ (66 mM) and low nascent chloride (96 mM) shown in Figure 1.23 are converted to the measured amounts observed in the posterior chamber, 21 mM and 125 mM, respectively (see Fig. 1.22). It can only be assumed that, in the largely anaerobic (glycolytic) metabolism of the lens, acid formation is sufficient to drive off a large fraction of secreted $HC0_3^-$. Note that the relative lens/posterior chamber volume ratio is on the order of 6, surely favoring such a scheme. The movement of chloride can be regarded as secondary, with Na^+ remaining constant, but no details can presently be furnished.

The enzyme carbonic anhydrase has been found in the ciliary processes of all vertebrates, and it is clear that inhibitors of this enzyme lower aqueous flow and intraocular pressure. This will be discussed below. In the present context of accession rates of $HC0_3^-$, and returning to Figure 1.23, it will be seen that inhibition of carbonic anhydrase by a full dose of the inhibitor acetazolamide reduces $HC0_3^-$ accumulation from 1.1 to 0.4 mM/min^{-1}. As will be shown in this next section, this enzyme performs a single function in the context of the type of secretion: the hydroxylation of $C0_2$ to form $HC0_3^-$. Therefore, the experiment of Figure 1.23 can have only one interpretation:

Figure 1.26. Result of Na,K-ATPase Inhibition on Fluid and Na^+ Movement and Electrical Measurements of Aqueous Humor in the Rabbit

	Control	After Ouabain*
Blood–aqueous, potential difference (mV)	-6.1	-1.7
Short-circuit current (μA)	435	85
Fluid entry (μl/min)	5.7	2.2
Sodium entry (μEq/min)	0.85	0.32

*Given by injection into lingual artery, 0.05 μmol/min x 40 min.
(From Cole DF: Electrochemical changes associated with the formation of the aqueous humor. *Br J Ophthalmol 1961;45:202.*)

$HC0_3^-$ is *formed* in the ciliary process from $C0_2$. The accession of $HC0_3^-$ in the aqueous (and other fluids) is thus entirely different in kind from that of the fixed ions Na^+ and Cl^-.

$HC0_3^-$ accession has a second attribute, which is that its movement (along with Na^+) attracts more fluid than does NaCl. Figure 1.23 shows that of the 2.7 mM/min^{-1} sodium being transported, 0.7 mM $HC0_3^-$ (control rate minus inhibited), or 26%, depends on the catalytic conversion of $C0_2 \rightarrow HC0_3^-$. On the other hand, the dependency of flow on the catalyzed rate is about 40%, i.e., the flow rate is decreased by inhibition.[107] This relation is found in other secretory systems for formation of $HC0_3^-$ catalyzed by carbonic anhydrase, i.e., cerebrospinal fluid and pancreatic fluid. There appears to be a special relation between the transfer of $NaHC0_3$ and fluid; perhaps this is the reason that important transport systems invoke carbonic anhydrase-mediated $HC0_3^-$ accession. The reason for this attraction between $HC0_3^-$ ion and water is not known, but surely is a worthwhile subject for further research.

A third attribute of $NaHC0_3$ is now being explored, which is that the undissociated molecule designated $NaHC0_3^\circ$ may be the transporting species.[108] It is known that ions are undissociated at low dielectric constant, such as in the region of cell membranes. Such an attribute would surely speed the passage of sodium and fluid.

CARBONIC ANHYDRASE (CA)

This enzyme is as different from the ATPases as can be imagined, yet they are complementary in function. CA is a soluble, single-stranded, nearly spherical protein of 30 kilodaltons, with a Zn atom at the active site center linked to three histidine molecules and water[100] (Fig. 1.27). The pK_a of the zinc-bound water is about 7, so the OH^- concentration at the active site is nearly seven

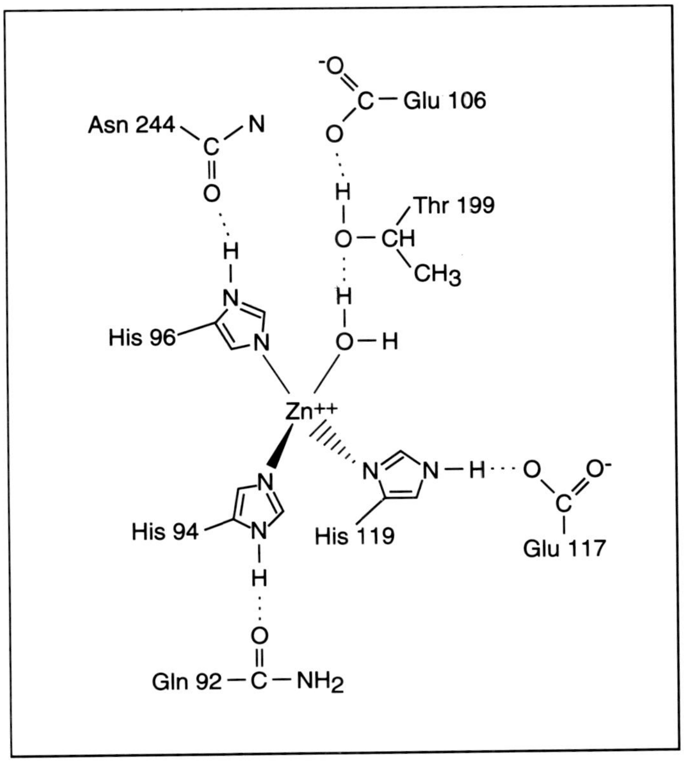

1.27 | Schematic drawing of the active site of carbonic anhydrase (II or IV) showing the central Zn atom and the water bonding network. The sulfonamide inhibitors bind directly to the Zn through the N in the SO_2NH^- group.

orders of magnitude greater than that of water (pK_a at 37°C is 13.6). The biologic role of the enzyme is the catalysis of the reversible reaction $CO_2 + OH^- \Leftrightarrow HCO_3^-$, and the enormous potential exaltation of the uncatalyzed rate, by over a millionfold, corresponds to this special ionization of water at the zinc site. All the known physiologic functions of the enzyme can be described in terms of this reaction, which include the carrier function of CO_2 (as HCO_3^-) in the red cells and the formation of acid (again from the ionization of water, followed by the buffering of OH^- by CO_2) in the renal tubule and stomach. In the present context we deal with HCO_3^- formation, as also is found in cerebrospinal fluid and pancreatic juice.

The biochemistry of carbonic anhydrase is complicated by the occurrence of a number of isozymes. In the present context we need to consider two of these, CA II and IV, each found in both pigmented (P) and nonpigmented (NP) epithelia[109] (P. Wistrand, personal communication). The first of these is found in cytoplasm, and the concentration and properties of CA II are used in the kinetic analysis to follow. CA IV is membrane-bound, usually at both basolateral and apical borders. In ciliary processes it has been identified histochemically in the basement membranes of NP and P epithelia.[109] Using sulfonamide inhibitors with a variety of chemical properties and measuring the transepithelial potential in isolated ciliary epithelia, the enzyme was localized to the basolateral membrane of NP epithelia.[110] An estimation of the contribution of the membrane-bound enzyme to HCO_3^- formation cannot be given. The calculated catalytic rate given in Figure 1.28 may be an underestimation, because it is based on total soluble enzyme in the tissue. This does not affect the general argument.

Figure 1.28 shows how the system is presumed to operate. The primary reaction is the protolysis of water to yield OH^- at the secretory cell surface. This reacts with CO_2 catalytically (or noncatalytically when the enzyme is inhibited) to form HCO_3^-, which passes into the aqueous humor along with sodium. The H^+ liberated from water passes into the blood and is buffered by proteins. Figure 1.28 footnotes show the theoretical HCO_3^- rates, based on the known constants, and some assumptions regarding cell volume and pH of the secretory region. The catalytic rate is 7 μmol/min, and the uncatalyzed is 0.07 μmol/min. (This hundredfold exaltation of the uncatalyzed rate is unusually low owing to the relatively low concentration of enzyme in the ciliary process.) These may be compared with the actual rates in monkey (see Fig. 1.28, right), derived from the molar rates of Figure 1.23 by adjusting to the volume of the posterior chamber, 60 μl. This yields 0.066 μmol/min for HCO_3^-. The Na^+ rate, also shown, is 2.5 times the HCO_3^- rate. It is likely that the Na^+ rate is all based on Na,K-ATPase, as discussed above. Note that the normal rate of HCO_3^- formation (0.066 μmol/min) is less than 1% of $V_{calc.\ cat.}$ the calculated catalyzed rate (see Fig. 1.28, footnote).

The uncatalyzed rate is found experimentally by inhibiting the enzyme in vivo by a large dose of the specific inhibitor acetazolamide. Such inhibition, when complete, should yield the uncatalyzed rate of HCO_3^- formation. In the present case, the observed inhibited rate (see Fig. 1.28, right, 0.024 μmol/min) is not far from the calculated $V_{calc.\ unc.}$ (see Fig. 1.28, footnote, 0.07 μmol/min). Considering the assumptions about pH and cell volume, the agreement seems reasonable, and we tentatively use the model of Figure 1.28. Demonstrated is the large excess of enzyme in this tissue, as has been found throughout nature. This is of great theoretical and practical interest; it ensures instant equilibrium between CO_2 and HCO_3^-. From a pharmacologic view, it means that to achieve a physiologic effect, >99% of the enzyme must be inhibited. That is the case for clinical doses of the sulfonamide inhibitors.

The sulfonamide carbonic anhydrase inhibitors have been in clinical use for treatment of glaucoma since 1955, when their action on the eye was discovered as an offshoot of their development as diuretics.[100] They have also been extremely useful in research on aqueous humor formation, because they are absolutely specific, having no other action at concentrations below 1 mM. The major compound is acetazolamide, but many discerning ophthalmologists prefer methazolamide, which acts on the eye in lower doses that

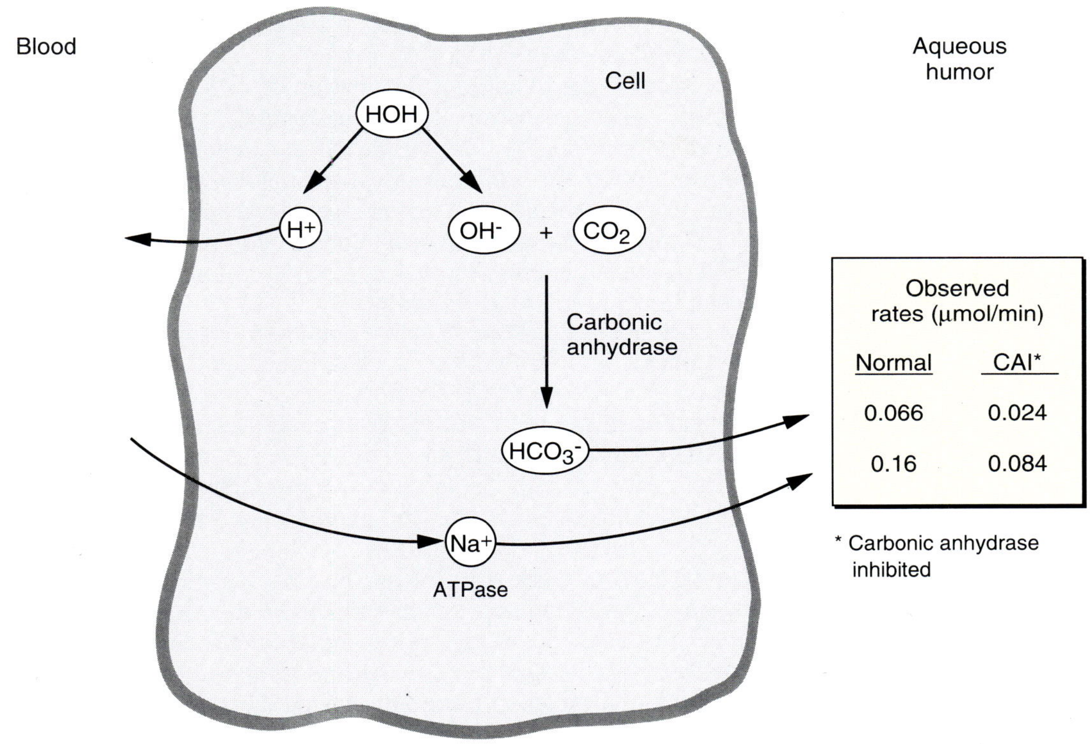

$$V_{calc.\ unc.} = (k_2)(OH^-)(CO_2)$$

$$= (23 \times 10^3\ M^{-1}sec^{-1})(10^{-5}\ M)(10^{-3}M)$$

for 5 μL secretory volume

$$= 0.07\ \mu mol/min$$

$$V_{calc.\ cat.} = \frac{(k_{cat})(E)(CO_2)}{CO_2 + k_m}$$

$$= \frac{(1 \times 10^6\ sec^{-1})(0.34\ \mu M)(1\ mM)}{1\ mM + 14\ mM}$$

for 5 μL secretory volume

$$= 7\ \mu mol/min$$

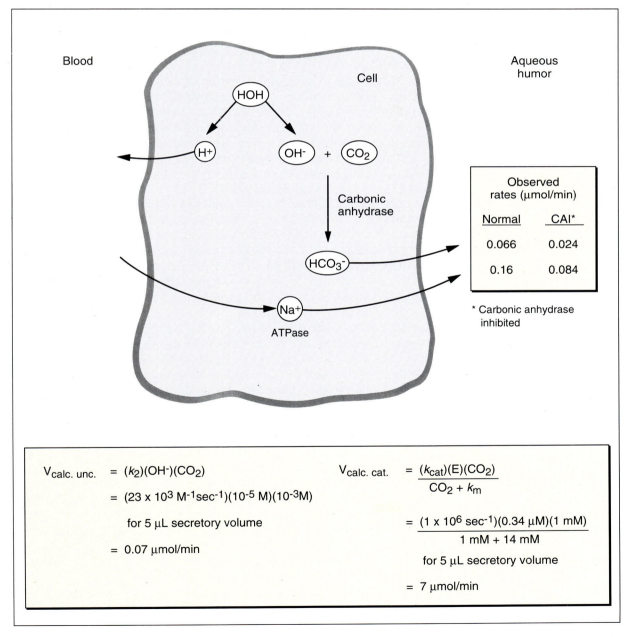

1.28 | Model for HCO_3^- formation linked to Na^+ transport in the ciliary process. Observed rates are for monkey. Chemical rate constants (37°) taken from the literature.[99]

have little or no action on other carbonic anhydrase sites in the body. This is due to the good fortune that, as mentioned above, the concentration of this enzyme in the ciliary process is much less than that of other tissues. The chief advantages of methazolamide are its ready diffusibility and its lack of concentration in the kidney.[107]

The cardinal characteristic of these compounds is the unsubstituted sulfonamide group $R\text{-}SO_2NH_2$, which exists at body pH in equilibrium with the anionic form $R\text{-}SO_2NH^-$. It is this molecule that attacks Zn at the active site of the enzyme (see Fig. 1.27), displacing water, or specifically OH^-. The link is tight, with dissociation constants reaching 10^{-9} M, but is entirely reversible. When such a drug is given orally or intravenously in therapeutic doses, it reaches the ciliary process at a concentration on the order of 10 μM (10^{-5} M) which for methazolamide, whose K_I against the enzyme is 10^{-8} M, means 99.9% inhibition. The effect on aqueous flow persists until this concentration drops to 1–2 μM.[107,111]

Despite the ubiquitous distribution of carbonic anhydrase, long-term chronic use of acetazolamide or methazolamide is only very rarely injurious. Details of treatment will be considered in Chapter 9, Section 2. However, a train of unpleasant symptoms, such as fatigue and depression, led over the years to diminished patient acceptance. It was feared that these would outweigh the clear-cut and now well-understood drop in pressure and flow in glaucomatous patients, so new research was undertaken to find topically active carbonic anhydrase inhibitors.[100,112]

The new generation of sulfonamides—the "topicals"—are characterized by elements of both lipid and water solubility and high activity against the enzyme. They permeate the eye from a single drop, across the cornea to aqueous humor, thence to iris and ciliary processes, and across conjunctiva and corneoscleral junction through ciliary muscle to the process.[113,114] Concentrations in the ciliary processes are as great as those following administration of parenteral sulfonamides, and the drop in intraocular pressure is comparable.[113,115]

CHLORIDE AND OTHER MECHANISMS

A great deal of work concerning secretory epithelia outside the eye has revealed several transport systems which are just now being investigated in ciliary processes. Such work is generally done in vitro, in vesicles formed from secretory cells or in tissue culture from such cells. Their discovery is largely due to the good fortune of having fairly specific inhibitors for each system. Using figure 1.29 (obtained from References 116 and 117), several systems are described, adding to carbonic anhydrase and Na,K-ATPase.

The $Na^+/2Cl^-/K^+$ cotransport system (#2 in Figure 1.29) is dependent on the ATPase pump for its driving force. When the pump keeps cell Na^+ low, Cl^- moves inward, accompanied by Na^+ and K^+. This is a powerful mechanism in the thick ascending limb of Henle in the kidney and in the shark rectal gland. This carrier is blocked by bumetanide and related "high ceiling" diuretics, which probably explains their mechanism of action.[118] Under special conditions in cultured pigmented epithelial cells, bumetanide does reduce Na^+ and Cl^- uptake. However, drugs of this class do not reduce the secretion of aqueous humor. Therefore, it is not clear whether this system plays an important role in aqueous formation.

$Cl^-\text{-}HCO_3^-$ exchange (#3 in Figure 1.29) is a system well known to occur in the red cell (band 3), and is studied by blocking with DIDS (4,4′-diisothiocyanatostilbene-2,2′-disulfonic acid) and other stilbene derivatives. In cultured pigmented epithelial cells of ciliary processes there is evidence for this system, but in vivo the net movement of Cl^- and HCO_3^- is in the same direction. Figure 1.29 shows how these facts can be reconciled; the *overall* movement of Cl^- (including step #2) is towards the aqueous. In vivo experiments with this class of compounds are limited by their toxicity and the necessity for high concentrations.

Na^+–H^+ exchange (#1 in Figure 1.29) is inhibited by amiloride, which reduces Na^+ uptake from the blood side to cultured pigmented epithelial cells of ciliary processes. However, the inhibitor is not entirely specific for this exchange system, and the high concentration used (1 mM) could not be approached in vivo. In the scheme depicted in Figure 1.29, there does not appear to be any necessity for Na^+–H^+ exchange.

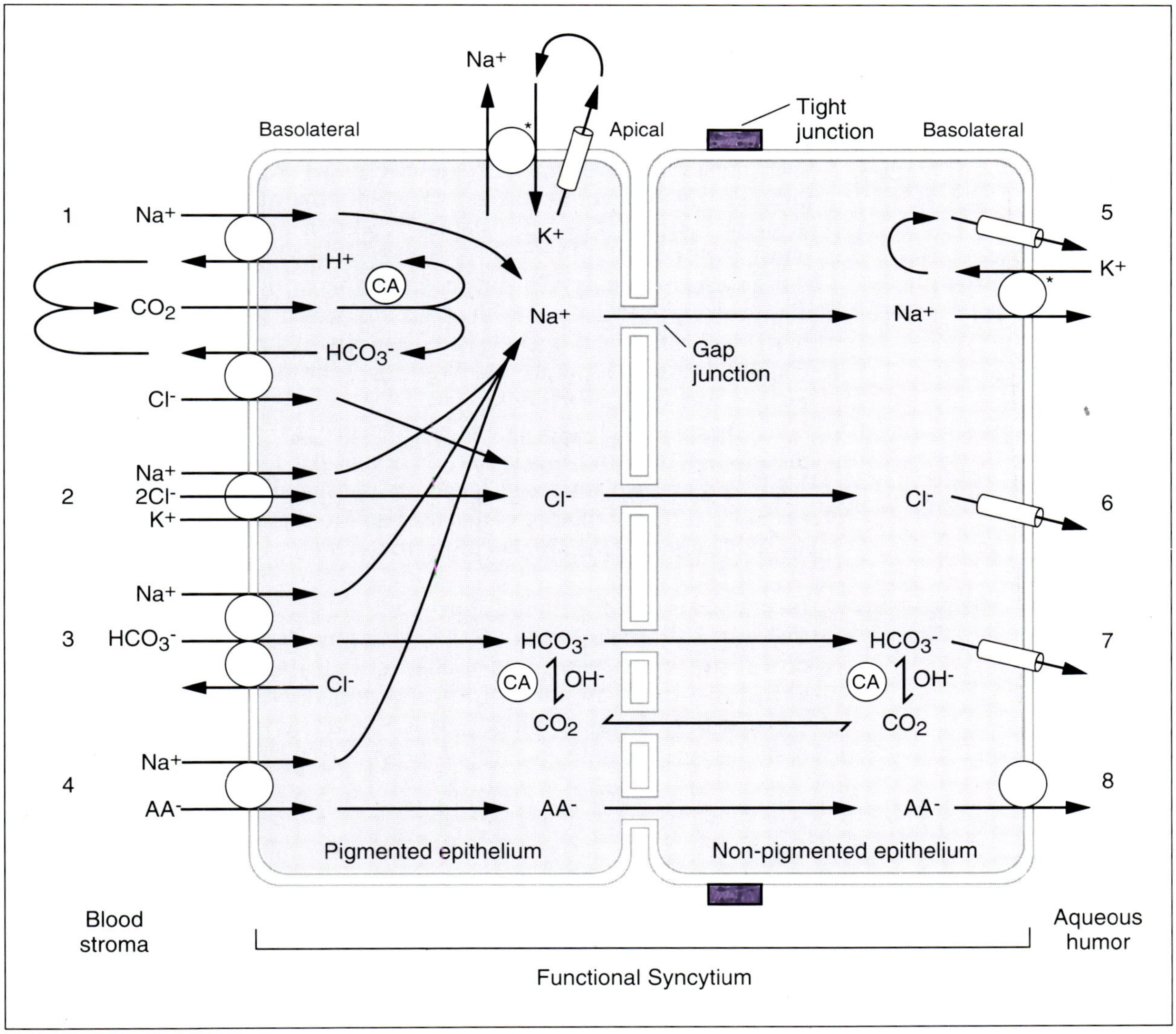

1.29 | Diagram of possible secretory pathways in the ciliary process, based on transport in isolated cells in tissue culture. *Na,K-ATPase. AA = ascorbic acid. CA = carbonic anhydrase. (Adapted from Wiederholt M, Helbig H, Korbmacher C: Ion transport across the ciliary epithelium: Lessons from cultured cells and proposed role of the carbonic anhydrase, in Botrè F, Gross G (eds): *Carbonic Anhydrase*. Cambridge, New York: Verlag-Chemie, 1992, 232–244.)

Despite the complexity of Figure 1.29, note that the final transport step, from nonpigmented epithelium to aqueous humor involves the accession of Na^+, Cl^- and HCO_3^-, just as observed in Figure 1.23.

It is clear that more work is needed in vivo on the transport of these ions when modified by ouabain, bumetanide, and amiloride and DIDS-type drugs.

A particular crux has been the connections between pharmacological actions of β-blockers or α_2-agonists and reduction of aqueous flow. It is by no means apparent how these autonomic effects might lower flow or, in view of the dependence of flow on Na^+ transport, how they may affect electrolyte movement. Preliminary study yielded the surprising result that timolol (the nonselective β-adrenergic antagonist) reduced flow in rabbit (as is well known for all species) but not Na^+ movement from plasma to posterior aqueous.[119] Further work is indicated on this vexing problem.

FLOW: POTENTIAL DIFFERENCE: ION MOVEMENT

Most body fluids are subject to wide variation in output, i.e., urine, pancreatic, salivary, and biliary secretion. The aqueous humor and cerebrospinal fluid are quite different in that they proceed at a relatively constant rate; there is no strong evidence for hormonal or metabolic control. There is some circadian rhythm, with aqueous flow (and intraocular pressure) diminished at night by some 40% (see Chapter 1, Section 2). Large increases in flow above the normal 3 µl/min are essentially unknown, so we can assume that during daytime the system runs continuously at (nearly) full speed. This is compatible with what is known about the two chief enzymes involved: carbonic anhydrase and Na,K-ATPase. The first is not subject to regulatory control; the second appears under control of the ions themselves, which normally do not change relations in vivo.

The aqueous humor potential difference is slightly negative to that of plasma (l–5 mV) and this is reduced somewhat by both ouabain (see Fig. 1.26) and acetazolamide.[120] These are considered to be HCO_3^- diffusion potentials. The cell interior is about -65 mV to the aqueous. These potentials are not considered the primary forces in secretion.

SUMMARY

In summary, aqueous humor flow is a consequence of sodium movement fueled by Na,K-ATPase and by HCO_3^- formation originating in the protolysis of water with the subsequent reaction of $OH^- + CO_2$ catalyzed by carbonic anhydrase. In a way not entirely understood, Na^+ and HCO_3^- engage in cotransport at the ciliary process, with osmotic forces generating the transfer of fluid to the posterior chamber of the eye.

Section IV

Biochemistry of Aqueous Humor Outflow

Ted S. Acott

The aqueous outflow pathway has not received the degree of molecular scrutiny that has been lavished on many larger and more accessible tissues. The human trabecular meshwork is small (~100–150 µg) with few cells (200,000–300,000 per eye). These cells are highly differentiated and moderately difficult to culture.[121–124] Human trabecular cells grow relatively slowly, undergo senescent changes between passage 5 and 10 in culture, and grow poorly from donors over 20 years of age. Human, nonhuman primate, bovine, cat, and pig trabecular meshwork extracts, cell suspensions and cell cultures, and human corneoscleral explant organ cultures have been the primary focus for molecular analysis of the outflow pathway.[125] In spite of the difficulty, several aspects of outflow pathway biochemistry and molecular biology have been studied in moderate detail and new methodologies are being applied with increasing frequency to expand our understanding of this tissue's molecular nature and behavior. Fortunately, many trabecular systems and processes are similar to those found in other tissues. Because the primary job of the trabecular meshwork is to maintain the appropriate aqueous humor outflow rate and conductance and, consequently, the appropriate ocular rigidity and intraocular pressure,[126,127] the primary focus of outflow pathway biochemistry has been on systems believed to modulate aqueous outflow.[128]

The Trabecular Extracellular Matrix

The trabecular meshwork's extracellular matrix (ECM) has since the 1950s been a strong candidate for the site of resistance to normal aqueous humor outflow. By inference, this ECM is also a likely site for the increased trabecular resistance, responsible for intraocular pressure elevation in open-angle glaucoma. Perfusion of the outflow pathway with glycosaminoglycan (GAG)-degrading enzymes produces approximately a doubling in outflow facility.[129,130] Similarities between in vivo and postmortem outflow facility, the lack of a thermal dependency of facility, and the inability of metabolic toxins to change facility provide evidence that outflow is a passive process not requiring trabecular cell metabolism or activity.[131–134] Trabecular cells are critically involved in maintaining and regulating outflow resistance, but they do not themselves appear to provide an active (energy-requiring) barrier to, or assistance with, outflow.

Light and electron microscopic observations, morphometric analysis, hydrodynamic modeling, and our knowledge of the roles and properties of GAGs and ECMs in other tissues (see below) support a role for the trabecular ECM in outflow resistance.[128,135–140] Trabecular cells are believed to regulate aqueous humor outflow, and consequently intraocular pressure, by cleaning and regularly replacing the molecular components of trabecular ECMs.[128] However, this has not yet been rigorously proven, and attractive alternatives have been postulated.[128,141–145]

There are several distinct trabecular ECMs (Fig. 1.30) including: basement membranes throughout the meshwork, basal to the trabecular cells; the bulk ECM, which forms the trabecular beams and sheets; the amorphous juxtacanalicular ECM (including basement membranes), which is immediately internal to the cells lining Schlemm's canal; and the cell surface ECM, which is apical to the trabecular cells and which protrudes into the intratrabecular flow channels. Of these, the two latter are most frequently singled out as the likely site(s) of the outflow resistance. Excellent transmission electron micrographs, showing strong GAG staining in these two regions, have been published and merit close examination.[128,146,147] No rigorous evidence establishing outflow resistance at either of these sites, or alternatives, has been presented.

MOLECULAR COMPONENTS OF TRABECULAR ECMS: STRUCTURE AND FUNCTIONS

ECMs are complex structures composed of many different proteins, most of which are glycoproteins or proteoglycans.[128,148–153] They are organized, and their structural integrity is maintained by a variety of specific interactions with each other and with cell surface receptors. It has become increasingly clear that ECM macromolecules and their interactions are critical to, and actually regulate, a wide variety of cell processes, including embryologic development programs and tissue organization, cell growth and differentiation patterns, gene expression profiles, tissue remodeling, and wound healing, as well as serving many specific functions that are directly dependent on their physical properties.[128,149,152,154–156]

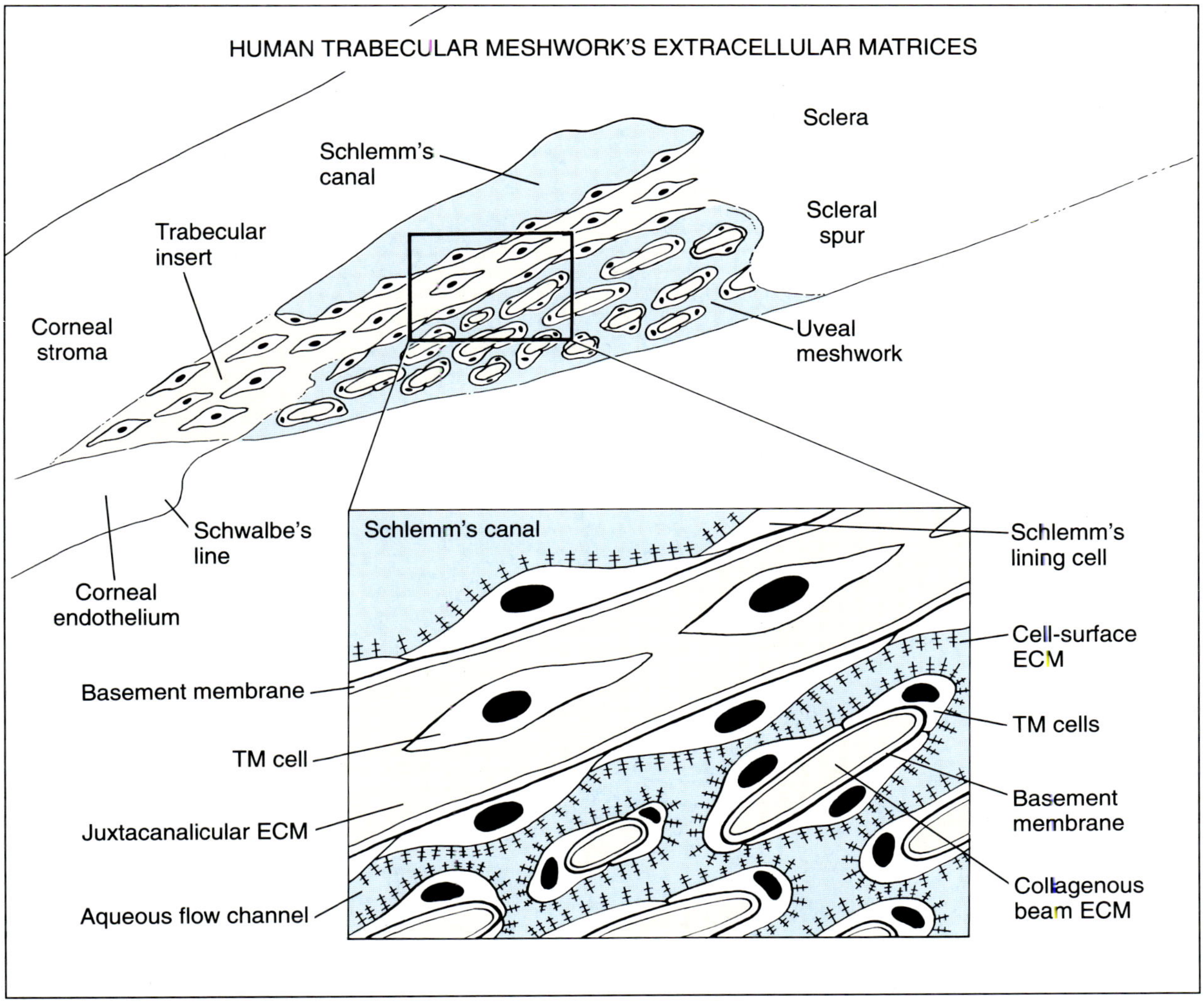

1.30 | Diagrammatic view of the ECMs of the human trabecular meshwork.[128] ‡ represents cell surface proteoglycans extending into the flow channels. Trabecular cell nuclei are shown in solid black.

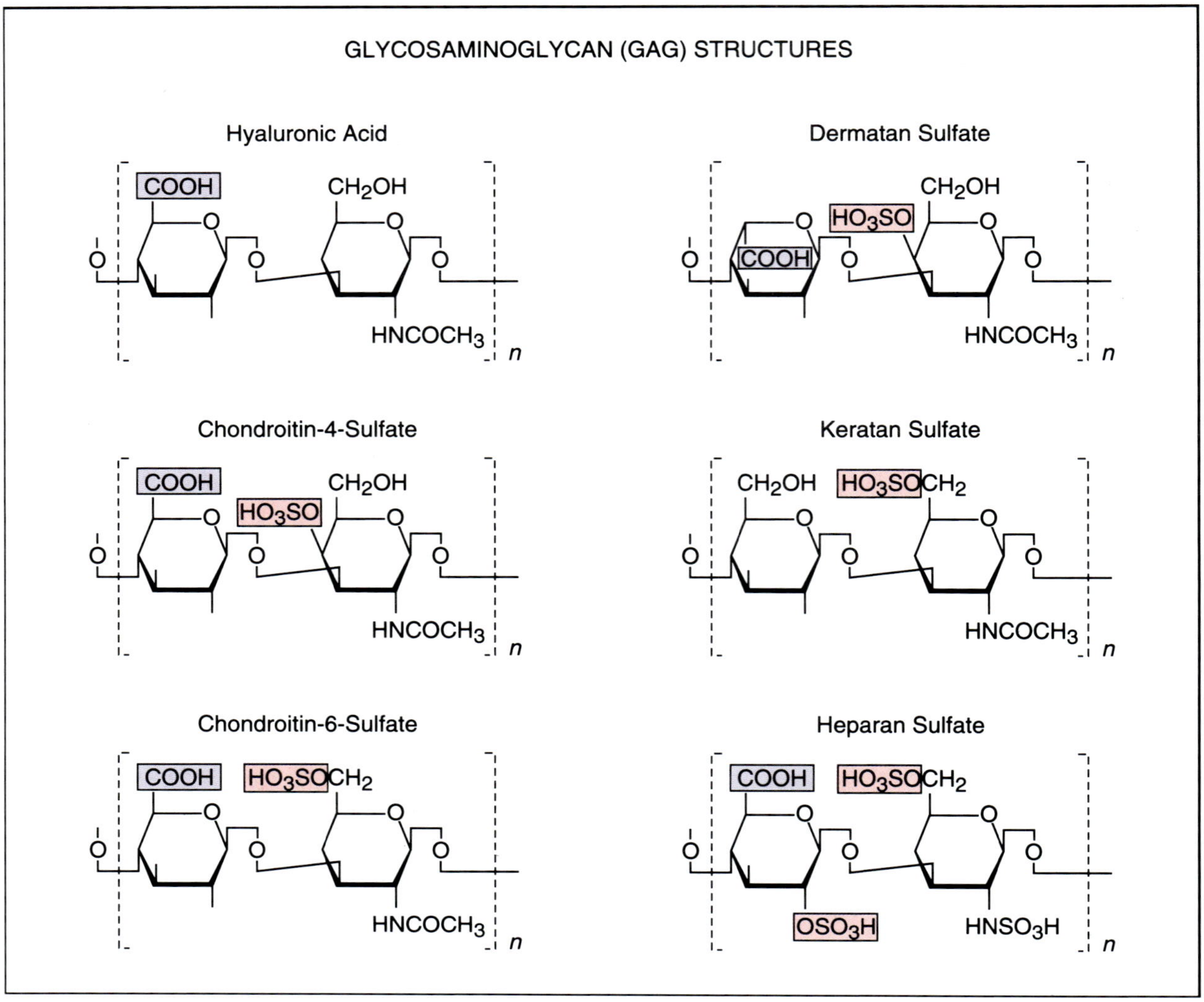

1.31 | Repeat disaccharide structures of the common glycosaminoglycans. Carboxyl and sulfate groups, which are negatively charged at physiologic pH, are highlighted.

GAGS AND PROTEOGLYCANS

GAGs are long carbohydrate chains composed of specific disaccharide repeat sequences (Fig. 1.31). They contain between one and four carboxyl and/or sulfate groups per disaccharide repeat. Both the carboxyl and the sulfate groups are ionized at physiologic pH, resulting in an extremely high density of negative charges. Many of their biological functions are dependent on this characteristic.

TRABECULAR GAGS

The GAG composition of the trabecular meshwork and the GAGs synthesized by trabecular cells have been determined[124,125,128,130,156–161] utilizing sequential enzymatic degradation with a series of enzymes specific for each type of known GAG. The trabecular meshwork glycosaminoglycan content shown in Figure 1.32 indicates the percentage of each type of GAG obtained by sequential enzymatic degradation from normal and primary open-angle glaucoma (POAG) eyes, organ cultures, and densely confluent cell cultures. The radiolabel experiments utilized glucosamine and sulfate precursor labeling. Histologic staining of the trabecular GAGs, coupled with this enzymatic degradation approach, allows their microscopic localization within the meshwork.[128,146,147,162–164]

Figure 1.32. Trabecular Meshwork Glycosaminoglycan Content

	Percentage of Total GAGs					
Type of Glycosaminoglycan (GAG)	Eye Bank Eyes			Organ Culture[125,342]		Cell Culture[51]
	Normal[157]	Normal[318]	POAG[318]	^{3}H-glu	^{35}S-SO_4	Confluence
Hyaluronic acid (HA)	25	11	<7	22 (20)	—	21
Chondroitin sulfates (CS)	14	60	71	28 (22)	33 (25)	39
Dermatan sulfate (DS)	21			21 (24)	35 (32)	14
Keratan sulfate (KS)	15	6	4	6 (14)	8 (13)	6
Heparan sulfate (HS)	18	22	16	18 (18)	14 (12)	21
Undegradable GAG-like material	9	1	2	5 (12)	11 (18)	—

PROTEOGLYCANS

With the exception of hyaluronic acid, GAGs are found as covalently attached linear sidechains added (posttranslationally) to the core protein of the proteoglycans (Fig. 1.33). The bonding is generally an O-linkage between serine or threonine of the protein and a xylose residue. The xylose is linked to two galactoses and a glucuronic acid before beginning the specific GAG disaccharide repeat.[155,165] The trabecular GAGs, except for hyaluronic acid, are found as sidechains of at least six different proteoglycans.[128,147,166–168] Only the large basement membrane heparan sulfate proteoglycan has been specifically identified within the meshwork;[169] some of the others undoubt-

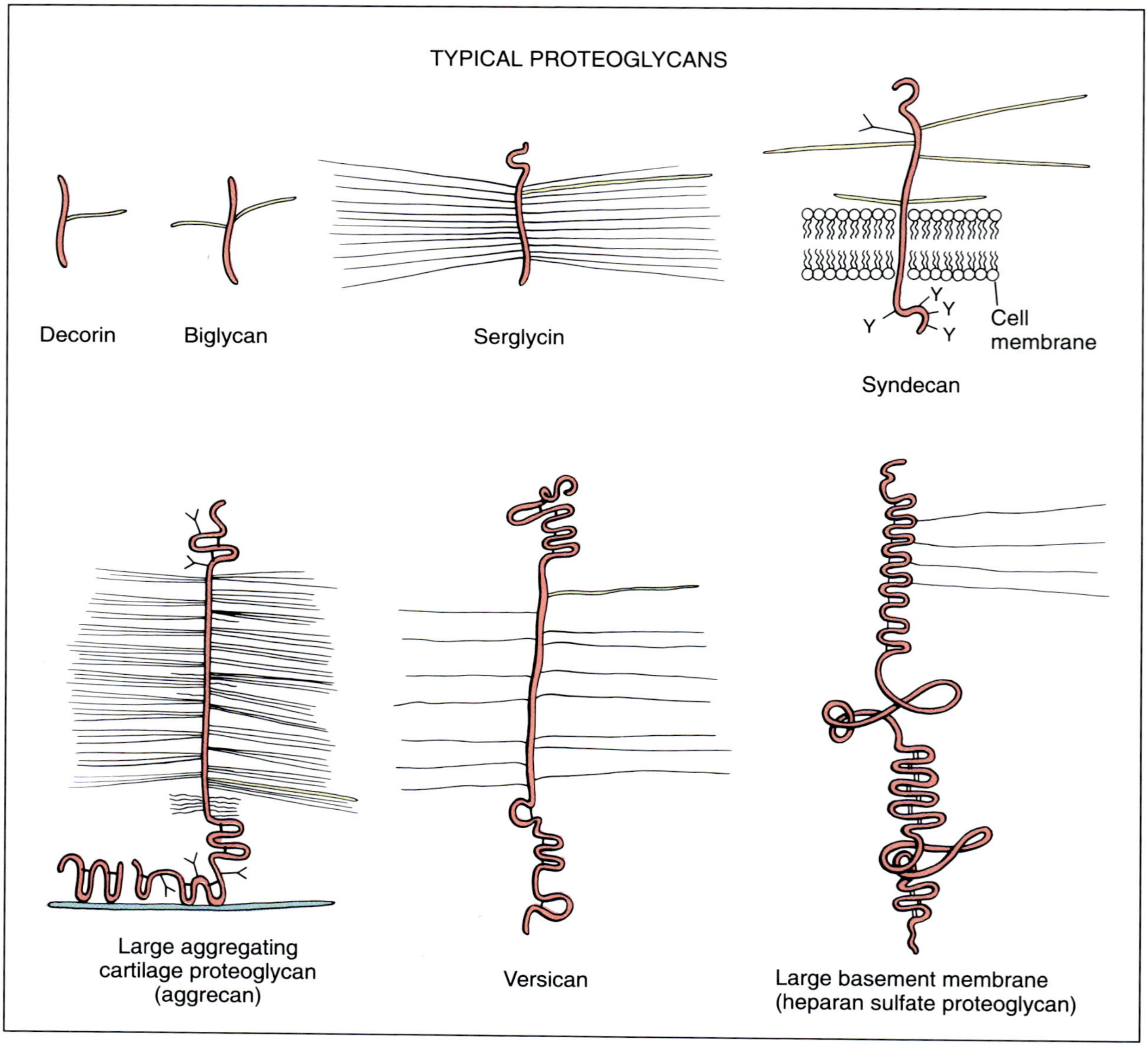

1.33 | Structural models of several typical proteoglycans.[128,149,140,152–156] Core proteins are highlighted in red and GAG sidechains are indicated by horizontal lines or are highlighted in yellow. Disulfide bonding is indicated by connecting loops in the core proteins in the specific cases where cysteine-rich folding domains are conserved. Tyrosines, which may be phosphorylated, are shown on the cytoplasmic portion of syndecan (Y). Oligosaccharides are shown in cases where their presence is known (—<) .

edly include the common proteoglycans found in other tissues, although trabecular-specific species cannot be ruled out at this time.

CORE PROTEINS

Several of the common proteoglycan core proteins have been cloned and sequenced in recent years.[128,149,152,154–156] These core proteins show a wide variety of sizes (11 to 400 kDa) and structures (see Fig. 1.33) with between one and over 100 GAG side-chains per core protein. Proteoglycan sizes range between 20,000 and several million Daltons. In addition to this diversity within the family of core proteins and in their GAG attachment patterns, considerable microheterogeneity is observed. Frequently, the number, length, degree of sulfation, ratio of glucuronic to iduronic acid epimers, and even the type of GAG chain found associated with a specific core protein is variable between tissues, within a tissue, and at different developmental stages. This variable microheterogeneity has hindered analysis of the structural characteristics of trabecular and other tissue proteoglycans. The microheterogeneity is assumed to have a functional significance (see below), but this is not well defined at this time.

Until recently, proteoglycans were named primarily for their size, tissue distribution, and type of GAG sidechain. With the recent availability of core protein sequence information, they are now commonly named for their core protein (see Fig. 1.33). Some characteristics of the more common proteoglycans are included in Figure 1.34.

PROTEOGLYCAN TYPES

Proteoglycans have also been divided into three categories based on their tissue location: (1) pericellular or cell surface proteoglycans, including those of basement membranes; (2) small intracellular granule proteoglycans; and (3) general extracellular matrix proteoglycans. Because of its diverse structure

Figure 1.34. Characteristics of Several Common Proteoglycans[128,149,150,152,154–156]

Proteoglycan	Proteoglycan Size	Core Protein Size	GAG Type	GAG Chain Number	Comments
Aggrecan	~2,500,000 Mr	220,952	CS KS	~100 15-40	Aggregates with HA; 80-90% carbohydrate; N- and O-linked oligosaccharides
Versican	>500,000	265,048	CS	~5-15	Homology to aggrecan
Syndecan	~190,000-280,000 Mr	32,868	HS CS	1-4 (14,000-36,000 Mr) 0-2 (11,000-17,000 Mr	Transmembrane cell-surface protein
Biglycan	~76,000 Mr	37,280	CS or DS	2 (40,000 Mr)	PG I; Leu rich
Decorin	74,000-100,000 Mr	36,383	CS or DS	1	PG-40; PG II
Serglycin	750,000-1,000,000 Mr 150,000 Mr	10,190 18,900	HS CS/DS	~49 ~14	In secretory granule; in ECM
Basement membrane HSPG	~500,000 Mr	~400,000 Mr	HS	2-4 (30,000-65,000 Mr)	29:71 protein:GAG; ~40% sequenced

(see Fig. 1.30) having both luminal and solid tissue regions, the trabecular meshwork is likely to contain proteoglycans from all three categories.[128,166,167] In addition to these common "dedicated" proteoglycans, a wide variety of other proteoglycans with diverse structures and functions have been defined. Among these are the transferrin receptor, the large or type III cell receptor for transforming growth factor-beta (TGF-β), type IX collagen, and fibronectin.[128,148–152,154–156]

GAG/ PROTEOGLYCAN FUNCTIONS

Until recently, the confusing heterogeneity of proteoglycan and GAG chain structures was interpreted as evidence that the primary function of proteoglycans was to provide a dense cluster of negative charges.[170–175] More recent studies have established high levels of functional specificity and have expanded the number of processes in which proteoglycans are involved.[128, 148–153,155,156] However, the physical property concept is clearly valid in many cases.

Hydration/ Water Traps

GAGs are heavily hydrated, trapping tremendous amounts of water and consequently filling very large hydrodynamic volumes. Proteoglycans act as shock absorbers in joints by resisting the release of trapped fluid under compression and reabsorbing the fluid after the compression is removed. They function in skin as a fluid trap, resisting dehydration. In the cornea, proteoglycan hydration forms aqueous "pools" between the collagen fibrils of the appropriate size to allow corneal transparency. Damage to the epithelial or endothelial membrane pumps allows increased corneal hydration with enlarged aqueous pools around the GAGs and results in opacity of the cornea. Several lysosomal storage diseases (mucopolysaccharidoses), in which the GAGs are inappropriately processed and build up in the cornea, are also associated with corneal opacity.[176]

Barriers/Filters

In the kidney's glomerular basement membrane, the large basement membrane heparan sulfate proteoglycan (HSPG) (see Figs. 1.33 and 1.34) provides the filtration barrier; removal or blockage of this HSPG dramatically increases porosity, allowing passage of large charged molecules which are normally retained by this barrier.[177–179] Basement membranes beneath vascular endothelium exhibit similar properties, resisting passage of both cells and select molecules.[152] In diabetes, in which the basement membranes become porous and thickened, HSPG is less prevalent and other basement membrane molecules appear to be overexpressed in an unsuccessful attempt to compensate.[180-182] Metastasizing melanoma secretes high levels of a specific enzyme, heparanase, which enables these migratory cells to penetrate the normally resistant endothelial basement membranes and subsequently to invade new tissues.[183,184]

MICROENVIRONMENTS/ ION TRAPS

Although perhaps less clearly defined, the basic properties of GAGs and their frequent location at cell surfaces ensure that they will produce microenvironmental domains with unique physical properties. The extreme density of negative charges created by GAGs will dramatically modify the passage of charged molecules, both small ions and large macromolecules, approaching and leaving cells. GAG-containing matrices have been shown to function much as do ion exchange columns, in that positively charged ions will tend to be trapped and negatively charged ions will tend to be repelled.[153,155, 170-175] The behaviors of small molecules in dilute aqueous solution, such as protons (pH), biologically active ions (Na^+, K^+, Ca^{2+}, Cl^-, OH^-, bicarbonate, etc.), and water must be dramatically modified by the binding and concentrating effects of the cell surface GAGs. Behavior of large molecules may also be dramatically modified, as discussed below.

SPECIFIC BINDING FUNCTIONS

Proteoglycans also serve a variety of functions, dependent on selective binding properties, usually contained in specific binding domains of the core protein and their GAG chains. Decorin, so named because it "decorates" type I collagen fibrils at regular 67-nm intervals, is necessary for normal collagen fibril formation. Several proteoglycans are critically involved in cellular adhesion and are concentrated in focal contact adhesions;[152,155,185-187] they also serve as the binding molecule for cell adhesion molecules and bind to fibronectin, laminin, type IV collagen, and a variety of other ECM components.[149,152,154-156,188] Heparin and heparan sulfate proteoglycans bind fibroblast or heparin-binding growth factors (FGFs or HBGFs), affecting their activity and sensitivity to degradation; they have been postulated to serve as an ECM reservoir for this family of growth factor molecules.[189-194]

ECM GLYCOPROTEINS

LAMININ, A BASEMENT MEMBRANE GLUE

Laminin, a large basement membrane glycoprotein (M_r 800–1,000 kDa), forms a floppy cross-like structure with three arms of approximately 37 nm in length and a fourth, longer arm approximately 77 nm long when viewed microscopically[195-197] (Fig. 1.35A). The major portions of the three subunit chains, A (400 kDa), Bl (220 kDa), and B2 (210 kDa), form a coiled coil of

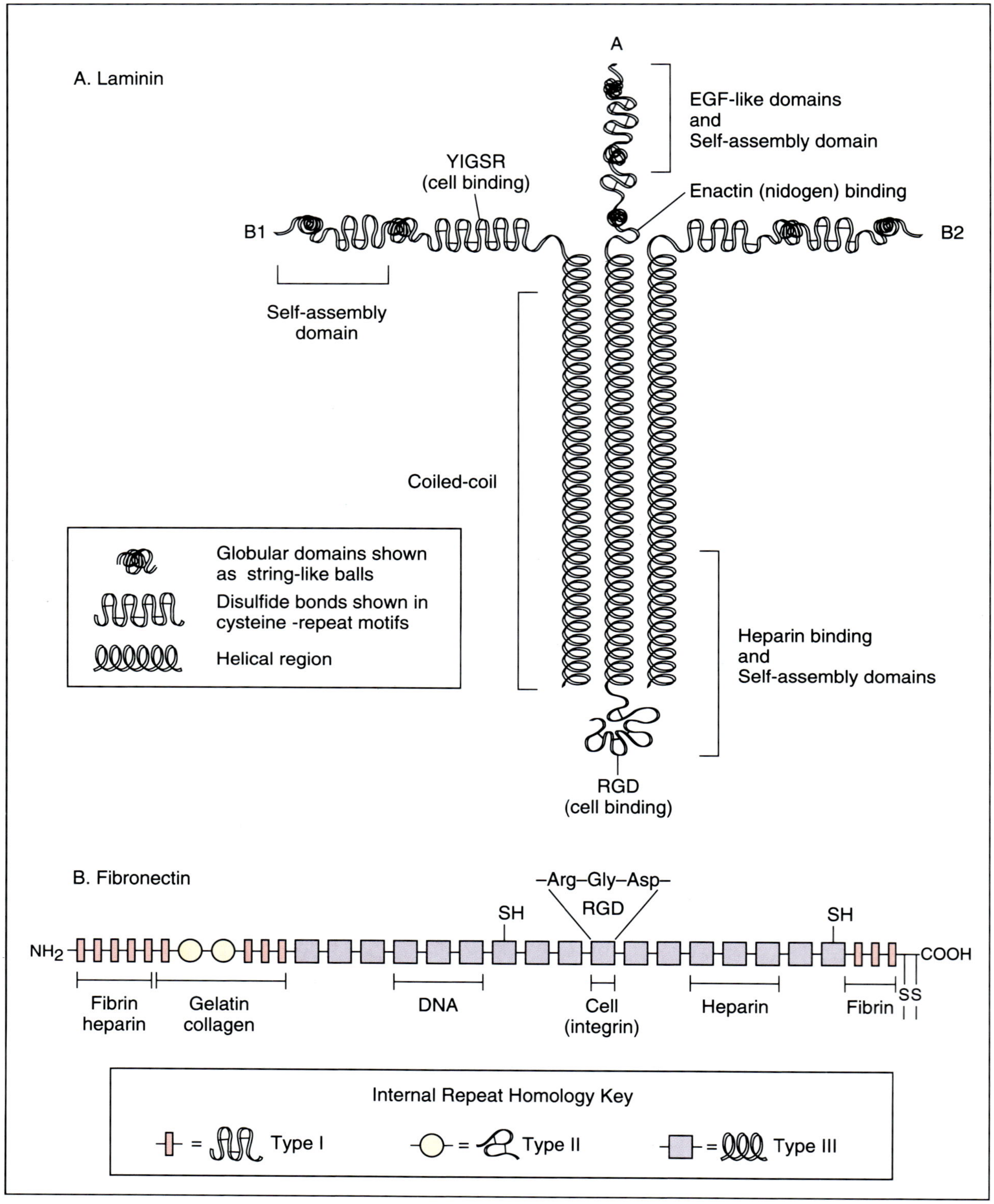

1.35 | Structural features of laminin[195,196,209] and fibronectin.[206–208] *A:* Laminin's YIGSR and RGD cell binding sequences are shown, as are other binding domains and motifs. Globular domains are shown as string-like balls; disulfide bonds are shown in the cysteine-repeat motifs. *B:* A single chain of fibronectin is shown, with the internal repeat homology patterns and various binding domains. The cell RGD binding domain is shown, as are terminal region disulfide bonds that hold two chains together.

three α-helices composing the long arm and then separate so that each forms one of the short arms. The A subunit forms a globular domain at the end of the long arm which contains the RGD, cell surface receptor, integrin, recognition signal (see below). The Bl chain contains another RGD sequence and the laminin-specific cell-receptor binding sequence, YIGSR. Several internal repeat sequences are found in each of these chains. Recently, structural variants, merosin and s-laminin, have been identified in several tissues.[198,199]

The three laminin chains, in the domains that form the three short arms, each contain multiple copies of an epidermal growth factor (EGF)-like motif with regular Cys repeat placement. This motif, as repeated in laminin, in the large basement membrane HSPG, in versican, and in a surprising number of other ECM proteins, is approximately 50 amino acids long and contains in several Gly and eight Cys, all spaced at conserved intervals. This EGF-like or growth factor-like motif may have regulatory significance, because proteolytic fragments of laminin have been reported to mimic EGF-induced mitogenic responses in fibroblasts.[200,201] This type of structure has also been implicated in receptor binding activities in several cases.

Functions of Laminin

Laminin's primary function appears to be as an ECM "glue," binding and organizing ECM molecular structure and attaching to cell surfaces. It has binding sites for the large basement membrane HSPG (mentioned above), type IV collagen, and at least two cell surface receptors, as mentioned above and discussed below. In addition, laminin self-associates in a calcium-dependent manner, and is involved in a variety of cell regulatory phenomena. In the trabecular meshwork, laminin has been identified by several investigators and may play critical roles in trabecular function.[123,169,202–204]

FIBRONECTIN, ANOTHER ECM GLUE MOLECULE

Another large ECM macromolecule, fibronectin, has been identified in the meshwork.[123,169,202–205] In contrast to laminin, which is believed to be present only in basement membranes and to be produced only by epithelium, endothelium, and some neuronal cells, fibronectin is present in some basement membranes and in many other ECMs.

Fibronectin is a long (200 kDa) chain which usually exists as a dimer, linked by disulfide bonds near its carboxyl terminus (Fig. 1.35B). Proteolytic cleavage produces fibronectin fragments, which have a variety of specific binding properties. One region contains an RGD cell surface binding motif (discussed later). Another interesting aspect of fibronectin's molecular arrangement is the presence of three types of internal structural motif repeats, thought to arise from gene duplication events during the evolution of this complex macromolecule. Although not completely resolved, they appear to reflect specific structure/function relationships. This type of behavior has been identified in many other ECM molecules and must represent a useful method for the evolutionary development of large molecules with multiple functions.

Alternative Splice Variants

Several forms of fibronectin have been identified as having various different-sized cellular mRNAs coded by the same gene.[206–209] This is due to alternative splicing of the transcripts from nearly 50 introns and exons, resulting in different mature mRNA forms with slightly different final amino acid sequences. One variation on this theme is the exclusion of the RGD cell binding domain, resulting in a fibronectin form that does not bind to cell surfaces. These variant forms have different binding properties, and consequently exhibit different functional behaviors.

Functions/Binding Domains

As with laminin, fibronectin has numerous binding domains along its length (see Fig. 1.35B) and serves as an ECM and cellular glue and organizer. As with laminin, modulation of fibronectin levels has dramatic effects on cell behaviors. Considerable evidence is accumulating that fibronectin receptors transduce signals from the ECM to the cell's interior, although the molecular mechanisms remain obscure.

COLLAGENS

Interstitial Collagens

Collagens are important components of ECMs,[210] and several types have been identified within the trabecular ECMs.[123,169,211,212] The classic interstitial collagens, types I, II, and III, have been studied in considerable detail and their properties are well understood.[210] The meshwork contains both types I and III, which form typical fibrils and are resistant to many proteinases. They are a major component of the trabecular beams and sheets, and their fibril patterns are distinctive and relatively easy to identify. Their amino acid sequence is predominantly Gly-Xaa-Yaa (where Xaa and Yaa are any amino acid). They contain considerable amounts of hydroxylysine and hydroxyproline, and they undergo various posttranslational modifications, i.e., proteolytic processing, glycosylation, disulfide bond formation, and cross-link formation. The basic unit of organization is a triple helix composed of three chains. This unit is responsible for supramolecular organization into fibrils with regular spacings that produce typical repetitive banding patterns, reflecting molecular overlap regions, and fibrils of uniform diameters.

Type IV (Basement Membrane) Collagen

Type IV collagen is found typically, and perhaps exclusively, in basement membranes, including those of the trabecular meshwork.[169,210] It resembles the interstitial collagens in many respects, with long, collagenous triple-helical domains, except that it also contains globular, noncollagenous (NC) domains that are susceptible to attack by various proteinases. Instead of forming the typical interstitial collagen fibrils, type IV collagen often forms a chicken-wire-like lattice. The noncollagenous domain, NC1, which is found on one end of the triple helix, undergoes self-association and the other end aggregates into a four-strand joint stabilized by disulfide bonds (Fig. 1.36). Models have been presented to explain the method of supramolecular organization that produces the lattice networks observed in several basement membranes. The complex organization of these networks in basement membranes is also dependent on the other ECM molecules that interact with type IV collagen, including laminin and the large basement membrane HSPG.

Type V Collagen

Although initially identified as another basement membrane collagen, more recent studies suggest that type V collagen is primarily an interstitial form or perhaps a cojoiner of interstitium to basement membranes.[210] It may also contribute to fibril formation. It shares characteristics of types I and III collagen, although it contains globular noncollagenous domains as does type IV collagen. It has been identified in the trabecular meshwork.[169]

TYPE VI COLLAGEN

Type VI collagen is considered an interstitial fibril-forming collagen, although it has unusual characteristics.[210] Only approximately half of its mass is involved in a short triple-helical domain, and it can be found as monomers and in assemblies as dimers and tetramers, rather than exclusively as trimers, as are observed with most other interstitial collagens. Globular domains are clearly present, and type VI collagen can be partially degraded by several proteinases. It forms fibrils that exhibit a 100-nm periodicity with 25-nm beaded internal repeats, thought to reflect molecular spacings. Although some controversy exists, it appears not to colocalize with basement membranes, types I or III collagens, or elastic fibrils. It has been identified in association with microfibrils and may serve as a nucleus for their formation. Type VI collagen has been identified in the trabecular meshwork.[213]

A variety of additional collagen types have been identified and studied in different degrees of detail; most have not thus far been reported to be present in the trabecular meshwork.

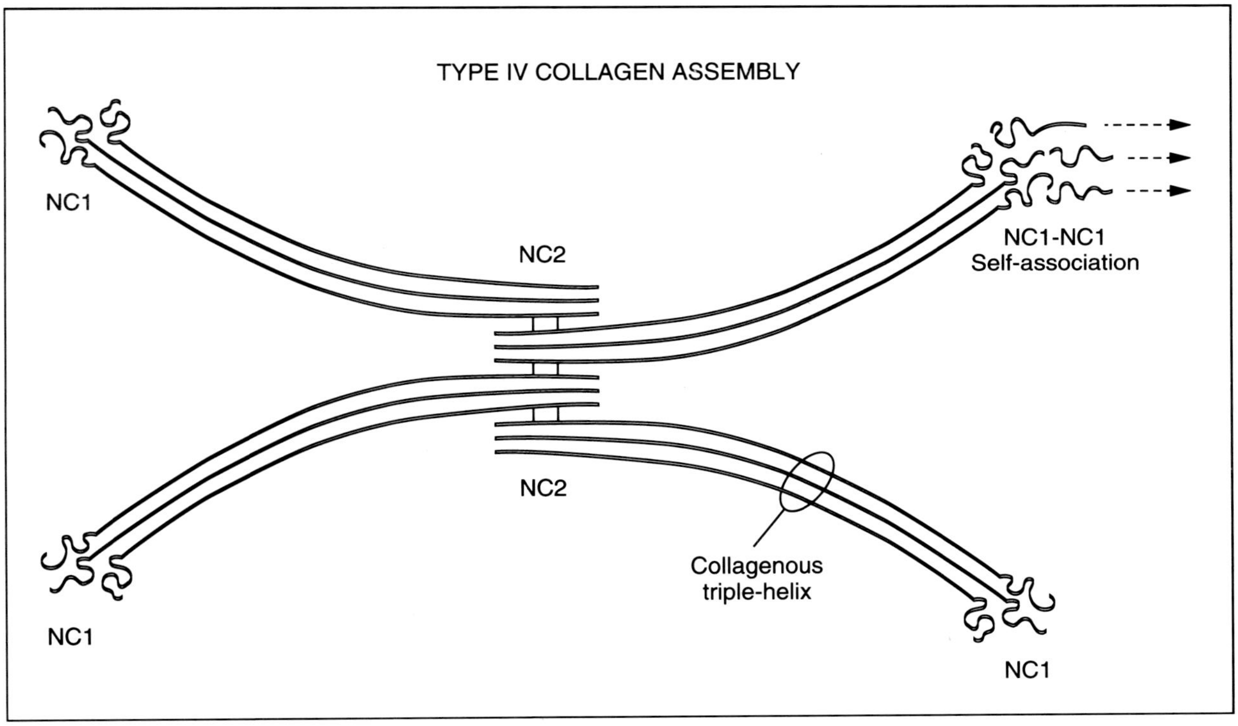

1.36 | Structural features of type IV collagen assembly.[210] Noncollagenous globular domains are shown with emphasis on their interactions and structural consequences; typical collagenous triple-helical regions and disulfide bonds in NC2 are as indicated.

ELASTIN

Elastic tissues are composed of the fibrous protein elastin and are formed around the microfibrillar protein fibrillin.[214–216] Elastin is rich in Gly and Ala, with frequent Lys residues that become covalently cross-linked to form an unusual structure called desmosine (Fig. 1.37). Four Lys groups are involved in this complex reaction, resulting in a desmosine bridge between elastin chains. This bridge is believed to account for the rubbery flexibility of elastin fibers. Fibrillin, a 350 kDa protein containing glucosamine but not sulfated, exhibits 10-nm diameter fibrils around the amorphous cores of elastic fibers. Fibrillin microfibrils are also found without elastin cores. At a molecular level, fibrillin molecules form a "beads-on-a-string" type of structure with a crab-like globular domain and many "legs" extending from it. Elastic struc-

1.37 | Desmosine structure forms cross-linkages in elastin.[165] Four molecules of elastin are cross-linked by the formation of the desmosine, in which a condensation occurs between four lysine groups.

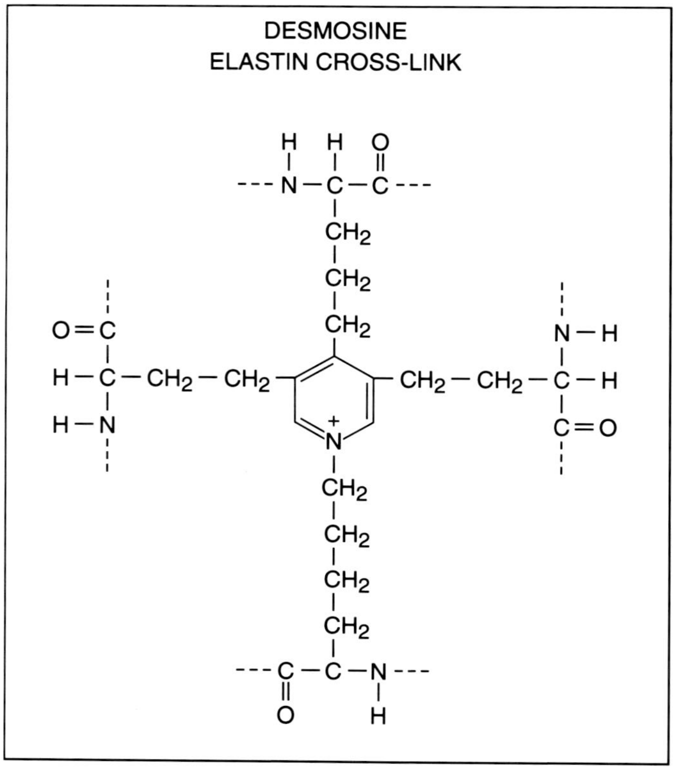

tures and elastin have both been identified in the trabecular meshwork and important roles have been postulated for their involvement in glaucoma.[217–222]

OTHER ECM MOLECULES

Although many other ECM molecules have been identified in other tissues, most have not been identified or studied in the trabecular meshwork.

ECM–ECM AND ECM–CELL INTERACTIONS

The functional properties of ECMs, undoubtedly including those of the trabecular meshwork, are dependent on many interactions among the various ECM molecules and between ECMs and cells. Essentially all components of ECMs are involved in interactions with other ECM components.[128,149,152–156,195–197,206–208,210] These interactions are generally very specific, occurring between discrete domains on each molecule. For example, in basement membranes interactions between laminin, type IV collagen, and the basement membrane HSPG have been defined and are partially responsible for the organization of this complex structure. As many as 100 other basement membrane peptides have been identified, although few have been studied in detail and their role in basement membrane organization is unclear. In addition, many ECM components bind to specific cell surface receptors, maintaining cell adhesion and regulating various cell functions. If the key binding and structural organizing protein(s) for the putative specific trabecular proteoglycan(s), postulated to be responsible for the outflow resistance, is defective or is present in inappropriate concentrations in the ECM, the outflow resistance could easily become impossible to regulate.

INTEGRINS

A variety of cell surface receptors for ECM molecules have been identified, including cell adhesion proteins (CAMs), cadherins, adhesion molecules from the immunoglobulin superfamily, homing receptors, lectin-like domain adhesion molecules (LEC-CAMs), and the integrins.[223–225] The latter, a flexible superfamily of cell surface receptors, are the most well studied.

INTEGRIN SUBUNIT STRUCTURE

Integrins are comprised of various combinations of α and β subunits, forming at least 16 specific heterodimers that bind a variety of ECM components (Fig. 1.38). Both types of subunit have large extracellular domains, a typical transmembrane domain, and small cytoplasmic domains. The cytoplasmic domains are unique. Some of these bind to actin-binding proteins such as talin, fibulin, vinculin, and α-actinin, forming a linkage between the cell cytoskeleton and the ECM. Some cytoplasmic binding is calcium-dependent, suggesting regulatory modulation. The subunits are between 95 and 200 kDa in size, and many have been cloned and sequenced.

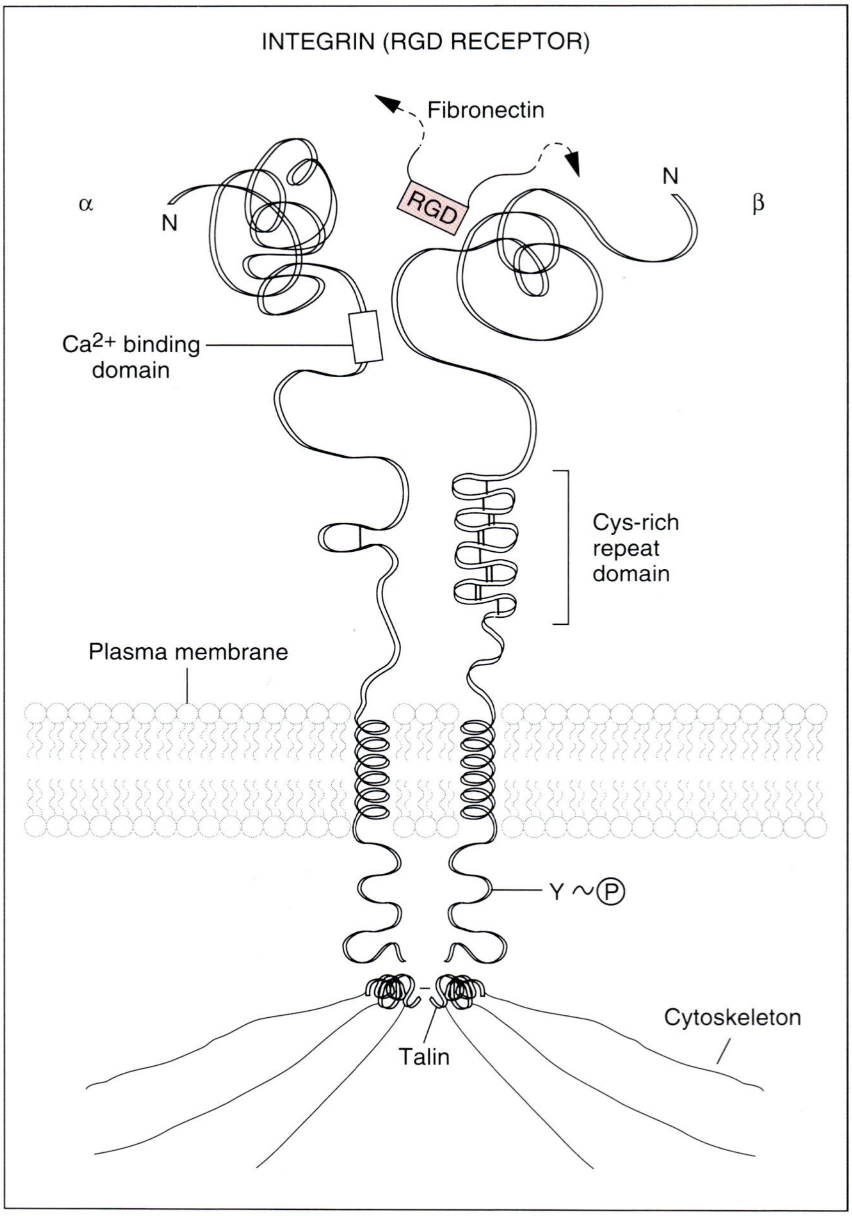

1.38 | Structural model of integrin, a cellular receptor for various ECM macromolecules.[206,208] Transmembrane helical regions separate the cytoplasmic and extracellular portion of this dimeric structure. The cytoplasmic region interacts with cytoskeletal components and probably participates in signal transduction to cell components. The extracellular domain of the β-chain contains a cysteine-rich repeat, while the α-chain contains a calcium-binding domain involved in binding. Globular domains near the amino terminal portion of both chains interact with the RGD recognition and binding motif of fibronectin or the many other integrin-binding ECM macromolecules. The amino terminal (N) of the peptides, tyrosine (Y) potential phosphorylation site (P), and Arg-Gly-Asp (RGD) sites are indicated.

INTEGRIN β SUBUNITS

Three subfamilies of integrins were initially identified on the basis of their β subunits, β_1, β_2, and β_3; more recently, three more types of β subunits have been identified. Each type of β subunit binds only a subset of the 11 or more identified α subunits, forming heterodimers with specific binding capabilities. The identified β subunits are quite similar, showing 40–48% sequence identity and very high conservation of the positional arrangement of 56 Cys residues found in the Cys-rich region near the middle of the molecule.

INTEGRIN α SUBUNITS

The α subunits are less similar to each other. They contain a conserved calcium-binding domain with moderately low affinity for calcium (Kd ~1 μM). Integrin–ECM binding is generally calcium dependent.

INTEGRIN–ECM BINDING

Portions of the extracellular domains of both α and β subunits form a specific binding site for the respective ECM ligand. Most of the ECM proteins bind to this site by a single linear sequence motif, Arg-Gly-Asp (RGD). The different integrin dimers apparently recognize this motif in a context-specific manner to produce the different ECM ligand-binding specificities.

Evidence for complex regulatory interactions of the ECM and cells, transduced via the integrin receptor system, make this an exciting area for future investigations of trabecular cell behavior. This would provide an excellent mechanism for cells to sense events occurring at their surface ECMs, and this type of information is clearly available to cells, as judged by their responses to extracellular events. Although trabecular integrins have not been studied, their ubiquitous distributions ensure that they are important in trabecular structure and function.

BIOSYNTHESIS OF OUTFLOW PATHWAY ECM COMPONENTS

Most ECM biosynthesis is similar to that which occurs for other proteins and carbohydrates.[128,165] This includes such processes as constitutive and regulated transcription of genomic DNA sequences into RNA (see below for a brief discussion of transcriptional regulation), processing of RNA by splicing out of introns and polyadenylation to form mature mRNAs, translocation of mRNAs to the cytoplasm, translation of RNA into proteins, post-translational processing steps, protein secretion, and extracellular processing events. All of these steps occur in specifically regulated patterns. Alternative splicing, in which several different mature mRNAs are generated from one gene by eliminating or including certain exons or parts of exons, appears to be a common occurrence in ECM genes (see above). Obviously, this flexibility in the use of genomic sequences provides a wide diversity of molecular options for cells and, of course, another avenue of regulatory controls to be unraveled.

Translation of ECM mRNAs into proteins also follows the standard patterns observed with other proteins regulated by the same types of mechanisms.[165] Post-translational processing of ECM macromolecules is more specific (see below), secretion tends to be rapid and only seldom involves storage vesicles, additional extracellular processing frequently occurs, and the processes of macromolecular self-assembly and supramolecular organization are poorly understood but clearly complex.

GLYCOSAMINOGLYCAN/ PROTEOGLYCAN BIOSYNTHESIS

GAGs are synthesized directly on proteoglycan core proteins (Fig. 1.39), primarily in the trans–Golgi.[128,149,150,152,155,165,226–229] The process includes GAG attachment, GAG chain elongation, and GAG modification. Xylosyltransferase is the first enzyme in most GAG additions and is a regulatory and rate-limiting enzyme in the pathway.[128,226,230–234] UDP sugars are used throughout as the donor substrates. In the first step, a xylose is added to a serine or threonine residue in the core protein, followed by addition of two galactoses, a glucuronic acid, and then the normal disaccharide repeat is begun. GAG attachment usually, although not exclusively, is to Ser-Gly-Xaa-Gly or (Asp/Glu)-Gly-Ser-Gly-(Asp/Glu) sequences.[128,237–240] All steps are catalyzed by specific enzymes (see Fig. 1.39). Of these enzymes, only

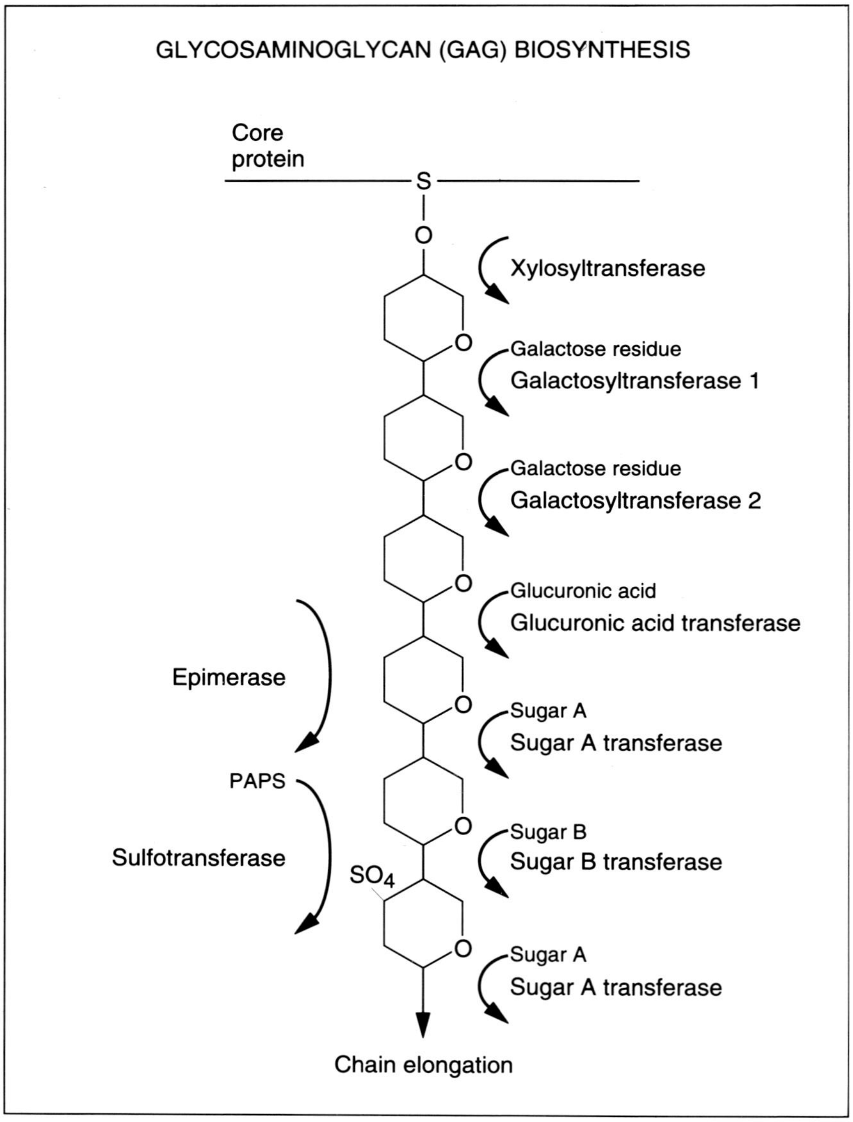

1.39 | GAG biosynthesis on a typical proteoglycan core protein. Unique aspects of the GAG biosynthetic pathway are depicted diagrammatically where a serine (S) of the core protein binds covalently to xylose. Two galactose residues are then added, followed by a glucuronic acid; chain elongation consists of the alternating addition of sugars A and B to form the repeating disaccharide pair of the specific GAG (see Fig. 1.31). During and after the chain elongation process, some glucuronic acids are epimerized to iduronic acids by a specific epimerase and sulfation occurs, catalyzed by a specific sulfotransferase using 3'-phosphoadenosine 5'-phosphosulfate (PAPS) as the sulfate donor. Carbohydrate additions utilize the UDP-derivative sugars, and the specific enzymes are as indicated.

xylosyltransferase has been studied in any detail. In the trabecular meshwork, xylosyltransferase exhibits kinetic and physical properties similar to those of this enzyme from other tissues.[128,235,236] The trabecular activity level is high compared with that of most other ocular tissues studied, either on a per cell or a per mg protein basis.

During GAG chain elongation, glucuronic acids are epimerized to iduronic acids by an epimerase and sulfation occurs. The sulfate donor is 3′-phosphoadenosine 5′-phosphosulfate and the enzyme is a specific sulfotransferase.[128,226,227,241] The selection of the possible site for epimerization and for sulfation is not completely understood, although groups of residues in which both are at high density are often found. Because the iduronate and sulfate pattern has very specific effects on proteoglycan function, e.g., heparin-binding growth factors bind only to specific patterns, this process must be critically regulated. To the extent that it has been studied,[235,236] trabecular GAG biosynthesis is not different from that observed in other tissues.

GLYCOPROTEIN BIOSYNTHESIS

In addition to GAG chains, many proteoglycans also have shorter O-linked and N-linked oligosaccharide chains, as do many other proteins.[165] Almost all ECM proteins are also glycoproteins with linear or branched oligosaccharide chains of various lengths. O-linked and N-linked oligosaccharide biosynthesis on proteoglycans follows a pattern similar to that shown on glycoproteins in general. Trabecular oligosaccharide additions are apparently the same as observed in other tissues.

TURNOVER OF OUTFLOW PATHWAY ECM COMPONENTS

Extracellular matrix turnover is an active and ongoing process, particularly when the ECM forms and is in a flow channel such as the aqueous outflow pathway through the trabecular meshwork. Trabecular GAG turnover is rapid compared with that of the neighboring tissues; trabecular GAG half-lives are 1–2 days, compared with 7–10 days or more for GAGs in the cornea and sclera.[125,128] ECM turnover usually (and the meshwork is no exception) is initiated by the regulated secretion of specific proteinases into the extracellular space. These proteinases selectively cleave a few ECM proteins and are then inactivated by proteinase inhibitors. The modified ECM components become disorganized and the overall structure of the ECM in that region degenerates. The cells then endocytose/phagocytose these disorganized ECM components, and they are degraded within the cell by the normal endosomal pathways (see below). The disintegrated region of ECM is then replaced by the trabecular cells using the biosynthetic pathways discussed above. Two families of secreted proteinases have been identified in the outflow pathway, the plasminogen activator family[242,243] and the matrix metalloproteinase family.[128,244]

PLASMINOGEN ACTIVATORS

Tissue plasminogen activator (tPA) has been identified in the outflow pathway by several investigators.[242,243] This serine proteinase (i.e., a covalent serine–substrate complex is formed as a reaction intermediate) is synthesized and secreted by trabecular cells in culture. Its primary function is the activation of plasminogen, another serine proteinase involved in the fibrin clot dissolution cascade, but it has been shown to exhibit some activity towards certain ECM components.[245–247] A specific tPA inhibitor, tPA-I, is also secreted by vascular endothelial cells in large excess over the tPA levels, ensuring that uncontrolled proteolytic damage will not occur in the surrounding tissue. In trabecular cell culture, the secretion ratio of inhibitor to enzyme is relatively low, and this has been interpreted to indicate that fibrinolysis is important in the anterior chamber to guard against the effects of blood reflux or blood–eye barrier disruption.[242]

MATRIX METALLOPROTEINASES (MMPs)

As with most tissues, the aqueous outflow pathway synthesizes, secretes, and appears to rely primarily on a family of zinc- and calcium-dependent endopeptidases to initiate and regulate ECM turnover.[128,244] This family includes several members[128,244,248–252]: an interstitial collagenase which makes only one cut at a specific Gly-Ile bond within native type I, II, and III collagens, resulting in two fragments, one quarter/three quarters the original chain length. These collagen fragments then disorganize or denature (into gelatins) and become a substrate for the other MMPs. The 72 kDa gelatinase (type IV collagenase) further degrades denatured interstitial collagens (gelatins) and is active against native laminin, fibronectin, and types IV and V collagen. The 92 kDa gelatinase (type IV collagenase) has substrate specificity similar to the 72 kDa form, although it is regulated quite differently and is clearly produced from a different gene. Stromelysin or proteoglycanase, which exhibits broader substrate specificity, cleaves gelatins and the globular domains of laminin, fibronectin, types IV and V collagen, many proteoglycan core proteins, and a variety of other globular proteins such as casein and transferrin. All four MMP family members are synthesized and secreted by trabecular cells.[244]

MMP Structural Features

These MMPs have been cloned and sequenced and are clearly from separate genes, although they share between 50% and 75% overall sequence similarity (Fig. 1.40A).[128] Recently, additional forms of stromelysin (stromelysin-2 and stromelysin-3) and a shortened interstitial collagenase with stromelysin-like activity (PUMP-l) have also been cloned; other members of the family have been observed, but their cloning has not been reported. The MMPs are all glycoproteins, have similar-sized signal peptides, are secreted in latent proenzyme forms, show regions of very high amino acid sequence homology, and have individual unique regions.

Activation of Latent Pro-MMP Forms

The "cysteine switch" activation of the proenzymes is interesting and common to all family members studied to date (Fig. 1.40B).[128,253,254] The active-site zinc is held by three chelation complex bonds and a fourth bond to a conserved Cys in the propeptide. Treatment with proteinases or mercurial agents disrupts the Cys–zinc bond, enabling it to bind a water molecule and to participate in the catalytic reaction mechanism of the enzymes. After this activation step, the proteinases autolytically cleave the propeptide or remaining fragments of it at a specific site, leaving the enzyme fully activated. Over time, the activated enzymes become further degraded to smaller active forms and then to inactive fragments, either by other enzymes or autolytically, thus limiting their active lifetime.

Tissue Inhibitors of MMPs

In addition to limitation by autolysis, a family of tissue inhibitors of metalloproteinases (TIMPs) is secreted by cells to limit MMP activity after their secretion and perhaps as part of an even more convoluted latency/actvation

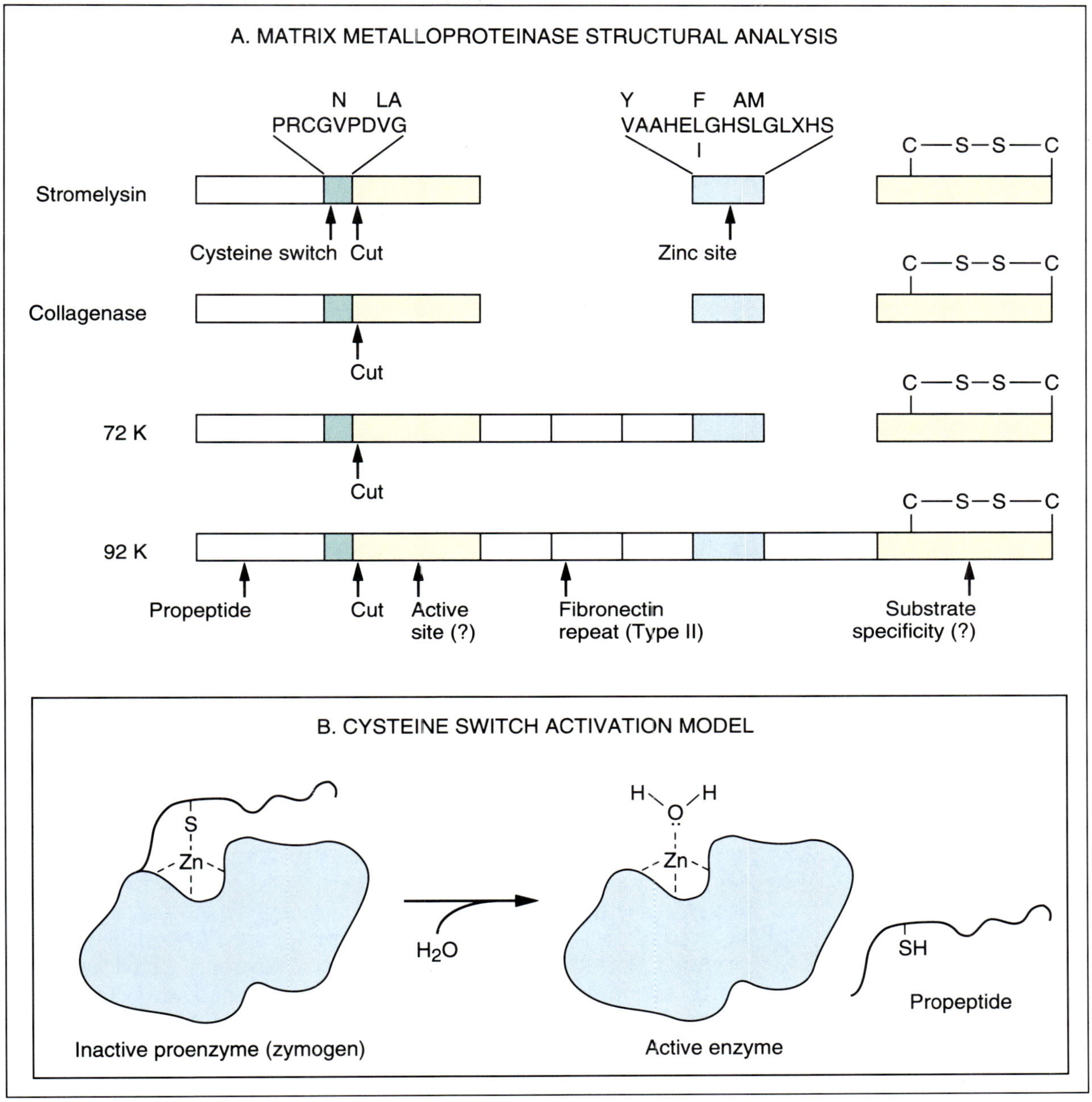

1.40 | Structural comparison and activation mechanism of matrix metalloproteinase family members. *A:* Comparisons of the sequences of the MMPs and several structure–function studies allow the tentative identification of several functional domains for the MMPs. The assignment and functions of the propeptide, the cysteine switch with the conserved activation cleavage site, and the (at least) two histidines in the metal binding site are relatively certain. The third zinc site residue has not been identified. Because fibronectin binds gelatin and collagen with its type II repeat region, it seems quite likely that the gelatinases use this domain for a similar binding recognition of this family of substrates. The carboxyl terminal portion is thought to be involved in dictating substrate specificity. The putative active site region, immediately to the right of the activation cut site, contains highly conserved amino acid placements. *B:* Model for metalloproteinase activation via the "cysteine switch."[253,254] The conserved cysteine comprises the fourth chelation point of the zinc in the latent proenzyme form. Activation can be produced by a variety of methods that share the common feature of removing the cysteine from the zinc complex, allowing a water to replace it. This pattern is commonly found in active zinc proteinases and plays an active role in the catalysis of proteolysis of select peptide bonds.

scheme.[128,244,248–251] TIMP-l and TIMP-2 have been cloned and are coded by separate genes. Both are glycoproteins ($M_r \approx 29$ kDa) with sequence-predicted protein sizes of ≈20 kDa. The aqueous outflow pathway synthesizes TIMP-l[244] and TIMP-2[255,256]; the latter is thought to be the major constitutive form in most tissues. Both TIMPs bind tightly to and inhibit the MMPs that have been activated; TIMP-2, but probably not TIMP-I, also binds to and inhibits the 72 kDa gelatinase when it has not been activated.[257–260] The extracellular temporal concentration ratio of the MMPs to TIMPs, and perhaps some regional distribution and activation factors, appear to regulate the net MMP activity in localized areas of ECM.

REGULATION OF OUTFLOW PATHWAY ECM COMPONENTS

REGULATION OF TRABECULAR ECM BIOSYNTHESIS

Although few detailed molecular studies of outflow pathway ECM biosynthesis have been conducted, some information has been obtained. Ascorbic acid modulates fibronectin, laminin, and GAG production by trabecular cells.[202,261] Dexamethasone differentially regulates GAG synthesis in several cell types, including trabecular meshwork cells.[204,262–265] Vitamin A also affects trabecular glycoconjugate biosynthesis.[266] Few other detailed molecular studies have been reported that focus on the regulation of outflow ECM biosynthesis, and virtually nothing is known about the cell mechanisms involved or about the physiologic significance of these or other regulators as they impact aqueous humor outflow resistance. In only a few cases have both proteoglycan/GAG biosynthesis regulation and outflow been investigated in concert.[262,263] Much can be inferred from the more detailed studies in other tissues, which probably utilize similar mechanisms, i.e., transcriptional activation as discussed below.

REGULATION OF MATRIX METALLOPROTEINASES

The expression of the matrix metalloproteinases and TIMPs is rigorously regulated, apparently individually, although often in concert, by a large variety of modulators of cell division, migration and ECM remodeling.[128,244,249–252,255] Growth factors, oncogene transformation, cytokines, tumor promoters, retinoids, dexamethasone, colchicine, and actin microfilament rearrangement are among the many modulators of these proteins. Trabecular meshwork secretion of these metalloproteinases and TIMPs and the levels of their trabecular cytoplasmic mRNAs are differentially regulated by several growth factors, interleukin-l, dexamethasone, a broad-spectrum phorbol ester mitogen, and by an unidentified medium-borne factor released by trabecular cells in response to laser trabeculoplasty.[128,244,255,256,267]

Transcriptional Regulation of Metalloproteinase and Other Genes

One primary mode of regulation of cell processes is the manipulation of mRNA or mature transcript levels available as templates for protein synthesis. This control can be achieved by regulating the rate and frequency of transcriptional initiation (see below): the rate of transcription by the RNA polymerase II complex, the rate of splicing and processing of the immature pre-mRNAs in the nucleus, the rate of polyadenylation and transport to the cytoplasm, the half-life of the mRNA in the cytoplasm, and the rate of utilization by the translation machinery.[268,269] Little specific information is available concerning these regulatory processes in the trabecular meshwork. However, some information on transcriptional regulation can be safely inferred from what is known about trabecular gene expression. This area is of considerable importance and current investigations promise to expand our understanding of the details of trabecular gene expression and regulation in the near future.

Transcriptional Complex and Promoters

RNA polymerase II and several other peptides form a preinitiation or transcription complex, while binding to a promoter sequence of the genomic DNA usually located just upstream from the transcription start site.[268,270] This process is followed by the transcription of heterogeneous nuclear RNA (hnRNA) or pre-mRNA. The transcriptional complex partially dissociates and additional peptides are added as the polymerase moves down the gene during transcription. The promoter site is bound by a specific factor, TFIID, which interacts with the polymerase and other members of the transcription complex to designate the exact point for beginning the pre-mRNA. The promoter usually allows initiation of transcription without assistance from additional factors, although usually at relatively low rates.

TRANSCRIPTIONAL ENHANCER SEQUENCES AND DNA-BINDING PROTEINS

Modulation of the initiation of specific gene transcription in eukaryotes is mediated by the interaction of regulatory DNA-binding proteins with short genomic DNA sequences called "enhancers."[271–277] Enhancers are usually located within a few hundred nucleotides upstream from the promoter sites, although they can be several thousand bases upstream or downstream or even within the gene itself. A few enhancer/transcriptional activator protein pairs of obvious and critical importance to the trabecular meshwork will be discussed briefly (Fig. 1.41).

TRE, AP-1, Jun, and Fos

Interstitial collagenase, stromelysin and the 92 kDa gelatinase are examples of the many genes regulated by the transcriptional activators, Jun and Fos.[270–273] A Jun/Fos heterodimer binds to an enhancer referred to as the TPA responsive element or enhancer (TRE). TRE-containing genes are modulated by the phorbol mitogen, TPA (hence the name) and by a variety of growth factors. The consensus palindromic DNA sequence for this enhancer (and several others discussed later) is shown in Figure 1.41 and is found approximately 70–80 nucleotides upstream from the transcription start site of these three metalloproteinases.[278–281] Some latitude in the consensus sequence of this and other enhancer sequences is apparently tolerated.

Figure 1.41. Characteristics of Several Enhancer/Transcriptional Activator Systems

Transcriptional Enhancers		Transcriptional Activators
Name	**DNA Consensus**	**Proteins**
TRE or AP-1	TGA(G/C)T(C/A)A	Jun (c-Jun); Jun B; Jun D Fos (c-Fos); Fos B; Fra 1
CRE	TGACGTCA	CREB
AP-2	CCCCAGGC	AP-2
GRE simple	TGTTCTnnnTCTTGT	Glucocorticoid receptor
GRE context-sensitive	GGTACAnnnTGTYCT	Glucocorticoid receptor

Mechanism of Transcriptional Activation

A current model of how transcriptional enhancement is achieved is depicted in Figure 1.42A.[271] The activator proteins, in this case a homodimer of Jun or a Jun/Fos heterodimer, bind to the enhancer sequence and increase the frequency of transcriptional initiation. Presumably this occurs by stabilization of the binding of TFIID to the promoter. This would facilitate the binding of another RNA polymerase molecule and, consequently, would increase the rate of transcriptional initiations. Although not clearly integrated into this model, recent evidence shows that Jun/Fos binding also produces significant bending of the DNA at the enhancer site. Several other models have been proposed and cannot be eliminated at this time.[274]

Jun and Fos Proteins

Originally studied as oncogenes, v-Jun and v-Fos are truncated portions of the cell genes (protooncogenes) c-Jun and c-Fos; these genes are apparently picked up by a retrovirus as a consequence of recombination in host cells and are transmitted by active virions to trigger oncogenesis. Jun and Fos dimerization is by a leucine zipper; an α-helical protein domain with five Leu residues spaced down one face is present in both proteins, and two such helices dimerize via hydrophobic bonding of these faces to form the "zipper" (Fig. 1.42B).[271–273,277] Near the end of these helical domains is another conserved α-helical region with similarly spaced Arg and Lys residues. These positively charged helix faces of the dimer are thought to bind to the enhancer sequence of the DNA. Additional regulatory domains serving some modulatory or interactive functions are present further up these proteins.

Regulation of Jun/Fos by Phosphorylation

Both Jun and Fos are phosphorylated rapidly and in a regulated manner by Ser/Thr protein kinases, thereby enhancing their dimerization.[271,272,279,282] TPA, a tumor promoter, activates protein kinase C and one effect is apparently the sustained phosphorylation of Jun and Fos. Another tumor promoter, okadaic acid, inhibits protein phosphatases 1 and 2A, which can dephosphorylate Jun and Fos, consequently sustaining Jun/Fos phosphorylation. Both mitogens stimulate interstitial collagenase expression. At least in some cases, it appears that both activator and inhibitory phosphorylations occur in domains of Jun/Fos responsible for these respective types of actions.[283]

1.42 | OPPOSITE PAGE: Model for transcriptional activation and for Jun/Fos dimerization via a leucine zipper. *A:* Model of TRE enhancer interaction with Jun/Fos transcriptional activator heterodimer and putative mechanism of increased initiation events with RNA polymerase II transcriptional complex.[271,272] The ability of Jun/Fos bound to the TRE site to stabilize the interaction of a transcriptional factor, TFIID, with the promoter site after the polymerase moves down the DNA during transcription is thought to increase the frequency of initiation complex formation and, therefore, mRNA synthesis. Recently, a role for the Jun/Fos dimer bending the template DNA has been hypothesized.[344] *B:* Model of Jun/Fos leucine zipper and DNA-binding domain.[271,272,290] Sequence homology is shown for the putative DNA-binding domain (left group) and the leucine zipper dimerization domain (right group) for several members of the Fos and Jun families. Below is a diagrammatic model for Jun/Fos dimerization and their interaction with a TRE site on a DNA template. The remaining helix and surrounding regions are thought to be involved in the phosphorylation and other activity-modulation events which control Jun/Fos activity. Helical spacing of groups at every 3–4 amino acids will result in their proximity along the face of a standard α-helix.

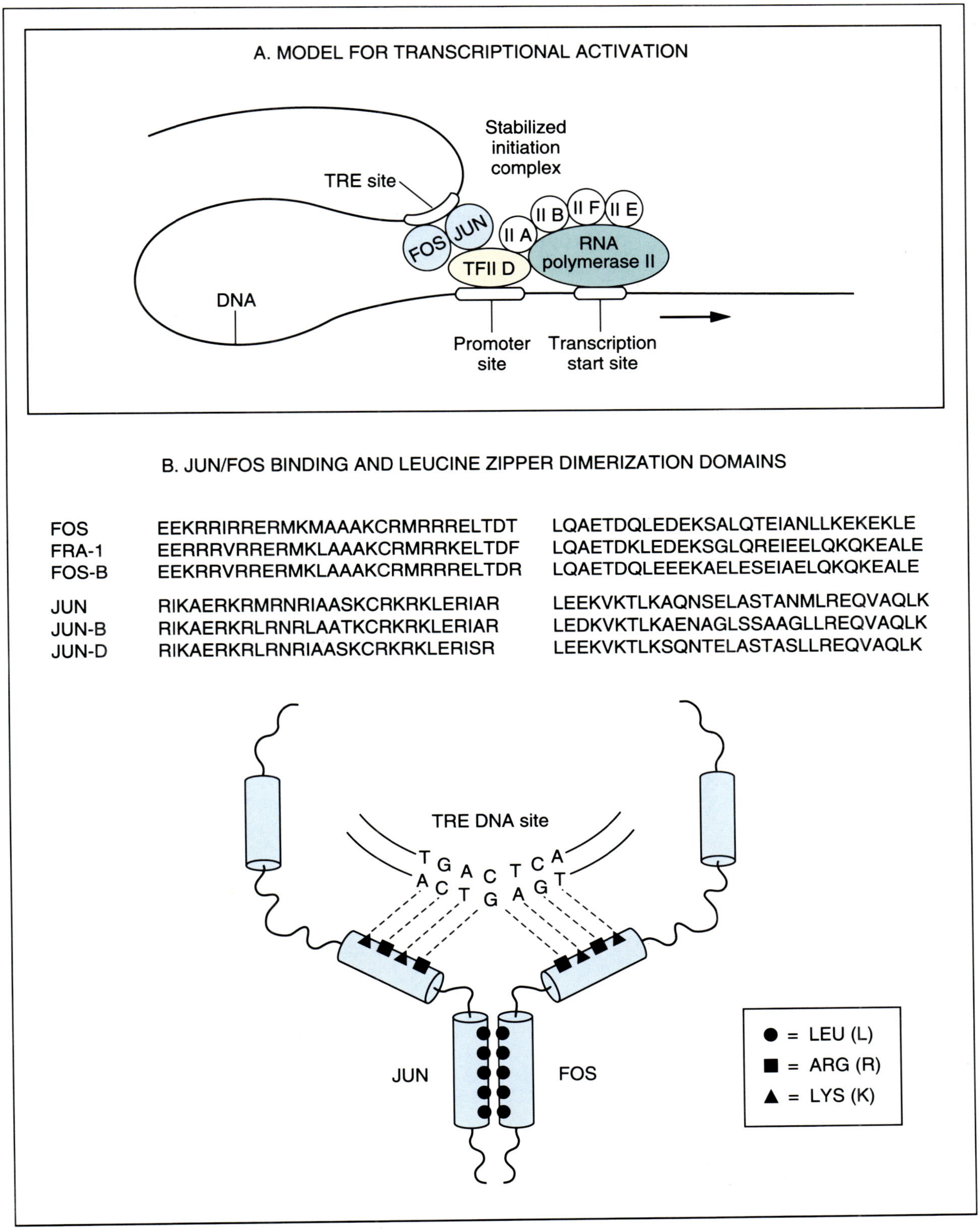
A. MODEL FOR TRANSCRIPTIONAL ACTIVATION
Stabilized initiation complex
TRE site
FOS
JUN
II A
II B
II F
II E
RNA polymerase II
TFII D
DNA
Promoter site
Transcription start site
B. JUN/FOS BINDING AND LEUCINE ZIPPER DIMERIZATION DOMAINS
FOS EEKRRIRRERMKMAAAKCRMRRRELTDT LQAETDQLEDEKSALQTEIANLLKEKEKLE
FRA-1 EERRRVRRERMKLAAAKCRMRRKELTDF LQAETDKLEDEKSGLQREIEELQKQKEALE
FOS-B EEKRRVRRERMKLAAAKCRMRRRELTDR LQAETDQLEEEKAELESEIAELQKQKEALE
JUN RIKAERKRMRNRIAASKCRKRKLERIAR LEEKVKTLKAQNSELASTANMLREQVAQLK
JUN-B RIKAERKRLRNRLAATKCRKRKLERIAR LEDKVKTLKAENAGLSSAAGLLREQVAQLK
JUN-D RIKAERKRLRNRIAASKCRKRKLERISR LEEKVKTLKSQNTELASTASLLREQVAQLK
TRE DNA site
T G A C T C A
A C T G A G T
JUN
FOS
● = LEU (L)
■ = ARG (R)
▲ = LYS (K)

Regulation of Jun/Fos Expression

In addition, transcription and translation of Jun and Fos mRNAs is induced rapidly (within a few minutes, reaching a maximum by 1 or 2 hours) by modulators that induce AP-l-regulated genes.[271,272,274,278,279] As is the case with most regulatory molecules, both of these proteins and their mRNAs have very short half-lives in the cell, allowing a rapid return to unstimulated cell behaviors on removal of the stimulatory signal. Their mRNAs have an AU repetitive sequence upstream from the polyadenylation signal, which triggers rapid shortening of the poly-A tail by cell nucleases and targets them for selective degradation.[269] This rapid removal of Jun and Fos increases the sensitivity of this regulatory process.

Negative Regulation by the Jun/Fos Family

Another aspect of this regulatory process has recently been identified; there are several forms of both Jun and Fos.[272,276,282] Jun B, Jun D, Fos B, Fra 1, etc., have recently been found. Although these proteins are quite similar in structure and binding behavior to c-Jun and c-Fos, some of these form heterodimers which are not stimulatory but actually block or repress transcriptional initiation of TRE-containing genes. This multifaceted regulation is complex and is not fully understood, but clearly it allows for considerable flexibility in the regulation of expression of these genes.

CYCLIC AMP, CRE, AND CREB

Another transcriptional activator system of considerable relevance to trabecular meshwork gene expression is the cAMP-responsive element or enhancer (CRE) and its transcriptional activator protein CREB.[271,275,276,284] Interleukin-l (Il-l), which owes much of its mode of action to the CRE/CREB system, stimulates trabecular stromelysin, 92 kDa gelatinase, and TIMP-l expression.[255] Other trabecular genes are also responsive to Il-l modulation and to other agents which modulate the CRE/CREB mechanism (see below).

The palindromic CRE enhancer sequence is almost identical to the TRE, and CREB is similar in several ways to Jun and Fos (see Fig. 1.41).[284] CREB has a DNA-binding domain, with sequence homology to Jun, containing primarily basic amino acids and dimerization via a leucine zipper. A third domain has a cluster of phosphorylation sites for protein kinase A, protein kinase C, and casein kinase II. Phosphorylation of Ser-133 by protein kinase A is apparently critical in transcriptional activation. A cluster of six Glu residues near the phosphorylation site is thought to be involved in the interaction of CREB with TFIID of the RNA polymerase II-transcriptional complex to stabilize their interaction with the promoter sequence, much as proposed for Jun/Fos. Both monomer and dimer forms of CREB have been shown to bind to CRE, although the dimer is apparently the active form.

GLUCOCORTICOIDS AND SIMPLE GREs

As discussed later, glucocorticoids are important regulators of trabecular function and of some of the matrix metalloproteinase/TIMP genes.[255,256] The glucocorticoid receptor (GR) is maintained in a latent form in the cytoplasm as a complex of one GR molecule bound to two molecules of a heat shock protein, HSP-90[271,275,285,286] (Fig. 1.43A). The free diffusion limit for proteins

1.43 | OPPOSITE PAGE: Diagrammatic models of the action and characteristics of the glucocorticoid receptor, a transcriptional activator. *A:* Model of glucocorticoid receptor interaction with a heat shock protein, HSP-90, and with the receptor ligand, depicted as G.[286] HSP-90 binding to the GR stabilizes it; binding of the ligand to the receptor allows dissociation of the HSP-90 molecules and dimerization of the receptor. The GR dimer with steroid attached is carried by a specific transporter to the nucleus, where DNA interaction is possible. *B:* Structural organization of glucocorticoid receptor shows the sequences of interest and the related functional domains.[286] *C:* The GR region binding to the GRE site on the DNA utilizes a common motif, the zinc-finger DNA-binding motif.

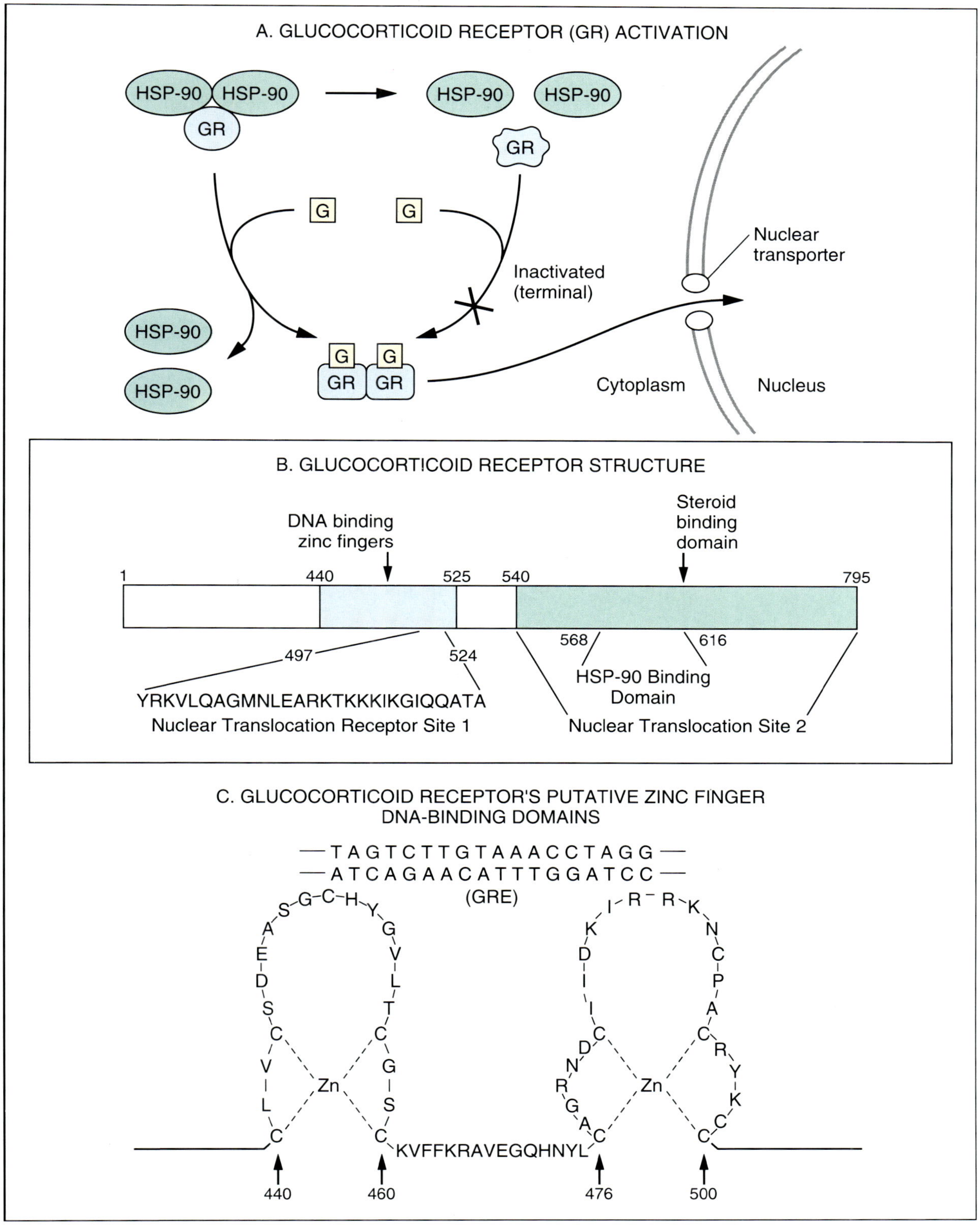
A. GLUCOCORTICOID RECEPTOR (GR) ACTIVATION
HSP-90
GR
G
Inactivated
(terminal)
Nuclear
transporter
Cytoplasm
Nucleus
B. GLUCOCORTICOID RECEPTOR STRUCTURE
DNA binding
zinc fingers
Steroid
binding
domain
1
440
525
540
795
497
524
568
616
HSP-90 Binding
Domain
YRKVLQAGMNLEARKTKKKIKGIQQATA
Nuclear Translocation Receptor Site 1
Nuclear Translocation Site 2
C. GLUCOCORTICOID RECEPTOR'S PUTATIVE ZINC FINGER
DNA-BINDING DOMAINS
—TAGTCTTGTAAACCTAGG—
—ATCAGAACATTTGGATCC—
(GRE)
Zn
KVFFKRAVEGQHNYL
440
460
476
500

through nuclear pores is ~70 kDa; the GR alone is 87.5 kDa, so it cannot enter the nucleus as a monomer and especially not as the ~300 kDa latent complex. On binding of the hormone or of an analogue, dexamethasone, the HSP-90 proteins are released and a GR homodimer forms. Hormone binding unmasks two specific short amino acid sequences in the GR which act as recognition signals for a nuclear pore transporter, and the GR dimer is translocated to the nucleus. In the simple case, the dimer binds to glucocorticoid-responsive element or enhancer sequences (GRE) and activates transcription of GRE-containing genes, including stromelysin, the 92 kDa gelatinase, and TIMP-l.[255,256]

GR Structure/Function

The GR has been studied in some detail and two important functional domains have been identified (Fig. 1.43B). The hormone binding domain is located between amino acids 540 and 795 (the carboxyl terminal) and the DNA binding domain is located between amino acids 440 and 525. The DNA binding is via a pair of putative "zinc fingers," a typical motif for this function, and requires zinc for activity (Fig. 1.43C).[271,273,277] The two nuclear localization signals, NLl between 497 and 524 and NL2 somewhere in the steroid binding domain, have also been identified. Interaction with HSP-90 is via residues between 568 and 616, in the hormone binding domain.

Interestingly, phosphorylation of GR by protein kinase C increases dimer formation but not transcriptional activation. Phosphorylation of a separate residue by protein kinase A is required for transcriptional activation but does not affect dimerization. Additional studies will be necessary to unravel the complete role of phosphorylation in GR behavior.

Context-Sensitive GREs

Glucocorticoids are frequently involved in negative or repressive transcriptional regulation, and this complex system has been studied in some detail.[285,286] Because trabecular metalloproteinase/TIMP and other protein expression are modulated both positively and negatively by dexamethasone, this type of regulation is of interest. Dexamethasone both enhances and antagonizes stromelysin induction by interleukin-l.[255]

Glucocorticoid receptor binds to a context-sensitive GRE site with a modified TRE contained within it (see Fig. 1.41). When GR and Jun/Fos are both present, a GR–Jun binding interaction occurs. Depending on either the Jun/Fos ratio or the absolute Fos concentration, a 70-fold enhancement or complete gene repression can be achieved. In a similar system, a slight overlap of a GRE and a CRE produces glucocorticoid repression of CREB enhancement of the gene. A somewhat similar condition has been demonstrated for retinoic acid mediation of stromelysin expression.[287] These types of complex regulation may explain some of the apparently conflicting observations in the literature.

Multiple Enhancers and Multifaceted Regulation

Frequently, several enhancer sequences are found in one gene's regulatory regions.[271,274,286,288–290] Combinations of transcriptional activators can produce dramatic synergistic effects many-fold larger than the sum of both acting alone. Multifaceted regulation has also been recently reported for the 72 kDa gelatinase,[291] and for trabecular stromelysin and TIMP-l.[255] Additional studies of this type will be necessary to unravel the mechanisms of their responses to the many different modulators mentioned earlier.[267] Considerable interest in this type of regulation is evident in the current literature.

IMPLICATIONS FOR AQUEOUS OUTFLOW REGULATION

Matrix metalloproteinase activity levels in the trabecular ECM are probably regulated by this multifaceted modulation of their expression/secretion, by extracellular matrix free calcium levels, which would activate the enzymes, and by the expression/secretion of trabecular TIMPs. The temporal pattern of the ratio of the levels of active metalloproteinases to TIMPs and their spatial patterns and activations in the ECM are probably key components in the regulation of trabecular ECM turnover. Coordinated with this ECM turnover, replacement ECM component biosynthesis is also apparent.[128] Very little detailed information is available on the coordination of these two processes in the meshwork or even in other tissues. A feedback coupling seems probable, e.g., biosynthesis occurs in response to prior turnover and turnover diminishes to allow biosynthetic ECM replacement, but minimal direct evidence and no mechanistic information are available.

Some type of higher-level regulation, by which trabecular cells somehow sense either the aqueous outflow rate or the intraocular pressure (IOP), can also be assumed.[128] Without some mechanism to couple IOP to ECM turnover and biosynthesis, glaucoma would probably be a very common condition.

LTP AND TRABECULAR ECM REGULATION: A MODEL SYSTEM

Laser trabeculoplasty (LTP), a common treatment of open-angle glaucoma, ameliorates the increased resistance to aqueous humor outflow by unknown mechanisms. Recent studies provide the framework for a hypothesis to explain this mechanism which is based upon transcriptional activation of trabecular matrix metalloproteinases.[128]

LTP induces trabecular cell division and a change in GAG production profiles within the first 48 hours following treatment.[292–294] The cell division is localized to a population of specialized cells found within the trabecular insert, the triangular portion of the trabecular meshwork anterior to Schlemm's canal where the meshwork "inserts" into the cornea (see Fig. 1.30).[295] Basal trabecular cell division is also localized to this insert region. By 1 or 2 weeks post LTP, the cells that divided within the first 48 hours have migrated from the insert and are found surrounding the LTP burn-sites.[295] By 10 days after LTP, restoration to a more normal GAG biosynthesis profile has also occurred.[293]

LTP treatment induces a rapid increase in the mRNA levels of the trabecular matrix metalloproteinases and their TIMPs,[267,296] followed by an increase in the expression of these proteins.[267,296,297] The induction of cell division and metalloproteinase expression occurs for the full 360° of the meshwork, whether 360° or only 180° are laser treated.[296] In addition, culture medium that is conditioned for 8 hours by LTP-treated meshworks induces identical responses in untreated meshworks.[267,296,297] This supports rather strongly the hypothesis that a medium-borne factor(s) is responsible for triggering these responses. Several growth factors and a cytokine can elicit similar responses, although the identity of the medium-borne factor has not been rigorously established.[255,267]

Localization of stromelysin mRNA and protein expression by in situ hybridization and immunohistochemistry[297] shows that the initial increases occur rapidly and are localized to the trabecular insert region and to the juxtacanalicular region. By 48 hours, stromelysin mRNA levels have declined in both regions. Stromelysin immunostaining is diminished in the insert but remains relatively high in the juxtacanalicular ECM, declining somewhat by

1 week post LTP. The stromelysin immunostaining is localized at the trabecular cell surface at 8–16 hours but becomes more diffuse throughout the adjacent ECM over the next week. It can be hypothesized[128,297] that the freshly divided cells migrate to the burn sites and restore normal outflow through the obstructed meshwork. Perhaps more relevant, is the more sustained elevation of trabecular stromelysin levels within the juxtacanalicular ECM, a putative site for glaucomatous obstruction of outflow due to chronically reduced proteoglycan turnover.[128] Although this explanation for the cause of glaucoma and the efficacy of LTP is not rigorously established, it clearly relies heavily on transcriptional activation mechanisms to modulate ECM turnover and biosynthesis.

OUTFLOW PATHWAY INTRACELLULAR BIOCHEMISTRY

TRABECULAR CELL CYTOSKELETAL COMPONENTS

The cytoskeleton of trabecular cells is undoubtedly of considerable importance to trabecular cell functions, including the maintenance of cell shape, maintenance of cell attachment to ECMs, cell division, cell migration in response to wounding or cell-density depletion, support of exocytotic/secretory activity, and support of phagocytosis/endocytosis.[298–302]

The microfilament protein F-actin, the intermediate filament protein vimentin (but not desmin or cytokeratins), and the microtubule protein a-tubulin have been identified and localized in trabecular cells.[298,303–306] Cells containing smooth muscle myosin have also been identified in the meshwork.[144] No detailed molecular studies have been conducted beyond these identifications, localizations, and some studies manipulating their subcellular distribution patterns with cytochalasin B, colchicine, taxol, and nocodozol.[304] Increased facility of aqueous outflow has been achieved by manipulation of the trabecular cytoskeleton by cytochalasin B.[307,308] Further detailed molecular analysis of the behavior and regulation of the trabecular cytoskeleton is of considerable importance.

OUTFLOW PATHWAY LYSOSOMAL ENZYMES

Enzymatic components of the lysosomes in the trabecular meshwork have been studied in some detail, and a variety of specific enzymes have been identified,[204,309,310] including acid phosphatase, alkaline phosphatase, hyaluronidase, *N*-acetyl-β-D-hexosaminidase, β-glucuronidase, acid lipase, cholesteryl esterase, acid esterase, β-D-glucuronidase, β-D-galactosidase, α-D-mannosidase, and α-L-fucosidase. In addition, the presence of mannose-6-phosphate receptors on trabecular cells has been demonstrated.[310] Presumably, the strong phagocytic/endocytic activity exhibited by trabecular cells, which is believed to enable the rapid ECM turnover and cleaning of outflow pathway structures, places a heavy load on the trabecular lysosomal system. Included in this load is the frequent release of pigment granules from other eye structures that must pass through the outflow pathway. Pigment buildup does occur within trabecular cells over time, and several studies have demonstrated that pigment granule phagocytosis can stimulate a migratory response in trabecular cells.[299] Except as outlined above, the actual biochemical details of the system are still necessarily inferred to be similar to those of other cell types.

ENZYMES OF TRABECULAR ENERGY METABOLISM

Trabecular cells resemble erythrocytes, lens, or sperm more than most other cell types in terms of their energy metabolism. They rely less on respiration (20%), and more on glycolysis (80%) and the pentose shunt, than most other tissues.[311] This is thought to be due to the meshwork's avascular nature, presumably experiencing less availability of oxygen than many other tissues. The PO_2 to which the meshwork is exposed is only ~47 mm Hg,[312] well below that of an average vascularized tissue.

Several trabecular enzymes with regulatory roles in energy metabolism have been identified and/or characterized. Both the adult and fetal forms of type I hexokinase and the type II form of the isoenzyme were found in trabecular cells; the adult forms exhibited kinetic parameters similar to those of other tissues and appear to pace entry of hexose sugars into glycolysis as in other tissues.[313] Trabecular phosphofructokinase, another key regulatory enzyme in glycolysis, was studied and exhibited similar characteristics to that of other tissues, although it did show an absolute requirement for ammonium ion in the range of 0.18 mM (its aqueous humor concentration).[314] Glucose-6-phosphate dehydrogenase and 6-phosphogluconate dehydrogenase activities (involved in $NADP^+ \rightarrow$ NADPH conversion and the latter perhaps in GAG biosynthesis) were analyzed, and isozyme banding patterns resembling the retina rather than the liver were observed.[315]

OUTFLOW PATHWAY OXIDATION/REDUCTION ENZYMES AND OXIDATIVE DAMAGE

One hypothesis put forth to explain reduced trabecular cellularity with aging and with glaucoma,[316,317] the increase in undegradable trabecular GAG-like material with aging and in glaucoma,[318,319] and the proposed inability of trabecular cells to maintain the appropriate resistance to aqueous humor outflow with age and in glaucoma is based on the long-term effects of oxidative/free radical damage to trabecular cells. Several groups have studied the trabecular levels of the enzymes, which might be involved in protection against such oxidative damage.[121,204,320] Catalase,[121,321] other peroxidases, glutathione reductase,[143] superoxide dismutase,[321] and glutathione peroxidase,[322] as well as glutathione, hydrogen peroxide, NADPH, and several related metabolites, have been all measured in trabecular cells. Age-related changes in their various levels make this hypothesis a viable possibility, although cause and effect are difficult to establish rigorously. Unlike cataracts, no solid epidemiological evidence has been reported linking glaucoma with lifetime light exposure or climate/latitude of residence. Oxidative damage, probably primarily due to membrane lipids, could easily compromise cell integrity and permeability balances and thus cell viability. Some type of sulflhydryl-reactive damage has also been postulated.[323–325]

OUTFLOW PATHWAY RECEPTORS AND REGULATORY PATHWAYS

Although not studied in great molecular detail, some trabecular meshwork regulatory mechanisms have been analyzed. In addition to the ECM modulation discussed earlier, several second-messenger systems appear to be involved in trabecular behavior.

Cyclic AMP in Trabecular Regulation

Cyclic AMP is present in the meshwork and its stimulation has been observed in response to dopamine receptor activation and vasoactive intestinal peptide (VIP), suggesting its coupling (no doubt transduced by some unidentified G-proteins) to trabecular adenylyl cyclase.[326–331] Adrenergic receptors of the β_2 subtype have also been identified on trabecular cells and stimulate cAMP increases.[326,332,333]

The cAMP Second Messenger System

Although not studied in detail, we can extrapolate from what is known of the meshwork and of this regulatory system in other tissues[165] to what can be expected in trabecular cells. None of the enzymes of this pathway has been studied specifically in the meshwork, e.g., adenylyl cyclase, cyclic nucleotide phosphodiesterase, cAMP-dependent protein kinases, or protein phosphatases. This is an extremely important regulatory system, and unraveling the details of its roles in the meshwork is of high priority.

Trabecular Glucocorticoid Responses

Trabecular cells in culture also exhibit ~60,000 high affinity (5–20 nM for dexamethasone) glucocorticoid receptors per cell which undergo translocation to the nuclei,[204,326,334,335] presumably interacting with GRE enhancer sequences on DNA, as discussed earlier. Induction and secretion of specific trabecular proteins, presumably triggered via this pathway, have been reported.[204,326,336–338] One particularly noticeable protein was elastin or an elastin-like protein.[336] Glucocorticoid regulation of induction of trabecular ECM enzymes, including the metalloproteinases and TIMPs, was discussed earlier. These effects have major implications on the etiology of steroid glaucoma. Cell differentiative glucocorticoid effects such as reduced trabecular cell division[122,340,341] have been observed.

Trabecular Prostaglandins

Much attention has been focused on the effects of eicosanoids/prostaglandins on aqueous outflow. Trabecular cell biosynthesis of prostaglandins has been studied briefly,[145,335,339] and the secretion of PGE_2, PGF_2, and 6-keto-$PGF_{1\alpha}$ demonstrated. Dexamethasone diminished their secretion at concentrations as low as 1 nM, presumably by GRE-dependent induction of proteins that inhibit phospholipases.[145]

Other Trabecular Regulatory Systems

Unfortunately, little information is available on the many other regulatory systems that could, and probably do, have major roles in trabecular behavior. Calcium signaling transients have been reported.[343] Basal calcium levels of 188 nM were observed and heterogeneous responses in approximately 25% of trabecular cells in culture were seen after adrenergic and cholinergic drug exposure. The inositol phosphates, calcium/calmodulin and related systems, protein kinase C and other serine/threonine protein kinases and phosphatases, growth factor and other tyrosine protein kinases and phosphatases, G proteins, intracellular pH, and other steroid receptors, just to name a few of the many other established regulatory systems, have either not been identified or not studied in any molecular detail in the meshwork.

PROSPECTS FOR AQUEOUS OUTFLOW PATHWAY BIOCHEMISTRY

As is presumably quite apparent at this point, with a few notable exceptions, the biochemistry of the aqueous outflow pathway has not yet reached even its infancy, and most major areas are virtually untouched. The increased accessibility of sophisticated molecular approaches that allow evaluation of events in small tissues should produce dramatic increases in our understanding of the biochemistry and molecular biology of the outflow pathway in the very immediate future. Considerable additional research seems necessary before a molecular understanding of the cause of glaucoma becomes available.

2 THE NORMAL POSTERIOR SEGMENT

SECTION I

ANATOMY AND EMBRYOLOGY OF THE OPTIC NERVE

Ronald L. Radius

EMBRYOLOGY

As an extension of the neurosensory retina, the optic nerve can be said to have its beginning during the third week of gestation. At that time the primary optic vesicle forms as an outpouching of cells from the region of the optic pit, the rudimentary eye spot located on either side of the primitive anterior forebrain[1] (Fig. 2.1). As this single layer of neuroectoderm expands in size, a central depression develops, converting the primary vesicle into the optic cup.[1,2] The invagination continues until the inner layer of cells approximates the outer layer, eliminating the intervening space that was previously the cavity of the primary optic vesicle. Simultaneously, the primitive optic stalk, connecting the primary optic vesicle to the forebrain, elongates and participates in the invagination, creating a medial and inferior groove extending the entire length of the optic stalk and into the rim of the primary optic cup anteriorly (Fig. 2.2). By the end of the seventh week this stage of morphogenesis is completed, with closure of this cleft.[2] Closure begins near the center of the optic stalk, proceeding anteriorly to the rim of the optic cup and posteriorly along the stalk towards the primitive forebrain. The hyaloid artery is included within the optic stalk and pierces the closing fetal fissure just posterior to the developing eye.

As the walls of the optic cup come together, the inner cell layers fuse, as do the two outer layers, eliminating any trace of the fetal fissure and creating two concentric layers of neuroectoderm within the optic vesicle. By the fifth week of gestation, granules of brown pigment begin to appear in what will become the retinal pigmented epithelium. Simultaneously, the anterior rim of this same outer layer extends beyond the optic vesicle to form the pigmented epithelial layers of the ciliary body and iris.

Development within the inner cell layer more closely parallels concurrent changes within the brain itself. Even before invagination is complete, the anterior layer of the primary optic vesicle shows intense mitotic activity. At approximately 4 to 5 weeks of gestation, two zones can already be

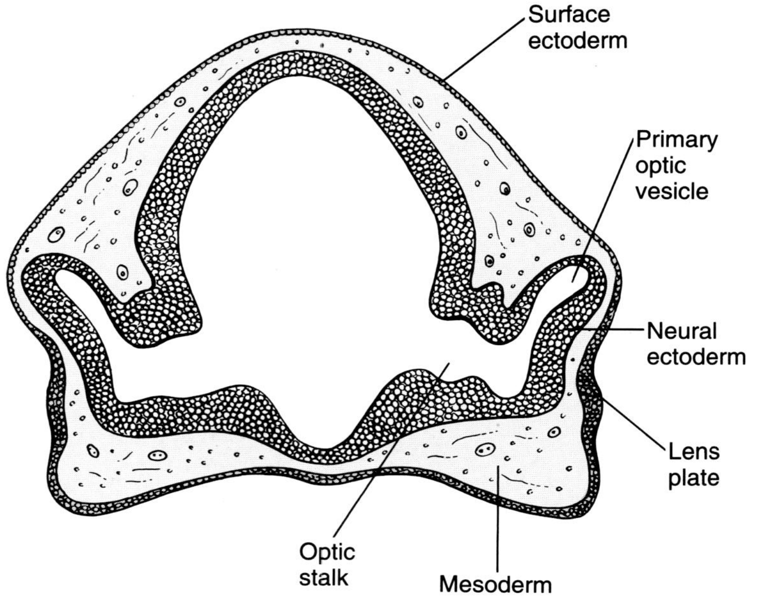

2.1 | Frontal section through the eye of a 5-mm (fourth week of gestation) embryo. (Adapted from Duke-Elder S: *System of Ophthalmology,* Vol III, part 1: Embryology. St. Louis: CV Mosby, 1963.)

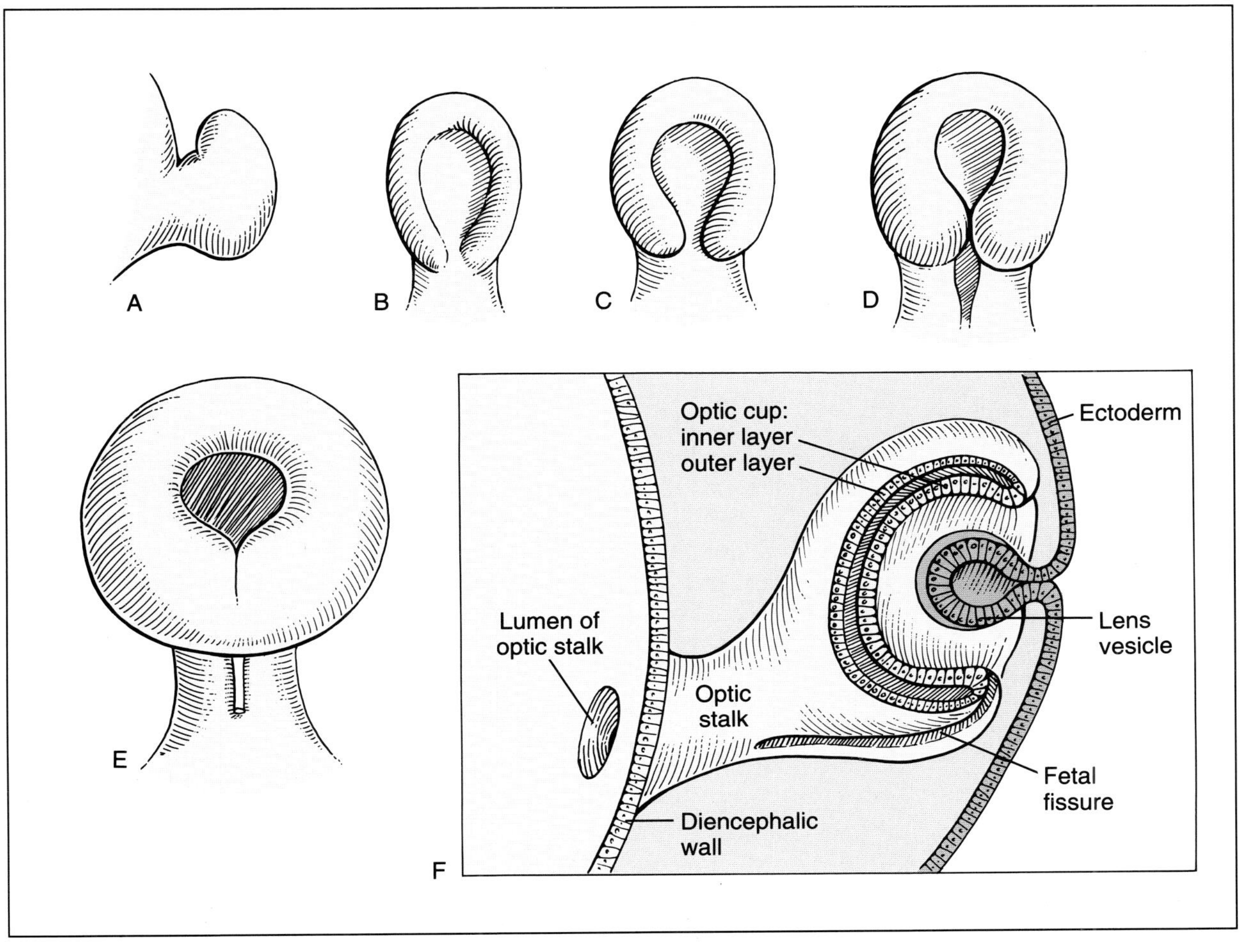

2.2 | The primary optic vesicle is connected to the primitive forebrain by the optic stalk *(A)*. Invagination of this structure creates the primary optic cup *(B)*. As the outer and inner layers of this vesicle fuse *(F)*, the invagination includes the edge of the cup and extends into the optic stalk *(B,C, and D)* forming the primitive fetal fissure. Ultimately, closure of the fissure occurs, beginning near the center of the optic stalk and proceeding anteriorly to the edge of the optic cup and posteriorly to the diencephalon *(F)*. The hyaloid artery is included within this closing fissure *(E)*.

appreciated[2] (Fig. 2.3). The outer zone, lying closest to the inner pigmented epithelium, contains eight or nine layers of actively dividing cells. The inner or marginal zone is devoid of cell nuclei. Throughout the remainder of the first trimester, the outer layer of cells splits into two layers, with the innermost layer migrating into the marginal zone.[1–3] This fission begins at the posterior pole and spreads slowly towards the equator and the ora serrata (Fig. 2.4). The innermost cells of this inner layer differentiate into retinal ganglion cells, beginning as early as the end of the second month of gestation. Migrating inward towards the retinal surface, these cells form the ganglion cell layer of the mature eye. Processes extending from them elongate into the more superficial retinal nerve fiber layer and towards the optic nerve stalk.

By the fifth month of gestation, formation of the retinal ganglion cell layer is complete. Development of the other retinal layers proceeds sequentially, with the outermost cell layers forming at later intervals during gestation. The inner nuclear layer arises from a fusion of the remaining inner cell layer and cells migrating through the marginal zone from the outermost portion of the primitive outer layer of cells. This process of migration and fusion during the fifth and sixth months of gestation eliminates the temporary fiber layer of Chevitz which previously separated the inner and outer layers of neuroblastic cells.[2,3] The cells remaining within the outer layer differentiate into the neural rods and cones whose nuclei comprise the outer nuclear layer of the mature retina. By the eighth month of gestation, formation of the retinal layers is complete, and little if any cell division occurs after birth.

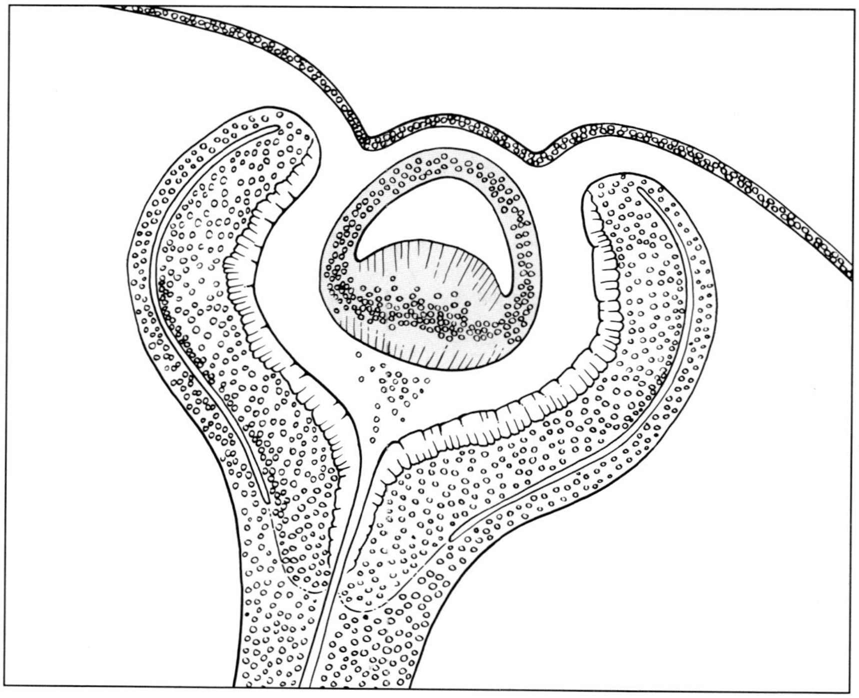

2.3 | At the 10-mm stage (approximately 4 to 5 weeks' gestation) the cavity within the primary optic vesicle is obliterated and formation of the optic cup is completed. Two retinal layers are clearly separated into the outer primitive zone containing eight to nine layers of nucleated cells and the inner marginal zone devoid of cell nuclei. (Adapted from Barber AN: *Embryology of the Human Eye.* St. Louis: CV Mosby, 1955.)

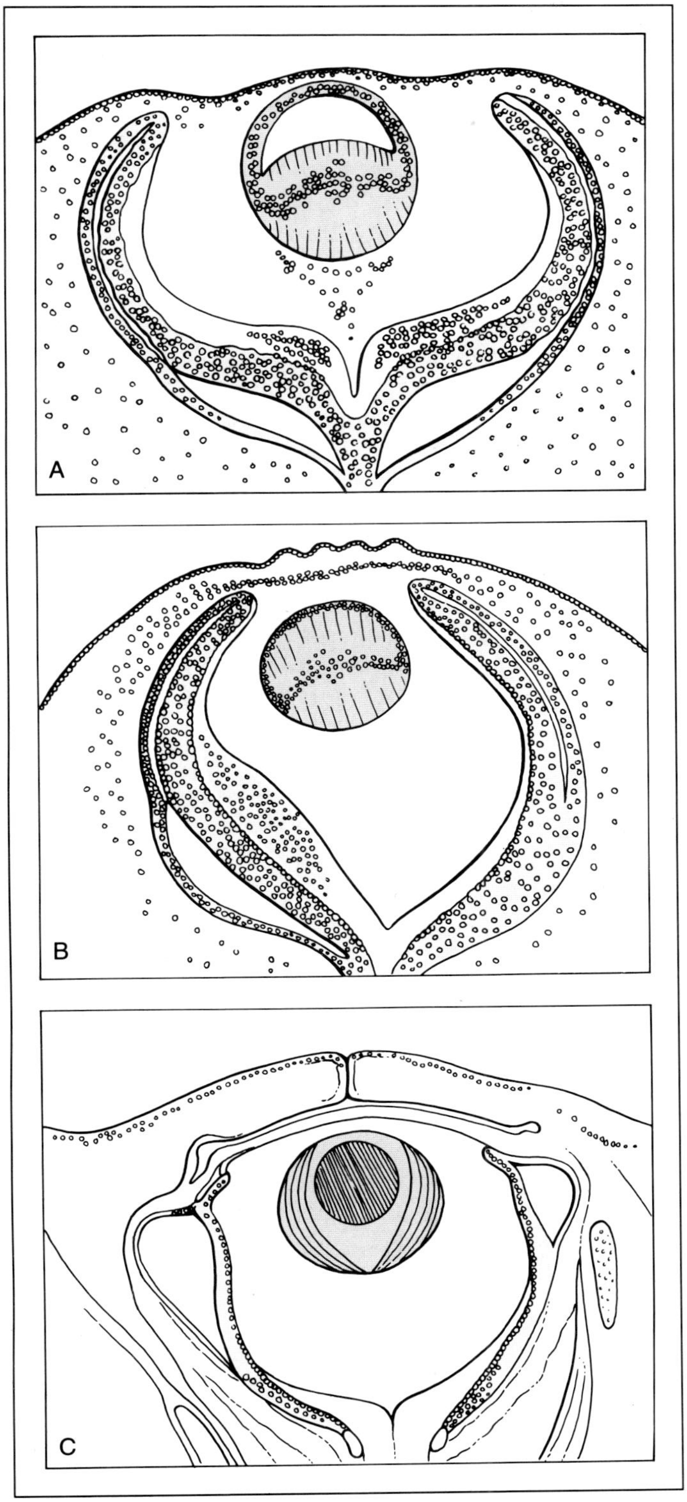

2.4 | During the third trimester, cells from the nucleated primitive zone migrate into the marginal zone, creating two cell layers. The process begins near the posterior pole at about the 13-mm stage *(A)*, proceeds anteriorly and reaches the equator at about the 26-mm stage *(B)* and is completed, extending from optic nerve head to ora serrata, by the 65-mm stage *(C)*. (Adapted from Barber AN: *Embryology of the Human Eye*. CV Mosby: St. Louis, 1955.)

Within the optic stalk, axons from the differentiating ganglion cell layer migrate into and essentially fill the tissue space within the primitive nerve by as early as the second month of gestation.[4] By the eleventh week of gestation, uncrossed fibers can be seen at the chiasm. By the thirteenth week, crossed fibers are present. As these neural processes elongate towards the brain, much of the primitive neuroectoderm within the optic stalk disappears. However, some of these original cells persist and differentiate into the neuroglia of the adult optic nerve.[4] Initially this glial tissue is scattered diffusely throughout the nerve substance. By the third month of gestation, however, longitudinal rows of glial cells appear, separating columns of ganglion cell axons within the optic nerve (Fig. 2.5). Some cells and associated processes orient themselves perpendicular to the axon columns within the most proximal portion of the optic nerve and form the early lamina cribrosa.

During the fourth and fifth months of gestation, astrocytes and oligodendrocytes differentiate from the primitive neuroglia. Oligodendrocytes produce elongated processes, enveloping individual axons within a multilaminated myelin sheath. Myelination of the optic nerve axons proceeds in reverse direction, from the lateral geniculate body towards the chiasm and globe. The process is first apparent by the fifth month of gestation at the lateral geniculate body, by the sixth month at the chiasm and by the eighth month within the optic nerve itself. This process is completed at or shortly after birth, with myelination of the optic nerve extending from the geniculate body to the level of the posterior lamina cribrosa. During the final 2 months of gestation, formation of the optic nerve structures is completed with the appearance of optic nerve microglia, optic nerve histiocytes, and ingrowth of blood vessels from the surrounding mesoderm. Mesodermal tissue forms septa between axonal columns and infiltrates the primitive lamina. The central retinal artery replaces the primitive hyaloid system as the nutrient artery to the inner layers of the retina and optic nerve head.

ANATOMY

RETINA

The optic nerve can be said to begin within the ganglion cell layer of the retina.[5] Each of the more than one million ganglion cells is, in turn, associated with its own receptor field. Receptor fields, generally circular in shape, contain the receptor elements and interneurons that ultimately impinge the

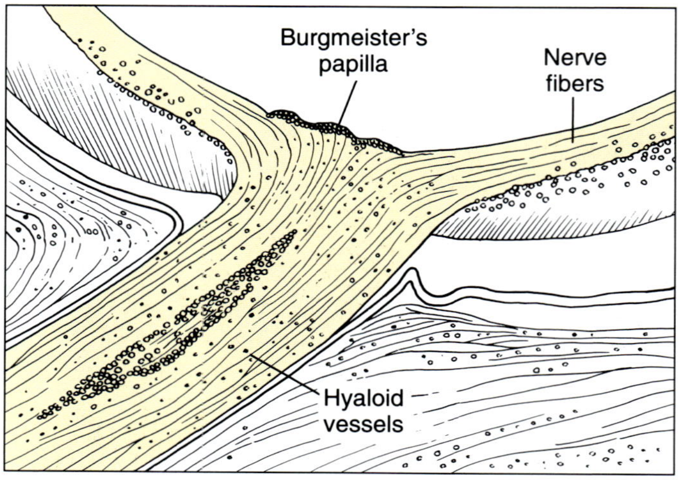

2.5 | By the second month of gestation, axons from retinal ganglion cells fill the nerve cross section immediately posterior to the optic nerve head. As early as the 45-mm stage (third month of gestation), longitudinal rows of primitive neuroglia appear, separating columns of axons within the nerve. (Adapted from Haden H: Development of the ectodermal framework of the optic nerve. *Am J Ophthalmol 1947;30:1205–1224.* Published with permission from the American Journal of Ophthalmology. Copyright by the Ophthalmic Publishing Company.)

ganglion cell's dendritic tree. There is considerable overlap of receptor fields between different ganglion cells, both at the receptor cell level and within the inner nuclear layer. In general, receptor fields are smaller within the posterior pole of the eye and larger in the more peripheral retina.[5,6]

The concentration of ganglion cells within the posterior pole of the retina corresponds to the variable sizes of these receptor fields. The ganglion cell layer decreases in thickness from a maximum of four to six cells surrounding the fovea to a single cell layer in the more peripheral retina (Fig. 2.6). Ganglion cells are absent within the most central portion of the fovea. Within the rest of the posterior pole, the area circumscribed by the major retinal vascular arcade, the ganglion cell layer is two to four cells thick.

Populations of ganglion cells can be characterized by their electrophysical response to changes in retinal illumination.[6] The "x-type" response is characterized by a sustained change in the firing rate of the ganglion cell when the corresponding receptor field is alternately illuminated by a light stimulus of proper orientation and frequency (see Section III). The "y-type" cell responds to a change in retinal illumination with an abrupt but transient change in the baseline firing rate. The baseline rate may be enhanced or reduced depending upon the region of the receptor field illuminated and the specific cell type involved. Processing of this complex pattern of increased and decreased ganglion cell firing by the lateral geniculate body, visual cortex and associated areas results in the final psychophysical response to light.

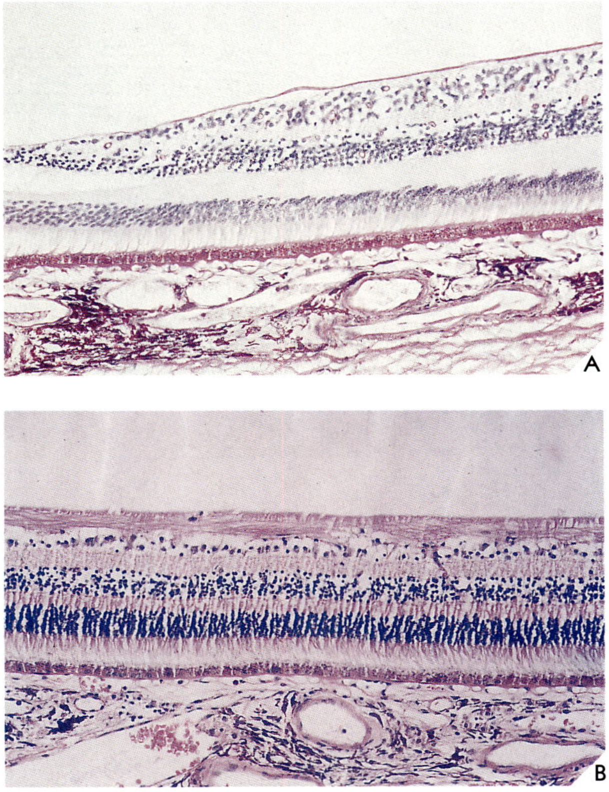

2.6 | The thickness of the retinal ganglion cell layer decreases from the maximum of six to eight cell layers in the parafoveal area *(A)* to one layer of nuclei in the retinal periphery *(B)*. (Courtesy of Dr. W.R. Green, Wilmer Institute.)

From each retinal ganglion cell, a single axon extends into the retinal nerve fiber layer towards the optic nerve head (Fig. 2.7). Within the nerve fiber layer, axons are grouped into individual channels formed by elongated glial processes of Müller cell origin[7] (Fig. 2.8). The cell bodies of the Müller processes are located deep to the nerve fiber layer within the inner nuclear layer. The extended processes of these specialized astrocytes and other glial cells within the retina envelop individual axons and ganglion cell bodies, separate neural tissue from retinal vasculature, and provide structural support for the various tissue elements within the inner retinal layers.[5,8,9] Most important, however, the retinal glia function to maintain the relatively constant microenvironment necessary for proper neuronal function by active participation in waste and nutrient exchange between the neurons and the microvasculature of the inner retina.[10–13] The terminal footplates of the Müller cells coalesce into a dense glial layer at the retina vitreous interface to form the internal limiting membrane of the retina.[6,14]

Nerve fiber bundles can be recognized clinically by routine ophthalmoscopy[15–18] (Fig. 2.9). The fine, silvery retinal striations, particularly obvious within the posterior pole and in the superior and inferior arcuate bundles where the nerve fiber layer is thickest, are the individual axon bundles.[19] The darker striations are the glial tunnels. The pattern is less obvious in the more peripheral retina where the nerve fiber layer is thinner, consistent with the reduced number of ganglion cells and larger retinal receptor fields

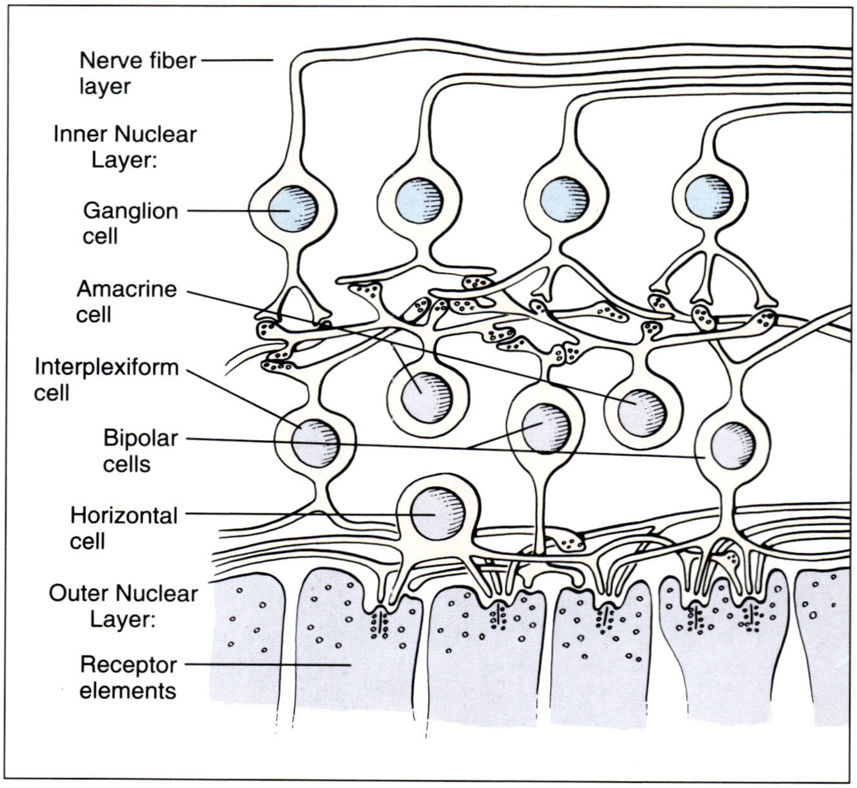

2.7 | The neural retina of the adult eye can be described simply as being composed of alternating nuclear and plexiform layers. The outer nuclear layer contains the cell bodies of the receptor elements, the rods and cones. The inner nuclear layer contains the amacrine cell, bipolar cells, horizontal cells, and the interplexiform cell. These interneurons modulate and relay the neural response to light originating within the outer nuclear layer to the innermost nuclear layer containing the retinal ganglion cells. From each ganglion cell a single axon extends into the more superficial retinal nerve fiber layer. Within this layer axons are grouped into fiber bundles and ultimately exit the eye at the optic nerve head. (Courtesy of Dr. J.E. Dowling, adapted from Miller NR: *Walsh and Hoyt's Clinical Neuro-Ophthalmology.* Baltimore: Williams and Wilkins, 1982.)

described earlier. Within the nasal retina, axon bundles follow a relatively direct course towards the optic nerve head. Within the temporal retina, axons from ganglion cells located nasal to the fovea also pass directly to the optic disc. Axons from the more peripheral ganglion cells, however, arc

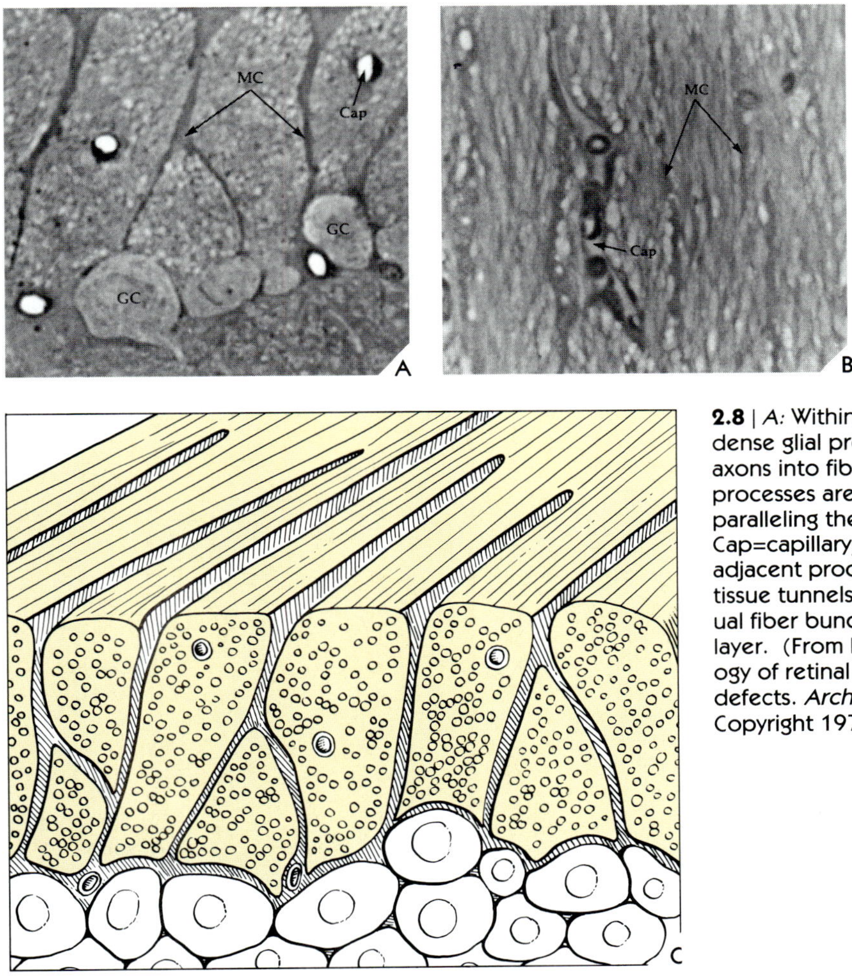

2.8 | *A:* Within the retinal nerve fiber layer, dense glial processes of Müller cell origin group axons into fiber bundles. *B:* These sheet-like glial processes are elongated in the plane of section paralleling the retinal surface. MC=Müller cell; Cap=capillary; GC=ganglion cell. *C:* Fusion of adjacent processes forms the walls of incomplete tissue tunnels that segregate axons into individual fiber bundles within the retinal nerve fiber layer. (From Radius RL, Anderson DR: The histology of retinal nerve fiber bundles and bundle defects. *Arch Ophthalmol 1979;97:948–950.* Copyright 1979, American Medical Association.)

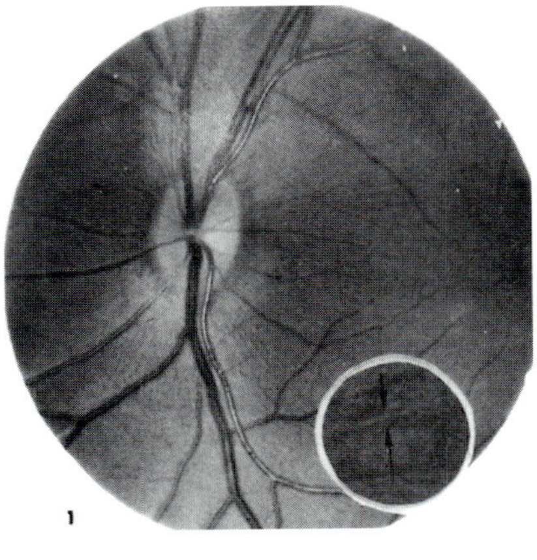

2.9 | Individual fiber bundles can be recognized clinically by routine ophthalmoscopy. The fine silvery striations at the retinal surface represent individual axon bundles (inset, arrows). The darker lines between bundles are the elongated glial tissue tunnels of Müller cell origin. (From Radius RL, Anderson DR: The histology of retinal nerve fiber bundles and bundle defects. *Arch Ophthalmol 1979;97:948–950.* Copyright 1979, American Medical Association.)

around the macular region and exit the eye near the superior and inferior poles of the optic nerve head[6,17,20–23] (Fig. 2.10).

There is no extensive exchange of individual axons between adjacent fiber bundles within the nerve fiber layer.[17] The pattern of vertical stratification of axons within the fiber bundles varies among different species.[17,24–26] In selected primates, axons from ganglion cells near the optic nerve head enter the nerve fiber layer, pass between axons from more distally located ganglion cells, and occupy the more superficial nerve fiber layer (Fig. 2.11). In other species, axons from the more proximal ganglion cells lie in the deeper strata of the nerve fiber layer. The anatomy in the human eye has not been defined.

The blood supply to the inner retina, including the nerve fiber layer, the ganglion cell layer, the inner plexiform layer, and part of the inner nuclear layer, is provided by the central retinal artery, a branch of the ophthalmic artery.[27–31] This vessel enters the optic nerve just posterior to the globe and splits into four main trunks that supply the inferior and superior temporal and nasal retina as it pierces the optic nerve head within the eye. At the nerve

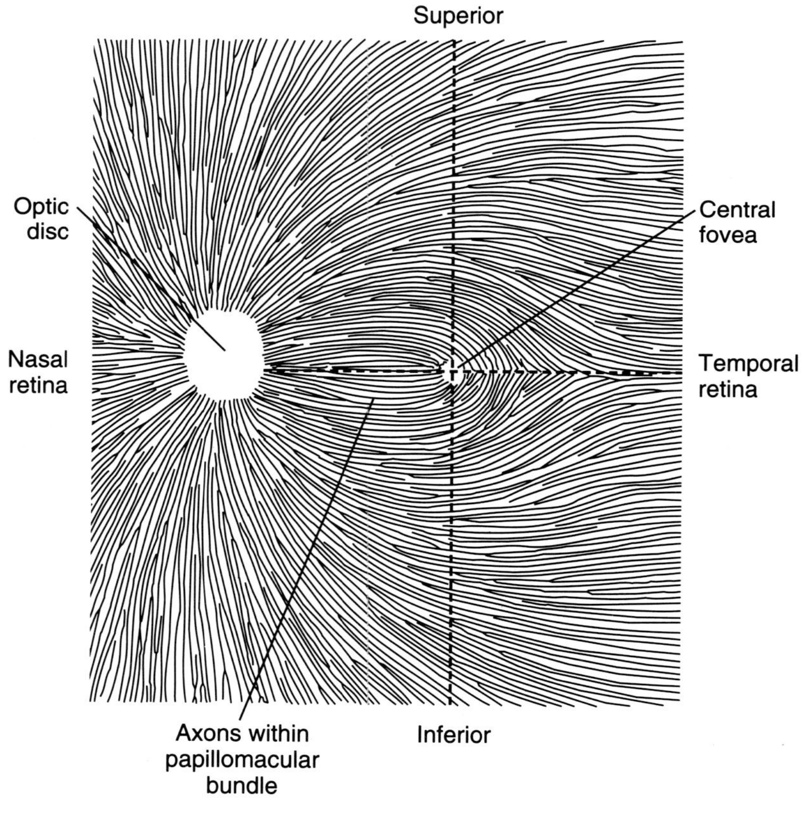

2.10 | Within the retinal nerve fiber layer, axons from the nasal retina travel directly towards the nerve head to enter along the nasal margin of the disc. Axons within the papillomacular bundle follow a relatively direct course to enter the temporal margin of the disc. Fibers from the temporal retina arc around the area centralis and fovea to enter the superior and inferior poles of the optic nerve head. Horizontal (small rectangle and dotted line temporal to the fovea) and vertical lines through the fovea divide the retina into superior and inferior as well as nasal and temporal halves. (Adapted from Hogan MJ, Alvarado JA, Weddell JE: *Histology of the Human Eye. An Atlas and Textbook.* Philadelphia: WB Saunders, 1971.)

head, this central vessel is a true artery with a complete muscular coat. Within the retina, however, the muscular coat is lost and the major branches of the central artery are really arterioles. All of the retinal vessels and capillaries that penetrate the inner retinal layers are confined within the structural glial tissue elements and are segregated from the neuronal tissue by processes of glial cell origin.[5,9] The endothelial cell wall and associated pericytes are characterized by tight cell junctions.[14,32–34] There is little collateral blood flow between separate retinal regions. The retinal circulation, however, demonstrates a considerable capacity to autoregulate blood flow within the retina under different physiologic conditions that may affect the eye.[35–39] Blood exits the eye through the retinal veins draining into the central retinal vein. Venous drainage roughly parallels the course of the retinal arterial supply.

OPTIC NERVE HEAD

At the optic nerve head, all axon fiber bundles turn to exit the eye through the scleral canal. The canal is not truly perpendicular, but instead runs from lateral to medial and slightly inferior as it traverses the eye wall. Consequently, axons from the nasal retina turn acutely at the nerve head, whereas axons from the temporal retina follow a more obtuse angle as they enter the

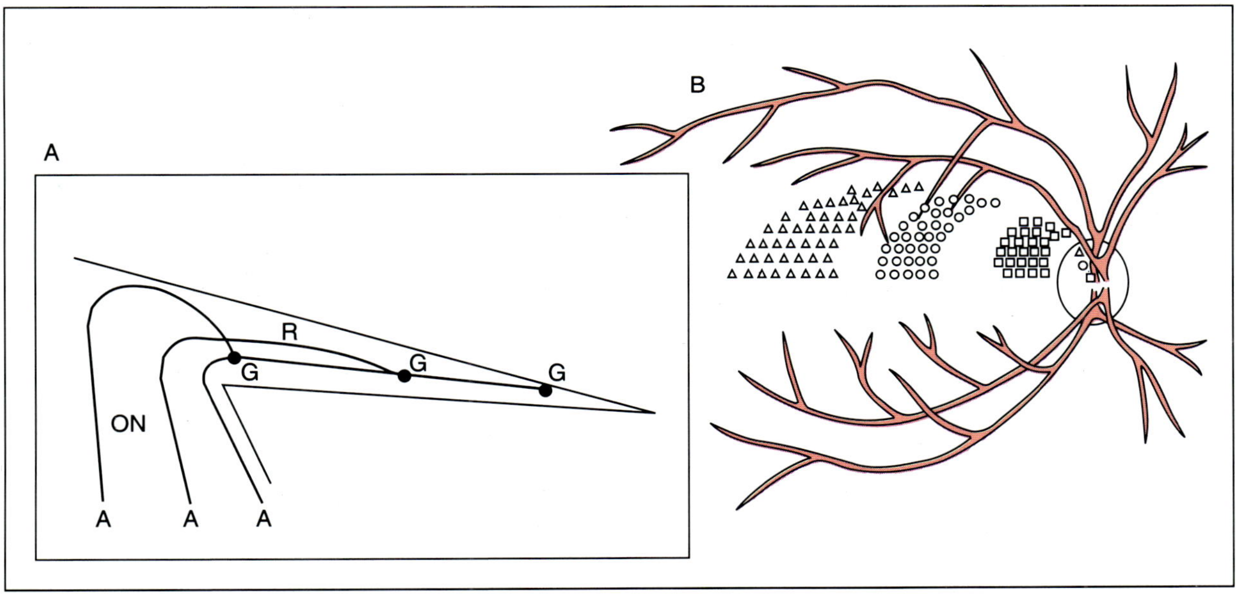

2.11 | Vertical stratification within the nerve fiber layer is species specific. *A:* In the Rhesus monkey, axons (A) from peripheral ganglion cells (G) assume a deeper position within the nerve fiber layer as subsequent axons from ganglion cells closer to the optic nerve (ON) head are added to the more superficial layers. *B:* Within the optic nerve head itself, fibers from more peripheral retina assume a more circumferential position (triangles), while fibers from peripapillary retina assume a more axial position (squares). Axons from more central locations (circles) assume an intermediate position. (Adapted from Minkler DS: The organization of nerve fiber bundles in the primate optic nerve head. *Arch Ophthalmol 1980;98:1630–1636.* Copyright 1980, American Medical Association.)

nerve[40,41] (Fig. 2.12). Fiber bundles occupy the margins of the nerve head, whereas the central retinal vessels and associated adventitia are near the core. The central nerve, devoid of tissue, is referred to as the optic cup. The size of this central cup depends on the actual number of neurons within the optic nerve (somewhat more than one million) and the dimensions of the scleral canal[40–43] (Fig. 2.13).

Within the anterior optic nerve head, which represents an extension of the retinal nerve fiber layer, Müller cell processes are absent. Their role is replaced by fibrous astrocytes.[10–13]

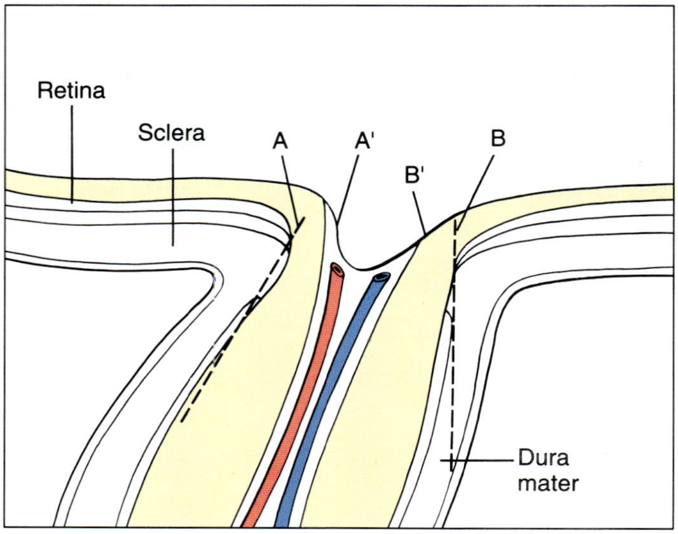

2.12 | The ophthalmoscopic appearance of the optic nerve head reflects the slant of the scleral canal through which the nerve exits the eye. If the canal traverses the posterior eye wall at an acute angle (A), then the nasal wall of the cup will be steep and often undermine the scleral edge (A'). In eyes with the scleral canal oriented more perpendicular to the eye wall (B'), the sides of the cup will slope more gradually (B) (Adapted from Anderson DR: The optic nerve in glaucoma, in Duane TD: *Clinical Ophthalmology.* Philadelphia: Harper & Row, 1985.)

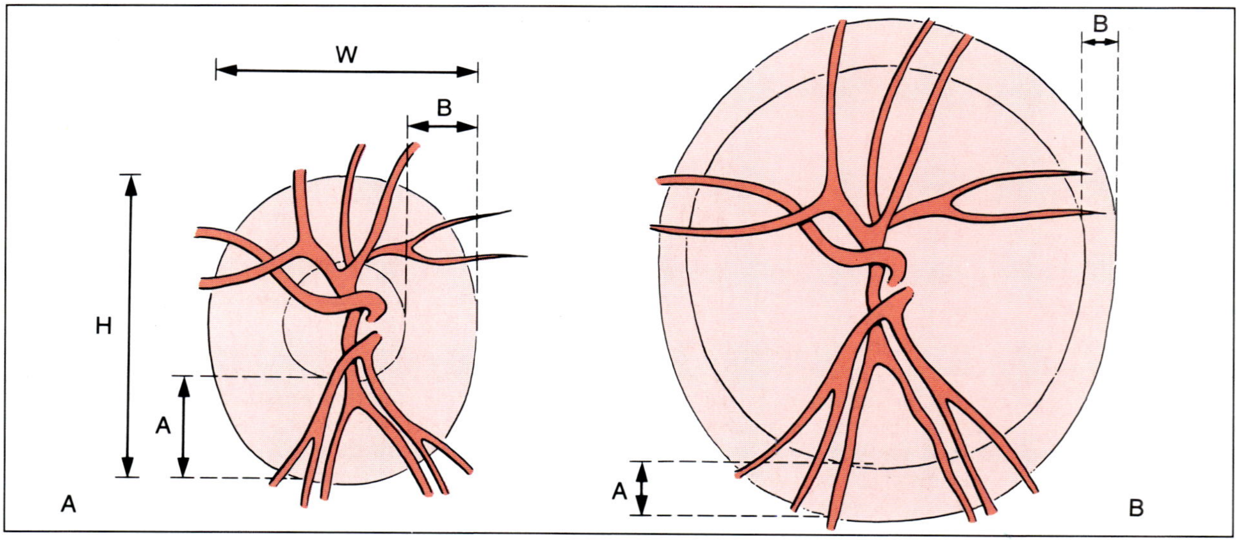

2.13 | In the normal optic nerve head *(A)*, the height (H) of the disc is somewhat greater than the width (W). Conversely, the superior and inferior neural rim (A) is somewhat thicker than the nasal and temporal rim. Consequently, the shape of the central cup is generally round. In eyes with a larger scleral canal *(B)*, the neural tissue rim (inferior and superior, A; nasal and temporal, B) will be thinner and the central cup correspondingly larger. (Adapted from Anderson DR: The optic nerve in glaucoma, in Duane TD: *Clinical Ophthalmology.* Philadelphia: Harper & Row, 1985.)

The amount of glial tissue within the anterior optic nerve is much reduced, however, in comparison with that in the retinal nerve fiber layer (Fig. 2.14). The axon bundles comprise nearly 90% of the tissue volume at the anterior optic nerve head.[44] Fiber bundle groupings of retinal axons probably parallel that in the adjacent retinal nerve fiber layer. Although the retinotopic anatomy of these groupings is not defined in the human eye, limited clinical information suggests that the axons from the more peripheral ganglion cells are located most circumferentially within the nerve head.[15,20,21] The glial cells and processes are vertically oriented, paralleling the course of the axons. Glial septa between axon bundles serve much the same support and nutrient functions within the nerve head as do the Müller cell processes within the retina (Fig. 2.15). Fusion of specialized endplates at the retina–vitreous interface forms the internal limiting membrane of Elschnig, replacing the much thicker internal limiting membrane of the retina.[45]

Deep to the anterior optic nerve head is the lamina cribrosa. The anterior lamina cribrosa, the lamina choroidalis, is at the level of the retina and choroid in the adjacent eye wall. The amount of glial tissue in this region of

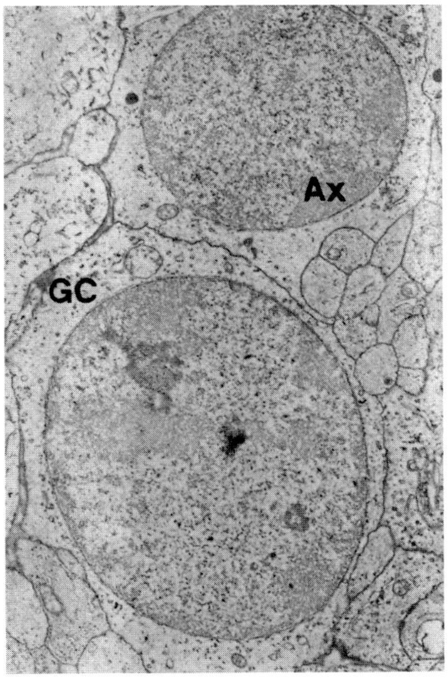

2.14 | Within the anterior optic nerve head, Müller cell processes are absent and processes from optic nerve fibrous astrocytes envelop and segregate axons and axon bundles. There is little extracellular space between axon cylinders (Ax) and these processes of glial cell (GC) origin. (From Anderson DR, Hoyt WF, Hogan MJ: The fine structure of the astroglia in the human optic nerve and optic nerve head. *Trans Am Ophthalmol Soc* *1967;65:275–303.*)

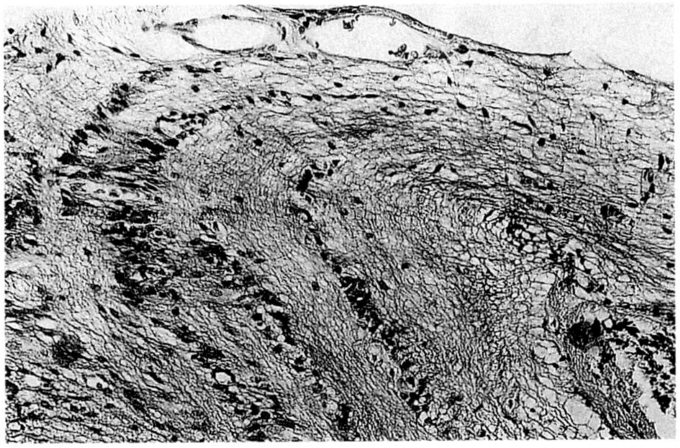

2.15 | Within the anterior optic nerve head, columns of glial cells and glial cell processes separate groups of axons into nerve fiber bundles. (From Anderson DR, Hoyt WF, Hogan MJ: The fine structure of the astroglia in the human optic nerve and optic nerve head. *Trans Am Ophthalmol Soc 1967;65:275–303.*)

the nerve is greatly increased over that seen more anteriorly.[10–13] However, connective tissue elements are largely absent and are confined primarily to the adventitia of the central retinal vessels located in the center of the nerve cross-section. Vertical columns of glial cells, increasing in thickness at deeper levels of the lamina, confine axons within individual fiber bundles (Fig. 2.16).

Within the more posterior lamina scleralis, the nerve is surrounded by the sclera of the posterior eye wall. At this level, the amount of connective tissue elements within these glial columns increases gradually but significantly until almost 50% of the nerve cross section consists of nonaxonal tissue.[10,11,13,44] The lamina is formed by parallel sheets of glial tissue alternating with lamellae of fibroblasts, collagen, ground substance, and basement membrane material, all oriented perpendicular to the course of the optic nerve.[10–13,44] The relative amounts of the connective tissue elements increase at deeper levels of the lamina (Fig. 2.17). Perforations within these parallel lamellae lie roughly in register, forming the pores through which pass the individual 200 or 300 axon bundles[10,11,13,46–49] (Fig. 2.18). Although the axon bundles are confined by this complex of glial and connective tissue tunnels, the tissue columns are incomplete. There is extensive branching of fiber bundles, with exchange of axons between columns within this region of the posterior optic nerve head.[10,11,13,44]

Throughout its course within the lamina cribrosa, the nerve is circumferentially enveloped by a sheath of glial tissue. Anteriorly, at the level of the lamina choroidalis, the border tissue of Kuhnt separates the fiber bundles from the adjacent retina and choroid.[10,11,13,50] More posteriorly, within the lamina scleralis, the border tissue of Jacoby, which is formed of both glial and connective tissue elements, lines the scleral canal.[10,11,13,51] Sheets of glial tissue also line the adventitia of the central retinal vessels as they travel within the optic nerve and ultimately exit from it approximately 1 cm posterior to the eye wall.

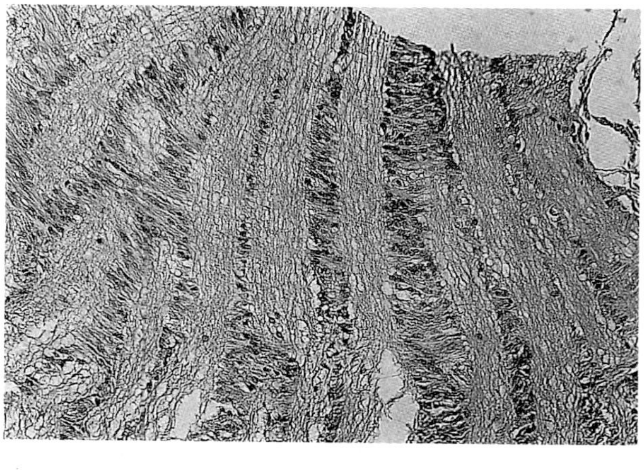

2.16 | The region of the anterior lamina cribrosa, the lamina choroidalis, is defined by the level of the retina and choroid in the adjacent eye wall. The amount of glial tissue in this region is greatly increased over that seen in the more anterior optic nerve. Columns of astrocyte nuclei separate axons into fiber bundles. (From Anderson DR, Hoyt WF, Hogan MJ: The fine structure of the astroglia in the human optic nerve and optic nerve head. *Trans Am Ophthalmol Soc 1967;65:275–303.*)

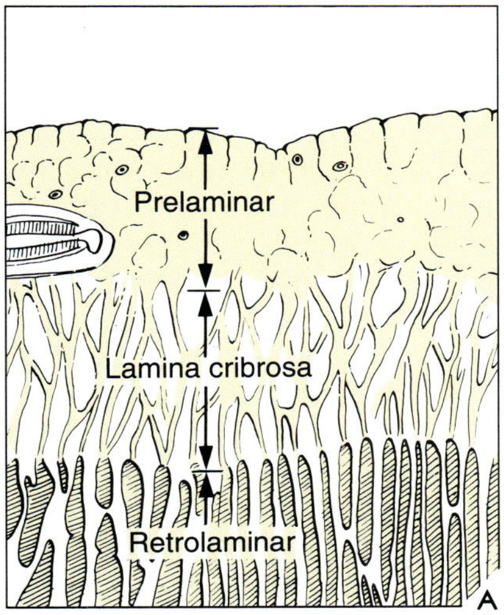

2.17 | *A:* With the exception of that associated with the microvasculature, connective tissue elements are absent in the prelaminar optic nerve. At all levels of the optic nerve, columns of glial cells segregate groups of axons into fiber bundles. *B:* Nerve head microvasculature (C) is confined to these tissue columns (top right). Within the lamina cribrosa, the glial columns become thicker and, at the level of the more posterior lamina scleralis, the amount of connective tissue present gradually increases as the nerve passes through the eye wall. A=fiber bundles; G=glial cells. *C:* Within the retrolaminar optic nerve, axons are reenveloped by a myelin sheath (M), significantly increasing the thickness of the extraocular optic nerve. A=fiber bundles; G=glial cells. (Courtesy of Dr. H.A. Quigley. Adapted from Miller NR: *Walsh and Hoyt's Clinical Neuro-Ophthalmology.* Baltimore: Williams & Wilkins, 1982.)

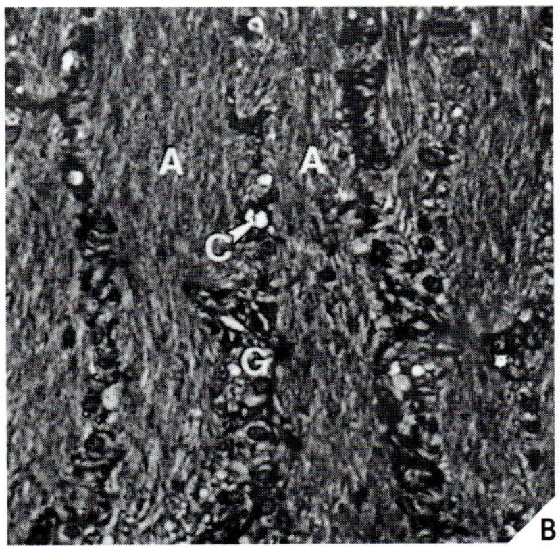

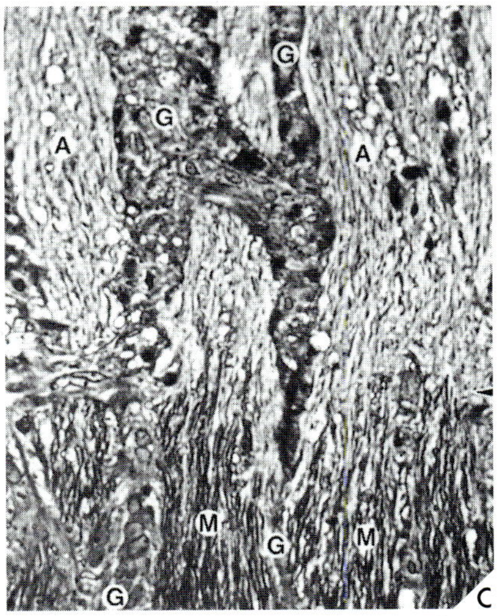

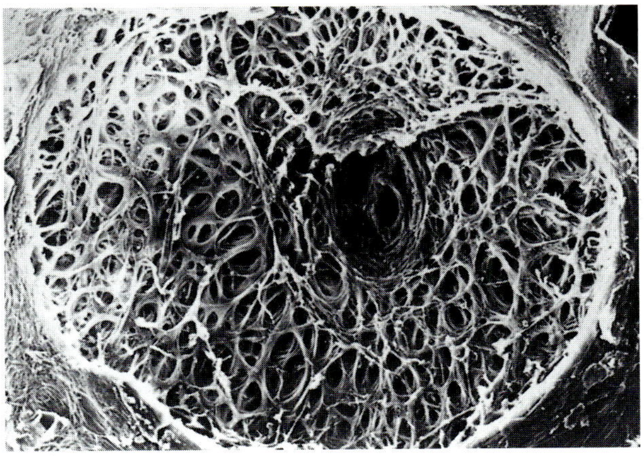

2.18 | At the level of the lamina scleralis, the scleral canal consists of several hundred irregular perforations through the sclera, through which pass the one million optic nerve axons as they exit the eye. (From Miller NR: *Walsh and Hoyt's Clinical Neuro-Ophthalmology.* Baltimore: Williams & Wilkins, 1982.)

Patterns of blood flow within the optic nerve head are quite complex[10–13,27,29–31] (Figs. 2.19 and 2.20). At all levels of the nerve head, arterioles penetrating the nerve tissue quickly distribute their blood flow to the extensive network of capillaries confined within the glial columns. The capillary lumen is isolated from the adjacent neural tissue by its own endothelial cell wall complete with tight junctions between cells, basement membrane material, and associated vascular adventitia. In addition, a syncytium of enveloping glial cell processes segregates the mesodermal from the neuronal tissue[10–13] (Fig. 2.21).

Within the anterior optic nerve head, blood flow to this microvasculature comes primarily from small branches of the central retinal artery.[27,29–31] At the level of the lamina choroidalis, the blood supply comes primarily from branches of the posterior ciliary arteries penetrating the adjacent choroid and sclera.[27,29-31] Within the lamina scleralis, blood flow also comes from branches of the posterior ciliary system, as well as from smaller vessels of pial origin penetrating the nerve tissue posterior to the globe. At all levels of the optic nerve head there are extensive anastomoses between capillary beds of adjacent tissue lying more anterior or posterior within the optic

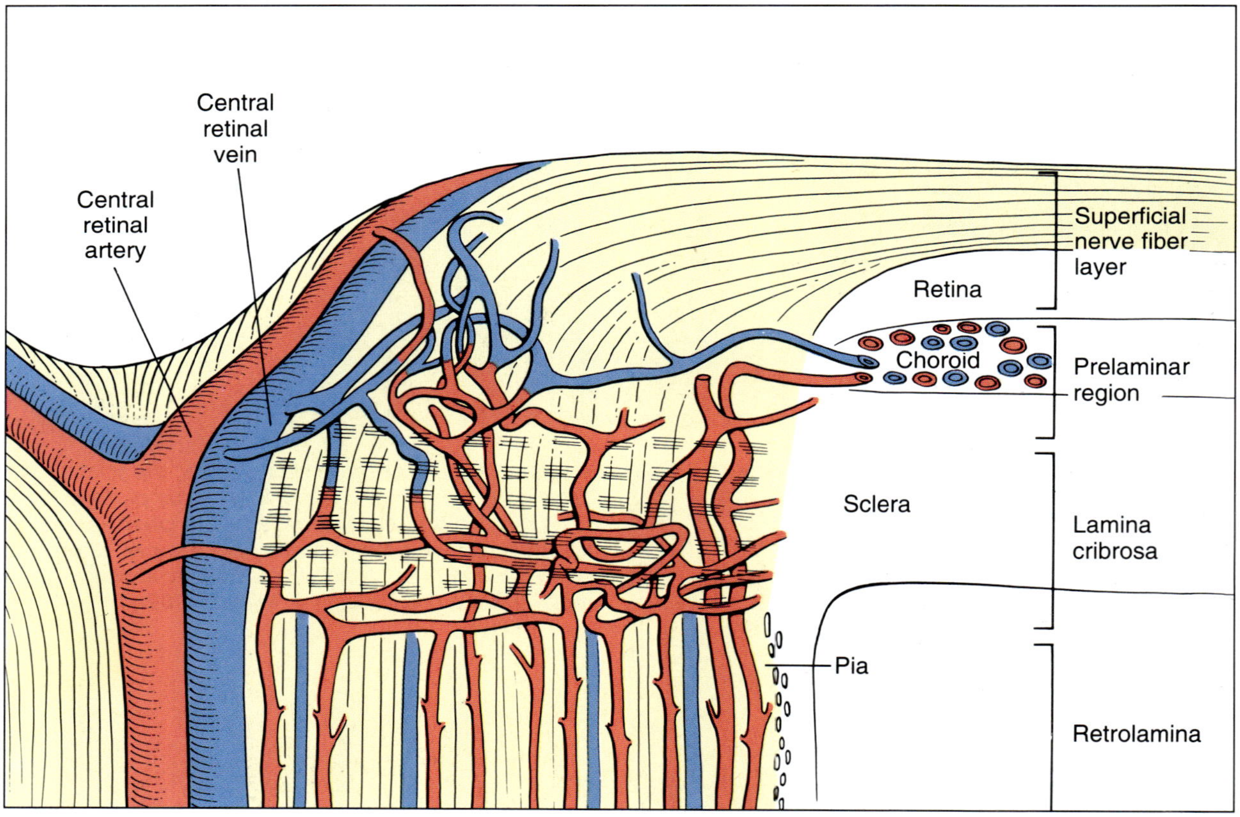

2.19 | There are complex anastomoses between capillary beds of anterior optic nerve head, lamina choroidalis, lamina scleralis and retroorbital optic nerve. In these drawings, the horizontal scale has been elongated and the three contiguous regions expanded to facilitate illustration of anastomoses. (Adapted from Lieberman MF, Maumenee AE, Green WR: Histologic studies of the vasculature of the anterior optic nerve. *Am J Ophthalmol 1976;82:405–423.* Published with permission from the American Journal of Ophthalmology. Copyright by the Ophthalmic Publishing Company.)

nerve.[27,29,31] Although the functional significance of these anastomoses is unknown, the nerve head itself has a capacity to autoregulate blood flow comparable to that seen in the retina.[35–37]

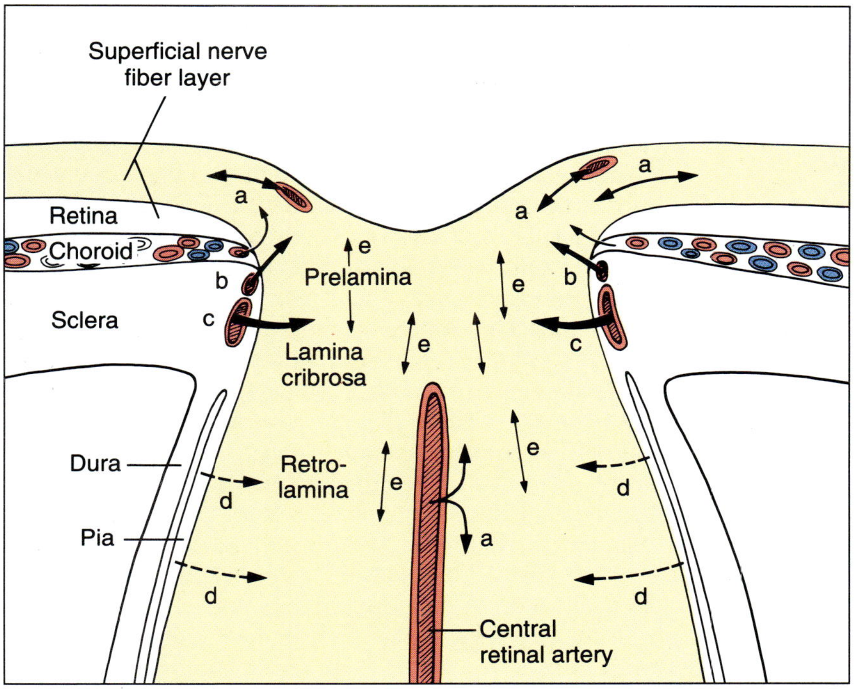

2.20 | Capillary beds of the anterior optic nerve head receive blood supply primarily from branches of the central retinal artery (double-headed arrows, a). The regions of the prelamina and lamina cribrosa receive blood flow primarily from branches of the posterior ciliary arteries (solid arrows, b + c). The retrolaminar optic nerve receives its blood supply primarily from branches of the pial vessels (single-headed arrows, d) and a small amount from branches off the central retinal artery (double-headed arrows, a). There are extensive anastomoses between capillary beds of anterior optic nerve, lamina cribrosa, and retrolaminar optic nerve (double-headed arrows, e). The functional significance of these anastomoses in eyes with elevated intraocular pressure or reduced nerve head perfusion remains to be demonstrated. (Adapted from Lieberman MF, Maumenee AE, Green WR: Histologic studies of the vasculature of the anterior optic nerve. *Am J Ophthalmol 1976;82:405–423.* Published with permission from The American Journal of Ophthalmology. Copyright by the Ophthalmic Publishing Company.)

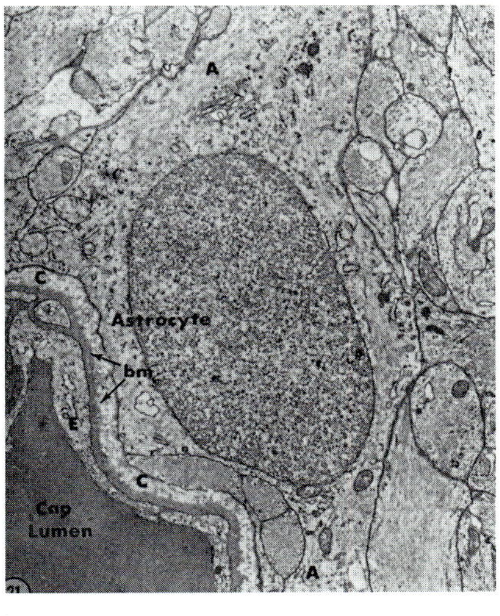

2.21 | Within the anterior lamina cribrosa as at all levels of the optic nerve, a syncytium of glial tissue segregates mesodermal tissue from axonal segments. The lumen of the nerve head capillary pictured here is encircled by endothelial cells (E) and their basement membrane (bm). A small amount of collagen (C) accompanies the capillary. Processes from a perivascular astrocyte (A) separate the vascular lumen and associated mesoderm from the adjacent neurons. (From Anderson DR, Hoyt WF, Hogan MJ: The fine structure of the astroglia in the human optic nerve and optic nerve head. *Trans Am Ophthalmol Soc 1967;65:275–303.*)

EXTRAOCULAR OPTIC NERVE

The intraorbital portion of the extraocular optic nerve, 2–3 cm in length, is enveloped by three vaginal sheaths. The outermost layer, the dense dura mater, fuses anteriorly with the sclera and posteriorly with the periosteum of the sphenoid bone where the nerve enters the optic canal. The other two layers, the arachnoid and the pia mater, are anterior extensions of the brain meninges. The subarachnoid space, continuous with that of the brain, ends as a blind pouch anteriorly at the posterior eye wall.

Connective tissue septa of pial origin pierce this portion of the optic nerve along its entire extent and continue within the nerve substance, oriented in a generally longitudinal direction and paralleling the course of the axon bundles.[10–13] These septa segregate the axons into fiber bundles much as the glial columns did in the more anterior optic nerve (Fig. 2.22). The microcirculation of the extraocular optic nerve is confined within these tissue columns and consists of capillaries and small arterioles of pial origin which enter the nerve within the tissue septa. The capillary lumen is formed by a nonfenestrated endothelium characterized by tight junctions between cells.

Separate but parallel to these septa are columns of glial cells including astrocytes and oligodendroglia.[10–13] Astrocyte processes extend towards and into the connective tissue septa. These glial processes envelope the capillary endothelium and associated connective tissue elements, segregating the tissue of mesodermal origin from the neuronal elements. The axons are, in turn, enveloped by extended, sheet-like processes from the oligodendroglia which form multilaminated wrappings around individual neurons within the fiber bundles[11–13,52,53] (Fig. 2.23). Addition of this myelin material to the nerve, extending from the level of the posterior lamina cribrosa to the optic nerve synapse within the lateral geniculate body, increases the nerve diameter to between 3 and 4 mm.

The optic nerve exits the orbit through the optic canal and enters the middle fossa. Here the nerves from opposite eyes undergo a hemidecussation at the optic chiasm. Ultimately, axons from both optic tracts terminate within the paired right and left lateral geniculate bodies.

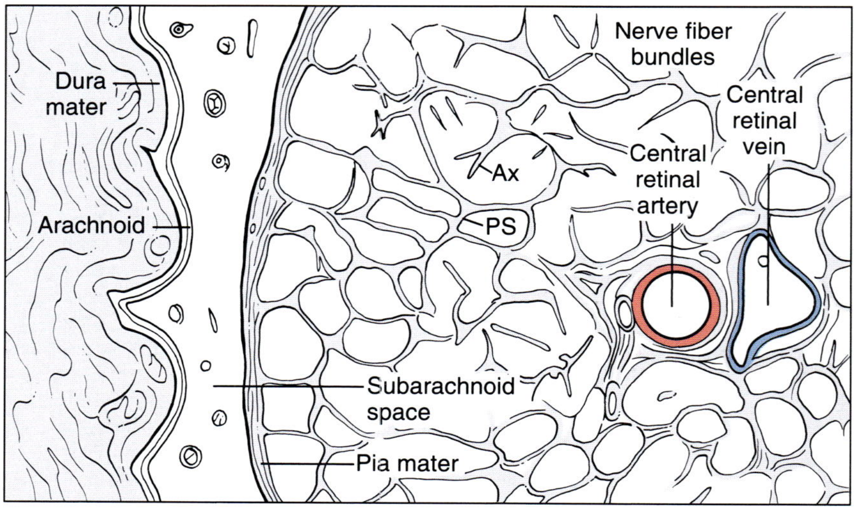

2.22 | In the retroorbital optic nerve, septa of pial origin (PS) enter the nerve substance separating axons (Ax) into fiber bundles. (Adapted From Miller NR: *Walsh and Hoyt's Clinical Neuro-Ophthalmology.* Baltimore: Williams & Wilkins, 1982.)

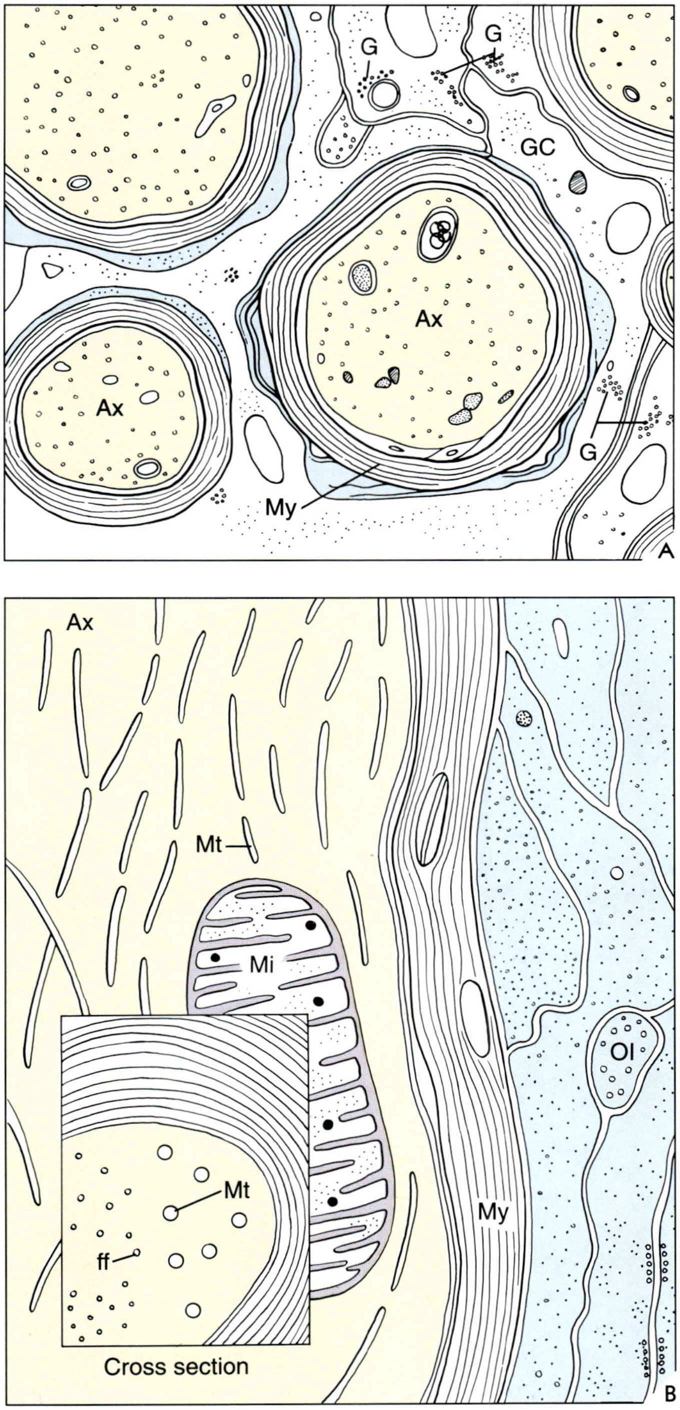

2.23 I *A:* Within the intraorbital optic nerve, cytoplasmic processes of glial cell (GC) origin fill most of the space between myelinated axons (Ax). *B:* Multiple wrappings of sheet like processes of oligodendroglia (Ol) around individual axon (Ax) cylinders, however, account for most of the increased thickness of the optic nerve at this level compared to that of the intraocular nerve. Mi=mitochondria; Mt=microtubuli; My=myelin; ff=microfilaments; G=Golgi body. (Adapted from Anderson DR, Hoyt WF, Hogan MJ: The fine structure of the astroglia in the human optic nerve and optic nerve head. *Trans Am Ophthalmol Soc 1967;65:275–303.* Copyright 1969, American Medical Association.)

SECTION II

EXTRACELLULAR MATRIX OF THE HUMAN OPTIC NERVE HEAD

M. Rosario Hernandez

Before 1985, few investigations focused on the extracellular matrix components of the connective tissue of the optic nerve head. A survey of scleral collagen types in bovine and human eyes gave a brief description of the lamina cribrosa.[54] In addition, a short report claimed an increase in the collagen content, and perhaps a change in its composition, in the lamina cribrosa of glaucomatous eyes compared with normal human eyes.[55] More recent studies of the biology of the lamina cribrosa have characterized the extracellular matrix components, the cells that are present and their roles in the maintenance of the target extracellular matrix materials, the age-related changes, and the response to elevated pressure as measured by biosynthetic parameters.

The extracellular matrix provides the structural support that enables groups of cells to function as a tissue. This matrix is made up of specific macromolecules that are assembled in geometric relationships to provide strength, flexibility, elasticity, and surfaces to the tissues that they serve. Study of the extracellular matrix has become a major objective in many laboratories because changes in this structure are related to changes during development, aging, disease, and various aspects of cell behavior.[56]

The development of immunohistochemical techniques has allowed the study of the distribution of the macromolecules of the extracellular matrix in different tissues. With this approach, a specific monoclonal or polyclonal antibody to the target macromolecule is reacted with tissue sections or cells in tissue culture. The antibodies used are able to distinguish among the different types of collagens as well as among the different types of attachment factors and other macromolecules present in the extracellular matrix. To visualize the antibody associated with the antigenic site in the tissue sections, a second antibody directed against the first antibody is tagged with a fluorescent or enzyme label and is reacted with the tissue sections or cells in culture.

NORMAL EXTRACELLULAR MATRIX

Immunofluorescent staining for extracellular matrix components in the human lamina cribrosa has provided new insights into the structure of this tissue. In the lamina cribrosa of young adults, the core of the cribriform plates contains substantial amounts of elastin in the form of long fibers (Fig. 2.24),[57] which is consistent with the ultrastructural demonstration of elastic fibers.[58] Collagen type III co-distributes with elastin, appearing as patches within the core. Collagen type I is present, disposed transversely as fine fibers in the core of the plates (Fig. 2.25).[57,59] These immunohistochemical findings are consistent with the ultrastructural demonstration of striated collagen fibers within this tissue.[58] Within the core of the cribriform plates, the blood vessels are delimited by collagen type IV and laminin, consistent with the distribution of their basement membranes, and are also surrounded by collagen type III and fibronectin. Fibronectin does not appear elsewhere in the cribriform plates of the human lamina cribrosa.[57,59]

Separating the core of the cribriform plates from the surrounding astrocytes is a well-defined, continuous layer composed of collagen type IV and laminin. These lamellar structures of collagen type IV and laminin are appar-

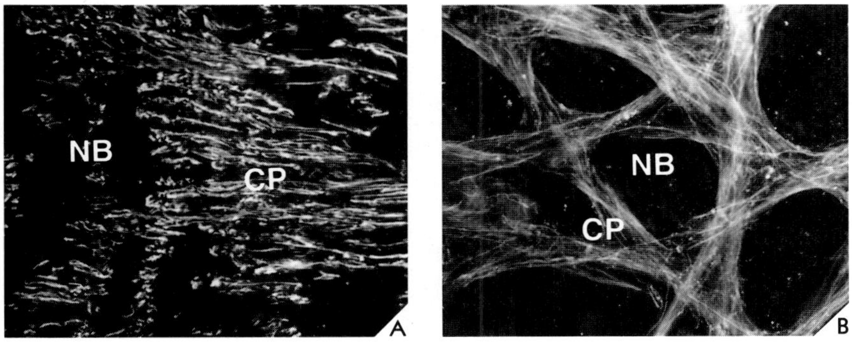

2.24 | Immunofluorescent staining for α-elastin in the lamina cribrosa. *A*: Thirty-six-year-old patient. Sagittal view of the cribriform plates showing fibers of elastin running across the lamina cribrosa (X370). *B*: Twenty-year-old patient. Cross-sectional view of the cribriform plates showing fibers of elastin running longitudinally in the core of the plates (X405). NB=nerve bundles; CP=cribriform plates. (From Hernandez MR, Neufeld AH: The extracellular matrix of the optic nerve, in Drance SM, Neufeld AH, Van Buskirk EM (eds): *Pharmacology of the Glaucomas.* Baltimore: Williams and Wilkins, 1992.)

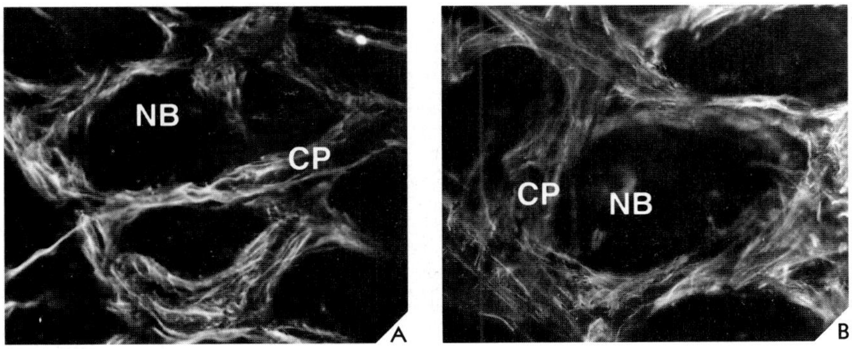

2.25 | Immunofluorescent staining for collagen type I in cross-sections of the lamina cribrosa (X450). *A*: Twenty-year-old subject. *B*: Seventy-year-old subject. Note the increase in collagen type I as the cribriform plates expand with age. NB=nerve bundles; CP=cribriform plates. (From Hernandez MR, Luo XX, Andrzejewska W, Neufeld AH: Age-related changes in the extracellular matrix of the human optic nerve head. *Am J Ophthalmol 1989;107:476–484.*)

ently part of the basement membranes of the astrocytes and extend linearly into the core of the cribriform plates forming a network of fibrillar material (Fig. 2.26).[57,60] A recent report using immunohistochemistry and electron microscopy describes a "mesh-like web of astrocyte processes" piercing the connective tissue of the cribriform plates.[60] This is consistent with the reported staining for collagen type IV inside the core of the cribriform plates.[57,61,62]

The extracellular matrix of the lamina cribrosa is quite different from that of the sclera. As an interstitial connective tissue, the extracellular matrix of the sclera is made up primarily of fibrillar forms of collagen, mostly collagen type I, surrounding fibroblasts. The sclera contains no collagen type IV and little elastin. In contrast, the core of the cribriform plates containing elastin, fibrils of collagen type IV, relatively little collagen types I and III, and surrounded by basement membrane macromolecules indicates that the lamina cribrosa is a specialized connective tissue of the central nervous system.

The insertion of the lamina cribrosa into the sclera is a specialized structure. Concentric, circumferential, tightly packed elastin fibers surround the laminar and prelaminar region of the optic nerve head (Fig. 2.27). Fur-

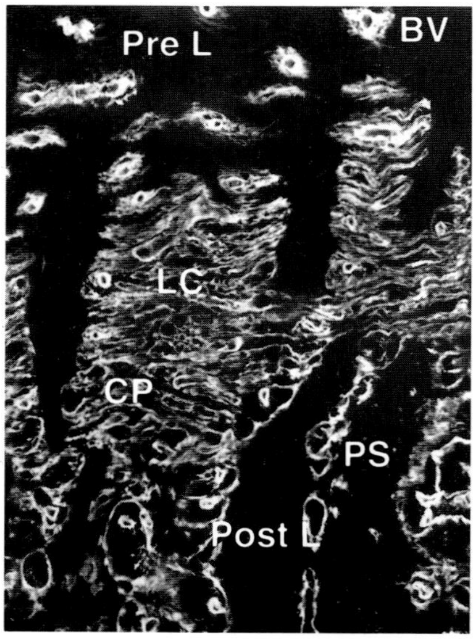

2.26 | Immunofluorescent staining for collagen type IV in a sagittal section of the optic nerve head; 49-year-old subject (X220). In the prelaminar region (Pre L), only the blood vessels (BV) show positive staining. In the lamina cribrosa (LC), staining for collagen type IV forms lamellar structures corresponding to the cribriform plates (CP). In the post-laminar region (Post L), staining for collagen type IV is observed lining the pial septa (PS) and around blood vessels. (From Hernandez MR, Neufeld AH: The extracellular matrix of the optic nerve, in Drance SM, Neufeld AH, Van Buskirk EM (eds): *Pharmacology of the Glaucomas.* Baltimore: Williams and Wilkins, 1992.)

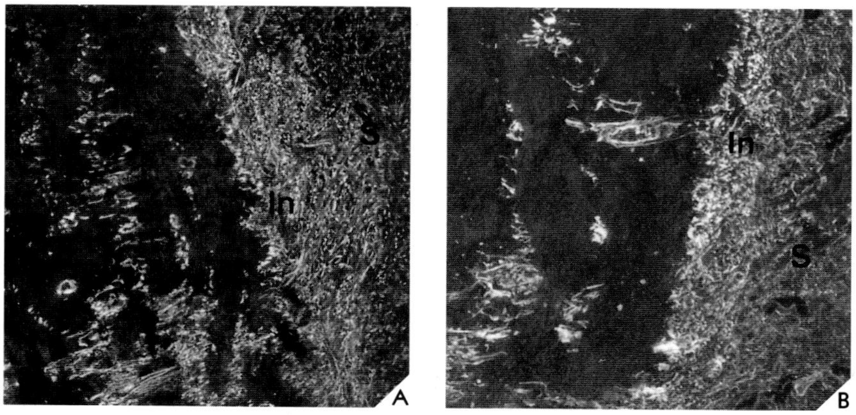

2.27 | Immunofluorescent staining for α-elastin in sagittal sections of the optic nerve head (X185). *A*: Newborn patient. *B*: Thirty-six-year-old patient. Tightly packed fibers of elastin form a wedge around the optic nerve head in the insertion region (In). Note that the fibers of elastin extend further into the sclera (S) in younger eyes. (From Hernandez MR, Luo XX, Andrzejewska W, Neufeld AH: Age-related changes in the extracellular matrix of the human optic nerve head. *Am J Ophthalmol 1989;107:476-484.*)

thermore, the elastin fibers of the cribriform plates, running perpendicular to the nerve bundles, are continuous with, and appear to originate from, those of the insertion. In the adjacent sclera, the elastin fibers are short and sparse and do not show any special orientation. Glial cell processes, which are covered by basement membranes, form an anchoring network through the bundles of elastin fibers in the insertion region; the basement membrane components extend beyond the glial cell processes into the sclera.[57,62]

Age-related changes in the extracellular matrix of the human optic nerve head are seen with fluorescence microscopy.[61] As the core of the cribriform plates enlarges with age, the apparent density of collagen types I and III increases markedly (see Fig. 2.25), indicating increases in interstitial and fibrillar forms of collagen. In tissues such as the sclera and corneal stroma, these types of macromolecules provide structural support, strength, and rigidity. In addition, a network of filamentous material which stains positive for collagen type IV within the cribriform plates (Fig. 2.28) and the elastin fibers also increase in density, as the plates expand with age.

The increased collagen and elastin presumably accounts for an age-related increase in connective tissue area.[63] Thus, as gradual loss of axons of the optic nerve occurs with age,[64,65] lost tissue is at least partially replaced with extracellular matrix material, including fibrillar forms of collagen and elastin. Therefore, little loss of volume of the optic nerve head may occur with age. Increases in extracellular matrix macromolecules such as collagen types I and III may make the tissue more rigid and less resilient, whereas collagen type IV and elastin may enable the tissue to retain some flexibility and resiliency as it ages. Perhaps the normal aging process in this tissue increases the ratio of these macromolecules in a way that maintains normal function. However, in certain individuals the aging process may alter the distribution of the macromolecules and thus alter the functions of the connective tissue of the optic nerve head.

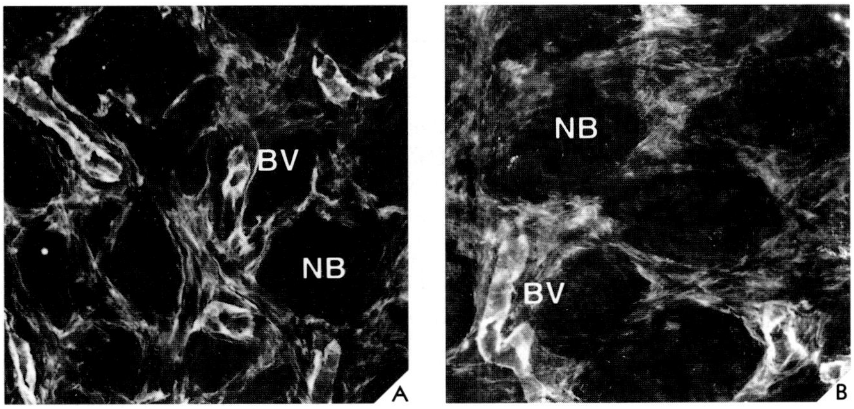

2.28 | Immunofluorescent staining for collagen type IV in cross-sections of the lamina cribrosa (X450). *A*: Thirty-one-year-old subject. *B*: Seventy-three-year-old subject. Collagen type IV is present inside the core of the cribriform plates. Note the increase with age in collagen type IV positive material. BV=blood vessels; NB=nerve bundles. (From Hernandez MR, Neufeld AH: The extracellular matrix of the optic nerve, in Drance SM, Neufeld AH, Van Buskirk EM (eds): *Pharmacology of the Glaucomas.* Baltimore: Williams and Wilkins, 1992.)

Section III

Physiology of Retinal Ganglion Cells

Scott E. Brodie

Glaucoma is ultimately a disease of the retinal ganglion cells and their axons.[66] Therefore, considerable effort has been directed towards the understanding of retinal ganglion cell function and the extent to which alterations in ganglion cell function can be monitored by electrophysiological and psychophysical procedures.

The retinal ganglion cells are the sole conduits through which visual information is transmitted from the eyes to the brain. Ganglion cell dendrites ramify in the inner plexiform layer of the retina, providing the final stage for intraretinal information processing. Visual information, encoded as sequences of action potentials, is then transmitted along the axons of the ganglion cells via the retinal nerve fiber layer through the optic nerve to the brain. The optic nerve fibers traverse the optic chiasm, where they are resegregated according to visual field, and synapse in the various layers of the lateral geniculate body in the thalamus.

The retinal ganglion cells have been intensively studied, both anatomically and physiologically.[67] This research has led to a bewildering proliferation of classifications of ganglion cells according to the presence or absence of many different attributes, such as on-center or off-center receptive field organization, presence and type of color opposition, dendritic field size and location, central projections, and response dynamics. During the last decade, many of these distinctions have been simplified by the recognition of two major classes of retinal ganglion cells, which reconciles many of the dichotomous distinctions that have been drawn. These two classes of ganglion cells, the M-cells and the P-cells, appear to function in parallel, simultaneously conveying different aspects of the visual sensation.

The M-cells are larger ganglion cells that project to the ventral, magnocellular layers of the lateral geniculate body (LGN). The P-cells are smaller cells that project to the dorsal, parvocellular layers of the LGN (Fig. 2.29). The M-cells comprise perhaps 10% of the ganglion cell population, while the P-cells comprise about 80%.[67] The remaining cells do not project to the LGN

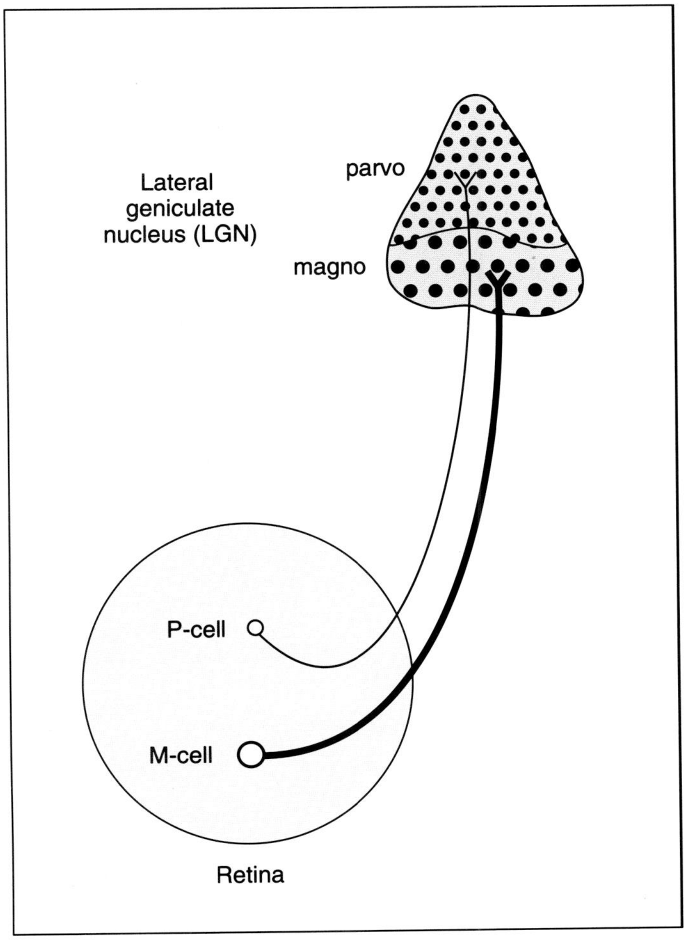

2.29 | Diagram of the central connections of M-cells and P-cells. The M-cells, with larger receptive fields and larger optic nerve fibers, synapse in magnocellular layers of the lateral geniculate nucleus. The P-cells, with smaller receptive fields and smaller optic nerve fibers, synapse in parvocellular layers of the lateral geniculate nucleus.

and therefore do not mediate cortical vision. Further distinctions between the M-cells and P-cells are listed in Figure 2.30.

The M-cells show little spectral (color) selectivity, have large receptive fields, large-diameter axons with higher conduction velocity, phasic responses to changes in light intensity, and frequently demonstrate nonlinear spatial summation (Fig. 2.30). Conversely, P-cells show greater sensitivity to chromatic contrast, have smaller receptive fields, smaller axons, slower nerve conduction, tonic (persistent) responses to changes in light intensity, and linear spatial summation.

The M- and P-ganglion cell axons terminate in synapses in the lateral geniculate nuclei. In humans, the LGN exhibits a laminated architecture composed of six layers. Axons from the ipsilateral eye synapse in layers two, three, and five (counting from ventral to dorsal), leaving layers one, four, and six for the axons from the contralateral eye. The two ventral layers contain larger (magnocellular) neurons than the four dorsal (parvocellular) layers; this dichotomy is the primary defining characteristic of the distinction between M- and P-ganglion cells.[68] The axons of the LGN neurons form the optic radiation, which conveys visual information to the visual cortex in the occipital region of the brain.

Clinical interest in the M-cell–P-cell dichotomy has been greatly stimulated by reports that the larger axons and ganglion cells (presumably M-cells) are preferentially damaged by the glaucomatous disease process, both in humans and in animal models.[69–71] This observation has suggested that psychophysical or other tests of ganglion cell function that depend most critically on aspects of visual function identified with the M-cell subsystem, therefore, might be more sensitive indicators of early glaucomatous damage than conventional perimetric procedures.[72]

Figure 2.30. Comparison of M-cells and P-cells

Property	M-cells	P-cells
Color sensitive	No	Yes
Receptive field size	Larger	Smaller
LGN projection	Magnocellular	Parvocellular
Axon diameter	Larger	Smaller
Conduction velocity	Faster	Slower
Cell size	Larger	Smaller
Response dynamics	Phasic	Tonic
Spatial summation	Mixed	Linear

3 Diagnostic Techniques of the Anterior Segment

Section I

Tonometry and Tonography

Eve Juliet Higginbotham

MEASUREMENT OF INTRAOCULAR PRESSURE: TONOMETRY

The clinical measurement of intraocular pressure (IOP) involves the application of a force or weight to the eye and subsequent indentation or flattening of a finite area of the ocular surface. Knowing the force applied and the area, the intraocular pressure can be derived.[1,2]

APPLANATION TONOMETRY

Applanation tonometry is based on the Imbert–Fick principle, which models the eye after a dry, thin-walled sphere; the pressure within the sphere is equal to the force necessary to flatten its surface divided by the area of flattening.

$P = F/A$
where P = pressure, F = force, and A = area.

Goldmann Applanation Tonometry

Goldmann applanation tonometry is the most common technique of measuring IOP. This technique measures the force necessary to flatten a circle of central cornea having a diameter of 3.06 mm. At this diameter, the additive forces of the tear meniscus and the resistance of the cornea to flattening are counterbalanced. Therefore, the Imbert–Fick principle more closely applies. A split-field device enables the examiner to determine the appropriate endpoint that is enhanced by fluorescein dye.

Because this technique displaces only 0.5 μl of intraocular fluid, scleral rigidity (which is a factor in high myopia and in infants) does not significantly alter the readings. However, the examiner should be aware of other factors that can affect the accuracy of the measurement: squeezing of the eyelids, improper positioning of the patient,[3] excessive or insufficient fluorescein, a tight collar, breath holding, marked corneal astigmatism or edema, and an uncalibrated tonometer. If there is marked corneal astigmatism, creating an elliptical pattern to the mires, the red line on the tonometer head should be aligned with the major axis. In general, this technique is not accurate when more than 3 diopters of astigmatism are present. The tonometer head should be sterilized, by wiping the tip or soaking in either 70% ethanol, 3% hydrogen peroxide, or 0.5% sodium hypochlorite (Figs. 3.1–3.3).

Hand-Held Applanation Tonometers

The Perkins and Draeger applanation tonometers both utilize a Goldmann-like prism but have the advantages of not requiring a slit lamp and being portable. Therefore, IOP can be measured in a supine position.

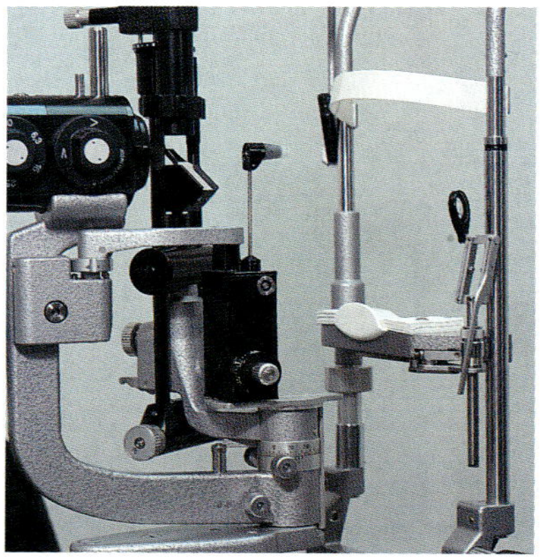

3.1 | Goldmann applanation tonometer, attached to a slit-lamp, is positioned before measuring the IOP. (Courtesy of C.L. Martonyi, C.O.P.R.A., W.K. Kellogg Eye Center, University of Michigan.)

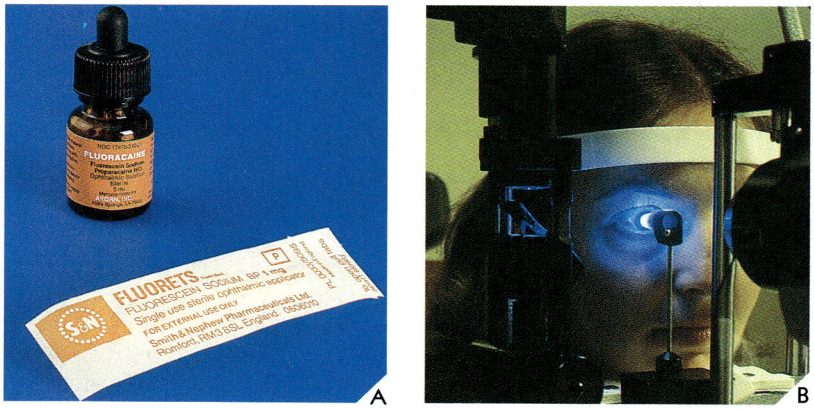

3.2 | *A:* Fluorescein dye and anesthetic drops are instilled before applanation. *B:* The blue light enhances visualization of the mires.

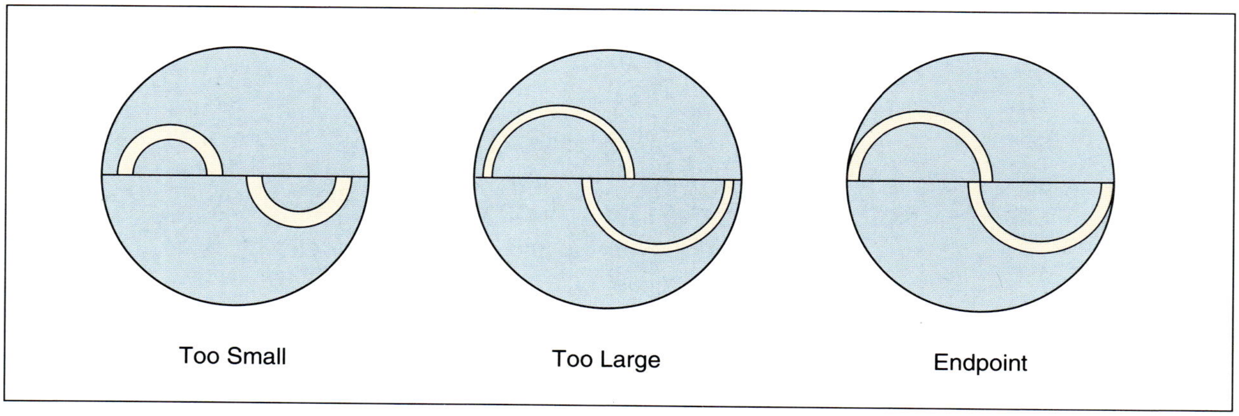

3.3 | The appropriate endpoint is visualized through the microscope. (Modified with permission from Kolker A, Hetherington J: *Becker–Shaffer's Diagnosis and Therapy of the Glaucomas,* ed 5. St. Louis: CV Mosby, 1983.)

Mackay–Marg Tonometer

This instrument is particularly useful when the cornea is edematous or distorted. It works by both applanation and indentation. The probe consists of a hollow tube within which sits a 1.5-mm movable plunger. When the probe comes in contact with the cornea, the force that is necessary to align the plunger with the surrounding probe is measured (Fig. 3.4).

Pneumatonometer

The pneumatonometer, like the Mackay–Marg tonometer, is useful when the cornea is distorted. This instrument works on principles of indentation and applanation. It consists of an air pressure-sensitive probe with an outer diameter of 0.25 inches. A central chamber is filled with pressurized gas, dichlorodifluoromethane (CCl_2F_2) and the tip is covered with a plastic diaphragm. The tip is applied to the cornea and the force necessary to flatten the surface is transmitted to a pressure transducer. The tip of the pneumatonometer should be cleaned with an alcohol wipe between uses (Fig. 3.5).

Tono-pen

The Tono-pen (Oculab, LaJolla, CA) is a portable, hand-held, battery-operated tonometer which measures IOP in a similar fashion to the Mackay-Marg described previously (Figs. 3.6A and 3.6B). A central plunger 1.02 mm in diameter is surrounded by a 3.22-mm annulus. The force needed to align the central plunger and the annulus is transmitted to a microprocessor which is encased within the instrument.[4]. The Tono-pen and the pneumatonometer both underestimate IOP greater than 30 mm Hg.[5,6]

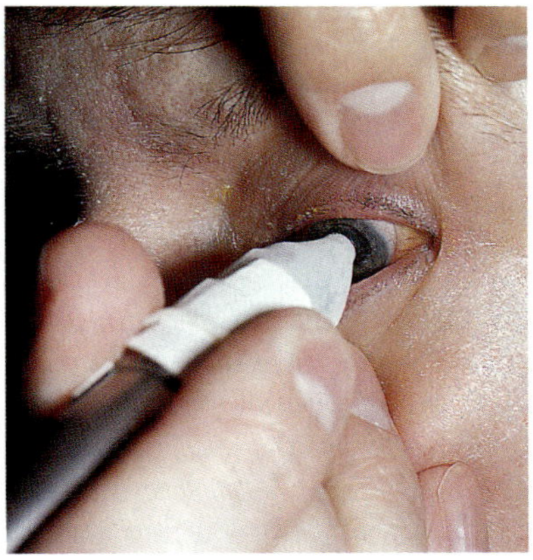

3.4 | A disposable plastic sleeve covers the head of the MacKay–Marg tonometer. (Courtesy of C.L. Martonyi, C.O.P.R.A., W.K. Kellogg Eye Center, University of Michigan.)

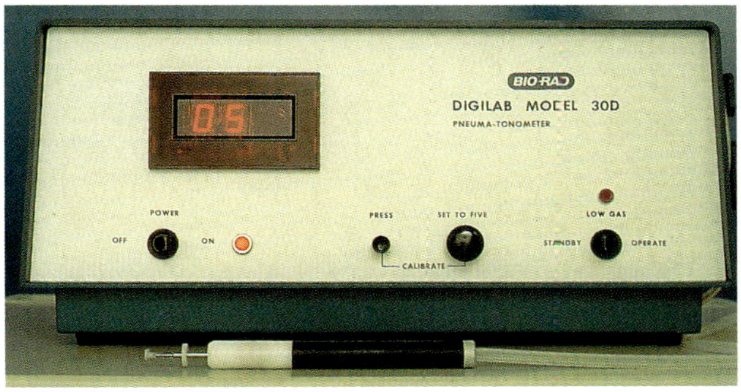

3.5 | The pneumatonometer is useful in measuring pressures in eyes with diseased corneas. (Courtesy of C.L. Martonyi, C.O.P.R.A., W.K. Kellogg Eye Center, University of Michigan.)

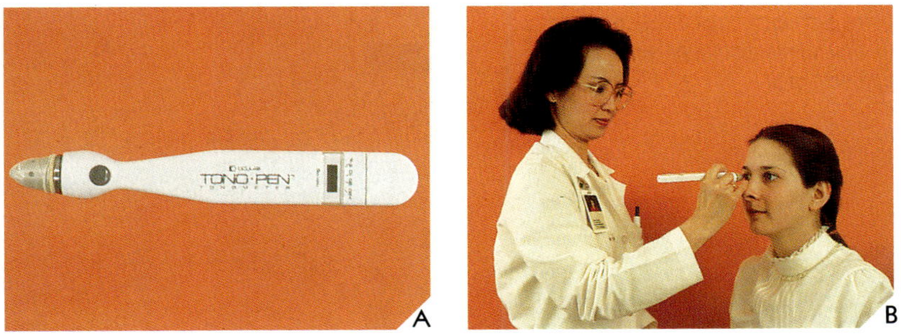

3.6 | *A:* The Tono-pen is very portable. *B:* It must be held perpendicular to the eye to obtain an accurate measurement. (Courtesy of C.L. Martonyi, C.O.P.R.A., W.K. Kellogg Eye Center, University of Michigan.)

Noncontact Tonometer

This method of measurement has the advantage of not requiring contact with the cornea. An aliquot of air of progressively increasing velocity is directed towards the cornea and flattens its surface, increasing the intensity of reflected light. The time required to maximize the reflected light intensity is proportional to the known force of the air puff and can therefore be converted to an IOP measurement.

INDENTATION TONOMETRY

This technique involves the application of a known weight to the eye, which indents the cornea to a degree proportional to the IOP. A number of factors, including scleral rigidity and corneal curvature, can interfere with the accuracy of this device.

Schiotz Tonometry

This instrument consists of a footplate, which approximates the corneal curvature, and a movable plunger, to which a 5.5-g weight is permanently affixed. This plunger engages a needle that sweeps across a scale. Essentially, the Schiotz tonometer is placed on the surface of the cornea while the patient is in a supine position. The plunger then indents the cornea and the amount of indentation is read off the scale. If the cornea is not indented, additional weights can be attached to the tonometer. The indentation reading is converted to IOP by referring to calibration tables. These tables (Friedenwald Calibration Tables, 1948 and 1955) assume two different values for ocular rigidity. It is generally assumed that the 1948 table more closely agrees with Goldmann applanation. The Schiotz tonometer is easy to use and portable (Fig. 3.7). However, measurement errors can occur when the ocular rigidity is significantly different from normal (such as in myopic eyes or those of infants) or, as can occur at low degrees of indentation, when the cornea protrudes into the hole of the footplate. Low ocular rigidity leads to an underestimation of the pressure, and protrusion of the cornea to an overestimation. A scale reading of at least 4 should be required when the IOP is measured.

MEASUREMENT OF OUTFLOW FACILITY: TONOGRAPHY

A noninvasive method to measure facility of outflow did not exist until the 20th century.[7] Tonography involves the application of an electronic Schiotz tonometer to the eye for a period of 4 minutes. The IOP initially increases and then decreases over time. The rate of IOP decay is related to outflow facility via a series of mathematical calculations. The rate of IOP decay is greater for normal than for glaucomatous eyes. Moreover, by measuring outflow facility and IOP, inferences can be drawn regarding aqueous production.[8,9]

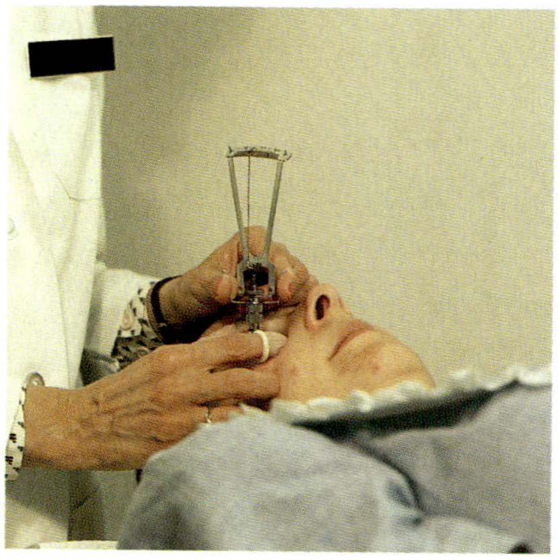

3.7 | The Schiotz tonometer is placed on an anesthesized eye with the patient supine.

Tonography assumes that trabecular flow is proportional to the pressure gradient across the aqueous outflow pathway. Outflow facility measured in microliters per minute per millimeter of mercury is defined as follows:

$$C = (DV)/4\ (P1\text{-}Po)$$

where C = facility of outflow, DV = change in scleral distension and corneal indentation during tonography, P1 = average IOP during tonography, and Po = IOP in the undisturbed eye. Corresponding values for corneal indentation, ocular distension, P1, and Po are available for all tonometric scale readings. This equation assumes that placing the tonometer on the eye causes no change in aqueous secretion, ocular blood flow, episcleral venous pressure, or facility of outflow.

These assumptions are not necessarily true in vivo. Aqueous formation decreases as IOP increases, resulting in an overestimation of outflow facility, termed pseudofacility, by up to 10% in normal eyes. The external pressure exerted on the eye by the tonometer also displaces choroidal blood and has been shown to increase episcleral venous pressure by 1.25 mm. Outflow facility itself varies slightly as a function of pressure, and scleral rigidity must also be taken into account if it differs significantly from average, as in high myopia.

Despite these assumptions tonography is an effective research tool for measuring outflow facility noninvasively, particularly for group comparisons. It is much less useful as a prognostic indicator in individual patients.

TONOGRAPHY TECHNIQUE

As a first step, Goldmann tonometry is performed in both eyes. The patient is then placed in a supine position and the machine is calibrated. The room should be quiet and free of interruptions, and the equipment clean. The patient must be cooperative and comfortable, should be encouraged to breathe normally, and blink the fellow eye when necessary. The cornea should be normal, without evidence of defects or edema. Because the patient's eye and tonometer should be vertical, a fixation device for the other eye may be beneficial. The tonographic technician should open the patient's lids gently and carry on a reassuring conversation.

Schiotz IOP measurements are recorded using appropriate weights. At least 4 scale units should be registered for best results. The patient is then asked to fixate, and the tonometer is held just above the eye for 15 to 30 seconds. The patient is encouraged to relax. The tonometer is then applied to the anesthesized cornea for 4 minutes in a vertical position. The test is then repeated in the fellow eye after rechecking the calibration (Fig. 3.8).

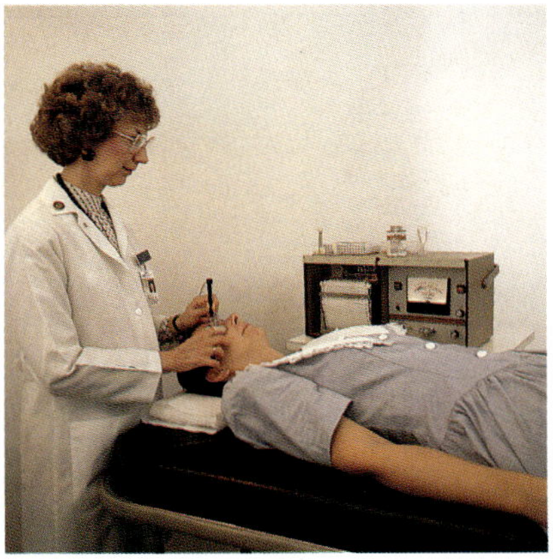

3.8 | The tonographer gently rests the plunger on the surface of the eye. (Courtesy of C.L. Martonyi, C.O.P.R.A., W.K. Kellogg Eye Center, University of Michigan.)

A smooth line is drawn through the middle of the tracing. The initial Schiotz IOP and the difference between 0- and 4-minute scale readings are used to obtain C (facility of outflow) from the table for the particular weight used. Average values for C range from 0.23 to 0.30. Above 0.20 is considered normal, 0.18 borderline, and 0.15 abnormal. A Po/C ratio greater than 100 suggests glaucoma, while a ratio of less than 100 is most likely normal (Figs. 3.9A and 3.9B).

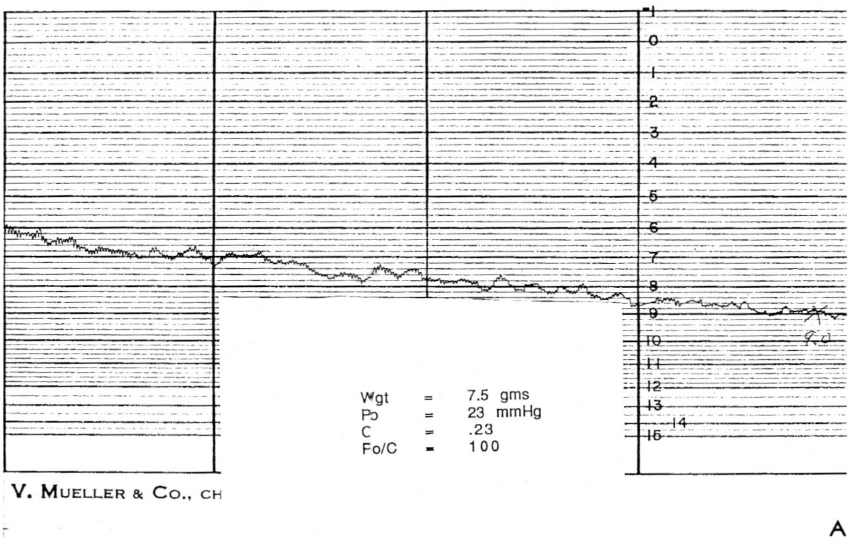

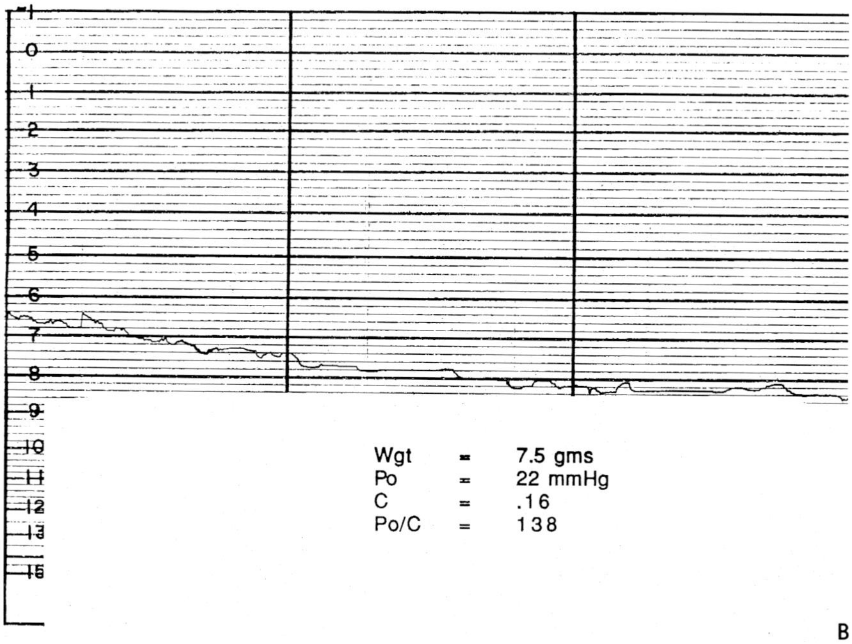

3.9 | Decay curves of a patient with asymmetric glaucoma. *A:* The right eye would be considered normal. *B:* The left eye represents impaired outflow facility. Although the entire tracing in *B* was not photographed, both *A* and *B* represent four-minute measurements. Furthermore, despite the differences in magnification between *A* and *B*, the slope remains the important parameter.

Section II

Fluorophotometric Measurement of Aqueous Flow

Richard F. Brubaker

Measurement of aqueous humor flow in humans is performed by fluorophotometry. This technique consists of the application of a fluorescent tracer to the eye, after which the rate of loss of the tracer is monitored over a period of several hours. Several kinds of fluorophotometric techniques have been devised, but the underlying principle of all of them is to measure the rate of clearance of the tracer from which the flow through the anterior chamber is derived.

FLUORESCEIN

The first investigator to quantify the rate of aqueous humor flow employing a fluorescent tracer was Goldmann.[10,11] Goldmann injected fluorescein intravenously and monitored the rate of accumulation and loss of the tracer from the aqueous humor in comparison with the concentration of the unbound dye in the plasma. From these data he was able to calculate flow. Goldmann's method is neither simple to perform nor to calculate, and it is complicated by the fact that fluorescein is converted to a weakly fluorescent metabolite which also enters the eye.[12]

In 1966, Jones and Maurice published a technique of measuring aqueous flow from topically applied fluorescein.[13] In this technique, fluorescein is forced through the epithelium by repeated application of a high concentration to the surface of the eye. Once in the cornea, the stroma serves as a depot from which the dye passes slowly into the anterior chamber through the endothelium. The half-life of fluorescein in this system is approximately four hours,[14,15] which enables an investigator to monitor aqueous flow over many hours without repeat application. The elegance and simplicity of this method, as well as its repeatability, have led to its wide acceptance. Almost all investigators who measure aqueous humor flow in human eyes use this technique, which will be described in the following paragraphs along with normal values and the effects of some drugs on aqueous flow.

APPLICATION OF FLUORESCEIN

Fluorescein must be applied to the eye 5 or 6 hours before measurements are to begin. This ensures that the tracer has time to become distributed uniformly in the stroma and that measurements of fluorescence in the center are representative of the concentration found elsewhere in the stroma.

One can instill concentrations from 0.2% to 10% sodium fluorescein.[16–19] Most commonly, 2% is chosen (2×10^{-2} g/ml) and is instilled three to five times into the cul-de-sac at 5-minute intervals. Younger subjects usually require more repetitions, and older subjects fewer. The optimal concentration in the stroma once fluorescein is uniformly distributed is 10^{-5} to 10^{-6} g/ml.

PHARMACOKINETICS OF TOPICALLY APPLIED FLUORESCEIN

Once in the stroma, fluorescein is trapped beneath the epithelium and finds its least resistive route of egress via the endothelium. Other routes of escape are the epithelium and the limbal stroma, but these are minor and can be ignored. Once in the aqueous humor, fluorescein can leave the normal eye either by flowing out with the aqueous or by diffusing into the blood vessels of the iris. These are the two major routes as long as the iridolenticular barrier is intact and convective or diffusional exchange with the posterior chamber (as after iridotomy) or the vitreous cannot occur. Of these two routes, loss by flow is at least 10 times greater than loss by diffusion in the normal eye.[19] For this reason some investigators consider that the clearance of fluorescein is equal to the rate of flow of aqueous humor through the anterior chamber, an assumption that is probably valid in uninflamed eyes.

DERIVATION OF FLOW FROM RATE OF DYE DISAPPEARANCE

Because the rate of flow is equal or very nearly equal to the rate of clearance of topically applied fluorescein from the eye, to obtain flow one must simply measure the clearance of fluorescein. This is accomplished by observing the rate of loss of fluorescein from the combined cornea and anterior chamber in proportion to its concentration in the anterior chamber:

Clearance = (rate of loss of fluorescein)/(concentration in chamber)

The concentration of fluorescein is measured in the stroma and the anterior chamber employing a fluorophotometer such as the Fluorotron Master (fitted with an anterior segment lens) or some other custom-built instrument.[14,18,20–22] If the volume of the stroma and the anterior chamber are known, it is simple to calculate from these concentrations and volumes the total amount of dye present in the eye at any time[23] (Fig. 3.10). If these measurements are repeated at intervals, the rate of loss is easily derived and the clearance can be calculated. For a more detailed treatment of the methods used to calculate flow, one can consult one of a number of publications.[13,19,24]

ADVANTAGES AND LIMITATIONS OF FLUOROPHOTOMETRY TO MEASURE FLOW

Fluorophotometric measurement of flow has become the accepted standard noninvasive method of measuring flow in human subjects, primarily because the technique can be accomplished with minimal disturbance of the eye and without altering IOP. In addition, no assumptions about constancy of outflow resistance, the route of escape of aqueous, or the constancy of aqueous humor formation are necessary. Quite unlike the measurement of IOP, the measurement of aqueous humor flow with fluorophotometry can be carried out over a period of time when the subject is participating in any activity whatever, including sleeping. The precision of the measurement is approximately ±15%. The accuracy of the measurement is more difficult to derive. There is good agreement between fluorophotometric measurements of flow and measurements using the rate of decay of radioactive tracers[25,26] and the rate of formation of a "pupillary bubble" as measured by photogrammetry.[27] These techniques depend on entirely different assumptions, and agreement among them is reassurance that all three are accurate.

Fluorophotometric measurement of flow has some disadvantages. First, it cannot be applied to eyes in which the posterior segment of the eye is in two-way communication with the anterior chamber. Therefore, aphakic eyes are not suitable for measurements. In addition, patients with severely inflamed eyes or with rubeosis iridis are not suitable subjects. This is because the fluorescence of fluorescein is altered in the presence of albumin,[28] and diffusional loss in patients with neovascularization of the iris may not be insignificant. Finally, persons with cloudy corneas cannot undergo accurate measurements of fluorescence.

The reader is also cautioned that, when data from this technique are interpreted, no conclusions can be drawn about IOP or outflow resistance. These parameters must be measured directly with tonometry or tonography.

AQUEOUS HUMOR FLOW IN NORMAL HUMAN EYES

The rate of aqueous humor flow through the anterior chamber of the normal human eye at the peak of its circadian rhythm is approximately 2.5 to 3.0 µl/min.[19] This information is based on measurements in adults; measurements in children are seldom performed, and measurements in infants are technically impossible. There is a slight decrease in the maximal daytime rate of flow with age,[29] but the regression with age is not clinically significant before extreme senility.[30] No difference in aqueous flow has been observed between men and women.[19]

There is a circadian rhythm of aqueous humor flow.[31] The most rapid rate is observed for several hours after awakening.[32] In the afternoon there is

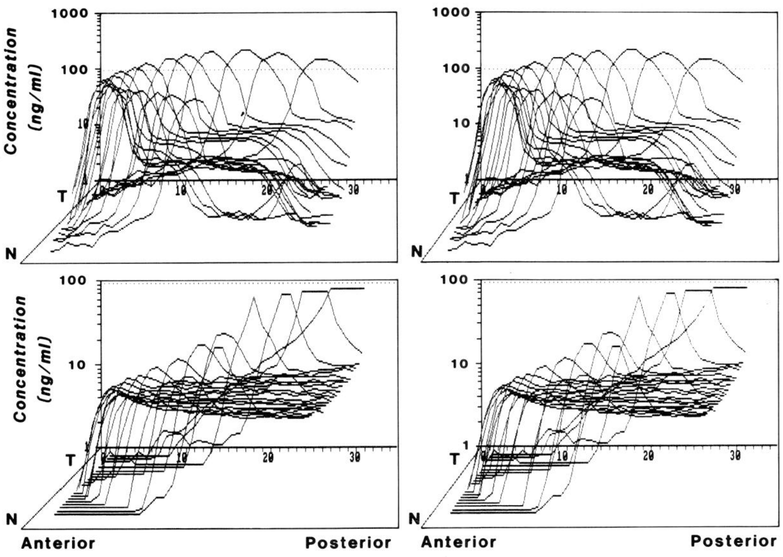

3.10 | Stereographic three-dimensional graphs of fluorescence in the cornea and the anterior chamber of the human eye obtained with a scanning ocular fluorophotometer.[22] Concentration is displayed on the vertical axis on a log scale. Horizontal axes represent axial dimension (0 in front of cornea, 30 in or behind anterior chamber) and frontal dimension (N = nasal, T = temporal). Upper pair illustrates fluorescence several hours after topical administration (note the "pupillary bubble"); the lower pair, several hours after oral administration (note the gradient of concentration from limbus to center). (Reproduced from McLaren J, Brubaker F: A two-dimensional scanning ocular fluorophotometer. *Invest Ophthalmol Vis Sci 1985;26:144–152.*)

approximately a 15% fall in aqueous flow.[33,34] During sleep the rate falls to half the rate observed during waking hours.[32] Lid closure or a recumbent position does not mimic the effects of sleep.[32] Bright lights do not block the effects of sleep,[35] and melatonin given during the day does not mimic the effects of sleep.[36] Sleep deprivation at the time of day when one would ordinarily sleep is associated with a modest fall in the rate of aqueous humor flow, but not to the lowest levels observed in sleeping subjects.[32] It is hypothesized that the circadian rhythm of aqueous humor flow is hormonally controlled, but the specific substance that regulates this cycle is not known.

EFFECTS OF PHARMACOLOGIC AGENTS ON FLOW

Most pharmacologic agents, administered either topically or systemically, have no effect on aqueous humor flow. Three classes of drugs are notable exceptions: carbonic anhydrase inhibitors,[34] β-adrenergic antagonists,[16,37] and α_2-selective adrenergic agonists.[33] All of these classes of drugs have been observed to lower the rate of aqueous flow by approximately 50% during waking hours. Interestingly, β-adrenergic antagonists have no effect on flow in sleeping subjects,[38] whereas the other two classes of drugs have slight effects in sleeping subjects.[39]

A number of other drugs have been tested and found to have no clinically significant effect on aqueous humor flow. These include corticosteroids,[40] α_1-adrenergic agonists,[41] cholinergics,[42] prostaglandin derivatives,[43] caffeine,[44] and melatonin.[36]

Virtually no pharmacologic agents have been discovered that are able to increase the rate of aqueous humor flow. The only exceptions are the adrenergic agonists, especially those with β-selective activity, including epinephrine,[45] salbutamol,[46] isoproterenol,[47] and terbutaline.[48] All these agents are more effective at increasing flow in sleeping subjects, but the effect is small and variable.

REGULATION OF AQUEOUS HUMOR FLOW IN HUMANS

The need to develop pharmacologic agents for the control of IOP in glaucoma and the successful development of agents that suppress aqueous humor formation have stimulated research into the physiology of its regulation. In humans, the dynamic range over which regulation of flow seems to occur is very narrow, merely a factor of two. Except during sleep and inflammatory responses, the rate of flow seems to remain unperturbed. Even moderate changes of intraocular pressure have no effect on flow.[49] Basic research has established a link between aqueous flow and the synthesis of the intracellular messengers cyclic AMP [50,51] and cyclic GMP.[52] These cyclic nucleotides are known to regulate a large number of cell functions and undoubtedly have a significant role in some of the functions of the ciliary epithelia. A clearer understanding of the cell mechanisms that govern the rate of aqueous formation would provide a rational basis for the design of new drugs to control IOP by down-regulating flow.

Section III

Gonioscopy

Alan H. Zalta

Gonioscopy is a clinical biomicroscopic technique used to examine the anterior chamber angle of the eye. Although not part of a routine eye exam, gonioscopy is integral to the evaluation of eyes with elevated intraocular pressure (IOP), glaucoma, suspected narrow angles using the slit lamp technique of Van Herick et al,[53] abnormal anterior segment anatomy, and after significant ocular trauma. Gonioscopy is the most important tool used to differentiate the open-angle glaucomas from the narrow-angle glaucomas and is essential to identification of the mechanism responsible for glaucoma. Because iridocorneal relationships can be altered by pharmacologic agents, surgery, or time, gonioscopy may need to be repeated periodically to detect changes or the emergence of secondary pathology. Mastering gonioscopy is also a necessary antecedent to the laser treatment of the open-angle glaucomas. Competent performance of gonioscopy is a demanding skill acquired only through experience. It requires considerable eye–hand coordination, knowledge of normal and abnormal anatomy, and the ability to avoid artifactual observations.

The anterior-chamber angle may be visualized using direct and indirect techniques of gonioscopy. Direct gonioscopy allows direct visualization of the chamber angle through a domed goniolens and is performed with a hand-held viewer, separate light source, and the patient in a supine position. Because direct gonioscopy is cumbersome, inconvenient, time consuming, and requires special equipment, it now is used rarely by ophthalmologists[54] except in the evaluation and surgical therapy of glaucoma in anesthetized infants. By contrast, indirect gonioscopy is conveniently performed at the slit-lamp biomicroscope and permits a rapid examination at high magnification with optimal control and flexibility of illumination. Indirect gonioscopy is an indispensable diagnostic and therapeutic skill for any ophthalmologist.

PRINCIPLE OF INDIRECT GONIOSCOPY

Indirect gonioscopy is performed at the slit-lamp microscope using a mirrored contact lens. The contact lens neutralizes the corneal refractive power and the mirror allows indirect visualization of angle structures that could otherwise not be seen by direct viewing of the anterior segment. Normally, light rays coming from the angle are totally internally reflected because they exceed the critical angle, about 46°, for the cornea–air interface (Fig. 3.11A). A contact lens with a similar index of refraction can eliminate the cornea optically and allow the light rays from the angle to pass through the new contact lens–air interface. A mirror positioned within the contact lens may reflect these light rays at nearly a right angle to the contact lens-air interface and allow a straight-ahead vantage point for viewing the angle structures with the slit-lamp biomicroscope (Fig. 3.11B). With indirect gonioscopy, the anterior chamber angle appears inverted as it is reflected in a particular goniolens mirror. The examiner's view is a reflection of structures 180° away, i.e., a goniolens mirror positioned superiorly views the inferior angle, a goniolens mirror positioned temporally views the nasal angle, and so on.

INSTRUMENTS FOR INDIRECT GONIOSCOPY

Two different styles of goniolenses, Goldmann-type and Zeiss-type, are used in indirect gonioscopy. Goldmann-type goniolenses (Fig. 3.12) are easier to use because they keep the globe stationary and afford better control during examination. These lenses require the placement of methylcellulose, an optically clear, highly viscous fluid, on their concave surface to act as a buffer between the cornea and the goniolens. The methylcellulose creates an innocuous suction cup adherence which provides the clinician with fine control of eye–goniolens–slit beam positioning. In contrast, Zeiss-type goniolenses (Fig. 3.13) utilize the precorneal tear film as an interface between goniolens and cornea. Because there is no adherence between goniolens and

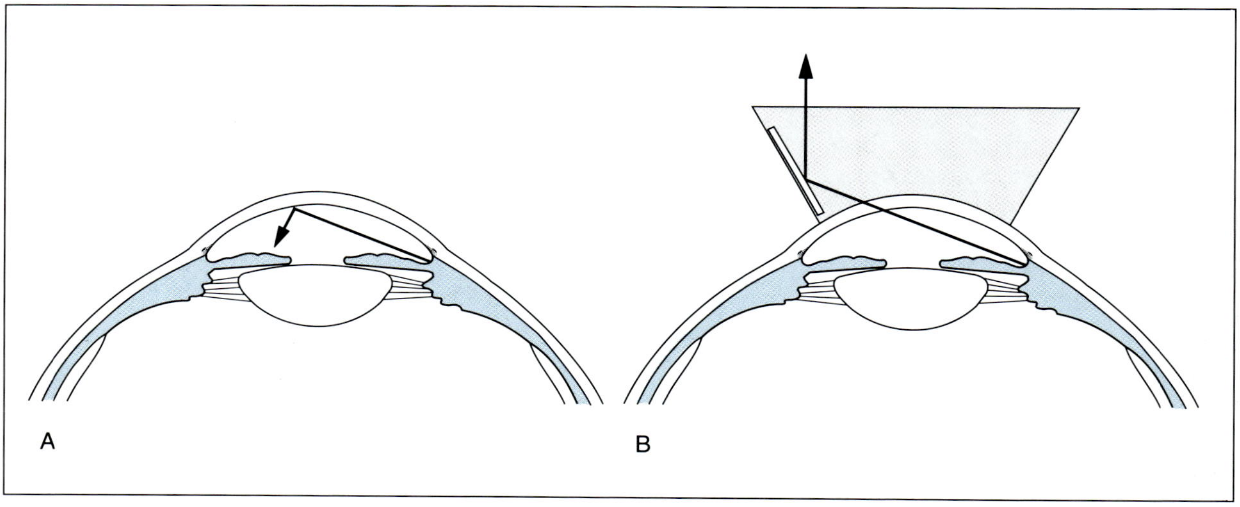

3.11 | Principle of indirect gonioscopy. *A:* Diagram of light ray which originates from the anterior chamber angle, exceeds the critical angle at the cornea–air interface, and is totally internally reflected. *B:* Diagram of light ray which originates from the anterior chamber angle, passes through the cornea–goniolens interface, and is reflected by a goniomirror.

cornea, greater patient cooperation is necessary to avoid ocular drift, prevent blepharospasm, and maintain optimal ocular positioning. An advantage to not using methylcellulose is that the cornea and tear film are not significantly disturbed. As a result, Zeiss-type goniolenses do not optically interfere with the examiner's or camera's view into the eye or with the patient's view out of the eye after gonioscopic examination. Although Zeiss-type goniolenses must be used with greater dexterity and skill to avoid unintentional distortion of the angle, they offer many advantages over Goldmann-type goniolenses. Specifically, they enable rapid examination, rapid transfer from one eye to the other for comparison purposes, and indentation gonioscopy for assessing angle-closure glaucoma. Because of the inherent differences in the Goldmann- and Zeiss-type goniolenses, each has advantages which merit their tailored use for indirect gonioscopy.

Goldmann-Type Goniolenses

The Goldmann-type lenses most commonly used for gonioscopy are the Goldmann three-mirror and Thorpe four-mirror (see Fig. 3.12). Whereas the Goldmann three-mirror lens has only one of the three mirrors inclined at 59° for gonioscopy, the Thorpe four-mirror has all four mirrors inclined at 62°, obviating the need for rotation to visualize the entire angle.

Zeiss-Type Goniolenses

All four mirrors in the Zeiss and Posner lenses (see Fig. 3.13) are inclined at 62° and 64°, respectively, allowing visualization of the entire circumference of the anterior chamber angle without rotation. Both lenses have handles that facilitate lens application to the eye.

Technique of Indirect Gonioscopy

Physical Positioning of Patient and Examiner

The physical positioning of patient and examiner during indirect gonioscopy is critical to avoid excessive eye, body, or head movement by the patient and to avoid technique artifact or fatigue-related hand tremor by the examiner. The table height of the slit-lamp must be adjusted so that the patient is seated comfortably with optimal chinrest and headrest support. Because many patients will pull away from the headrest once a goniolens has been placed on their eye, they should be instructed to keep their forehead firmly

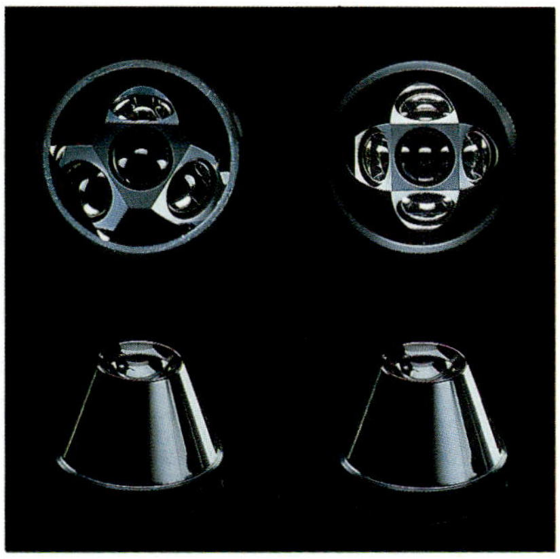

3.12 | The Goldmann three-mirror *(left)* and Thorpe four-mirror *(right)* goniolenses with front/anterior view *(top)* and back/posterior view from an oblique angle *(bottom)*.

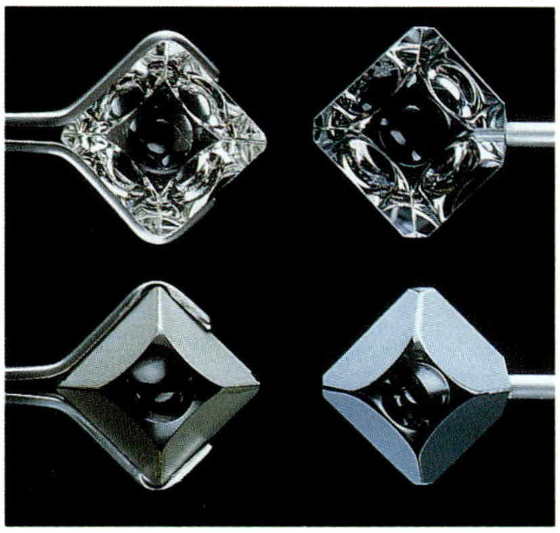

3.13 | The Zeiss *(left)* and Posner *(right)* goniolenses with front/anterior view *(top)* and back/posterior view *(bottom)*.

against the headrest throughout the examination. The patient's eye should be positioned to allow maximal vertical range of the slit lamp microscope via the joystick. This allows the superior and inferior angles to be viewed without having to adjust the chinrest during examination. The examiner should sit at a comfortable height for viewing and for supporting the elbow and hand holding the goniolens.

Goldmann-Type Goniolenses

A topical anesthetic solution is placed on all eyes prior to gonioscopy. Methylcellulose is placed in the concave surface of the Goldmann-type lenses, with care taken not to introduce any bubbles. Bottles of methylcellulose should be stored upside down so that the methylcellulose drops are free of air bubbles. The air that replaces spent methylcellulose rises to the bottom of the bottle if it is stored in the inverted position. The Goldmann-type goniolens is held with one hand while the free hand elevates the upper eyelid. The lower lid is depressed with either hand and the patient is instructed to look up. The lower edge of the lens is placed in the lower fornix (Fig. 3.14A) and the lens is rotated against the eye. Air bubbles between the cornea and goniolens occur rarely when it is properly inserted. If air bubbles are present, they can usually be removed by tilting and turning the lens. To stabilize and rotate Goldmann-type lenses on an eye, the lens rim may be grasped using either a two- or three-finger technique (Fig. 3.14B). To prevent examiner fatigue and tremor, the fingers not holding the lens are placed on the patient's cheek, the slit-lamp headrest, or the vertical bar attached to the silt-lamp headrest, and the elbow is supported by the slit-lamp tabletop, the slit-lamp roller guards, or an elbow rest. The free hand manipulates the joystick to focus the reflected image of the anterior chamber angle in the goniomirror. With the Goldmann three-mirror lens, the goniomirror must be rotated, usually in 90° segments, to examine the entire angle for 360°. If Descemet's folds are present in a nonhypotonous eye, they are most likely caused by excessive rotatory pressure on the lens. With the Thorpe four-mirror lens, the slit-lamp joystick is manipulated to refocus in each of the four goniomirrors without rotating the lens.

Zeiss-Type Goniolenses

Zeiss-type goniolenses are placed directly on an anesthesized eye using the precorneal tear film as the lens–cornea interface. The lens is grasped by the holding fork or stem using a two-, three-, or four-finger technique (Fig.

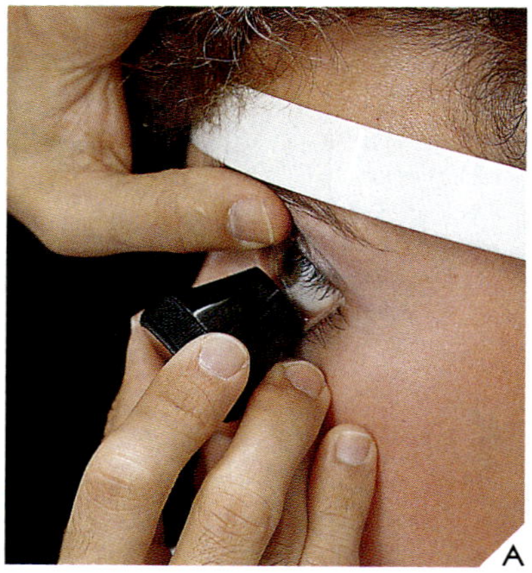

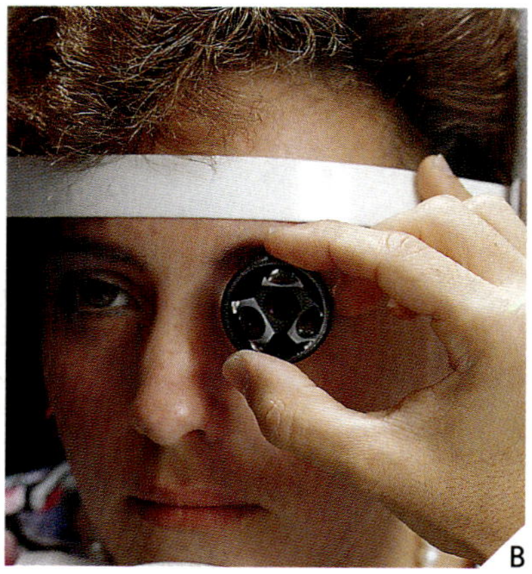

3.14 | Technique of Goldmann goniolens insertion and stabilization. *A:* Separation of eyelids and placement of the lower edge of the lens in the inferior cul-de-sac with the patient looking upward. *B:* Three-fingered grasp on rim of lens with goniomirror in 12 o'clock position and hand supported by vertical bar attached to headrest.

3.15A). The ring finger can be used to support either the handle of the lens (Fig. 3.15B) or the little finger, which is steadied against the patient's cheek or adjacent headrest. Optimizing arm and hand support is critical to enable dextrous placement and manipulation of these lenses on the cornea (see Fig. 3.15A). The small posterior diameter of the lens minimizes lid contact. If reflex blinking or blepharospasm interferes with lens positioning, the eyelids can be manually separated to facilitate lens placement. The Zeiss-type lenses should be applied with the eye in primary gaze and should touch the corneal surface sufficiently to create a fluid level without producing folds in Descemet's membrane. When the lens is optimally positioned, a slight reduction in application pressure allows intrusion of an air bubble under the lens. If air bubbles accumulate during gonioscopy, they are easily eliminated by slight rocking, rotation, or removal and reapplication of the lens. Inadvertent pressure on the eye or malpositioning of the lens will distort the angle configuration. Because there is no suction adherence between the cornea and the goniolens, some eyes have a tendency to drift away from the primary gaze position. However, these lenses can be easily repositioned or removed and quickly reapplied. While holding the goniolens in position with one hand, the slit-lamp joystick is manipulated with the other hand to refocus each of the four mirrors without rotating the lens.

NORMAL GONIOSCOPIC ANATOMY

CLASSIC LANDMARKS

Usually, angle structures are easiest to identify in the inferior quadrant because of its greater depth and its increased pigmentation compared with the other quadrants. Whichever goniolens is used, the inferior angle is visualized by focusing in a goniomirror positioned at the 12 o'clock position. With the Goldmann three-mirror lens, the gonioscopy mirror should be aligned to the 12 o'clock position prior to lens placement on the eye. This will avoid the need to rotate immediately the lens in order to visualize the inferior angle. After examination of the inferior quadrant, the remaining quadrants should be viewed sequentially in a clockwise direction. This convention will reduce potential confusion about the location of the goniomirror and the examiner's reflected view of structures 180° away.

From an anterior to posterior direction, the classic anatomic structures in the iridocorneal angle that should be identified include Schwalbe's line, the trabecular meshwork, the scleral spur, and the ciliary body band

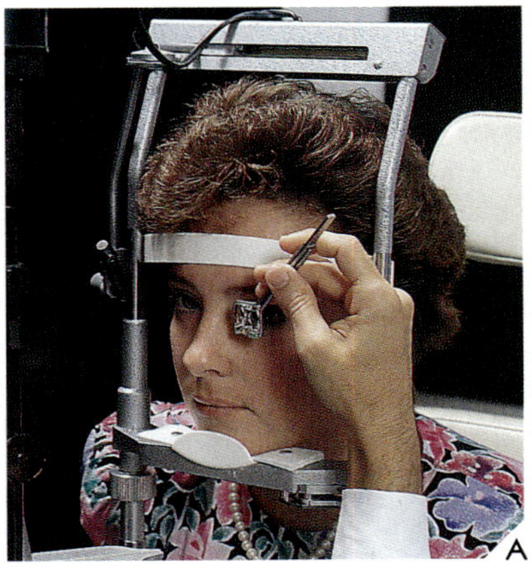

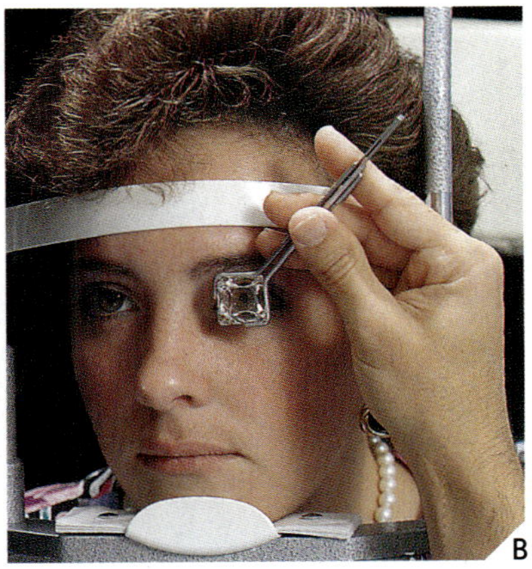

3.15 | Technique of Zeiss goniolens placement onto the cornea. *A:* Elbow is supported by slit-lamp roller guard, arm and wrist are supported by vertical bar connected to headrest, and hand is supported on patient's cheek while the goniolens is grasped by three-fingered technique. *B:* Goniolens horizontally aligned and supported by four-fingered technique during placement on eye in primary gaze.

(Fig. 3.16). Schwalbe's line, also known as the anterior border ring of the filtration angle, is a translucent or white ledge which marks the most anterior extension of the trabecular meshwork and the termination of Descemet's membrane. The trabecular meshwork, located between Schwalbe's line and the scleral spur, is a band of variable color which increases from faint tan to dark brown with age. The trabecular meshwork typically has a ground-glass appearance and represents the perforated layers of connective tissue through which aqueous humor flows to Schlemm's canal. The scleral spur, also known as the posterior border ring of the filtration angle, is a prominent white line between the trabecular meshwork and the ciliary body band which marks the most anterior projection of the sclera internally and the insertion site of the anterior portion of the ciliary body. The ciliary body band, formed by the anterior ciliary face, is usually a gray, tan, or dark brown band which extends from the scleral spur to the iris root. The ciliary body band is of variable width, depending upon the level of iris insertion, and tends to be wider in myopic and narrower in hyperopic eyes.

Termination of Corneal Light Wedge at Schwalbe's Line

When angle landmarks are not readily apparent, finding the termination of the corneal slit beam wedge becomes an invaluable method of identifying structures. When a thin slit beam of light is projected at a 10–15° angle into the iridocorneal angle, the two reflections of the optical cross-section of the

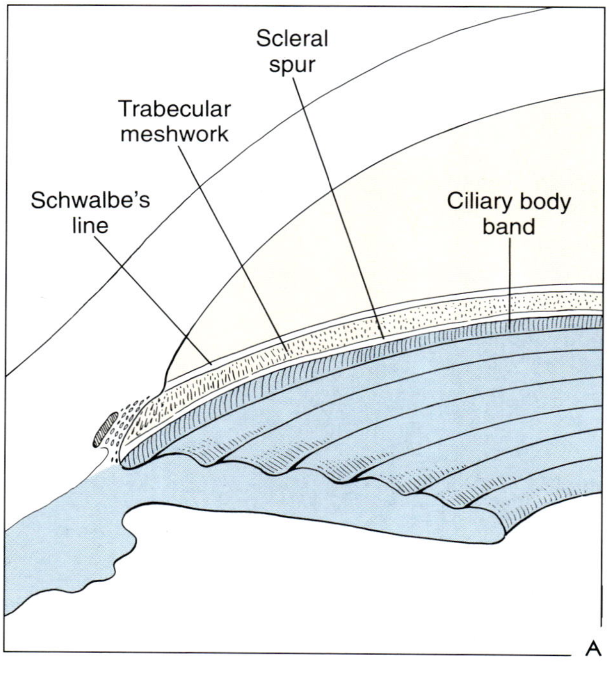

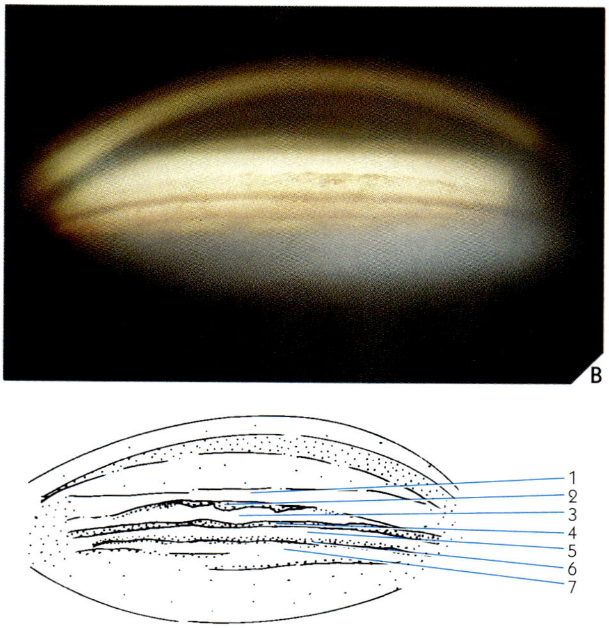

3.16 | Gonioscopic anatomy. *A:* Diagrammatic view. *B:* Clinical view. Structures include (1) cornea, (2) Sampaolesi line, (3) Schwalbe's line, (4) trabecular meshwork, (5) scleral spur, (6) ciliary body band, and (7) iris root.

cornea meet at Schwalbe's line (Fig. 3.17). At Schwalbe's line, the external and internal reflections of the three-dimensional parallelepiped of light seen through the cornea merge into a two-dimensional single line with a brighter luminance, which extends in a perpendicular direction across the trabecular meshwork. The termination of this corneal light wedge identifies the anterior limit of the trabecular meshwork. This method of identifying anatomic landmarks is invaluable in the absence of angle pigment, the presence of multiple pigmented bands, narrow angles, and angle-closure glaucoma. Special care must be taken to use dim illumination when projecting the slit beam into the iridocorneal angle. Bright illumination will artifactually deepen the anterior chamber by inducing pupillary constriction and may lead to the mistaken classification of an angle as more widely open instead of narrow. If anatomic landmarks cannot be readily differentiated in dim illumination, alternately increasing and decreasing the illumination will dynamically deepen and shallow chamber depth via pupillary movement and will facilitate identification of angle structures.

VARIATIONS OF NORMAL GONIOSCOPIC ANATOMY

Sampaolesi Line

An important practical consideration in adult gonioscopic anatomy is a Sampaolesi line, i.e., a line of irregular pigment deposition on Schwalbe's line in the inferior quadrant (see Fig. 3.16). A dense Sampaolesi line may be mistaken for the trabecular meshwork in an eye with a narrow or closed angle and has clinical significance in the diagnosis of pigmentary glaucoma and exfoliation glaucoma (see Chapter 8). Compared with the trabecular meshwork, the pigmentation in a Sampaolesi line is deposited in a discontinuous fashion resembling salt and pepper and is usually confined to the inferior quadrant. Although normally there is no pigment in the angle at birth, pigment deposition in the inferior angle at 6 o'clock is present in 90% of indi-

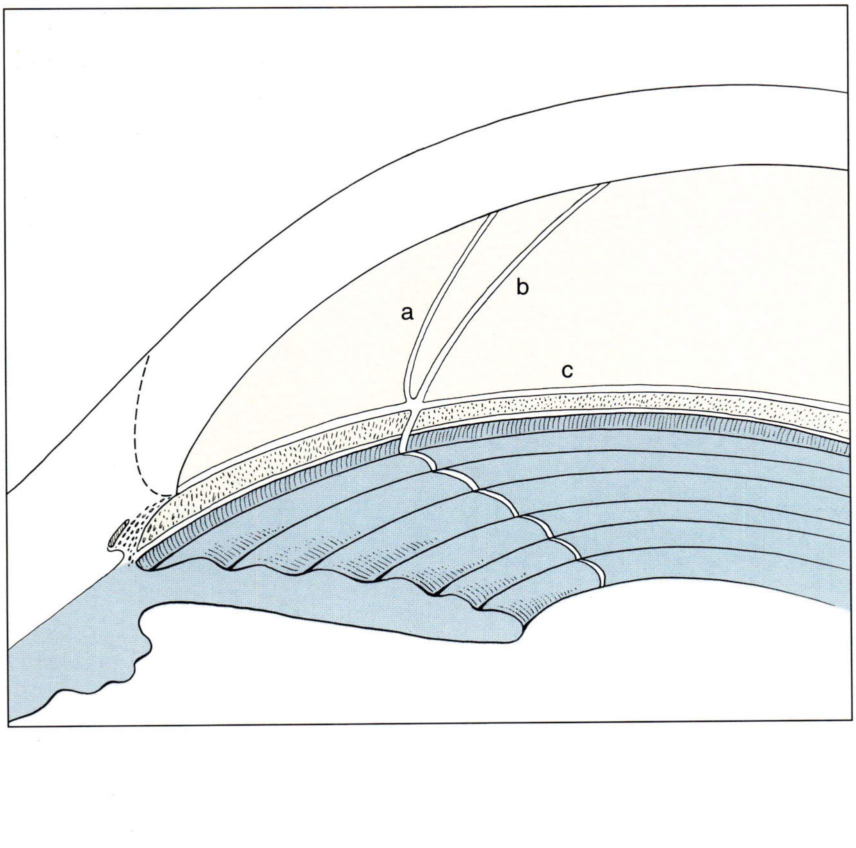

3.17 | Diagrammatic representation of termination of corneal slit beam wedge at Schwalbe's line. External (a) and internal (b) light reflections of corneal parallelepiped merge at Schwalbe's line (c), identifying the anterior limit of the trabecular meshwork.

viduals over the age of 50.[55] In contrast, in the superior angle at 12 o'clock, 88% of individuals have at most trace pigmentation and less than 3% of individuals have moderate to dense pigmentation of the trabecular meshwork.[55] In most instances where marked pigmentation of the superior angle is pathologic, a dense Sampaolesi line is present in the inferior quadrant.

Iris Processes

Iris processes can be found in 78% of brown eyes, 48% of hazel eyes, and 17% of blue eyes,[55] and are not indicative of any disease process. Iris processes are usually seen as gray or brown lacy, finger-like extensions of the peripheral iris which bridge the angle concavity to insert into the scleral spur or posterior portion of the trabecular meshwork (Fig. 3.18). Less frequently, iris processes are seen lining the inner, deep portion of the angle recess. Iris processes most commonly occur in the nasal quadrant and are mild in density.[56] Because the appearance of iris processes may vary considerably, they are on occasion mistaken for pathologic peripheral anterior synechiae which are broader, tent-shaped, and abut the trabecular meshwork concealing angle landmarks.

Angle Vessels

In the normal anterior chamber angle, blood vessels may be visible in 51% to 62% of blue eyes and in 9% to 16% of brown eyes.[57,58] Four distinctly different types of vessels have been noted: circular ciliary body band, radial iris

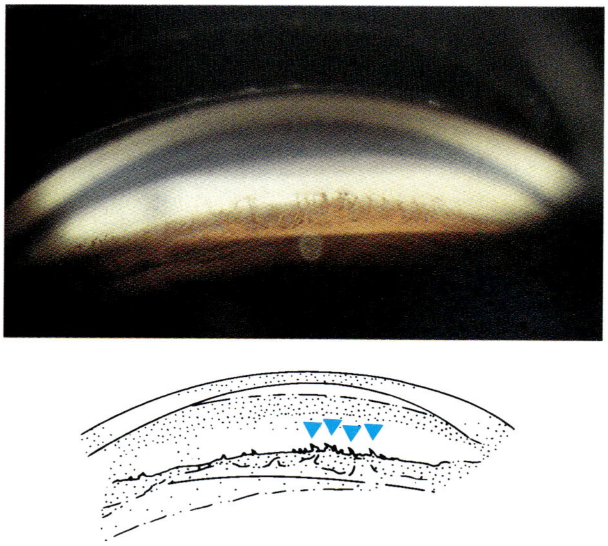

3.18 | Many iris processes (arrows) in anterior chamber angle extend to a prominent scleral spur and to the posterior trabecular meshwork.

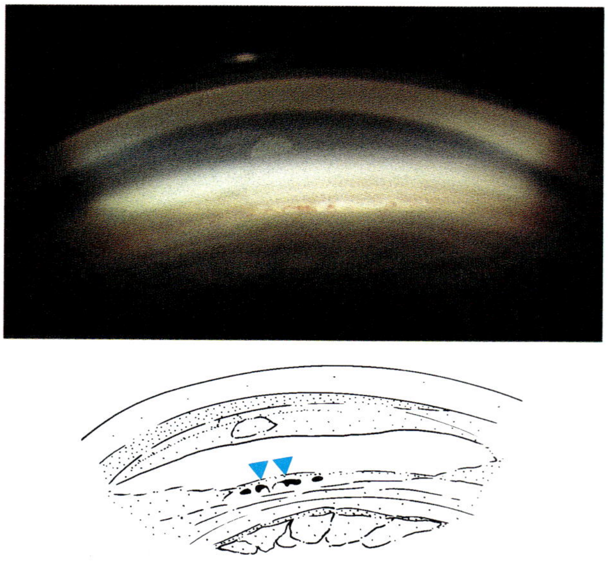

3.19 | The most commonly seen angle vessels, the circular ciliary body band vessels (arrows), take a sinuous course circumferentially in the angle recess.

root, radial ciliary body band, and circular iris root. The circular ciliary body band vessels and radial iris vessels occur most frequently (Fig. 3.19). The circular ciliary body band vessels are most easily visualized, take a sinuous course in the angle recess, and represent prominent segments of the major arterial circle of the iris. The radial iris vessels are arterioles emanating from the major arterial circle of the iris which appear at the iris root, hook over the last iris roll, and disappear into the peripheral iris stroma. The radial ciliary body band vessels appear as thin, linear red streaks which lie deep within the ciliary body and course perpendicular to the iris plane. The circular iris root vessels are seen least frequently and appear as short circumferential segments at the iris root. In contrast to pathologic angle neovascularization, normal angle vessels are typically broad in character, appear in short segments, do not extend anterior to the scleral spur, and do not arborize in the trabecular meshwork.

ASSESSMENT OF ANTERIOR CHAMBER DEPTH AND ANGLE CONFIGURATION

The most common purpose in gonioscopy is to permit characterization of the angle configuration in patients with glaucoma, i.e., to differentiate between an open, narrow, and closed angle. The anterior chamber-angle width is genetically determined,[59] varies inversely with ocular refractive power[60] being wider in myopes and narrower in hyperopes, and decreases with age[55,60] owing to growth of the crystalline lens and an increase in relative pupillary block. Eyes predisposed to angle closure should have gonioscopy repeated at regular intervals.

PRIMARY GAZE

Anterior chamber angle width should be initially evaluated in primary gaze with all types of goniolenses positioned centrally on the cornea. A thin slit beam and reduced illumination should be used to avoid constricting the pupil and artificially widening the angle. With the Goldmann-type lenses, care must be taken to avoid indentation of the peripheral cornea, as this may artifactually narrow the iridocorneal angle. With the Zeiss-type lenses, care must be taken to avoid undue pressure against the central cornea, since this may artifactually widen the iridocorneal angle. Inadvertent pressure creates folds in Descemet's membrane and shifts the iris–lens diaphragm posteriorly. If these signs occur, a slight withdrawal of the Zeiss goniolens away from the cornea without losing the tear interface will correct the artifact. Each quadrant should be inspected.

The best examination is achieved using direct focal illumination. A narrow beam is used for precise examination and localization. In contrast, a wide beam is used for diffuse illumination and a general view. Retroillumination and proximal sclerotic scatter illumination may occasionally be needed for internal illumination and identification of the scleral spur. Examination and optimal ocular alignment may be aided by positioning of the fixation light in front of the patient's fellow eye.

EXTREME GAZE

In eyes with narrow iridocorneal angles, additional manipulations may be necessary to evaluate chamber depth, the degree of angle occludability or closure, and the presence of peripheral anterior synechiae or other pathology. A more tangential viewing of a narrow or closed angle will facilitate identification of angle structures obscured by prominent iris convexity (Fig. 3.20). A tangential approach may be achieved by having the patient look in the direction of the goniomirror being viewed. This maneuver can be facilitated by shifting the fixation light, which is positioned in front of the fellow eye, in the same direction, i.e., the direction of the goniomirror being viewed. The examiner can produce a similar effect by moving the lens towards the part of the angle to be examined, e.g., by displacing a goniolens nasally when examining the nasal quadrant. Often, examination in extreme gaze is the only way to appreciate any anatomic landmarks in an extremely narrowed or partially closed angle. Once angle structures are visualized, it may be necessary to use the slit-beam wedge sign to help identify or differentiate these landmarks.

INDENTATION GONIOSCOPY

A major advantage of Zeiss-type goniolenses is their ability to indent the central cornea and artificially widen the anterior chamber angle. Because the smaller radius of curvature allows these lenses to come into direct contact with the anterior corneal surface, central depression of the cornea will displace aqueous humor peripherally and the iris root posteriorly. When this maneuver is performed dynamically during gonioscopy, the postion of the iris relative to the angle structures may be altered during examination. This technique is known as *pressure, indentation,* or *dynamic gonioscopy.* When the

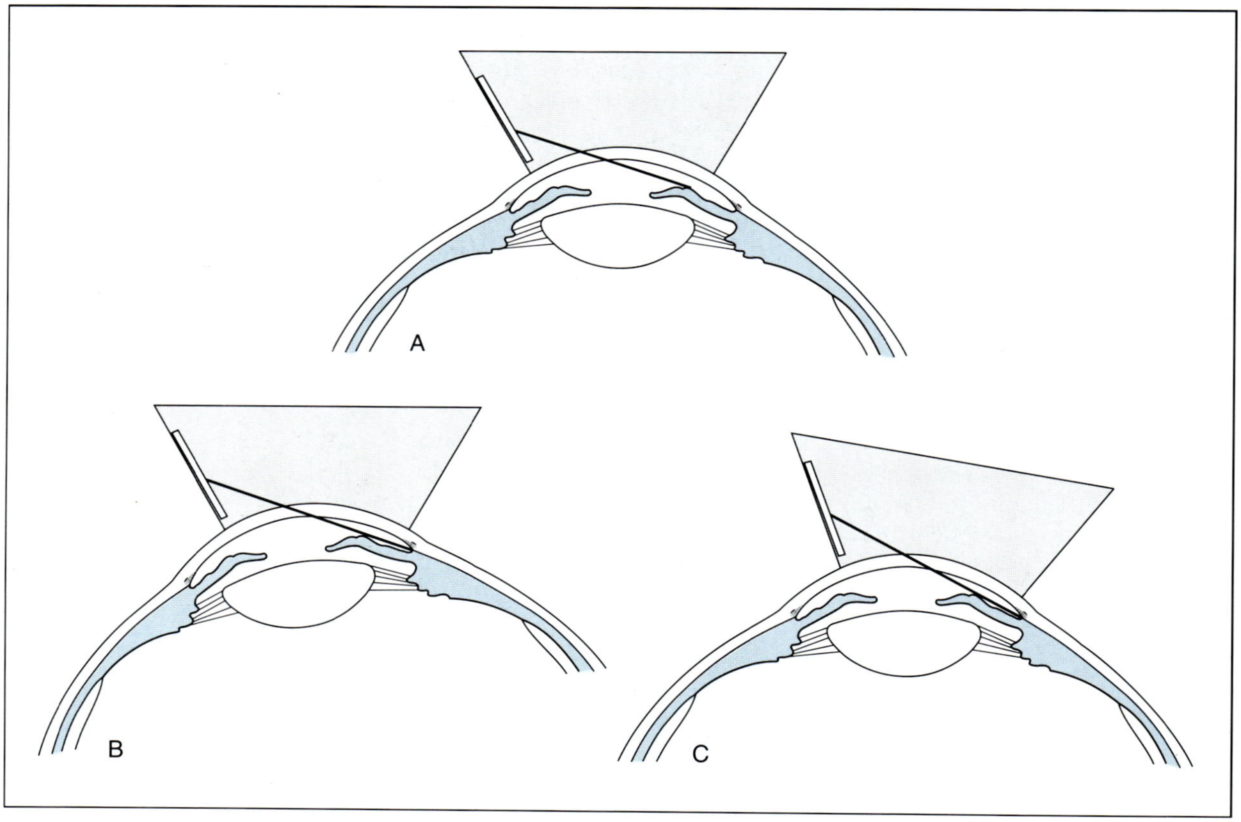

3.20 | *A:* Tangential viewing of the iridocorneal angle may be necessary to identify angle structures obscured by a prominent iris convexity. *B:* A tangential approach can be achieved either by having the patient look in extreme gaze towards the goniomirror being viewed, or *C,* by moving the goniolens towards the part of the angle to be examined.

iridocorneal angle is optically narrow, indentation gonioscopy facilitates identification of angle structures. When the iridocorneal angle is optically closed, indentation gonioscopy enables differentiation of reversible appositional from irreversible synechial angle closure[61] (Fig. 3.21). In performing this technique, the angle is first assessed without (Fig. 3.22A) and then with corneal indentation (Fig. 3.22B). Folds in Descemet's membrane will be present during indentation and may distort, but not obscure, the view of the iridocorneal angle. The angle configuration is observed and angle structures are identified as pressure is applied and withdrawn in repeated sequence. With this technique, areas of appositional closure are readily opened and adhesions are clearly exposed. If angle anatomy is not readily apparent, the slit beam corneal wedge sign may be used during indentation to identify Schwalbe's line. Other refinements of this technique to maximally displace aqueous or improve the viewing angle include decentration of the goniolens

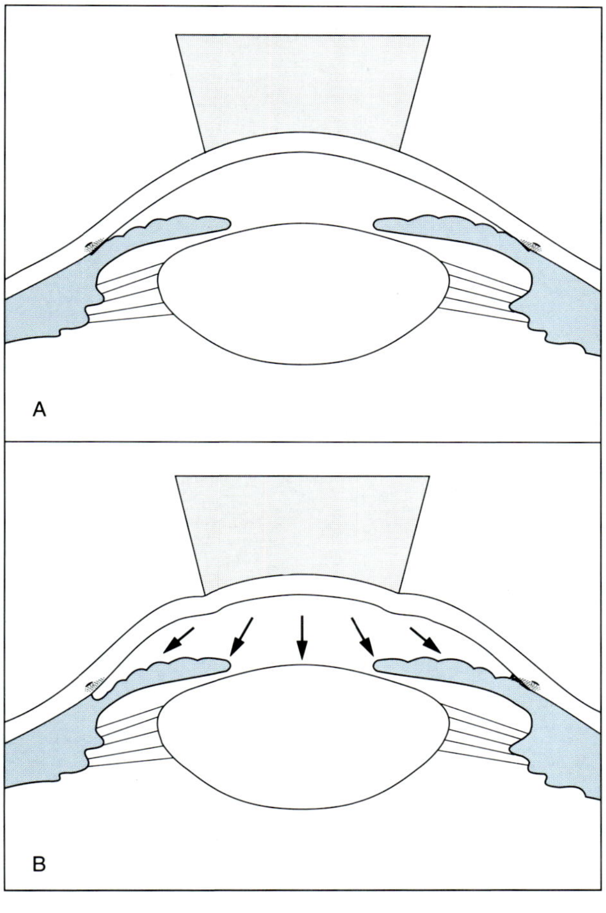

3.21 | Indirect gonioscopy using Zeiss-type goniolens without *(A)* and with *(B)* indentation. During indentation, areas of iris apposition open *(B, left)* and areas of peripheral anterior synechiae remain closed *(B, right)*. (Adapted from Forbes M: Gonioscopy with corneal indentation. *Arch Ophthalmol 1966;76:488–492.*)

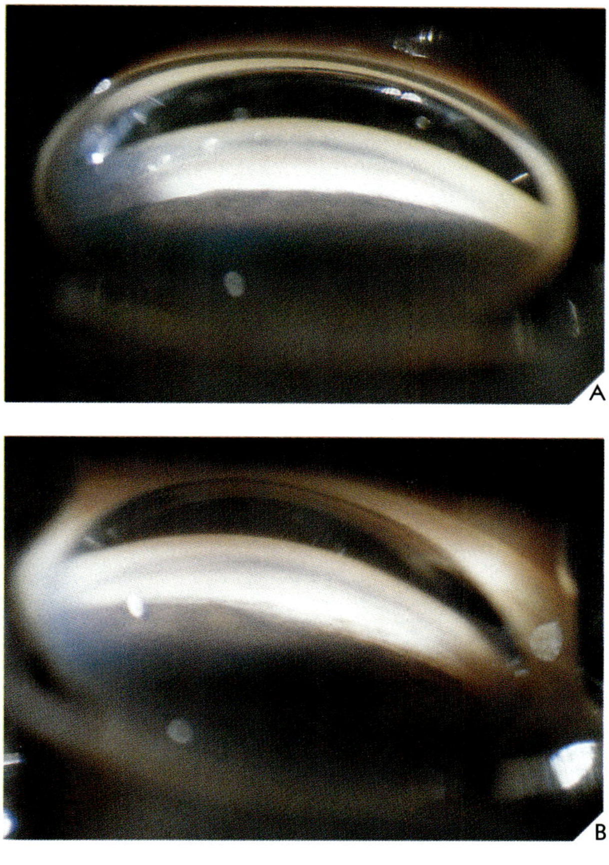

3.22 | Angle appearance seen through a Zeiss goniolens without *(A)* and with *(B)* dynamic depression. Without dynamic indentation *(A)*, a thin, irregular pigment line is seen in the anterior chamber angle, but no structures are clearly identifiable. With dynamic indentation *(B)*, the peripheral iris is flattened and the anterior chamber deepened, revealing a previously obscured trabecular meshwork and scleral spur below a Sampaolesi line on the right half of the figure. Peripheral anterior synechiae caused by primary angle-closure glaucoma occlude the left portion of this anterior chamber angle.

on the cornea, extreme gaze in the direction of the mirror, and lifting of the goniolens while pressing inward. The most common errors in performing indentation gonioscopy include unintentional depression of the cornea, improper positioning of the goniolens, and excessive illumination.

GONIOSCOPIC DOCUMENTATION, INTERPRETATION, AND CLASSIFICATION

Using descriptive words or drawings, certain gonioscopic findings should be documented in a standardized fashion. This is especially important for angle findings that may change over time, particularly depth, degree of pigmentation, and presence or extent of peripheral anterior synechiae and neovascularization.

In an effort to correlate anterior chamber-angle width with the potential for angle closure, numerous grading systems have been proposed. The most common classification system, that of Shaffer,[62,63] correlates an angle and numeric grade with the angular width of the angle recess and a clinical interpretation of the potential for angle closure (Fig. 3.23). An angular width of grade 3 and grade 4 is present in 98.6% of a normal population, whereas grade 2 occurs in 1% and grade 1 occurs in only 0.64%[62] (Fig. 3.24).

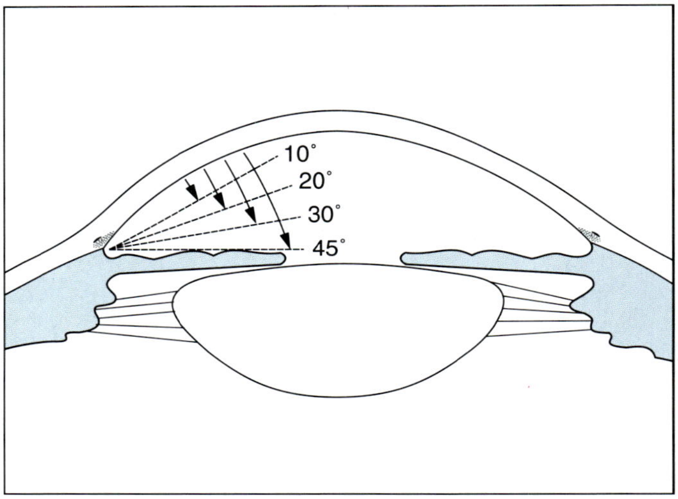

3.23 | Shaffer's classification system for grading anterior chamber angle depth. (Adapted from Shaffer RN: Gonioscopy, ophthalmoscopy and perimetry. *Trans Am Acad Ophthalmol Otolaryngol 1960;64:112–125,* and Hoskins HD, Kass MA (eds): *Becker-Shaffer's Diagnosis and Therapy of the Glaucomas,* ed 6. St. Louis: CV Mosby, 1989, 106,107.)

Figure 3.24. Shaffer Classification System

Angle Grade	Numeric Grade	Angular Width of Angle Recess	Clinical Interpretation
Wide open angle	3–4	30–45°	Closure improbable or impossible
Moderately narrow angle	2	20°	Closure possible
Extremely narrow angle	Slit-1	Few–10°	Closure probable eventually
Partial or complete angle closure	0	0°	Closure present

Spaeth's classification system is based on the angular width of the anterior chamber recess as well as the curvature of the peripheral iris and the site of iris insertion (Figs. 3.25 and 3.26).[55,59] The angle width is determined by constructing a tangent to the anterior iris surface about one-third of the distance from the most peripheral portion of the iris. The most common anatomic configuration combines an angular width between 30° and 40°, a relatively flat peripheral iris configuration, and iris insertion into the anterior portion of the ciliary body. Marked anterior convexity of the peripheral iris may be one of the important attributes of eyes predisposed to the development of primary angle-closure glaucoma.[59]

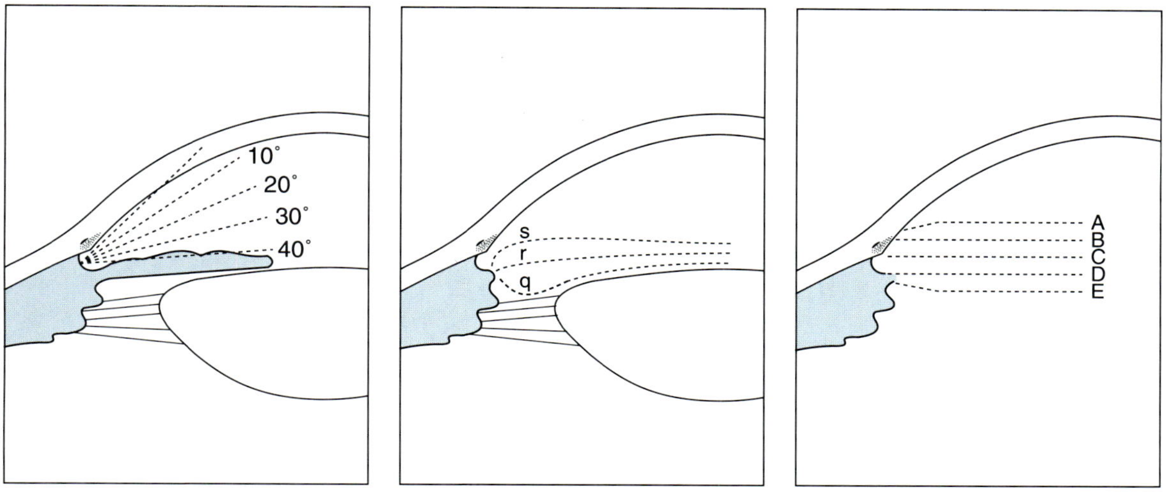

3.25 | Spaeth's classification system for describing angle configuration. (Adapted from Spaeth GL: The normal development of the human anterior chamber angle: A new system of descriptive grading. *Trans Ophthalmol Soc UK 1971;91:709–739* and Spaeth GL: Gonioscopy: Uses old and new. The inheritance of occludable angles. *Trans Am Acad Ophthalmol Otolaryngol 1978;85:222–232.*)

Figure 3.26. Spaeth Classification System

Angle Width	Peripheral Iris Curvature	Site of Iris Insertion
10°	Concave = q	Anterior to trabecular meshwork = A
20°	Flat = r	Behind Schwalbe's line = B
	Convex = s	At scleral spur = C
30°		Normal deep angle recess = D
40°		Extremely deep angle recess = E

Scheie's grading convention[64] is opposite to that of Shaffer's system and is based on the extent of anterior chamber angle structures visualized. Because of the potential for confusion, it is important to specify which grading scheme is being used when communicating with other ophthalmologists.

Descriptive words or drawings are preferred by many clinicians over an arbitrary classification system. Regardless of format used for gonioscopic documentation, the purpose is to record findings pertinent to the diagnosis and management of particular types of glaucoma.

ASSESSMENT OF SECONDARY ANGLE PATHOLOGY

Gonioscopy is also essential to the identification of secondary mechanisms responsible for glaucoma. Among the more common angle abnormalities are peripheral anterior synechiae, neovascularization, excessive pigmentation, angle recession, clefts, mass lesions, membranes, and congenital or developmental anomalies. The gonioscopic discovery of these conditions is critical to their management approach both therapeutically and prognostically.

ACKNOWLEDGMENT

Earl Choromokos, FOPS, provided expert photographic assistance during the preparation of this section.

4 Diagnostic Techniques of the Posterior Segment

Section I

Ophthalmoscopy: Examination Techniques

Eve Juliet Higginbotham

GENERAL APPROACH

Whichever examination technique is employed, the examiner should keep in mind the characteristics of glaucomatous optic disc cupping and retinal nerve fiber layer loss (see Higginbotham, Chapter 6). The discs should be compared for asymmetry. When each disc is examined individually, the presence of any disc hemorrhage should be noted. The observer should judge the relationship of the vertical diameter to the horizontal diameter of the cup. Is the vertical diameter larger? What is the relationship of the cup to the entire area of the disc? Are there any focal areas of thinning? It may be helpful to compare the four quadrants to each other. For example, the contour of the superior temporal quadrant can be compared to the inferior temporal quadrant. Particular attention should be paid to the inferior temporal quadrant, because changes often occur in this location first.[1] The course of the vessels exiting the nerve, as well as the presence or absence of circumlinear vessels (which may have been obliterated due to glaucomatous atrophy), should be noted. Special filters can be used in the direct ophthalmoscope or slit lamp illumination systems to enhance visibility of the retinal nerve fiber layer and any glaucomatous defects (see below).

DIRECT OPHTHALMOSCOPY

The direct ophthalmoscope (Fig. 4.1) is the most commonly used instrument for ophthalmoscopy. This instrument is extremely portable and the technique requires less patient cooperation compared with other techniques. Although the examiner is at a disadvantage due to the small field of view and the lack of stereopsis, a skilled observer can develop monocular clues over time by examining patients initially using both direct ophthalmoscopy and stereoscopic techniques. By moving the light across the disc margin, the examiner can appreciate a change in depth. If the patient has a miotic pupil, a Koeppe gonioscopic lens can be applied to the eye, and with high plus on the direct ophthalmoscope the nerve can more easily be examined. The nerve fiber layer can sometimes be seen by switching to the green or blue filter. The superior pole should be compared with the inferior pole. Slit defects or wedge defects in the nerve fiber layer should be noted. If vessels can be more clearly distinguished in one area compared with another, a defect may be present. However, visualization of the nerve fiber is more easily seen photographically, and requires clear media and a widely dilated pupil. It is also more difficult to visualize the nerve fiber layer in a lightly pigmented fundus.[2]

SLIT LAMP

Slit Lamp with a Hruby Lens

A high-minus Hruby lens is usually available with most slit lamps. This technique requires dilated pupils and a cooperative patient. The advantage of this technique over the direct ophthalmoscope is stereopsis, which facilitates the appreciation of the contour of the disc. Corneal contact is not required (Fig. 4.2).

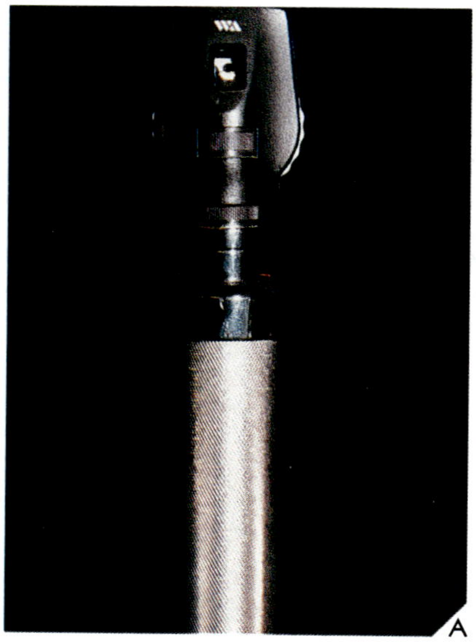

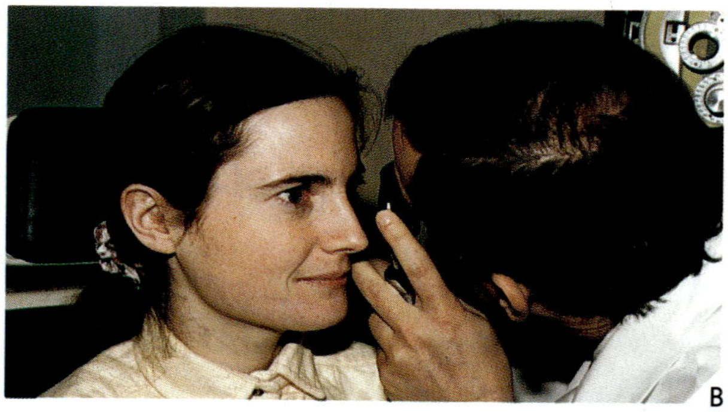

4.1 | *A:* Direct ophthalmoscope. *B:* Examination of patient with direct ophthalmoscope.

Slit Lamp with a Contact Lens

A Goldmann, Zeiss, or similar contact lens (see below) can be used to visualize the optic nerve. Again, stereopsis is an advantage and the examiner has greater control of the eye because the lens is in contact with the cornea. However, disc photography will be compromised after this examination. Alternatively, these high-minus lenses can be used without contacting the cornea, analogous to the Hruby lens (Fig. 4.3).

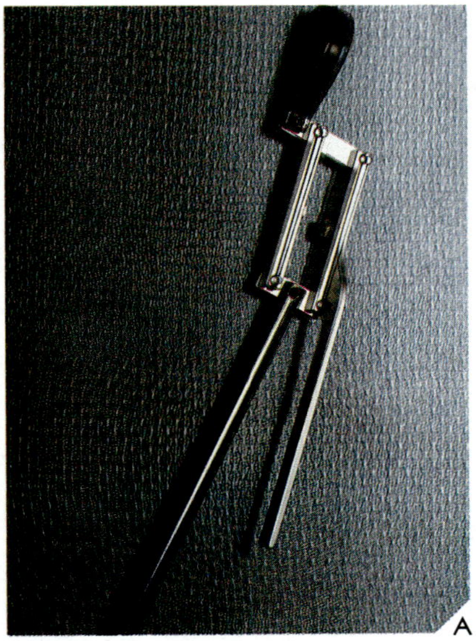

A

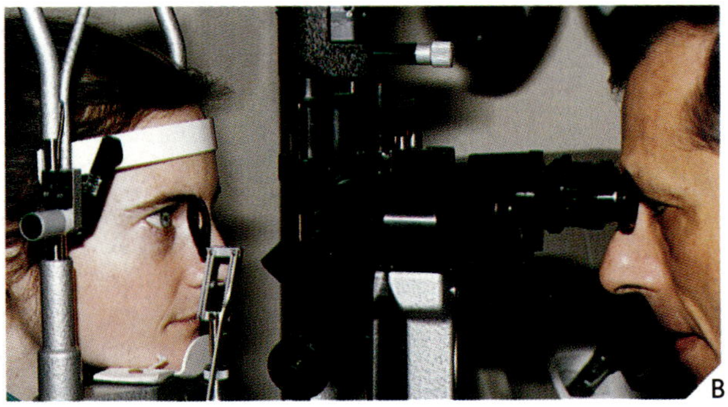

B

4.2 | *A:* Hruby lens. *B:* Examination of patient with slit lamp and Hruby lens.

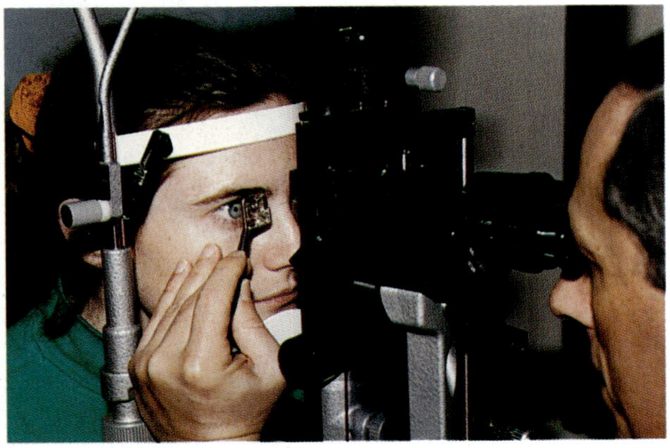

4.3 | Examination of patient with Zeiss lens, without contacting the cornea.

Slit Lamp with a High-Power Convex Lens

A +60, +78, or +90 diopter lens offers a three-dimensional view without requiring corneal contact; however, the image is inverted and dilation of the pupils may be necessary (Fig. 4.4).

INDIRECT OPHTHALMOSCOPY

Because of the low magnification, indirect ophthalmoscopy is generally an undesirable method for carefully evaluating the optic nerve head.

DOCUMENTATION

After examining the optic nerve, it is extremely important to document the appearance so that comparisons can be made in the future. As noted earlier, the cup-to-disc ratio is an imprecise method of describing the nerve. More specific observations are more helpful, particularly relating to the appearance of the neuroretinal rim. A sketch of the nerve is more helpful than a cup-to-disc ratio. However, the best method is stereophotography of the optic disc. These photographs should be included in the patient's chart and compared to examinations in the future. If there is a question in the clinician's mind regarding changes, photographs can be repeated. It is sometimes easier to note disc changes by comparing photographs taken at different times. Photographs should be repeated periodically.

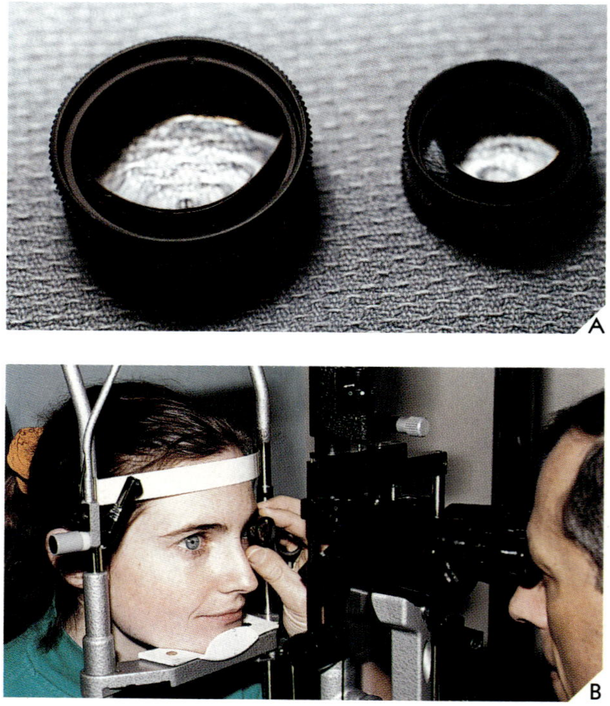

4.4 | *A:* +60 (left) and +90 (right) diopter lenses. *B:* Examination of patient with slit lamp and +90 diopter lens.

Section II

Optic Nerve Photography

Bernard Schwartz

THE NEED FOR PHOTOGRAPHY

Observations of the optic disc have been classically performed with the direct ophthalmoscope. With the introduction of fundus cameras, objective recordings of the optic nerve head and fundus could be obtained.[3] Photography allows the archival storage of an image which can be evaluated or measured by different observers and used as a baseline for observing or recording further changes in a patient, especially with progression of the disease. A number of fundus cameras have been commercially available for the last few decades. Their clinical use has constantly increased, so that photography of the optic nerve has become a standard clinical procedure.[4–6]

Large variations can occur between experienced observers in their evaluation of the optic disc, particularly using the direct ophthalmoscope and evaluating optic disc photographs in glaucomatous eyes.[7,8] Furthermore, observations that are fairly obvious, such as optic disc hemorrhages, can be missed frequently (Fig. 4.5). Review of optic disc photographs indicates optic disc hemorrhages that were missed with observation by direct ophthalmoscopy.[9–11]

Photography is particularly important when a patient is moving to another geographic location. In such cases it is appropriate for the ophthalmologist to supply photographs to the ophthalmologist who will now care for the patient, particularly the initial and most recent photographs of the optic disc.

FUNDUS CAMERAS

Photographs of the optic disc can be obtained as single photographs or as stereophotographs under a variety of conditions.[4–6] Single photographs are usually taken with the disc centered in about a 30° field. Increased magnification can be utilized so that the disc occupies almost the entire frame (see Fig. 4.5). Photographs are usually taken with fairly high resolution color film, such as ASA 25 or 64, and are mounted as 35-mm transparencies or slides. High-resolution black and white film can be used for nerve fiber layer photography[12–15] (see Airaksinen, this chapter and in Chapter 6), and Polaroid® film for slides and prints. For florescein angiography of the optic disc, high-resolution black and white film is also used[16] (Fig. 4.6).

Stereophotographs of the optic disc can be taken in either a nonsimultaneous or a sequential mode in time, or as simultaneous stereophotographs. Sequential stereophotographs involve shifting the camera between photographs so that the photographs are taken at different angles.

Obtaining simultaneous stereophotographs involves taking both photographs at the same instant at a fixed angle. Fundus cameras can be designed so that two optical light paths are present, each obtaining an image at a different angle.[17,18] Simultaneous stereophotographs can also be obtained by the use of a twin set of prisms mounted in front of a fundus camera.[19] When sequential stereophotographs are obtained, a number of artifacts can occur, particularly eye movements between photographs. As a result, a set of sequential photographs is not reproducible from one instance to another for observing and measuring the optic disc.[20]

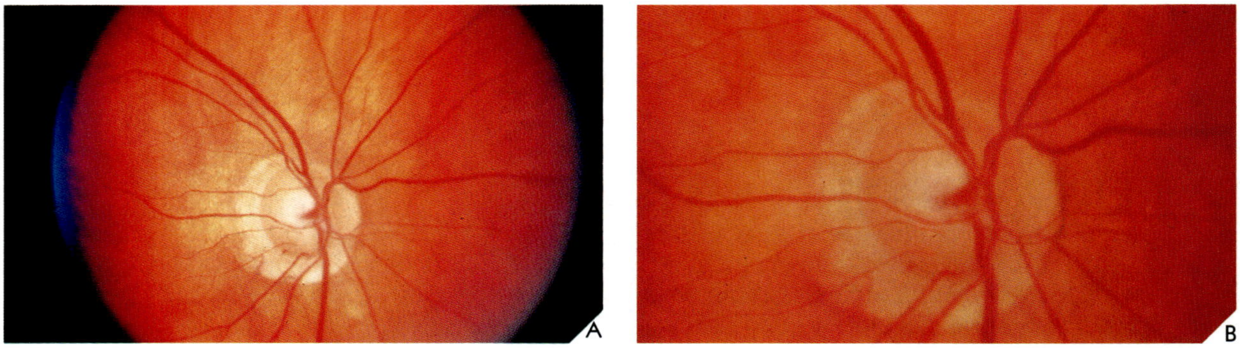

4.5 | *A:* Barely noticeable optic disc hemorrhage at 7 o'clock in photograph taken without 2x magnification lens. *B:* Same optic disc photographed with 2x magnification lens, showing a more visible disc hemorrhage.

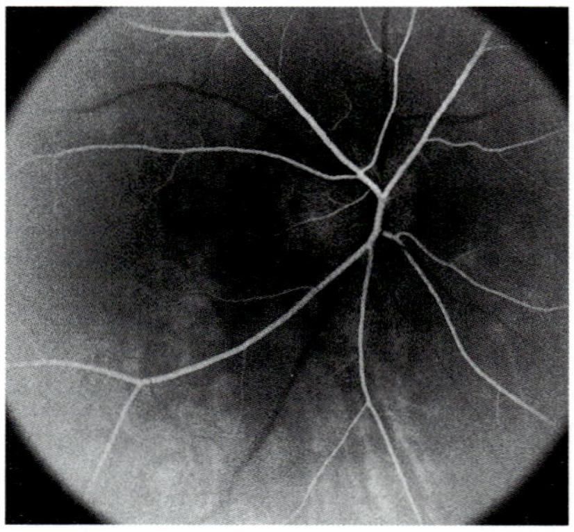

4.6 | Fluorescein angiogram of optic disc. Photograph is in retinal arterial phase, showing filling defect of optic disc superiorly.

For fluorescein angiography of the optic disc, any camera that has fluorescein capability and the appropriate interference filters can be used.[16]

OBTAINING AND USING PHOTOGRAPHS CLINICALLY

Photographs of the optic disc are best obtained with widely dilated pupils. Pupil diameters of 5 mm or more are required. The application of 2.5% phenylephrine drops plus 1% tropicamide drops is usually sufficient to obtain adequate enlargement of the pupil. However, several applications of the drops may be necessary. Ten percent phenylephrine drops should be avoided, particularly in elderly patients, because of possible systemic side effects.[21] The most detailed high-resolution photographs are obtained when the corneal surface is as smooth as possible. Therefore, procedures other than applanation tonometry, such as gonioscopy, should be avoided before obtaining optic disc photographs. If there has been excessive damage to the corneal epithelium, particularly with excessive fluorescein staining, as the result of applanation tonometry, adequate photographs of the disc may not be obtainable.

When the ocular pressures are markedly elevated, it may not be appropriate to dilate the patient's pupils, because even with an open angle 1% tropicamide drops may further elevate the pressure to a considerable degree.[22] The pupils should especially not be dilated when angle-closure glaucoma is suspected. When ocular pressures are elevated, one should determine by gonioscopy if the angle is open before dilation of the pupil.

Optic disc photographs should be taken of every patient in whom the diagnosis of glaucoma is suspected or confirmed on the initial examination. Color photographs are most useful. They should be taken at a similar magnification, preferably with a 2x magnification lens to obtain greater details (see Fig. 4.5). If a simultaneous stereofundus camera is available, then simultaneous stereophotographs should also be obtained at the same examination. It is preferable to obtain several photographs of each type, to compensate for errors (e.g., inadequate exposure, eye movements, poor focus).

The disc should always be centered on the film frame, as there is more distortion at the periphery of the film.[23] The focus of the camera should be on the surface of the disc for relatively small cups. However, when cups are relatively deep, the photographer may need to take several photographs focused at different depths (Fig. 4.7). If only one set of photographs is

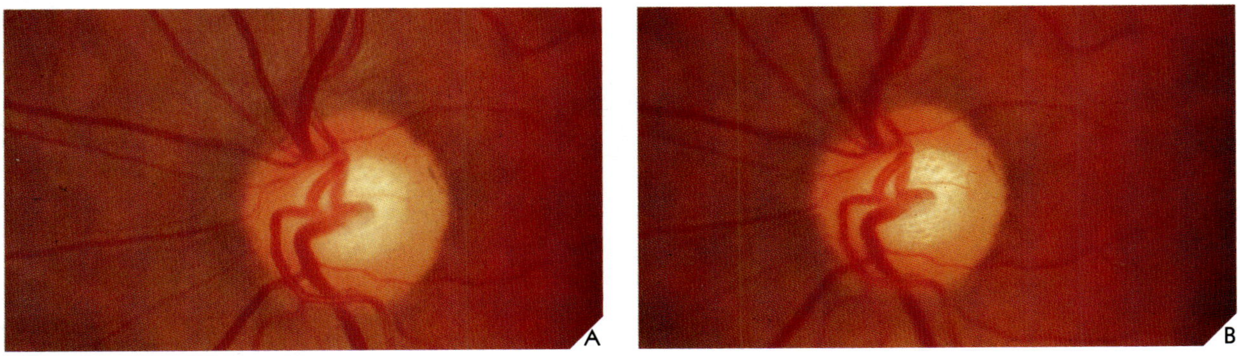

4.7 | *A:* Photograph of optic disc taken with focus on surface of disc; lamina cribrosa is barely visible. *B:* Same optic disc as in *A* but photograph taken with focus on bottom of cup; details of lamina cribrosa are clear.

obtained, they should be focused about halfway between the bottom and the top of the cup.

Photographs of the optic disc for a patient with glaucoma or suspect glaucoma should be repeated at intervals of 1 to 2 years. When photographs are returned from development, mounted as 35-mm slides, the slides should be labeled with the patient's name, date, and eye, as well as with other appropriate information such as medical record number or date of birth. Photographs of both right and left eyes can be stored in plastic sleeves, labeled for that particular date, and filed with the patient's chart. Storing of the photographs in plastic sleeve folders allows them to be examined on an X-ray viewbox in the clinical examination room with the 20- or 30-diopter retinal fundus lens (Fig. 4.8) or a stereoviewer.

When a patient returns for a follow-up examination of the optic disc, the photographs should be reviewed. The appearance of the optic nerve, as evaluated with the direct ophthalmoscope or the slit-lamp biomicroscope, should then be compared with the previous photographs. The clinical examination and recent set of photographs should be particularly compared with the earliest photographs to determine if any change has occurred.

For more detailed review of the photographs, two slide projectors should be set up. The left-hand screen should show the first (baseline) photograph, and the right-hand screen subsequent photographs obtained of the optic disc. The baseline or earliest photographs and the follow-up photographs can thus be compared side by side in great detail under high magnification to detect any change.

Appropriate stereoviewers are available for observing photographs obtained with simultaneous or sequential stereo cameras. It is difficult to compare stereophotographs by projection unless special stereo projectors are available and appropriate Polaroid® or red and green glasses are utilized. Such stereoprojection is utilized for research or for detailed teaching purposes.

INTERPRETATION OF PHOTOGRAPHS

The availability of photographs allows the detection of optic disc abnormalities. In two-dimensional photographs this would require an evaluation of the area of cupping as designated by the bend of the vessels over the edge of the cup, and the area of pallor as determined by the area of color contrast compared with the color of the rim of the optic disc or the retina.[24] Other abnormal signs can be observed, such as localized thinning of the disc rim, under-

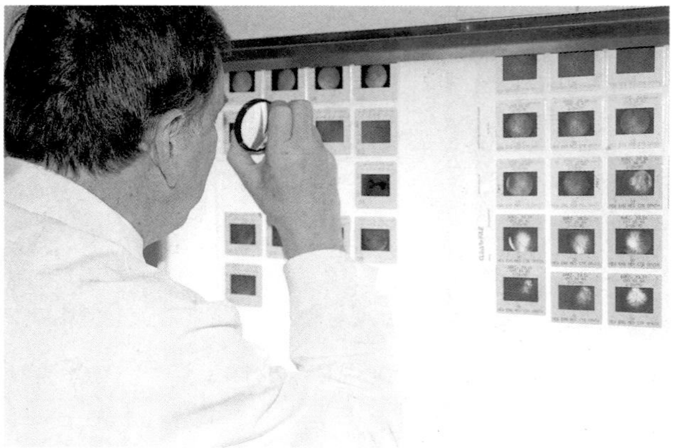

4.8 | Evaluation of optic disc photographs with 20-diopter lens. Photographs are mounted in plastic slide holders and placed on viewboxes in examining room, for comparison with ophthalmoscopic examination of the patient.

mining of the cup edge, and shifting of the vessels nasally. Asymmetry within or between discs for cupping and pallor (i.e., extension of cupping and pallor more superiorly or inferiorly) is a particularly useful sign[25–27] (Fig. 4.9). Disc hemorrhage is also an important sign, because the probability of visual field loss appears to increase with the presence of disc hemorrhages.[28] Occasionally, with a more pigmented fundus, retinal nerve fiber layer defects can be detected, with or without disc hemorrhages (Fig. 4.10). The presence of the lamina cribrosa in the photograph depends on the depth of the cup and also on the focus of the photograph. A photograph obtained by focusing on the surface of the disc will provide an inadequate estimate of the depth of the cup, as indicated by the absence of the appearance of the lamina cribrosa (see Fig. 4.7).

Stereophotographs are especially helpful in evaluating the amount of cupping in relation to the pallor of the disc. Some investigators also use stereophotographs routinely in determining retinal nerve fiber layer loss.[29]

In evaluating changes over time, the ophthalmologist should particularly look for extension of cupping, especially in a vertical direction, with resultant narrowing of the disc rim.[26,27] Increase in cupping may be more obvious as an increasing shift of the retinal vessels nasally with a narrowing of the nasal disc rim. Other changes may occur, such as increasing asymmetry of cupping and pallor between right and left discs, especially if asymmetry was present previously. New disc hemorrhages will also be apparent, because they come and go over time.[11] On fluorescein angiography of the

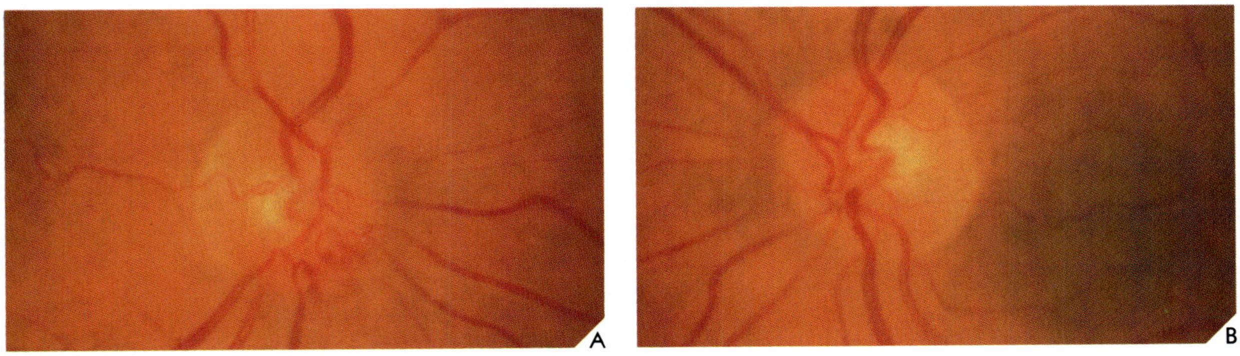

4.9 | Optic disc photograph of right eye *(A)* and left eye *(B)* in same patient shows asymmetry of cupping and pallor.

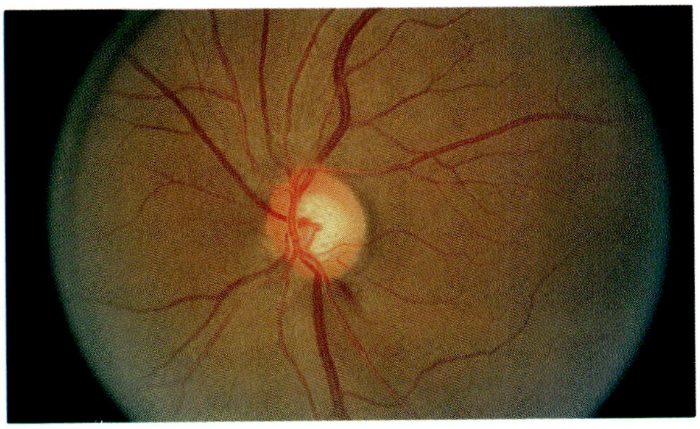

4.10 | Optic disc photograph shows hemorrhage at disc rim at 5 o'clock, associated with wedge-shaped retinal nerve fiber layer defect.

optic disc, the presence of absolute filling defects, i.e., areas that do not fill in the arterial phase and remained unfilled throughout the fluorescein angiogram, may increase with time [30] (Fig. 4.11).

Because areas of cupping and pallor and neuroretinal rim area are correlated with disc size or area,[31–33] some estimate should be obtained of the disc size during direct ophthalmoscopy and when viewing optic disc photographs. This can be done by planimetry of the disc from a projected photograph and calculation of the disc area in conjunction with determination of the patient's refractive error, using the formula of Bengsston and Krakau,[34] or, for more precision, using Littmann's magnification correction formulae.[35] A small disc may exhibit very little cupping and pallor but may still show visual field loss. A large disc, however, may show substantial cupping and pallor with relatively little or no visual field abnormality (Fig. 4.12).

For fluorescein angiography of the optic disc, the usual precautions should be taken before fluorescein is administered. In particular, fluorescein injection should not be done when there is a history of reaction to fluorescein, multiple significant drug or other types of allergies, or significant cerebrovascular or cardiovascular disease. The side effects of and the reactions to fluorescein injections have been well documented.[36] Appropriate drugs and equipment should be available in the photography area to treat any significant reactions to fluorescein.

To perform fluorescein angiography of the optic disc, sequences of photographs at intervals of 0.75 second or less are obtained. The first photograph should be taken about 15 seconds after completion of the fluorescein

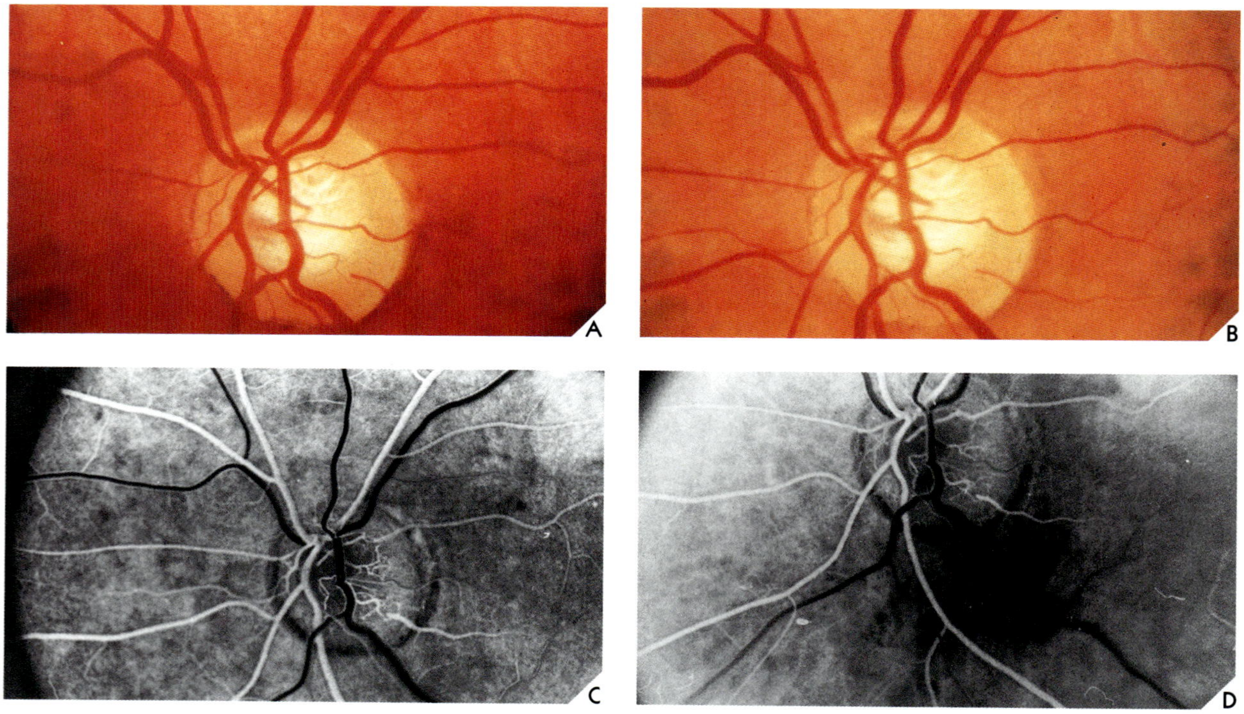

4.11 | Increase in area of fluorescein defect in ocular hypertensive eye without apparent change of disc or loss of visual field. *A,B:* Color photographs of optic disc on 3/6/79 *(A)* and 2/2/82 *(B)*. *C,D:* Early retinal arteriovenous phase of fluorescein angiograms on 3/6/79 *(C)* and 2/2/82 *(D)*, show further drop-out of vessels during the three-year interval.[30]

injection. A set of 20 early photographs, and several at about 20 minutes after the injection, should be obtained. The latter will identify any leakage of dye at the disc, indicating increased vascular permeability. Leakage can also be observed at locations of absolute fluorescein angiographic defects.[37,38]

OTHER MEANS OF OBTAINING IMAGES OF THE OPTIC NERVE

In addition to photographic films, video images can be obtained of the optic nerve, particularly during fluorescein angiography.[39] Instruments are also available for obtaining images from which measurements can be made.[40] Such instruments as the Rodenstock Optic Nerve Head Analyzer, the Topcon ImageNet, which utilizes a Topcon simultaneous fundus camera, and the Humphrey Retinal Analyzer use high-resolution CCD cameras to provide simultaneous images. A scanning laser ophthalmoscope that can provide a digital image has also been developed.[41] In general, images obtained with video tape may not have the same resolution as film images; however, images obtained with CCD cameras are usually equivalent in resolution to those obtained by film.

MEASUREMENTS OF PHOTOGRAPHS AND IMAGES OBTAINED BY INSTRUMENTS

Images obtained by photographs can be measured as single photographs for optic disc pallor[42] and retinal vessel width,[43] and as simultaneous stereophotographs for retinal nerve fiber layer thickness[44] and optic nerve cupping (volume, depth, area, and slope).[45] Images obtained by instruments are used to measure cup volume, area, depth, pallor density, and nerve fiber layer contour and thickness.[40,46] Studies are being pursued to determine the clinical usefulness of these techniques (see Weinreb and Caprioli, this chapter, and in Chapter 6).

SUMMARY AND CONCLUSION

Evaluation of the optic disc is only one facet of the evaluation of the patient for glaucoma. However, images of the optic disc provide an objective record that is probably less variable than the measurement of intraocular pressure or the evaluation of the visual field. Images of the optic disc provide a reference baseline for following patients and can be archived for comparison over time.

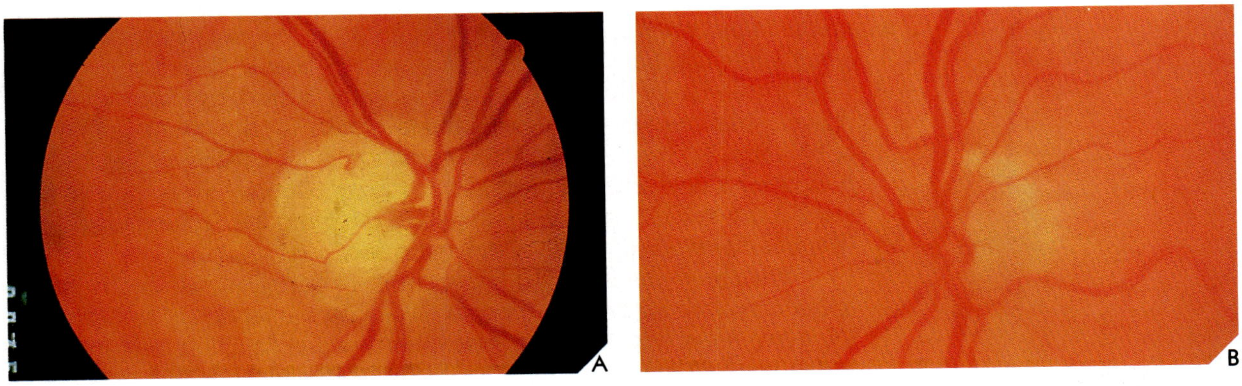

4.12 | *A:* Large disc (3.95 mm^2) with large area of cupping and pallor in ocular hypertensive eye without visual field loss. *B:* Small disc (1.39 mm^2) in a glaucomatous eye with visual field loss but essentially no cupping and pallor.

SECTION III

FUNDUSCOPY AND PHOTOGRAPHY OF THE RETINAL NERVE FIBER LAYER

Anja Tuulonen
P. Juhani Airaksinen

NORMAL RETINAL NERVE FIBER LAYER

The retinal nerve fiber layer (RNFL) is formed by the ganglion cell axons and represents the innermost layer of the fundus. It is separated from the vitreous by the internal limiting membrane. The retinal ganglion cell axons conduct visual information from the photoreceptors to the next synapse, in the lateral geniculate body.

In the retina the axons are spread out as a thin layer and appear as opaque striations (axon bundles) located in glial tunnels formed by Müller cells[47] (Figs. 4.13 and 4.14). Papillomacular bundles have an almost straight horizontal course, whereas the upper and lower temporal fibers form an arch around the macula and are bounded by the temporal raphe. Nasal nerve fiber bundles proceed radially to the optic disc.

The three-dimensional organization of ganglion cell axons in the retina may vary in different primate species. In humans, it is probable that the nerve fibers originating from peripheral retinal ganglion cells are closer to the pigment epithelium and are located peripherally in the optic nerve head. The fibers originating from more proximal ganglion cells traverse them

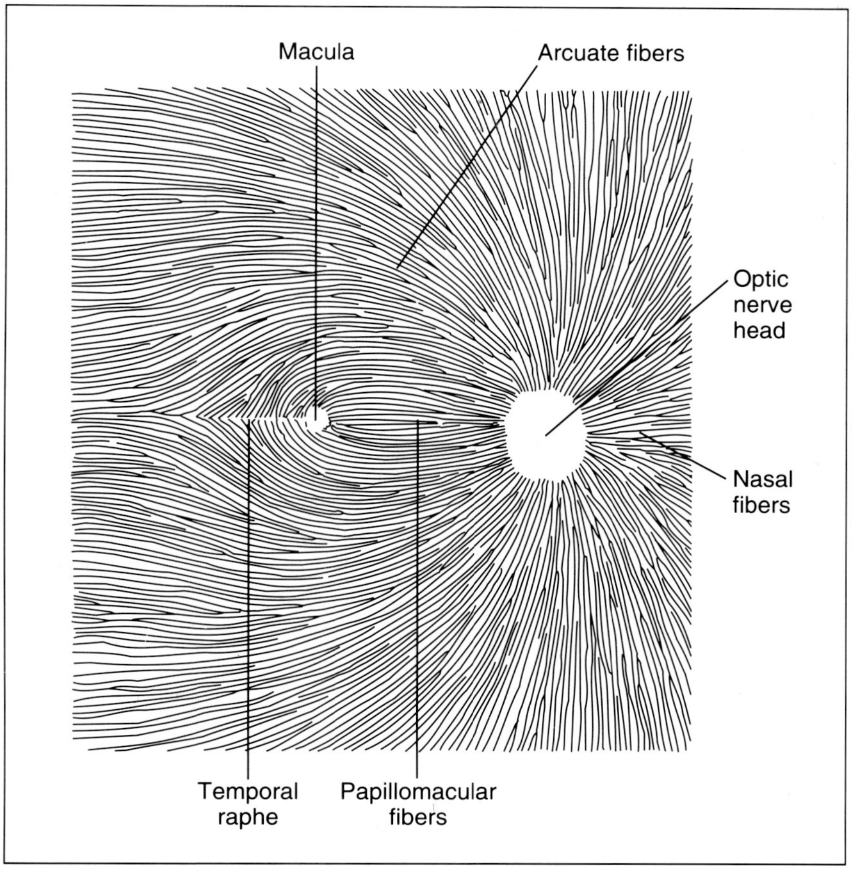

4.13 | Arrangement of axon bundles in the retinal nerve fiber layer.

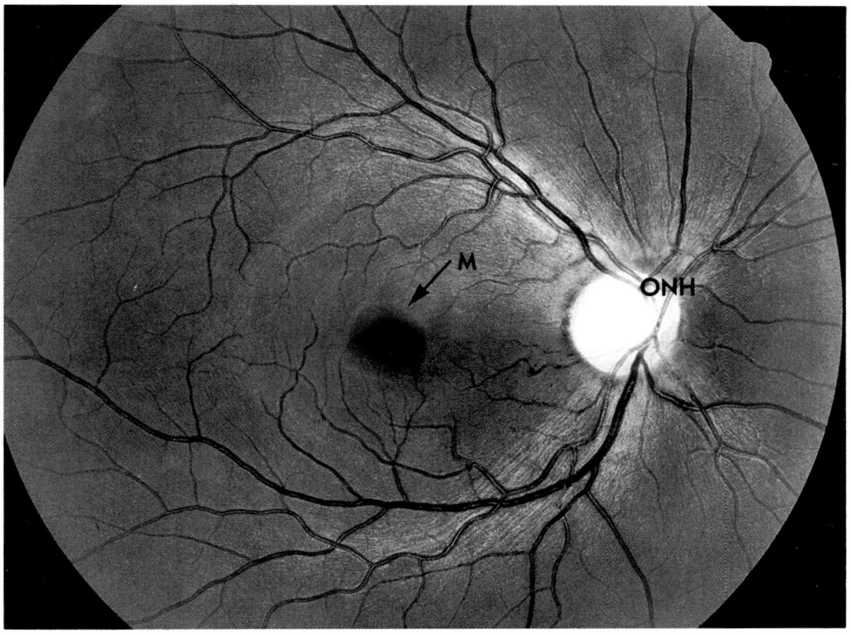

4.14 | Normal retinal nerve fiber layer (fundus photograph). Note prominence of superior and inferior arcuate fibers. ONH = optic nerve head; M = macula.

and proceed closer to the vitreous and more centrally in the optic nerve head[47–50] (Fig. 4.15).

The thickness of the RNFL increases towards the optic disc (see Fig. 4.15), with the best axon bundle visibility at the upper and lower temporal arcuate regions[51] (see Fig. 4.14). In these areas the RNFL is up to 300 µm thick and the nerve fiber bundles contain several axons per bundle.[52] The nerve fibers are more difficult to visualize in the nasal and papillomacular area (see Fig. 4.14) where the nerve fiber layer thickness is only one fifth of that in the upper and lower temporal regions. In nasal and papillomacular areas the striations consist of one axon per nerve bundle.

At the optic disc the axons bend backwards approximately 90°, pass through the scleral canal, and form the neuroretinal rim of the optic nerve head (Fig. 4.16). Optic disc cupping represents the area that does not contain nerve fibers. The width of the neuroretinal rim and the size of the optic disc cup are dependent on the size of the optic disc itself and on the number of nerve fibers passing through the scleral canal.

RETINAL NERVE FIBER LAYER PHOTOGRAPHY

Photographic documentation of the RNFL findings is essential for the diagnosis and follow-up of glaucoma. The thin and subtle structure of the RNFL becomes visible in the photographs because light reflects back from the nerve fiber bundles and separating glial septa (Fig. 4.17). In defective areas the light is absorbed by the underlying pigment epithelium and such areas therefore appear darker and more monotonous, as they show fewer fine details.[53]

The visibility of different retinal layers can be enhanced by changing the filters of the fundus camera.[54] Longer wavelengths give better visualization of the deeper retinal layers, while shorter wavelengths are reflected back

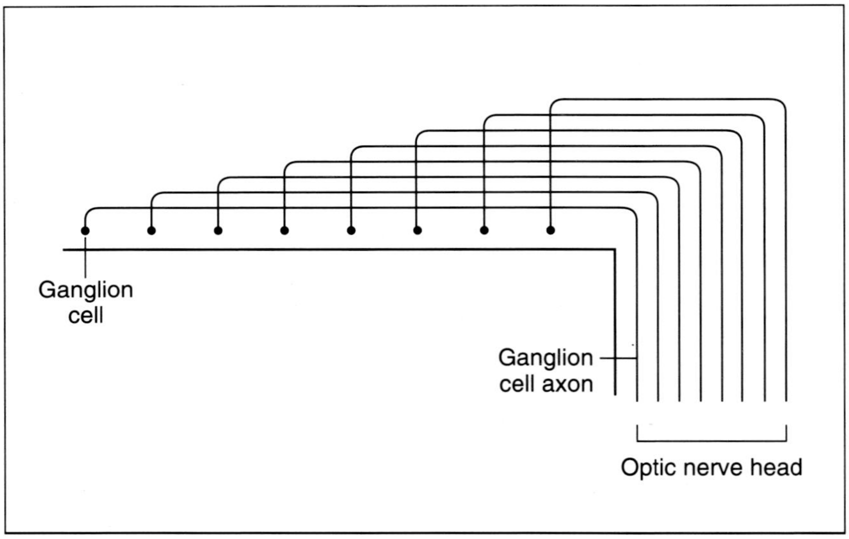

4.15 | Three-dimensional structure of the RNFL. RNFL thickness increases with proximity to optic nerve head. (From Airaksinen PJ, Alanko HI: Effect of retinal nerve fibre loss on the optic nerve head configuration in early glaucoma. *Graefe's Arch Clin Exp Ophthalmol 1983;220:193–196.* Copyright Springer-Verlag, Heidelberg.)

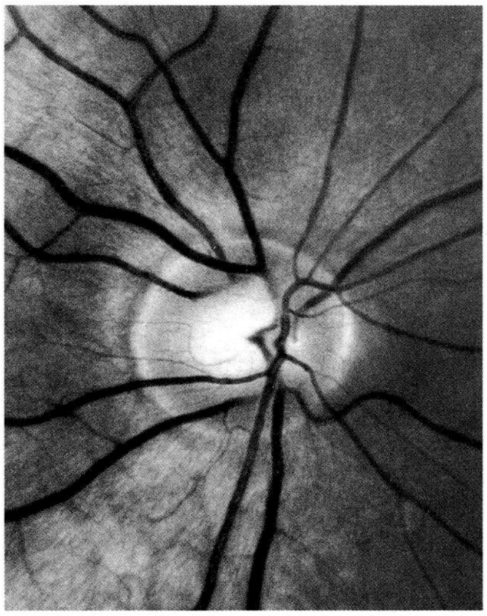

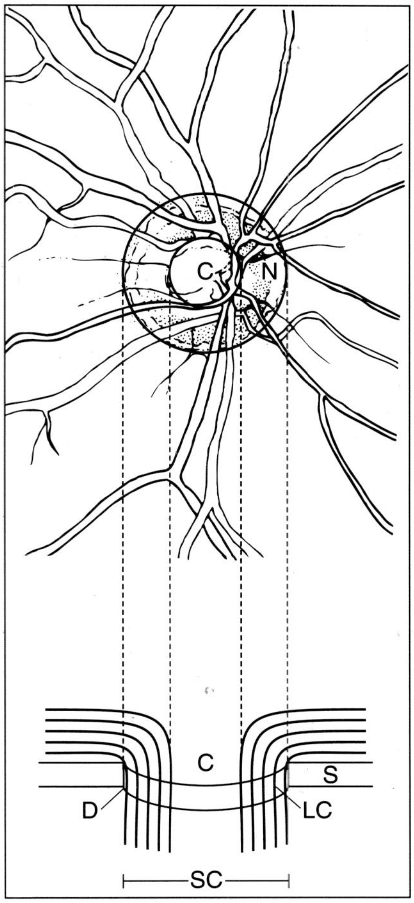

4.16 | The nerve fibers form the neuroretinal rim of the optic nerve head. N = neuroretinal rim; C = optic disc cupping; S = sclera; SC = scleral canal; LC = lamina cribrosa; D = optic disc margin.

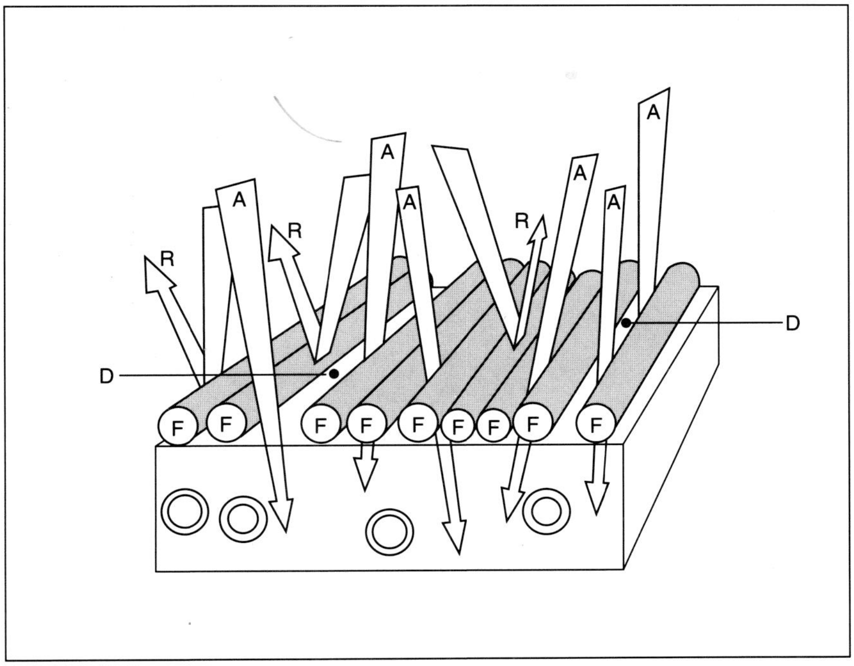

4.17 | Reflection of light from retinal nerve fibers. R = reflected light; A = absorbed light; F = retinal nerve fiber bundle; D = RNFL defect.

from the superficial layers (Fig. 4.18). Therefore, the blue, narrow-band interference filter (peak transmittance at 495 nm) is best suited for RNFL photography.[55,56] With this filter, the best results have been obtained using low-sensitivity, high-resolution black and white film. This technique was used in the RNFL photographs of this chapter. Other wavelengths and films have also been used successfully.[54,56] Photographs can also be taken as color slides, using white light, and then reproduced on black and white film through a green filter.[53,57]

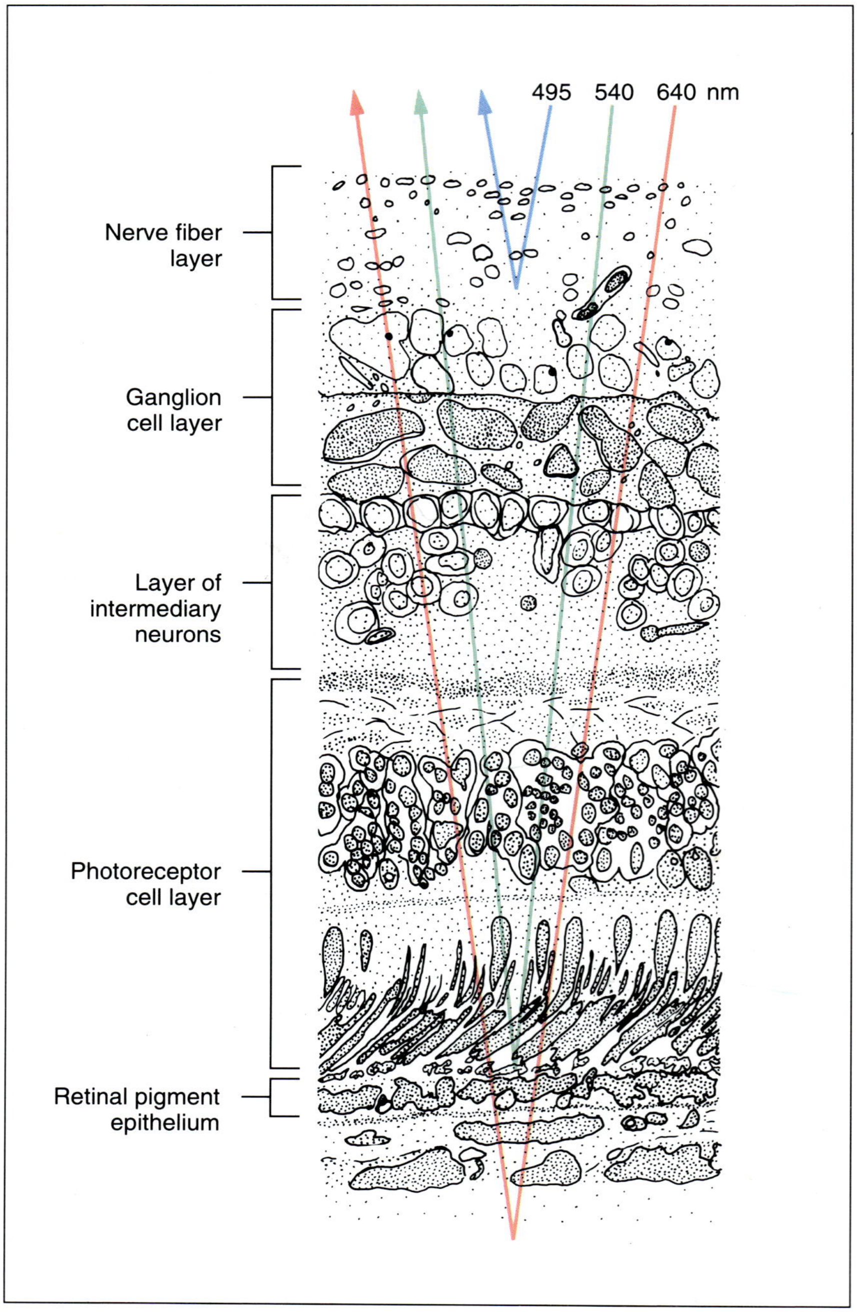

4.18 | Reflection of different wavelengths of light from the retinal layers. Because shorter wavelengths are reflected from the superficial layers, blue light is most suitable for RNFL visualization and photography.

With the wide-angle fundus camera, proper dilatation of the pupil is essential. Therefore, patients should be instructed to interrupt miotics for a day or two before photography. It is important that IOP not be measured with fluorescein before photography, because the fluorescein exciter filter used for photography would lead to a gray, poor-contrast image.

RNFL FUNDUSCOPY

The retinal nerve fiber layer can also be made visible during funduscopy (Fig. 4.19). With the white light of an ophthalmoscope (Fig. 4.19B), the healthy nerve fiber bundles are seen best as silvery striations at the peripapillary retina. RNFL atrophy appears as a darker red area in which visibility of the normal striation pattern is reduced or missing.[58] The nerve fiber layer and its defects stand out better, however, with green light [59] (Fig. 4.19C). Defective areas now appear as darker green and with less detail than the healthy areas.

With an ophthalmoscope, RNFL evaluation is limited to the peripapillary area. The use of a Volk lens, either 60D or 90D, or a contact lens will give a better binocular overview of the RNFL after dilatation of the pupil. The visibility can be enhanced by adjusting the light of the slit lamp, increasing its width and reducing its height to almost quadratic in shape, and using a very bright light.

RNFL EVALUATION

Wide-angle photography gives an overview of the fundus and the opportunity to identify subtle changes in RNFL density in different areas.[55] It is helpful to compare the visibility of superior and inferior fibers within the same

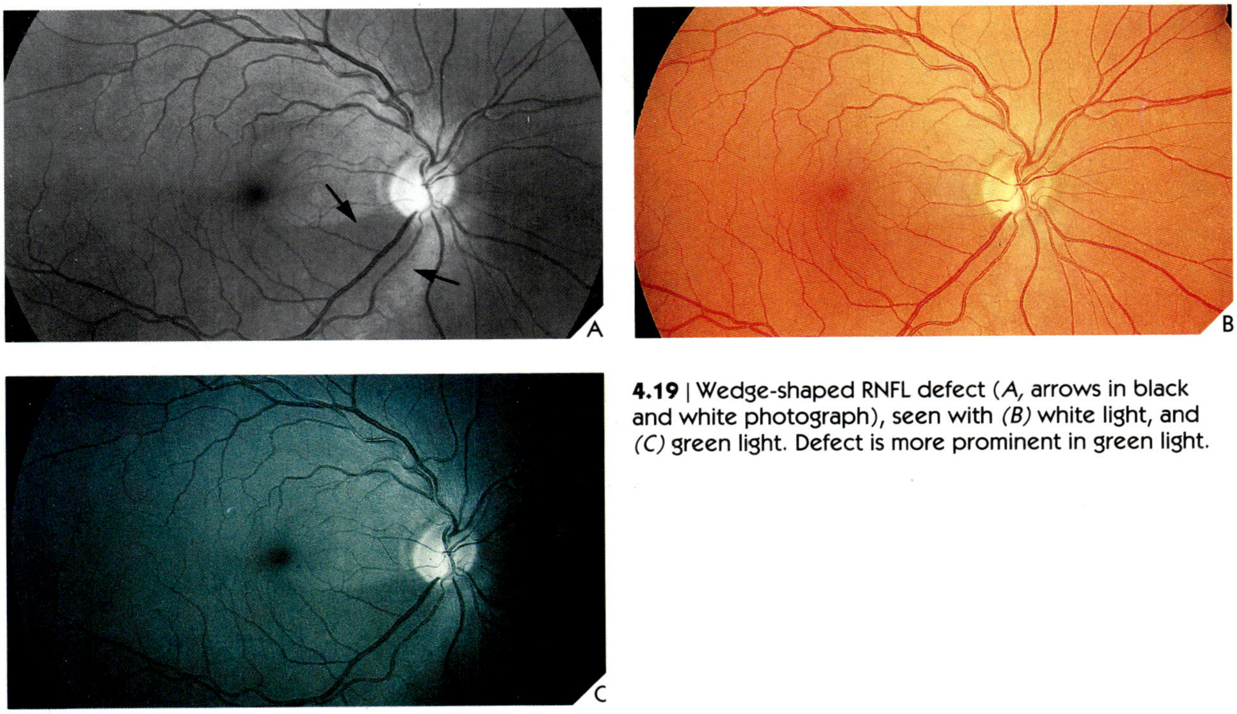

4.19 | Wedge-shaped RNFL defect (*A,* arrows in black and white photograph), seen with *(B)* white light, and *(C)* green light. Defect is more prominent in green light.

eye or, even better, to use the fellow eye for comparison (Fig. 4.20). In addition, the visibility of small blood vessels should be evaluated. In healthy eyes the small blood vessels appear blurred and cross-hatched because they are buried within the thick nerve fiber layer (Fig. 4.21A). Because the nerve fibers are missing in defective areas, the contrast of the naked vessel wall is sharp (Fig. 4.21B).

In addition to wide-angle photography, it is also useful to look at the peripapillary RNFL stereoscopically in optic disc stereophotos taken with a green filter (Kodak Wratten #58) (see Fig. 4.21). In this way both the optic disc and the adjacent RNFL can be observed simultaneously in detail. It is important to note that RNFL photographs taken with a 495-nm filter are unsuitable for optic disc evaluation because the film processing makes the optic disc look pale.

When no nerve fibers are visible in photographs, there are several possibilities to be considered. First, the patient may suffer from advanced loss of nerve fibers due to an eye disease (see Fig. 4.20A). Second, media opacities may obscure the visibility of the nerve fibers. In this case the photograph looks gray and fuzzy rather than dark (compare Fig. 4.22A with Fig. 4.20A). In addition, the large vessel trunks are poorly seen through a cataract (see Fig. 4.22A), whereas in advanced glaucomatous RNFL damage they stand out distinctly (see Fig. 4.20A). Finally, light pigmentation of the fundus (Fig. 4.22B) may also be a reason for poor visibility of nerve fibers, because a darkly pigmented epithelium as a background greatly enhances visibility of the axon bundles.

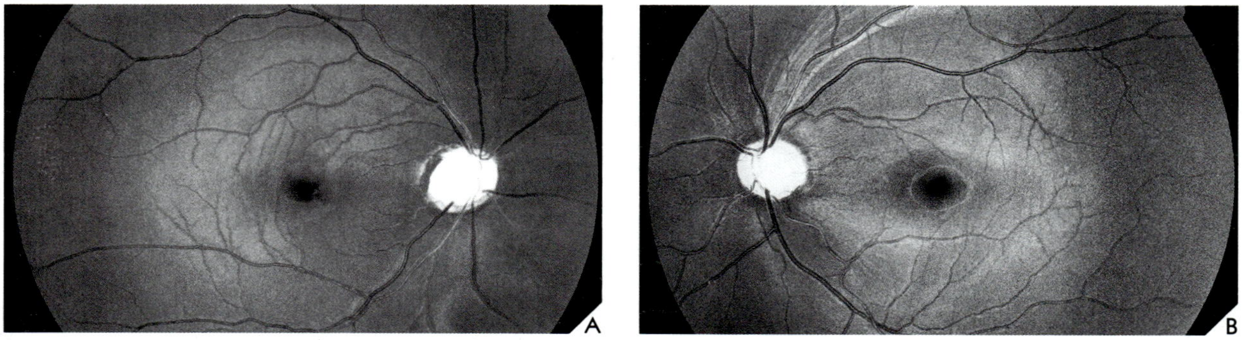

4.20 | RNFL evaluation. *A:* Right eye. Total loss of nerve fibers. Compare the visibility of nerve fibers in the right eye to those of the left. *B:* Left eye. Diffuse and localized RNFL defects. Compare the RNFL appearance in the upper and lower temporal regions of the left eye.

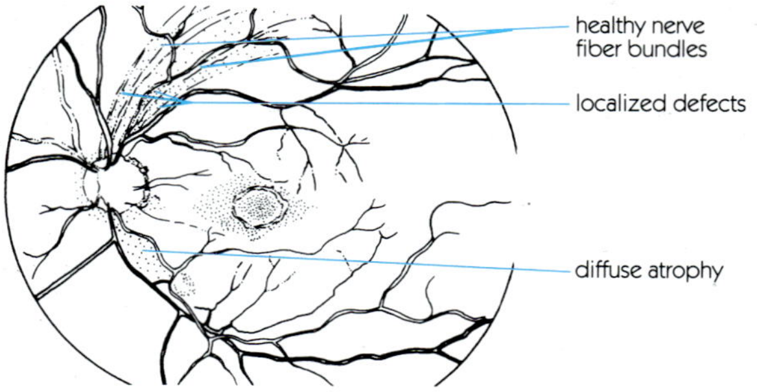

4.21 | Hints for recognizing diffuse RNFL atrophy. *A:* Normal RNFL. *B:* Subtotal RNFL atrophy.

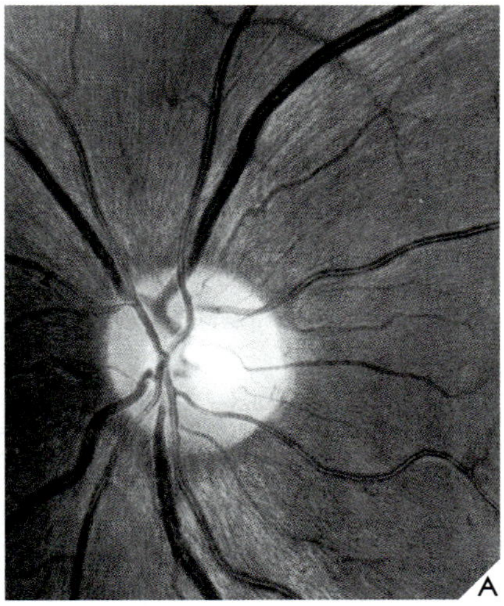

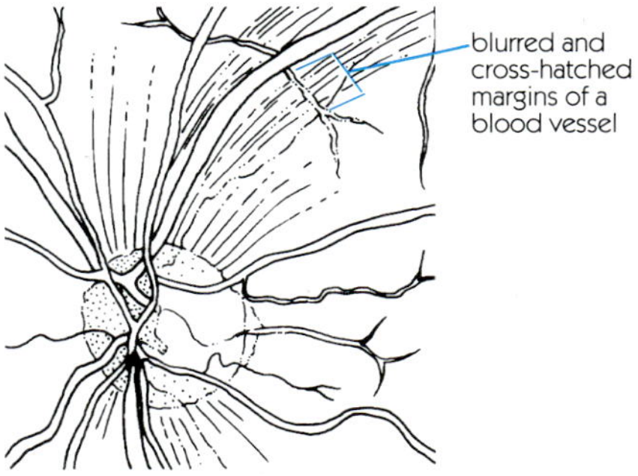

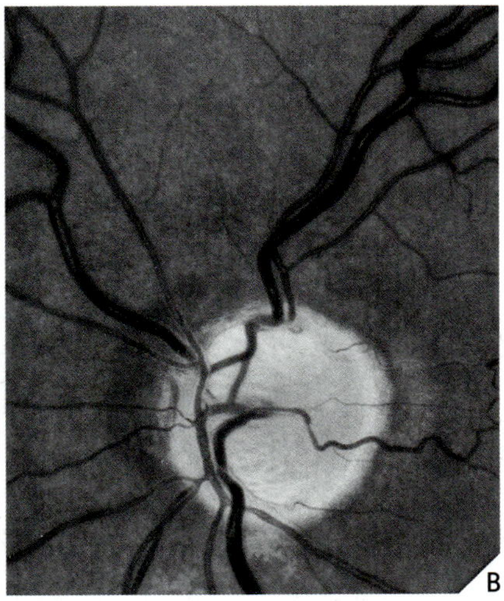

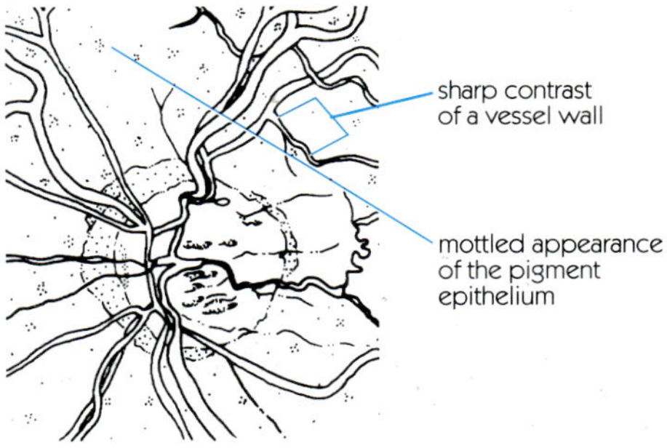

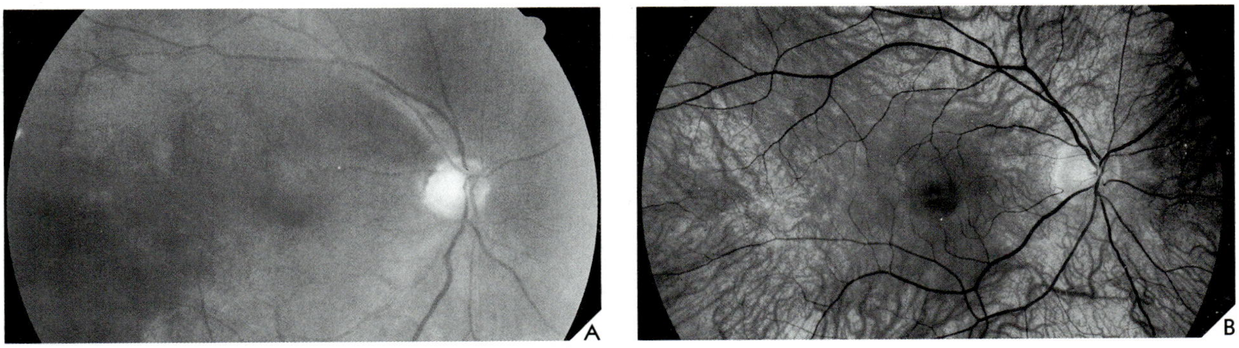

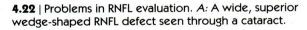

4.22 | Problems in RNFL evaluation. *A:* A wide, superior wedge-shaped RNFL defect seen through a cataract.

B: Poor visibility of RNFL due to lightly pigmented fundus. Normal optic disc.

Section IV

Image Analysis of the Optic Nerve Head and Retinal Nerve Fiber Layer

Robert N. Weinreb
Joseph Caprioli

OPTIC NERVE HEAD

Clinical assessment of optic nerve head size and shape (topography) has been of interest since the introduction of the direct ophthalmoscope over 100 years ago. Cup–disc ratio can be measured with direct ophthalmoscopy, binocular contact lens examination evaluation, and with qualitative or quantitative evaluation of fundus images. Most clinicians record estimates of cup–disc ratio to describe the appearance of the optic nerve head to determine if there is glaucomatous damage. By comparing these estimates with similar measures obtained at previous visits, one can also evaluate whether glaucoma damage is progressive. Although useful, estimates of this structural parameter are subjective and have been shown to have considerable interobserver and intraobserver variability, even when high quality serial stereoscopic optic nerve head photographs are employed.

Diagnosing or excluding the diagnosis of glaucoma is particularly difficult when the nerve head is examined only on a single occasion, because there is considerable overlap in cup–disc ratios among normal, glaucoma suspect, and glaucomatous eyes. Hence, there is a compelling need to define new structural parameters of the optic nerve head for diagnosing and monitoring the progression of glaucoma. In this regard, there has been considerable interest in developing objective measures of optic nerve head topography that delineate normal, glaucomatous suspect, and glaucoma eyes more clearly.

Although several computer-assisted techniques have been developed for quantitating measurements of optic nerve head topography,[60–74] only two will be considered here as representative approaches.

With one technique, fundus images are recorded with an image-intensified video camera.[63–66,72,73] The resulting digitized data are processed by a microcomputer to obtain a topographic map with quantitative depth measurements of the optic nerve head.

For these measurements, parallel stripes are projected on the fundus, some of which overlap an optic nerve head of average diameter, and a simultaneous stereoscopic pair of video images is recorded (Fig. 4.23). Deformations of the stripe patterns contain depth information. The computer selects stereoscopic images in which the vertical stripes are most evenly spaced, and an operator superimposes two pictures to create single-paired images. The computer analyzes disparity between corresponding positions of the bright stripes on the stereoscopic images at various points to generate the topographic map.

To determine the disc margin, the operator places four cardinal points on the television screen with a light pen, and the computer uses this information to fit an ellipse that outlines the disc. The cup margin is then automatically determined by the computer. The cup edge is identified as the locus points, one on each of many radial profiles, which lie a fixed distance (in mm) below and nearest the disc edge. The definition (level) of the cup can be changed by the operator. A series of such points for 360° are connected to create the arbitrary limits of the cup. The computer calculates certain summary parameters, which include: cup–disc ratio; neuroretinal rim area (area between disc margin and cup margin); disc area; cup volume; area of disc elevation; and disc diameter. These measurements are corrected for optical magnification with axial length or keratometric and refractive measurements.

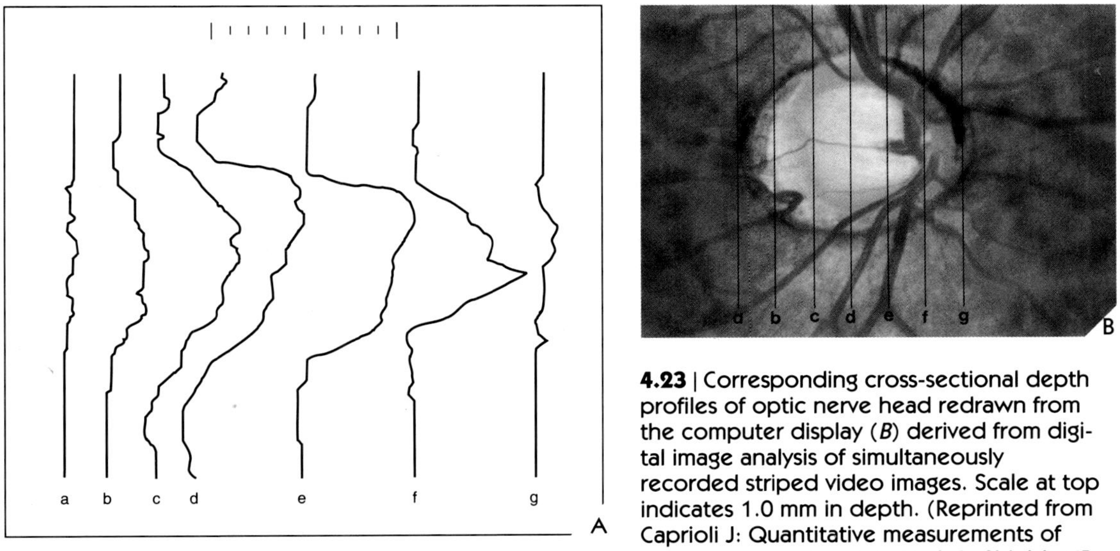

4.23 | Corresponding cross-sectional depth profiles of optic nerve head redrawn from the computer display (*B*) derived from digital image analysis of simultaneously recorded striped video images. Scale at top indicates 1.0 mm in depth. (Reprinted from Caprioli J: Quantitative measurements of the optic nerve head, in Ritch R, Shields MB, Krupin T (eds): *The Glaucomas.* St. Louis: CV Mosby, 1989, 500.)

Although this technique is automated, it is only computer-assisted, because the operator is required to focus and align the images on the video monitor during acquisition and to mark the edge of the disc before analysis. Other limitations include the need for imaging eyes of patients with reasonably clear media (e.g., 20/40 or better) and pupils that can be dilated to 5 mm or more to obtain images suitable for analysis. The greatest source of variability associated with this technique appears to be instrument variability. This relates to obtaining different images of the same eye at different times. The only important nonrandom effect relates to having different observers mark the disc margin.

Another technique which has been developed for quantitating measurements of optic nerve head topography employs the principle of confocal imaging to focus a laser beam on the optic disc and peripapillary retina and measure the reflected light[68,71,74] (Fig. 4.24). This ensures that reflected light is

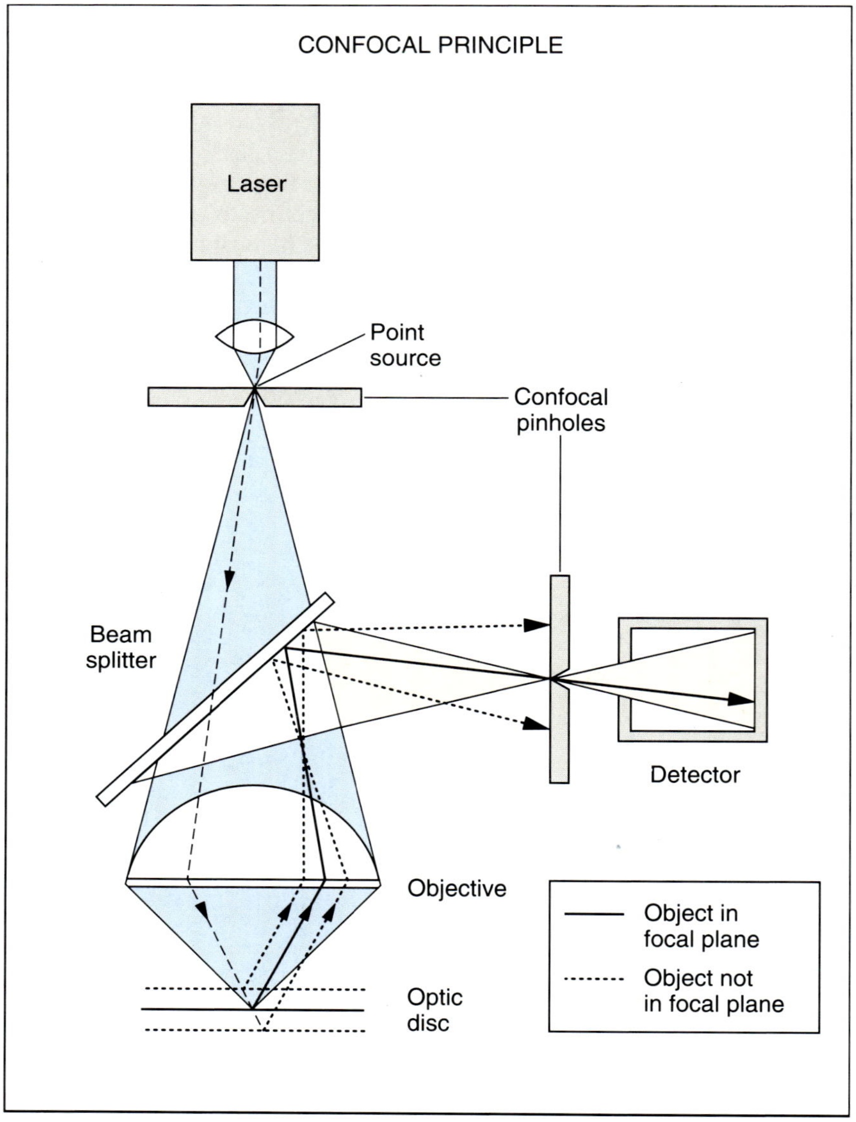

4.24 | Confocal principle: the optics, represented by the objective in this diagram, are moved to change the focal plane. The pinhole remains stationary and always corresponds to the given focal plane. The same illuminating beam also illuminates the out-of-focus plane. However, these are not imaged by the pinhole but are reflected from the aperture. The selected pixel is imaged through the pinhole. By moving the beam across the optic disc and retina using an x–y scanning system, a pixel-by-pixel image is obtained.

detected only when it originates from a very small region around the focal plane of the special optics. Consequently, images with high spatial resolution in all directions are obtained.

The laser beam enters the eye and is focused on a periretinal plane. The beam is moved raster-like across the plane by an x–y scanning system. At each point of the scan, the light reflected is detected confocally and is displayed as one pixel on the video monitor. To measure optic nerve head topography, the focal plane is moved posteriorly at consecutive step-like intervals which can be selected by the operator. The interval between consecutive images can be adjusted (e.g., between 30 and 60 μm). Section images are reduced to include only those pixels at which the reflection is maximum for the designated pixel throughout the image planes. Optic nerve head depth values are calculated from the measurements of confocal reflected light (Fig. 4.25). These values are optically corrected for magnification by

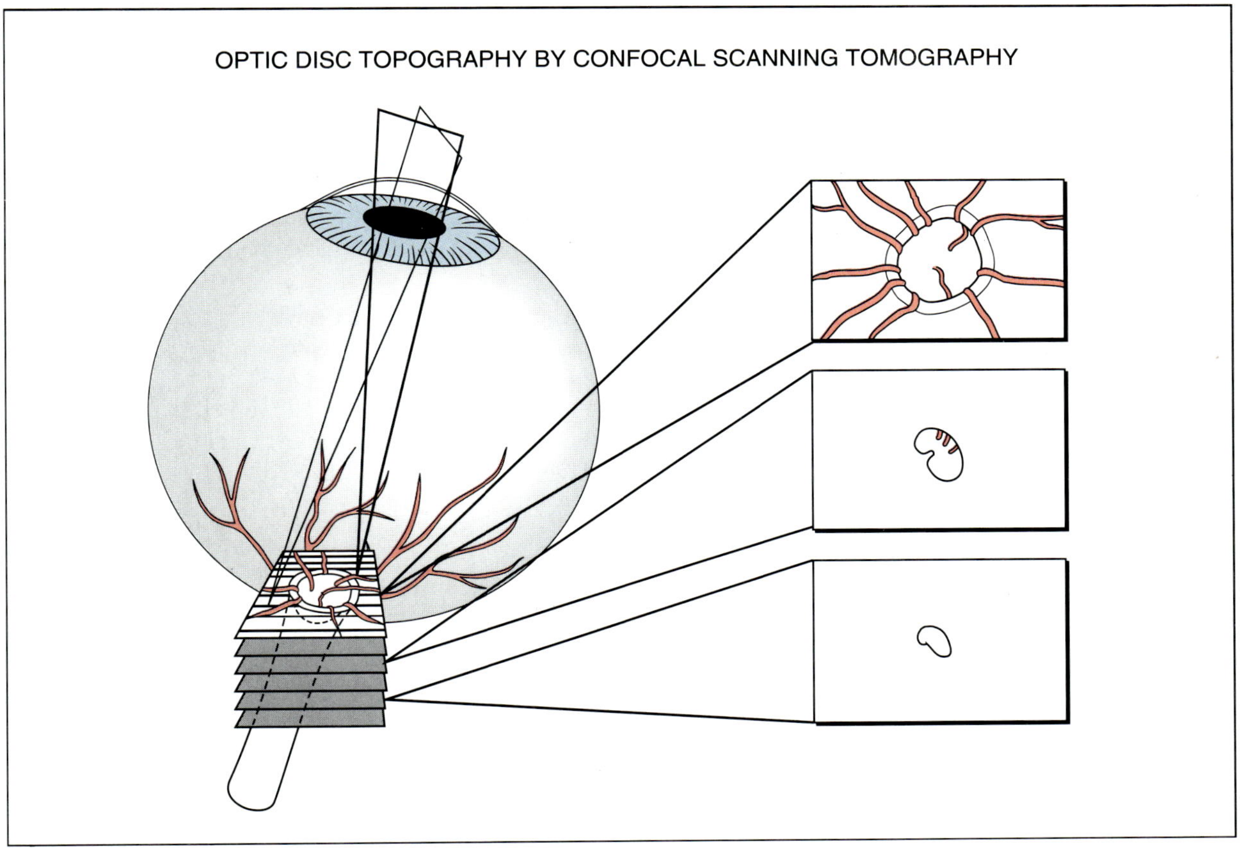

4.25 | Optic nerve head sectioning with retina tomograph (Heidelberg Engineering GmbH, Heidelberg, Germany). To measure optic nerve head topography, the focal plane is moved posteriorly at consecutive stepwise intervals which can be selected by the operator.

normalizing for axial length using keratometric, A-scan ultrasound, or refractive readings. The height of each of 65,536 locations (256 x 256 pixels) is determined. Topographic data are represented by a 16 x 16 matrix of height values, each corresponding to the average height of an array 16 x 16 pixels in the area of interest (Fig. 4.26).

This technique is computer-assisted, because the operator must focus and register the images as well as mark the edge of the optic nerve head. However, compared with other imaging systems for evaluating optic nerve head topography, the retina tomograph may have certain advantages. First, images often can be obtained with miotic pupils less than 2 mm. Second, the clarity of media is not as important as with conventional optical systems. With even small levels of cataractous change, images obtained with these latter systems degrade sufficiently so that useful topographic analysis is not possible. The retina tomographic system employs low light intensity, whereas more conventional optical methods require high light intensities for illumination of the optic nerve head.

Summary

Quantitative structural parameters that conform to descriptions of the optic nerve head employed in clinical practice can be obtained with several computer-assisted imaging instruments. However, these parameters may not be sensitive enough to detect small changes in surface contour of the optic nerve head. With novel structural parameters, such as quantitative serial point-by-point comparisons of surface contour, it may be possible to detect more effectively early structural damage from glaucoma.

RETINAL NERVE FIBER LAYER

Clinical signs describing the optic nerve head have not enabled glaucomatous eyes to be distinguished from normal eyes with sufficient sensitivity and specificity, and there is considerable variability and overlap of these values in normal and glaucomatous populations. Because the retinal nerve fiber layer (RNFL) thickness decreases in glaucoma (see Radius, Chapter 6), objectively measuring the earliest changes in peripapillary retinal nerve fibers might facilitate the diagnosis of glaucoma and improve the ability to assess progressive glaucomatous damage.

Previously, several methods for clinically evaluating the retinal NFL in glaucoma have been reported.[75–82] With both red-free ophthalmoscopy and photography with black and white film, slit-like defects and large wedge-shaped defects of the retinal NFL can be visualized (see Airaksinen, Chapters 4 and 6). These techniques are largely qualitative and lack precision. Although helpful in certain situations, they can be beneficially employed in clinical practice only with considerable experience.

Computerized densitometry of red-free photographs,[76] measurements of retinal thickness obtained with a slit-lamp biomicroscope modified with a green helium–neon laser (543 nm), and contrast enhancement[75] have also been evaluated. Enhancement may facilitate analysis by performing mathematical operations on images to obtain better visibility of features of interest. Although many of these techniques have been available for several years, they have not been widely utilized. This may in part be related to poor image quality and difficulties in compensating for media opacities.

With all of these methods, the NFL appears as a series of striations that emanate from the optic nerve head and spread over the surface of the retina (see Fig. 4.14). In areas where the NFL is thin, each bright striation corresponds to light reflected from a bundle of nerve fibers, and it is possible that each dark striation corresponds to a Müller cell septum separating the bundles. The discrimination of these methods appears to be improved with red-free (green or blue) illumination to enhance the contrast between the NFL and the reddish background of the fundus. However, few quantitative data are available to support these clinical observations.

In the cynomolgus monkey, reflectance of the NFL has been determined by subtracting the reflectance of a spot on the fundus in which the NFL is absent from the reflectance of the adjoining fundus with intact NFL.[78] The NFL is obliterated by photocoagulating a small area near the optic nerve head to cause nerve fiber atrophy. With this model, it has been found that NFL reflectance is relatively constant in red light and rises sharply with blue light. This rise towards the blue suggests Rayleigh scattering (scattering by particles much smaller than the wavelength of light) as the cause of the NFL reflectance. It also suggests that the reflectance spectrum of the NFL is from intracellular organelles rather than from the more obvious axons. NFL reflectance can be characterized by a spectrum that has the same shape at all points along an arcuate region of the NFL but decreases in absolute

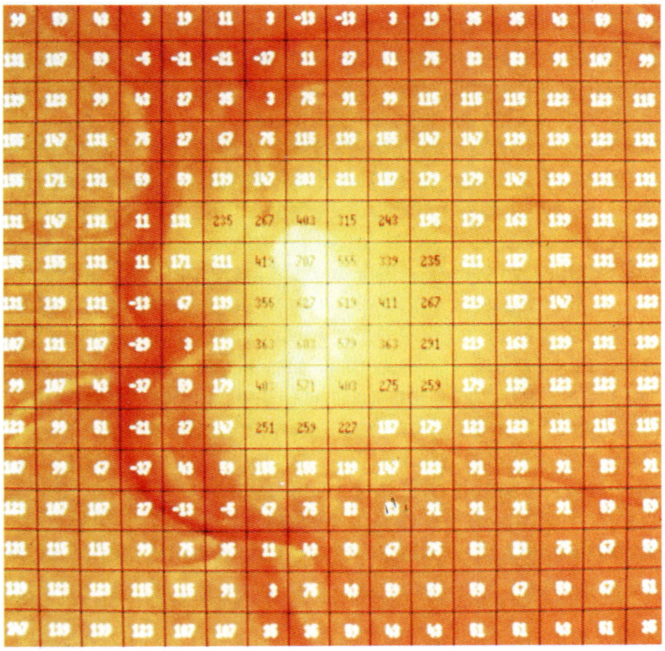

4.26 | Topography of the optic nerve head and peripapillary retina is presented as a matrix of 256 values, each value representing the average of 16 x 16 pixels in the area of interest (256 x 256 total pixels).

reflectance as the thickness of the NFL decreases. These data provide a quantitative understanding of empirically determined methods for enhancing the visibility of the NFL and have implications for retinal densitometry. Two promising techniques for quantitative measurement of the retinal NFL will be discussed.

One approach calculates relative NFL surface height (contour) from magnification-corrected surface contour measurements of the peripapillary retina made with computerized image analysis of simultaneous stereoscopic videographic images.[77,80,81] This technique measures the average height of NFL surface at 64 separate locations (16/quadrant) within a circumference 100 μm outside the disc edge, as detected with narrow-band green light (540 nm), with respect to a standardized reference plane. The heights of three areas of the retinal surface at the periphery of the image (located temporally, inferonasally, and supranasally) are used to construct a standard reference plane to which all images are registered (Fig. 4.27). This plane has a defined height of zero. Positive measurements lie above the plane in negative images and negative measurements lie below. Those portions of the image chosen to construct the retinal reference plane lie away from the normally thick superior and inferior nerve fiber bundles, and are in the most peripheral portion of the usable image. When these measurements are plotted against location, the resultant profile has a typical double-hump configuration in normal eyes. The elevations at the superior and inferior locations correspond to the thick areas of NFL at the superior and inferior poles of the disc.

Another approach employs a technique known as Fourier ellipsometry to measure the thickness of the retinal NFL.[79] This method is based on the assumption that the NFL has birefringent properties similar to those found for the Henle fibers in the macular region. An ellipsometer, an optical device used to measure the change in polarization of light (retardation), is implemented in a confocal scanning laser ophthalmoscope to obtain polarization data. With in vitro studies, there is a good correlation between the retardation as determined by Fourier ellipsometry and histopathologic measurement of retinal NFL thickness. This confirms the assumption that the polarization shifts are produced by the NFL and not by the remainder of the retina.

Summary

Quantitative measurement of retinal NFL height and thickness has potential for providing new objective means for diagnosis and follow-up of glaucoma eyes which may complement the quantitative data of optic nerve head topography.

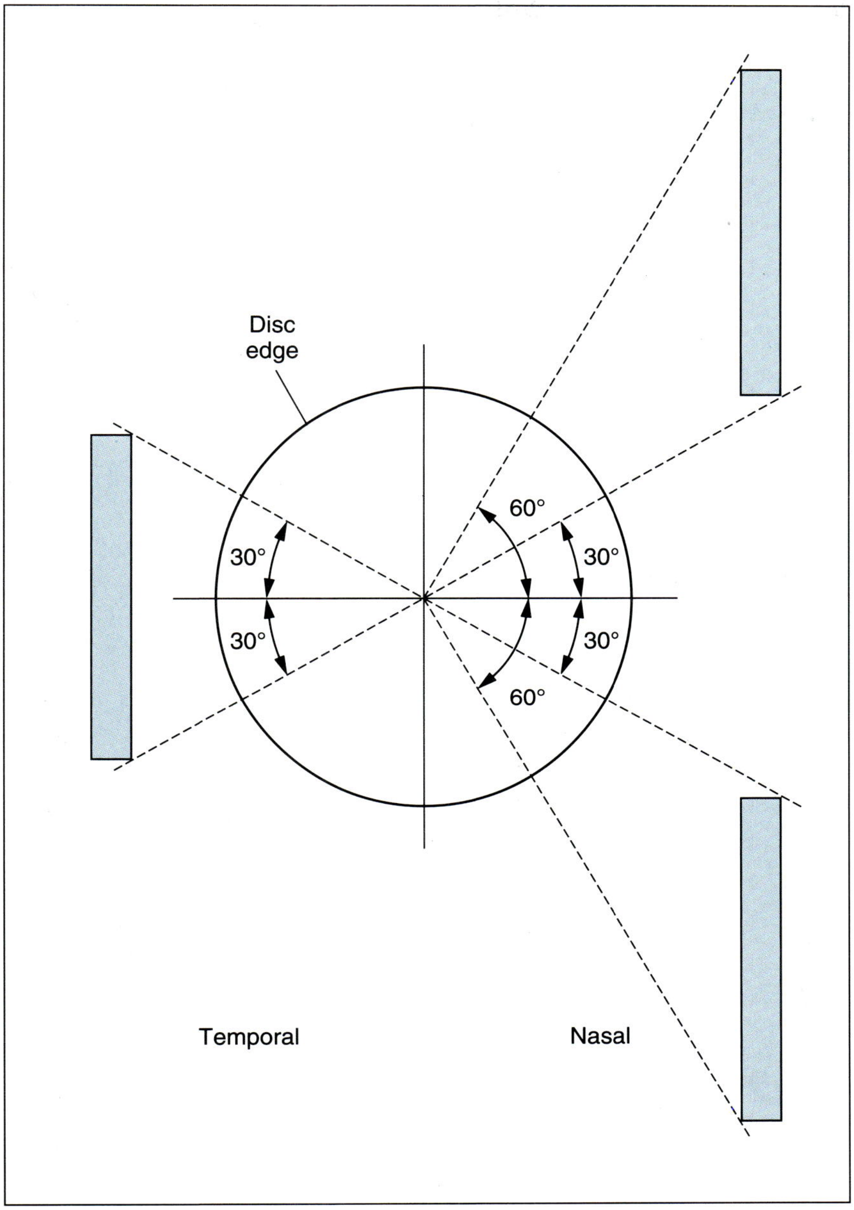

4.27 | Calculation of nerve fiber layer height from surface contour measurement of the peripapillary retina made with computerized image analysis of simultaneous stereoscopic videographic images. The heights of three areas of the retinal surface at the periphery of the image are used to construct a standard reference plane to which all images are registered. This plane has a defined height of zero. Positive measurements lie above the plane and negative measurements lie below. (Adapted from Caprioli J, Miller J: Measurement of relative nerve fiber layer surface height in glaucoma. *Ophthalmology 1989;96:633–641.)*

5 Visual Function

Section I

Perimetry

Anders Heijl

Visual field defects are widely regarded as the most important and definite sign of glaucoma, and perimetry is a vital technique in the diagnosis and management of the disease. It is important to realize, however, that when sensitive perimetric techniques are employed visual field defects are not rare in a supposedly healthy population.[1] Such defects are often due to small retinal lesions, tilted discs, or neurological disease; therefore, one must try to rule out nonglaucomatous field defects even in patients with elevated IOP, particularly when optic disc anatomy appears normal.

The roles of other psychophysical tests are not as well defined. Glaucoma usually does not influence visual acuity until late in the disease process. Alterations in color discrimination, contrast sensitivity, and pattern ERG have all been reported to precede visual field defects, but such changes are not always consistent or well understood.[2,3]

It is not uncommon for glaucoma to be diagnosed before the appearance of field loss. For instance, many glaucoma eyes exhibit transient but repeated disc hemorrhages before field defects are found.[4–6] Eyes with localized retinal nerve fiber defects usually have corresponding field defects, which are detected by standard computerized perimetric techniques.[7] Concentric enlargement of the optic cup certainly precedes the development of those types of obvious field loss that are regularly detected by manual kinetic perimetry,[8] but there seems to be a much closer correlation between the detection of morphologic changes at the disc and the appearance of field defects when sensitive perimetric techniques and optic disc analysis techniques are used simultaneously.[7,9,10] The relative diagnostic values of perimetry and disc morphology therefore depend on the quality of the techniques used, and in early stages they are complementary techniques. In late stages of the the disease, with little remaining neural tissue at the level of the disc, progression or stability can usually be better judged from repeated field testing than from disc photographs.

QUALITATIVE AND QUANTITATIVE PERIMETRY

Visual field testing can be performed in many different ways. Qualitative tests, such as confrontation techniques or testing of color saturation, are usually quite insufficient in glaucoma management. Early glaucomatous field defects infrequently involve the periphery and are, therefore, not detected by peripheral testing. They are also likely to be too irregular and shallow to be revealed by color saturation testing. Confrontation methods are more suitable in neuro-ophthalmic practice when the purpose of field testing often is to detect or rule out hemianopic defects.

Instead, in glaucoma management quantitative perimetry is most important. In quantitative perimetry, actual measurements of the sensitivity are performed at various locations in the visual field. Such quantitative techniques are, of course, mandatory in follow-up, but these types of tests are also most suitable for early detection.

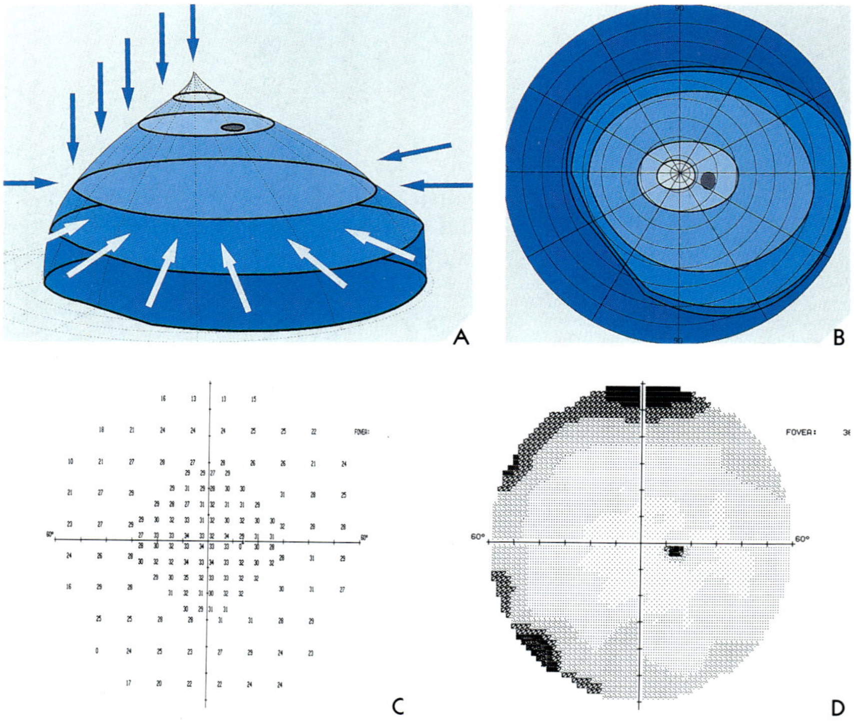

5.1 | *A:* Traquair's Island of Vision in a Sea of Darkness is a well-known and instructive representation of the visual field. The altitude above sea level represents sensitivity; the peak of the island thus corresponds to the point of fixation. Distance from this peak represents eccentricity. *B:* Kinetic testing (horizontal arrows in *A*) results in traditional isopter field charts. Such isopter charts are therefore maps of the Island of Vision seen from above. Static testing (vertical arrows in *A*) results in sensitivity measurements at predetermined locations in the field. *C:* These locations are usually distributed in a grid-like pattern in automated perimetry, with test results represented as numerical sensitivity in decibels (DB) at each tested location (*C*), or as an interpolated gray scale where sensitivity varies inversely with darkness (*D*). *E:* In manual static perimetry tested locations often follow one of the meridians through the point of fixation. *F:* Such static cuts can also be performed with computerized techniques. Static field charts *C* and *D* are maps of the Island of Vision as seen from above, while the static cuts (*E* and *F*) are profiles through the island seen from one side.

KINETIC AND STATIC PERIMETRY

Traquair's representation of the visual field as an Island of Vision in a Sea of Darkness (Fig. 5.1A) is a useful concept,[11] particularly when static and kinetic techniques are compared. The high peak of the island represents the central fovea, where visual sensitivity is highest. Distance from the peak represents eccentricity.

Visual field charts can present various views of the island of vision. The isopter charts of manual kinetic perimetry (Fig. 5.1B), and the gray-scale (Fig. 5.1D) and numerical sensitivity maps of computerized perimeters (Fig. 5.1C) are representations of the island as seen from above. Profile perimetry charts (Fig. 5.1E,F) are trans-sectional cuts through the island, seen from one side. Perimetric static cuts usually follow one of the meridians in the field, thus passing through the point of fixation.

5.1 | (Continued)

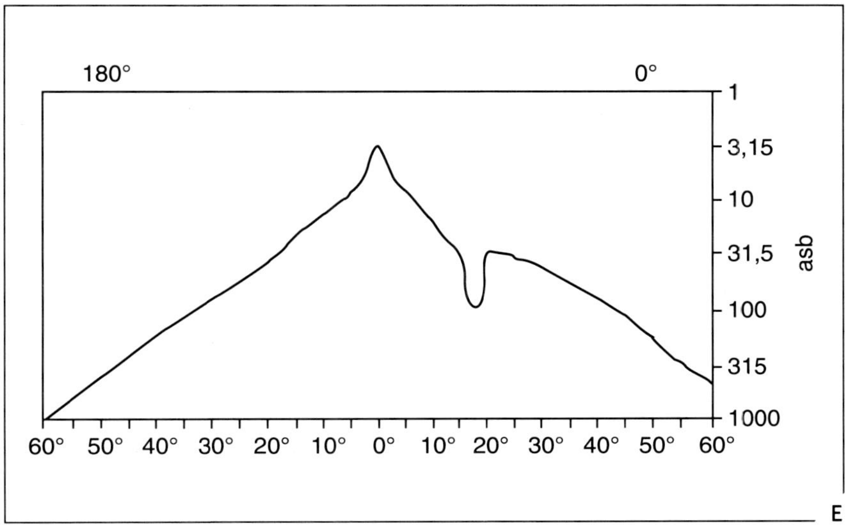

E

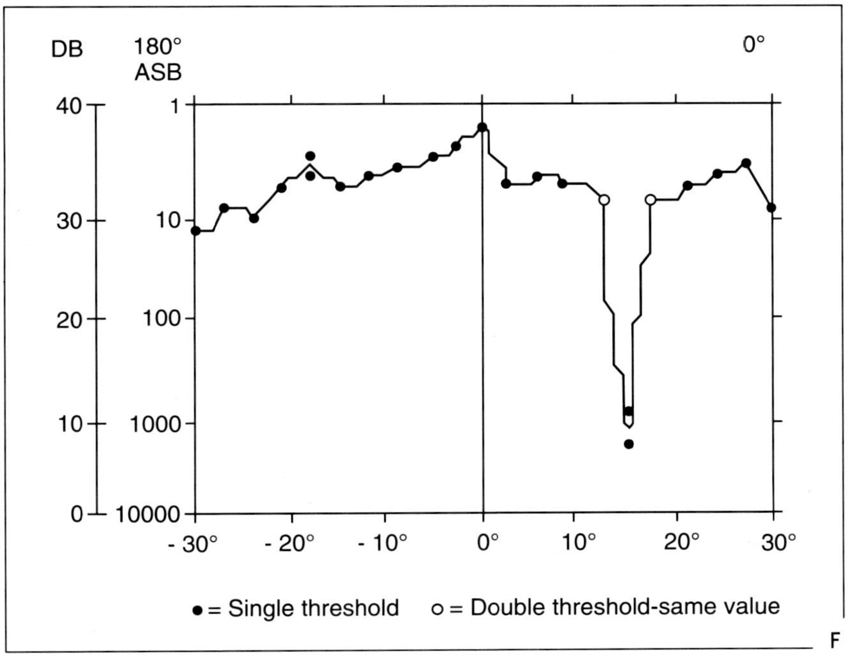

F

In kinetic perimetry a constant stimulus is moved from various directions in the periphery towards the central field until it is perceived (horizontal arrows in Figure 5.1A). The resulting isopter connects points with the same sensitivity. Larger or stronger stimuli are used to test more peripheral parts of the field; smaller and fainter stimuli are used for central field testing. Two to four isopters are plotted to map the island of vision.

Kinetic perimetry can rapidly provide an overview of the examined hill of vision. It is important to realize, however, that the areas between isopters really have not been tested. Even sizeable scotomas may pass undetected between isopters when only two or three isopters are used, and particularly when one of them is in the periphery (Fig. 5.2).

Manual kinetic perimetry usually is not difficult for the patient. Because the stimulus is always moved centrally until it can be seen, the patient is rewarded regularly by perceiving the stimulus. However, with this type of perimetry the patient can usually anticipate where the stimulus will appear. This sometimes makes it difficult to control fixation.

Quantitative static perimetry, on the other hand, involves the measurement of threshold sensitivities at specific predetermined locations in the visual field. Threshold sensitivities are determined by varying the intensity of the stimuli at each location in a step-wise fashion to find in each case the dimmest stimulus that the patient can see.

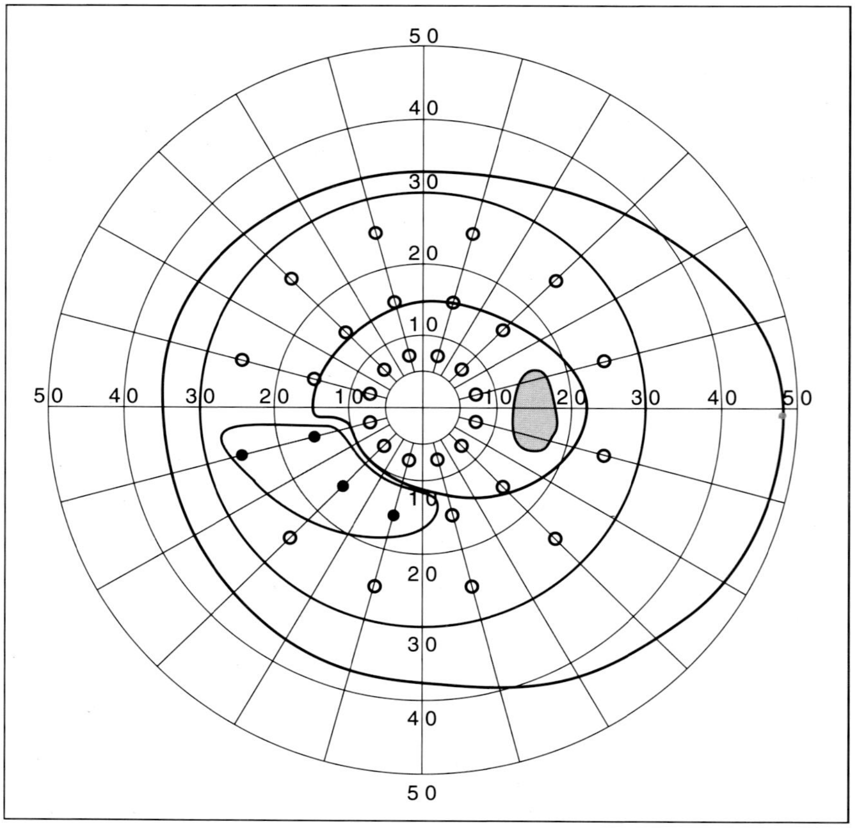

5.2 | In kinetic perimetry areas between isopters have not been tested. A paracentral defect was only revealed as a small central shifting of one isopter with kinetic testing. Static spot-checking readily detects the same defect; open circles represent stimuli detected, solid circles indicate stimuli missed.

Static perimetry is a more exact and often a more exacting type of visual field examination than kinetic testing. Test loci are predetermined, and standard grids of test points usually prevent small scotomas from being missed. Manual static threshold perimetry is quite difficult and time consuming and is, therefore, seldom used clinically, except that static spot checking between isopters is a valuable complement to manual kinetic perimetry (see Fig. 5.2). As an automated computerized test, on the other hand, static threshold perimetry has become the new perimetric standard. The repeated thresholding of exactly the same set of predetermined test points at every test is a particular advantage in follow-up.

Kinetic testing may be the only option in very advanced field loss because of the presence of statokinetic dissociation (Riddoch's phenomenon).[12] This is the name given to the common phenomenon in which a patient can perceive a moving stimulus but cannot see the same stimulus when it is presented in a static fashion. Therefore, in severely disturbed fields maximum-luminosity stimuli may not be seen until moved; kinetic perimetry may then still yield some quantitative measurements that may serve as a basis for further follow-up at a stage when static examinations fail to yield enough such information because the strongest available stimulus cannot be seen when statically presented.

AUTOMATED AND MANUAL PERIMETRY

Automated perimetry is almost always performed with static techniques, and manual perimetry with kinetic testing. The advantages of computerized and manual perimetry, therefore, are largely the same as those of static and kinetic field testing, respectively. Thus, for example, computerized perimetry regularly detects field loss at an earlier stage than manual examination.[13–15] This is partly, but not entirely, due to the tight grids and randomized stimulus presentations that are typical of computerized tests, but it also has to do with errors introduced by the examiner in manual perimetry (see below). The advantages of kinetic perimetry in late-stage disease are due not only to the presence of an encouraging human perimetrist but also to the kinetic test mode and stato-kinetic dissociation (see above).

There are other pros and cons associated with automated and manual approaches, apart from the kinetic and static aspects. Automation eliminates the errors introduced by the perimetrist. Examiner bias may be due to preconceived ideas of the tested field. Certainly, previously normal test results must introduce a bias for the perimetrist to disregard early and/or nonreproducible irregularities. This is particularly understandable when uncertain test results may lead to requests for extended and more detailed examinations, often difficult to comply within a busy clinical setting.

The lack of operator bias in computerized perimetry is a main reason for the better sensitivity of the automated techniques. At the same time, the soothing effect of the human perimetrist is lost; the large physiologic threshold variability becomes quite obvious in results from automated instruments. These irregularities lead to problems of interpretation, problems that are difficult to eliminate without thorough experience or computer-assisted interpretation.

One should not forget that the operator also has a large and positive influence. Proper patient instruction and support during the test is of great importance for reliable results. Only the most experienced patients can be left alone during automated perimetry; in most instances the operator should be close to the patient and the instrument during the entire procedure, to follow test results and test reliability parameters as they unfold and to provide positive and negative feedback.

For a more complete discussion of modern perimetric techniques in glaucoma, see Heijl, Chapter 7.

TWO PERIMETERS

Many factors influence the visibility of a perimetric stimulus, e.g., size, brightness, distance, background luminosity, stimulus blur, and color. It is important to keep as many as possible of these factors constant in quantitative perimetry.

The Goldmann perimeter (Fig. 5.3), first described in 1945,[16] was the first instrument to provide such stability and became the world standard for perimetry in the 1960s. It provided standardized conditions for testing, with well-defined background and stimulus properties among other advantages. The instrument is a manual projection bowl perimeter primarily intended for kinetic perimetry. The stimulus is moved with the help of a "self-registering" pantographic system. The point of the pantographic level always indicates the stimulus position directly on the field chart. Stimulus size can be varied from a large 64 mm^2 (size V) to a small 1/16 mm^2 stimulus intensity from 1,000 asb downwards. The bowl has a radius of 30 cm and background luminosity is fixed at 31.5 asb.

The Humphrey Field Analyzer[17] (Fig. 5.4) is an automated computerized projection perimeter (Fig. 5.5). It has become a world standard in computerized perimetry, because of the large numbers of instruments presently in use. Stimulus sizes and background luminosity are the same as in the Goldmann perimeter, but stimulus intensity can be varied up to a maximum

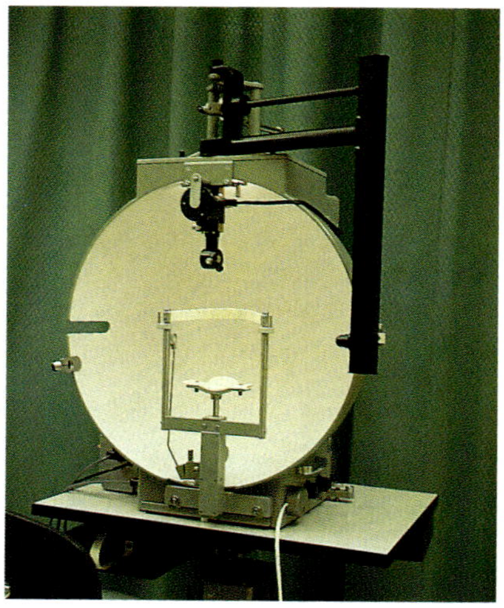

5.3 | Goldmann perimeter, a projection perimeter operated manually by a technician, primarily for kinetic perimetry.

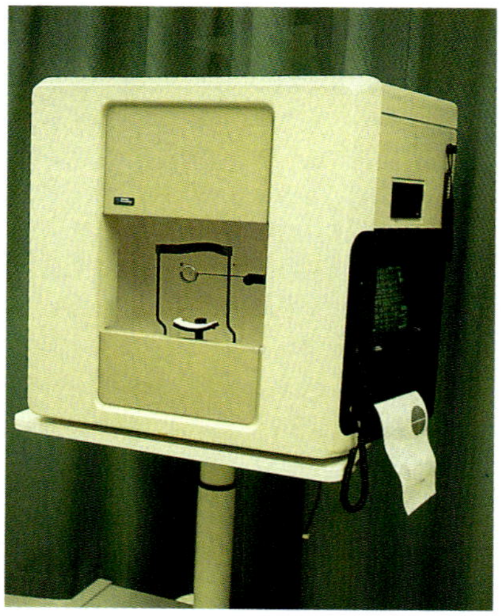

5.4 | Humphrey Visual Field Analyzer, a computer-controlled projection perimeter, primarily for static perimetry.

of 10,000 asb (as compared with 1,000 asb in Goldmann's instrument). The Humphrey perimeter, like other computerized perimeters, is mainly intended for static perimetry. It is mostly used for automated threshold determination within the central 30° field using the 30-2 and 24-2 programs. The interpretation programs Statpac 1 and 2 are used in most instruments.[18,19]

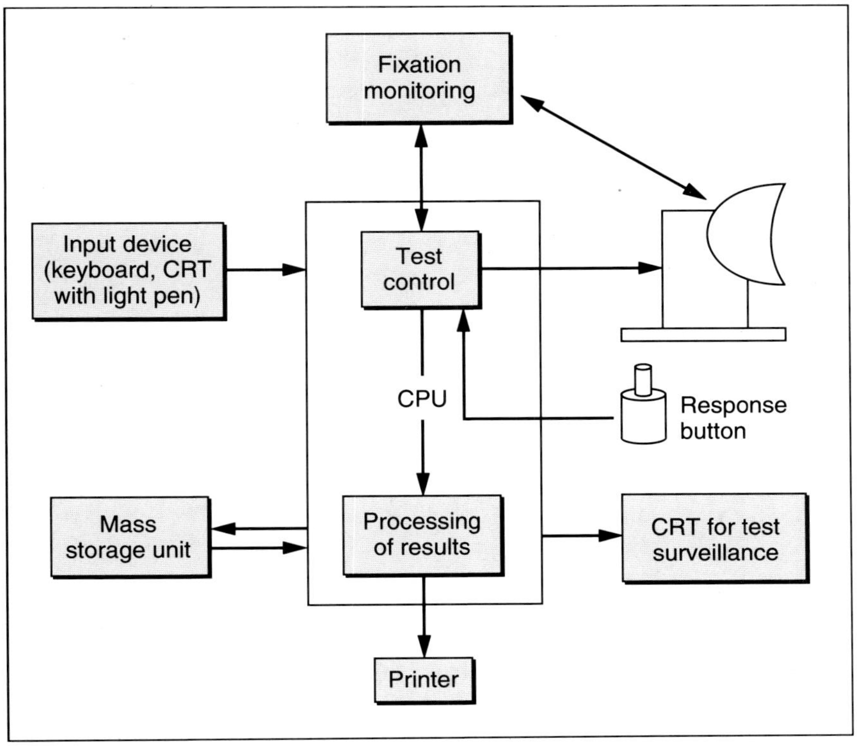

5.5 | Schematic diagram of an automated perimeter.

SECTION II

CONTRAST SENSITIVITY TESTING

Ivan Bodis-Wollner

Since its first use in 1972,[20] contrast sensitivity (CS) testing has emerged as an adjunct technique in the clinical evaluation of visual loss. This chapter describes the technique; a later chapter summarizes the current diagnostic value of CS testing in primary open-angle glaucoma and ocular hypertension.

CS is primarily a test of functional integrity of the central visual field. Although it is widely held that central defects are uncommon in glaucoma, evidence of various electrophysiological and, foremost, color vision abnormalities[21–23] challenge this concept.

VISUAL ACUITY AND CONTRAST SENSITIVITY

Visual resolution relies on the observer's ability to describe or indicate some feature of the smallest target presented. The minimum contrast required for an observer to detect a pattern is the measure of contrast threshold. CS is the reciprocal of contrast threshold. Contrast threshold can be tested for a target of any shape; however, the use of sinusoidal gratings is preferable when precise information is sought concerning CS for various target sizes. With these stimuli it has been shown that CS may be affected to low but not to high spatial frequencies. Spatial frequency is the number of alternating dark and bright bands of the pattern, subtended in 1° of visual angle at the eye. Analytically, any stimulus can be synthesized from a set of sinusoidal gratings of the appropriate orientation, contrast, and spatial frequency (Fig. 5.6). The graphic representation of CS as a function of spatial frequency of sinusoidal gratings is termed the contrast sensitivity function[24,25] (Figs. 5.7–5.9).

Sinusoidal gratings, the traditional visual targets used in vision research and in the original clinical tests of CS, are usually presented on television or

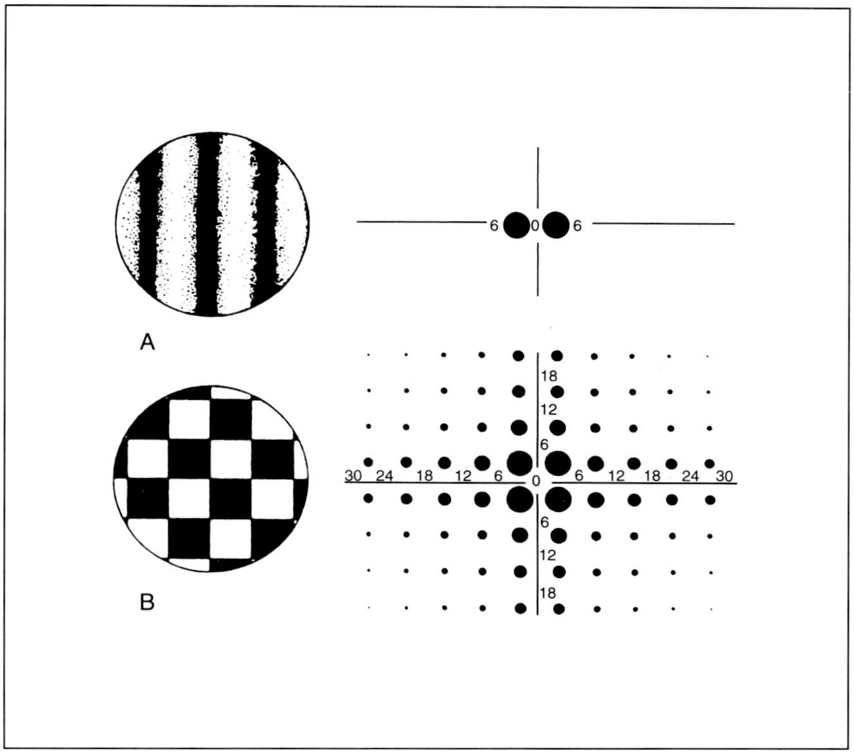

5.6 | Fourier spectra of a sine wave grating (*A*) and a checkerboard (*B*) (zero term omitted). These are polar plots in which radial distance from the origin indicates the spatial frequency (numbered). Azimuth indicates the orientation of the spatial frequency components. The area of each spot indicates the magnitude of each component. *A:* Note the absence of components parallel to the sides of the checks. *B:* The numbers are cycles per degree for a pattern of 10 arc min checks. Note that this figure does not imply that a checkerboard can be synthesized by superimposing sine wave gratings. (Adapted from Bodis-Wollner I, Ghilardi MF, Mylin LH: The importance of stimulus selection in VEP practice: the clinical relevance of visual physiology, in Cracco R, Bodis-Wollner I (eds): *Evoked Potentials.* New York: Alan R Liss, 1986, 15–27.)

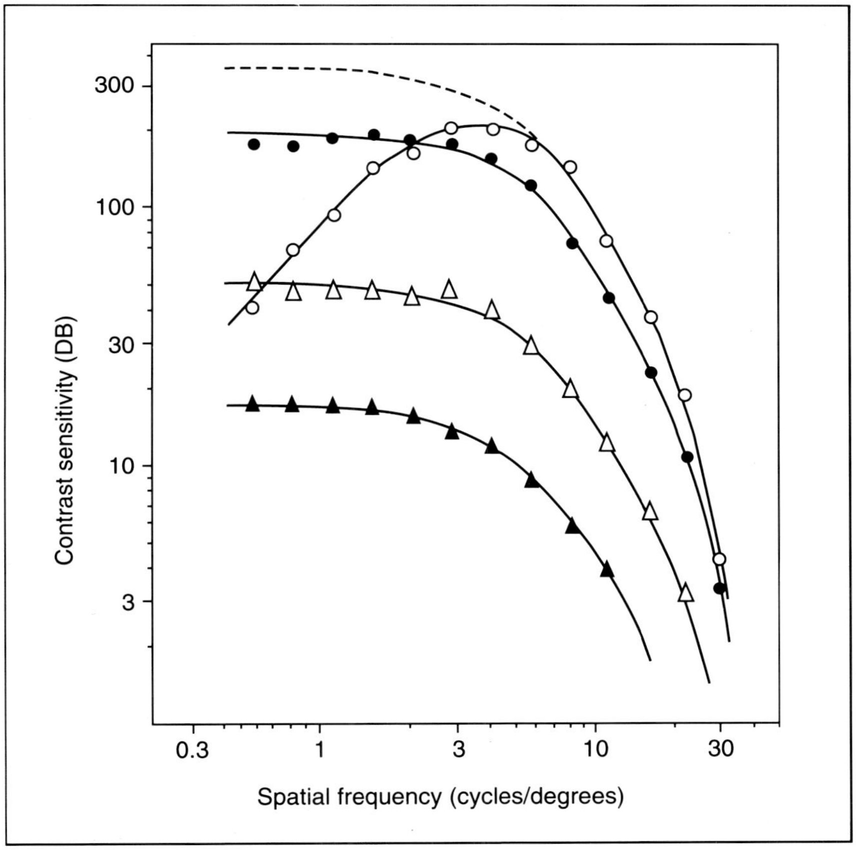

5.7 | Spatial contrast sensitivity curves obtained at different rates of modulation. The curves were obtained using sinusoidal grating patterns at different spatial frequencies modulated at various temporal rates. The observer had to indicate the minimal contrast at which patterns could be still detected. The inverted U-shaped curve (open circles) was obtained using a quasi-steady presentation. Note that at low spatial frequencies (below 2 cycles/degree) sensitivity is higher for the temporally modulated curve (8 Hertz, dark circles), whereas at higher spatial frequencies the converse is true. (After Robson JG: Spatial and temporal contrast sensitivity functions of the visual system. *J Opt Soc Am 1966;56: 1141.)*

on oscilloscopic-type displays, and testing devices are commercially available. Printed charts using either gratings or optotypes have also been developed and they too are commercially available. For some purposes printed charts are more convenient, but experience shows that although chart-type displays can serve as screening tests,[26–31] they often "detect" a large number of false positives.[32] Although the usefulness of a given chart may also depend on the testing method (such as alternative forced-choice or simple detection),[33] there are also noteworthy differences depending on the type of chart used. Nevertheless, CS charts using optotypes are most useful for screening rather than for specific diagnostic purposes. Especially in glaucoma, the printed charts presently available are not optimal, and oscilloscopic displays of extended patterns are recommended for reasons summarized below (see also Bodis-Wollner, Chapter 7).

THE VISUAL FIELD (VF) AND CONTRAST SENSITIVITY

The contrast threshold has been shown to decrease with stimulus area when stimuli are sinusoidal gratings, i.e., as the number of grating cycles increases the minimal contrast needed to detect the grating decreases.[34] The threshold decrease is not infinite; rather, there is a roughly constant critical *number* of cycles, irrespective of spatial frequency. Hence, for maximal detectability, coarse gratings (low spatial frequency) need a larger stimulus area than do fine gratings.[35] Conversely, therefore, a given restriction of the central field should affect low spatial frequency detection more than fine grating detection. The relationship between CS and VF area is of special importance to the diagnosis and possibly to the early treatment of glaucoma.

The definite diagnosis of chronic open-angle glaucoma includes the presence of VF defects. This diagnostic assumption has never been com-

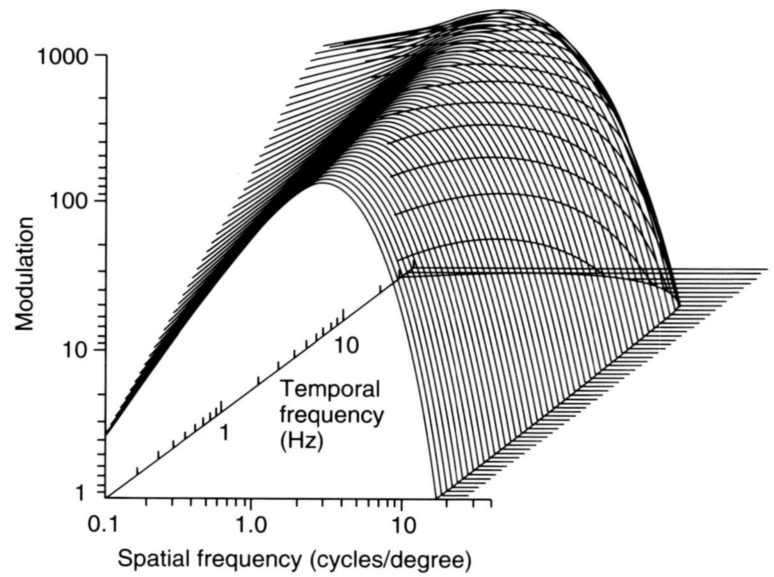

5.8 | An idealized spatiotemporal surface of contrast sensitivity (ST-CS) in normals. It provides a qualitative picture of the combined effect of spatial and temporal frequency on contrast sensitivity as a transformation of the data in Fig. 5.6. Each curve represents the CSF at a fixed temporal frequency. The neighboring curves are separated by a constant increment of 0.05 log in temporal frequency; modulation in this figure stands for contrast sensitivity because the scale is inversed and is equivalent to the Michaelson constant. Note how CS increases at low spatial frequencies as a function of temporal frequency. (Adapted from Kelly DA: Motion and vision. *J Opt Soc Am 1979;69:1340.)*

pletely satisfactory: by the time a discernible VF defect appears, half of the optic nerve fibers may already be lost.[36,37] Hence, the search for diagnostic techniques that reveal damage before irreversible losses have occurred is of great therapeutic importance, and extended stimuli may offer more hope than single optotypes.

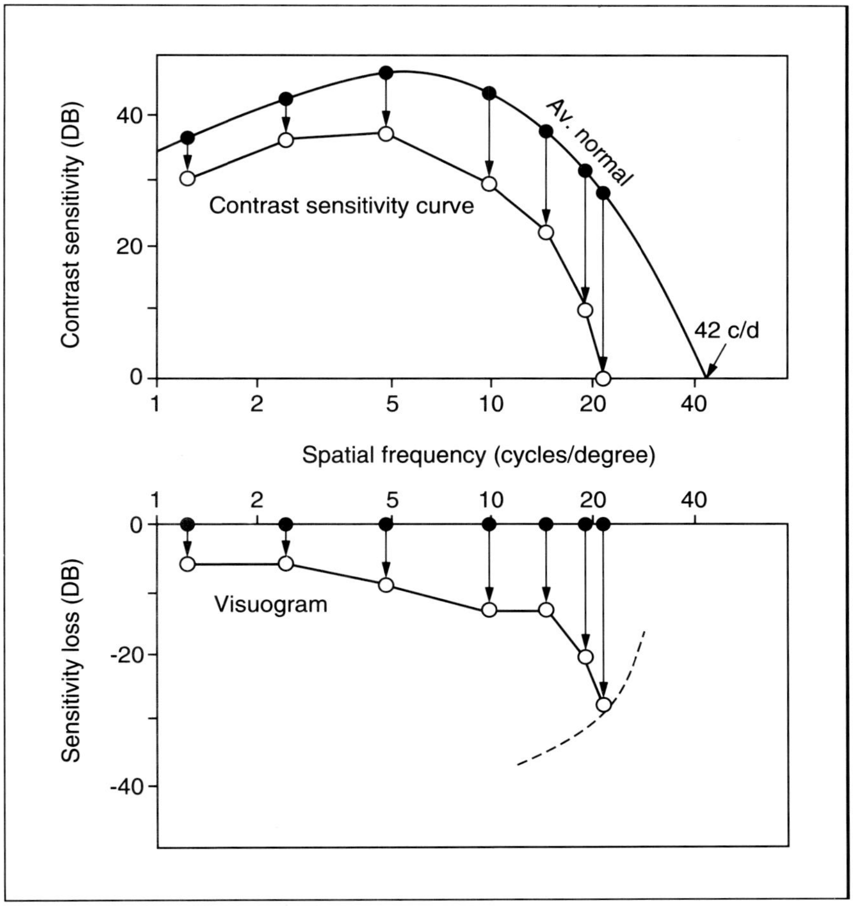

5.9 | Contrast sensitivity curve (above) and visuogram (below). Upper plot shows two contrast sensitivity curves: the average CS curve of normal subjects with 20/20 vision (smooth curve), and a CS curve of a patient with visual deficits (open circles). Contrast sensitivity (ordinate of upper plot), the inverse of the contrast threshold, is specified on a logarithmic scale in decibels (DB). The abscissa, spatial frequency, expressed in cycles (dark-light bar pairs) per degree of visual angle, specifies the coarseness or fineness of the grating. The cut-off frequency (CO), the spatial frequency at which the contrast sensitivity curve intercepts the abscissa, is a measure of maximal visual resolution at 100% contrast. In the average normal subject with 20/20 Snellen acuity, the cut-off is 42 cycles per degree (c/d). For the curve shown here the cut-off is 21 c/d. The lower plot is a visuogram, showing the CS deficit (Ø) at each of the tested spatial frequencies for the patient whose CS curve is shown above. A loss of 6 DB signifies twofold reduction of CS; a loss of 20 DB signifies a tenfold reduction. The spatial frequency scale (abscissa) of the visuogram is the same as that of the CS plot above it. (Adapted from Wolkstein M, et al: Contrast sensitivity in retinal disease. *Ophthalmology 1980;87:1140–1149.)*

SECTION III

COLOR VISION TESTING

Ruth D. Williams
Robert L. Stamper

The diagnosis of early glaucoma is a challenge for ophthalmologists. With expanding medical and surgical treatment options, it is increasingly important to identify patients with glaucoma and those who are likely to develop glaucoma. Historically, ophthalmologists have relied largely on the visual field to document glaucomatous damage. However, up to 50% of optic nerve fibers are lost in glaucoma before an abnormality is detected by Goldmann kinetic perimetry.[38] Therefore, earlier detection of visual loss is desirable. Practical and sensitive measures of visual function are needed to detect nerve fiber damage before perimetry is affected. Color vision testing offers this potential, since color vision abnormalities may precede standard perimetric ones in glaucoma (see Drance and Williams/Stamper, Chapter 7). However, for color vision testing to be valuable clinically, it must be easy to use, quickly administered, and diagnostically specific. Several color vision tests are available, and each has advantages and disadvantages.

CLINICAL COLOR VISION TESTS

THE ANOMALOSCOPE

The anomaloscope (Fig. 5.10A) presents a small circular field, the bottom half of which is yellow, neutral, or blue-green. The top half is a mixture of the two primaries of the color at the bottom (Fig. 5.10B). The patient controls two knobs; one varies the ratio of the two colors on top until it matches the bottom color and the other varies the brightness of the bottom color. The patient uses the two knobs to match the color of the two halves. The Nagel anomaloscope only evaluates red-green matches, whereas the Pickford-Nicholson anomaloscope[39] measures green-blue and yellow-blue matches as well.

The anomaloscope is considered the gold standard for color vision testing in research. The anomaloscope requires only a few minutes of testing.

However, evaluation of the results is complex, and calls for a skilled examiner trained in psychophysical techniques in order to provide a proper interpretation. In addition, the anomaloscope is expensive. Therefore, this method of color vision testing is rarely used clinically.

COLOR CAP TESTS

Although several variations are available, the most frequently used color cap tests are the Farnsworth-Munsell 100-Hue test, the Farnsworth D15 test, and the Lanthony desaturated Farnsworth D15 test. Each requires the subject to arrange a series of color chips in order of progression from one hue to another. These tests should be performed at 16 inches with controlled lighting; at this distance, the caps subtend a visual angle of 2°.

The Farnsworth-Munsell 100-Hue Test

The Farnsworth-Munsell 100-Hue test consists of 85 color discs of equal saturation and brightness which vary only in hue and are arranged on four trays.[40] One tray contains chips progressing from red shades through orange and yellow, the second progresses from yellow through green and green-blue, the third progresses from blue to purple, and the fourth progresses from purple to red. The patient arranges the chips in one tray at a time, so the gradation in color is continuous. The test takes about 30 minutes to administer in cooperative patients, but is often too cumbersome for routine clinical use. In addition, scoring may be complicated.

The Farnsworth D15 Test

The Farnsworth D15 test (Fig. 5.11) contains 15 color discs taken from the Munsell color circle and a reference disc. The patient begins with the reference chip and arranges the discs in order of the progression of hues. The test typically takes less than one minute, but is less sensitive for subtle defects and for some types of defects than the Farnsworth 100-Hue. The sensitivity of this test is increased significantly when the definition of a test failure is changed. Conventional test failure requires that two "major errors" be made, resulting in colors across the circle being placed side by side. When test failure is defined by one single-place error, the sensitivity of this test is enhanced.[41] The D15 color vision test is probably the most useful clinical test because it is simple to use, quickly administered, and easy to interpret.

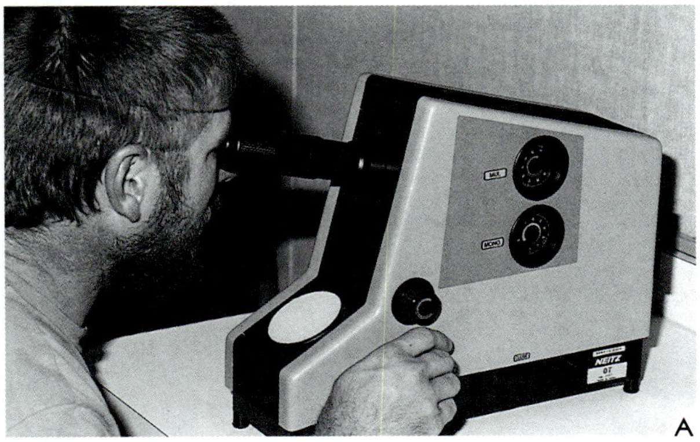
A

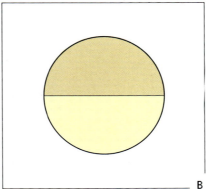
B

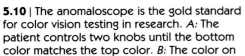

5.10 | The anomaloscope is the gold standard for color vision testing in research. *A:* The patient controls two knobs until the bottom color matches the top color. *B:* The color on the top half of the circular field is a mixture of the two primaries of the color at the bottom half.

The Desaturated Farnsworth D15 Test

The Lanthony desaturated Farnsworth D15 test has the same format as the Farnsworth D15 except that the color samples are paler and lighter by two Munsell units.[42,43] Although the test is more sensitive for color defects, it is less specific.

PSEUDOISOCHROMATIC PLATES

Several pseudoisochromatic plate tests are available, including the Ishihara, AO-HRR, and Tokyo Medical College color tests. Each consists of colored dots arranged to produce a figure hidden in a background of different colored dots. Most of the pseudoisochromatic plates were designed to detect inherited red–green defects. The AO-HRR plate (Fig. 5.11C) is one of the few that are useful for detecting acquired defects, because it can identify some blue–yellow defects.

The AO-HRR plates are easy to use, take little time, are relatively inexpensive, and can be used on naive subjects, illiterates, or children. However, there are no scoring criteria for classifying color defects. These plates have been discontinued by the manufacturer and may be difficult to obtain.

COLOR PERIMETRY

The color vision tests discussed above all evaluate central macular function. Color perception of the peripheral field can also be tested, even though fewer cones are present in the retinal periphery than in the center. In white-light perimetry the visual field defects found in glaucoma occur first in the Bjerrum region.[44–46] Color perimetry may offer advantages over conventional achromatic perimetry if it is found to be more sensitive in mapping defects of the peripheral visual field.

Color perimetry utilizes colored test objects to map the visual field and was introduced over 60 years ago.[47] Since then, many researchers have evaluated the use of color perimetry for a variety of ophthalmic diseases. Physical variables, however, have complicated the interpretation of color perimetry. For example, the luminance and saturation of the colored test objects are changed by the lighted background. It is important to achieve a background illuminance which is high enough to eliminate contribution from the rod

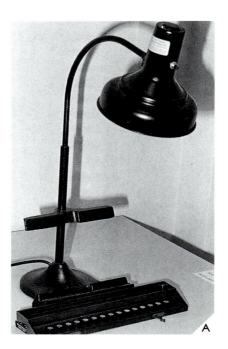

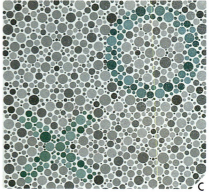

5.11 | Color vision testing should be administered in a standard fashion using proper lighting. *A:* The Farnsworth D15 test is positioned 16 inches from the light source, a Macbeth easel lamp. *B:* The patient arranges the 15 color discs in order of the hue progression to complete the Farnsworth D15 test. *C:* An AO-HRR plate consists of a background of dots in which a colored figure is hidden.

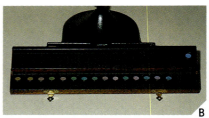

system.[48–50] Indeed, it has been questioned whether the visual fields obtained actually measure a separate color (chromatic) mechanism or instead measure the equivalent of a dimmer white test object (achromatic mechanism).[51,52]

Other factors complicating the use of color perimetry include intra- and interobserver variability,[53,54] threshold variability,[55] and adaptation variability.[54] The expense, the limited availability of the equipment, and the complexity of color perimetry discourage its use in the clinical setting. Further studies are needed to determine if color perimetry is more sensitive than conventional perimetry in detecting and following visual field changes.

FACTORS AFFECTING EVALUATION

The interpretation of color vision testing is complex. Variables such as small pupil size, aging, cataracts, background illumination, and IOP are difficult to control, and data regarding the effect of each are limited.

PUPIL SIZE

A small pupil size (2.0 mm) impairs performance on both the 100-hue test and the anomaloscope.[56] Pupil size is commonly affected in the population in question by miotics and aging. It is especially important to consider pupil size when comparing color vision changes over time in ocular hypertensives who develop glaucoma and may subsequently be using miotics. In addition, miosis reduces the overall color sensitivity at a given light level.

AGE

Color vision declines with age.[57,58] Most of the loss is blue–yellow and is attributed to the yellowing of the lens with its increased absorption of blue light.[58] Studies using color vision testing must control for pupil size and expected age-related changes to validate interpretation.

ILLUMINANTS

The type of background lighting, called the illuminant, can affect the apparent color of the test objects. Most color vision tests specify for standard illuminant C, an artificial illuminant, which is bluish-white and approximates the average spectral distribution of natural daylight.[59] When different illuminants are used, color vision testing results may change. In clinical and research settings, the background lighting should be carefully standardized.

The Macbeth easel lamp (Fig. 5.11A) uses a tungsten bulb which is modified with filters and was designed for use with screening plate tests. It is a good source of light which approximates standard illuminants. This lamp is also designed to place the source, the color vision test, and the subject at the correct distances.

LEVEL OF ILLUMINATION

The level of illumination is not specified for many color vision tests. The AO-HRR plates should be administered with an illumination of 100–650 lux and the 100-Hue with 270 lux.[60] Although screening tests are not altered by changes between approximately 100 and 1,000 lux,[61,62] 2,000 lux is recommended for research in color vision testing.[57]

TINTED LENSES

The examiner must inquire about tinted glasses or contact lenses, as either can alter color perception.

ACKNOWLEDGMENTS

This work was supported in part by Pacific Vision Foundation and Research to Prevent Blindness, Inc.

Section IV

Electroretinography

Scott E. Brodie

Electrophysiologic correlates of ganglion cell damage in glaucoma could serve to substantially clarify the glaucomatous disease process. The use of the visual evoked potential for this purpose is discussed in Chapters 5 and 7 (Stodtmeister and Pillunat). Recent applications of electroretinography (ERG) to the study of glaucomatous injury are discussed below.

The traditional "ganzfeld" ERG, obtained by recording the electrical potential at the cornea in response to uniform stimulation of the entire retina with a strong flash of light, is generally held to be of little value in the demonstration of glaucomatous damage.[63,64] Although careful study of large numbers of patients has demonstrated statistically significant reductions in ERG amplitudes in glaucoma patients compared with age-matched normal subjects,[65] these reductions are too small to be of clinical value when compared with the large variation within and between subjects inherent in the ganzfeld ERG. This lack of sensitivity to ganglion cell damage reflects the primarily circumferential orientation of ganglion cell processes, which prevents

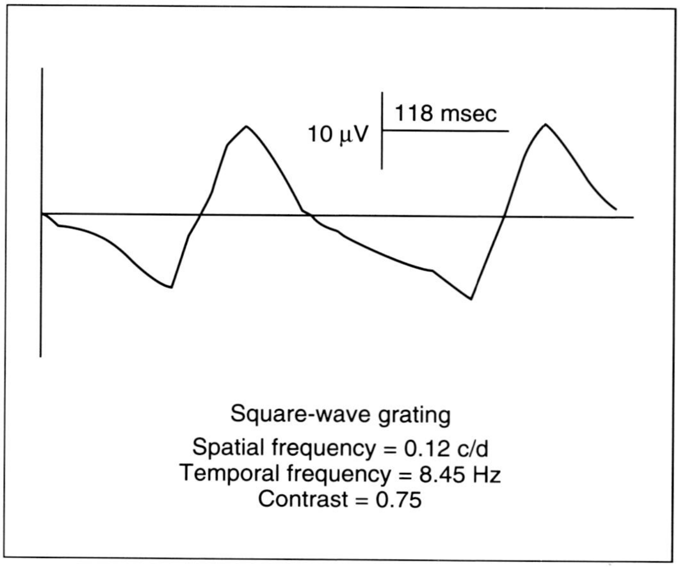

5.12 | Steady-state PERG from a normal individual. (Adapted from Conte M, Brodie SE: Altered contrast and luminance contributions to the pattern ERG in glaucoma. *Invest Ophthalmol Vis Sci 1987;28(suppl):129.)*

summation of individual cell contributions into a net electrical vector detectable at the cornea.

Recently, two novel electroretinographic approaches have shown great promise in the detection of damage to the innermost retina.

A small signal, the "pattern ERG" (PERG), can be recorded at the cornea in response to a reversing checkerboard stimulus similar to that commonly used to elicit the visual evoked potential. Recording the PERG is difficult. The pattern stimulus must be carefully calibrated so that there is no inadvertent variation in mean luminance associated with the pattern reversal. A check size (or stripe width) of about 0.5 to 1.0 degree is optimal. The choice of corneal electrode remains controversial. Many investigators recommend the use of a gold foil or conductive fiber electrode in an attempt to interfere as little as possible with the eye's natural optics. The PERG signal is typically less than 5 μV in amplitude, necessitating careful signal averaging and artifact rejection. Many researchers have advocated using a modulation frequency of 2 Hz (4 reversals per second), which allows analysis of a transient response to the pattern reversal. Alternatively, a modulation frequency of 8 Hz (16 reversals per second), which yields a robust steady-state response, may be just as informative and easier to implement (Fig. 5.12).

An alternative approach, based on standard ganzfeld ERG recording techniques, is the measurement of the oscillatory potentials (OPs). The OPs are small wavelets that are superimposed on the a-wave and b-wave of the ganzfeld ERG response.[66] OP recordings are usually performed under scotopic conditions, using standard contact lens electrodes and ganzfeld stroboscopic flash stimuli. The OPs are enhanced when a conditioning flash precedes the recording by 30–60 seconds or when the responses are averaged at a rate of one flash every 30 seconds. Optimal recordings can be obtained by raising the cutoff of the low-frequency filter of the ERG amplifier to approximately 75 Hz and increasing the amplifier gain tenfold compared with standard scotopic settings. This suppresses the a-wave and b-wave features of the ERG, leaving the OPs displayed to advantage (Fig. 5.13). Measurements can be made of the amplitude of each individual wavelet, or the magnitude of the entire wave train can be estimated by summing the individual wavelets or by Fourier analysis.

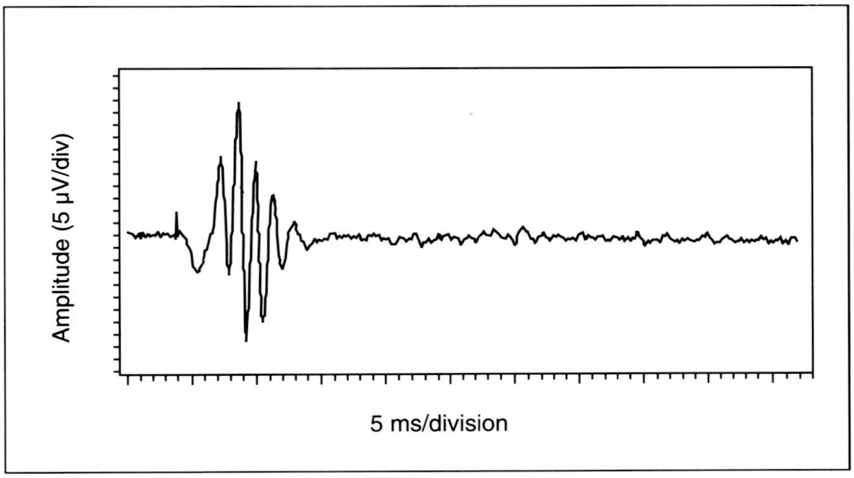

5.13 | Oscillatory potentials from a normal eye.

SECTION V

VISUALLY EVOKED CORTICAL POTENTIALS

Richard Stodtmeister
Lutz E. Pillunat

Visually evoked cortical potentials (VECP) are changes in electrical current recorded on the scalp above the calcarine cortex. They are *objective* signs of the function of the visual pathways rather than *subjective* methods such as perimetry, contrast threshold measurements, and color testing. In clear-cut glaucoma cases with a pale and widely excavated disc, large scotomas, and intraocular pressure (IOP) above 30 mm Hg, the latencies and the amplitudes of the VECP show pathological values, but such information is superfluous. However, even by use of the most subtle clinical and experimental methods it is quite difficult to make the diagnosis in borderline cases showing an IOP above 24 mm Hg but with no changes in the visual fields, contrast measurements, and color testing. About 30% of these people will develop glaucoma and require treatment during their lifetime, while 70% will not. Because the current clinical methods are not accurate prognosticators, alternative methods, such as VECP recordings, are needed.

The mean latencies and amplitudes of the VECP differ significantly between glaucoma patients and normal subjects,[67–69] but the ranges of the values overlap widely. Therefore, VECP recordings at spontaneous IOP are of little practical diagnostic value. However, it is a general principle in physics and biology that valuable information about a system can be obtained by testing under stress conditions. This principle has been applied in glaucoma diagnosis by carrying out perimetry at artificially increased IOP,[70] but the method was too tedious for routine clinical use. This may not be true for VECP recorded at artificially elevated IOP, a procedure called the "pressure tolerance test."

The circulation in the prelaminar part of the optic nerve head is a part of the ciliary circulation.[71] The small vessels that go to the prelaminar part of the optic nerve head stem from vessels that also feed the choroid. The resistance to flow in the choroid is lower than in the optic nerve head (Fig. 5.14). Therefore, the blood tends to flow to the choroid. Under normal conditions the optic nerve head receives enough blood for its well-being despite the higher resistance of the vessels that nourish it.

ANATOMIC AND PHYSIOLOGIC BASIS OF THE PRESSURE TOLERANCE TEST

A determining characteristic for the flow in a vessel is the pressure head. This pressure head is defined as the difference between the arterial pressure and the venous pressure and is called *perfusion pressure.* In most human organs the tissue pressure is lower than the venous pressure. In the eye, however, the tissue pressure—which is the IOP—is higher than the venous pressure. Therefore, the perfusion pressure in the eye is arterial pressure minus IOP

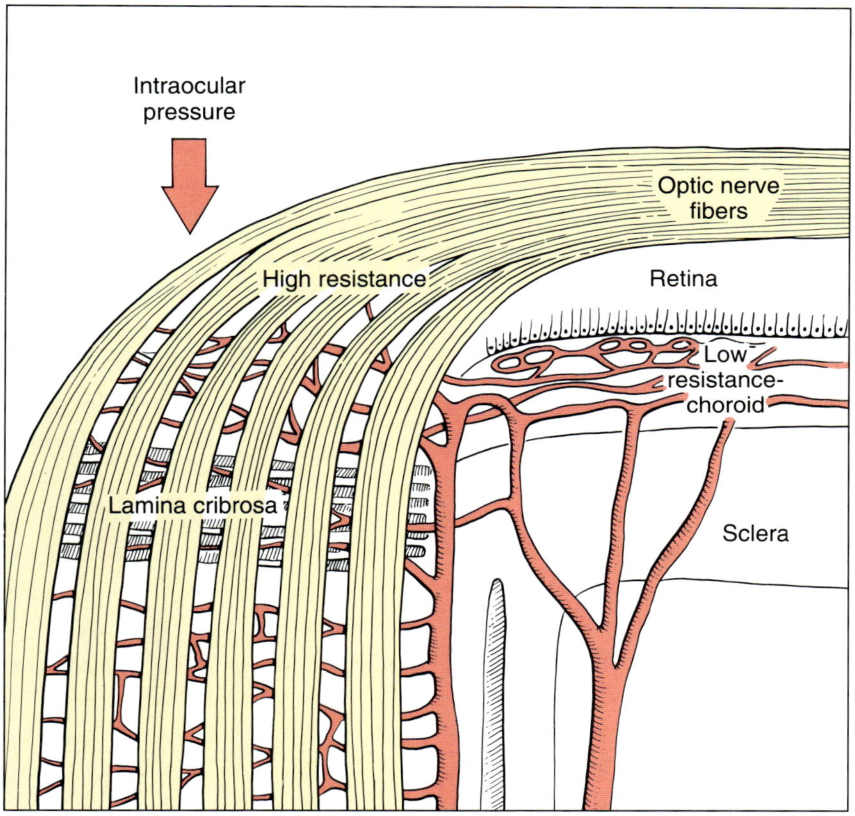

5.14 | Simplified schematic diagram of the circulation at the optic disc. The choroid has a low resistance to blood flow. The vessels in the optic disc have a high resistance. An increase in IOP influences blood flow at first in the optic disc. (Adapted from Hayreh SS: Structure and blood supply of the optic nerve, in Richardson K, Heilmann K (eds): *Glaucoma—Conceptions of Disease.* Stuttgart, New York: Thieme, 1978, 78–96.)

(Fig. 5.15). The pressure in the arteries entering the eye cannot be measured at the point of entry but only outside the eye, where the vessels branch from the ophthalmic artery[72] (Fig. 5.16) by methods such as ophthalmodynamometry,[73] ophthalmoplethysmography,[74] or their modification.[75] These methods are not clinically useful for the diagnosis of glaucoma[76,77] except in normal tension glaucoma, in which the ciliary perfusion pressure is significantly lowered in relation to the retinal perfusion pressure.[77]

The suction cup method used to determine ocular blood pressure and in the pressure tolerance test is the same. However, while ocular blood pressure is a characteristic distinct from (albeit in some way related to) glaucomatous optic nerve head damage, the pressure tolerance test artificially induces and records a reversible functional change in the nerve.

Anatomic and physiologic studies[71] have demonstrated that the vessels in the optic nerve head can be regarded as a backwater of the ciliary circulation. Therefore, a decrease in the ciliary perfusion pressure can cause deleteri-

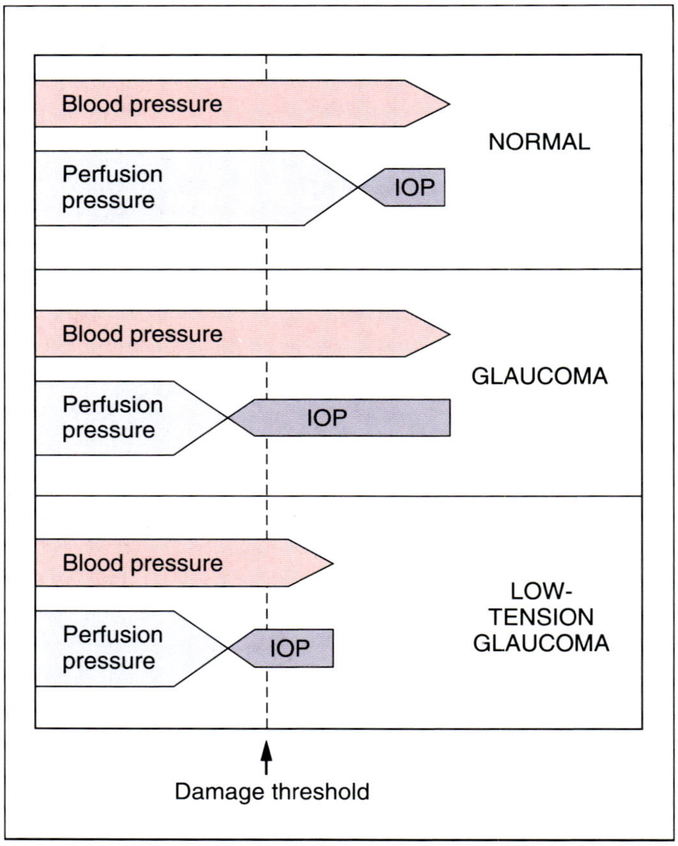

5.15 | Dependence of perfusion pressure on blood pressure and IOP. Perfusion pressure may be low due to high IOP, as in "typical" glaucoma, or to low local blood pressure, perhaps as in low-tension glaucoma. The relevant blood pressure is in the vessels entering the prelaminar part of the optic nerve head. In both conditions the perfusion pressure is below a supposed damage threshold.

ous effects in the optic nerve head (see Fig. 5.14). The vessels in the optic nerve head are end vessels[71] and are not arranged like a network. It can be assumed that there are regions in the optic disc in which only a small increase in IOP results in a perfusion pressure that falls short of the pressure head necessary to force the blood through the capillaries. The consequent decrease of blood flow may not be linearly dependent on the perfusion pressure, because blood is a non-Newtonian fluid and does not obey the same physical laws as water. Small changes in perfusion pressure may result in a complete stoppage of blood movement in a vessel. Stasis may occur in small regions of the optic nerve head and lead to small hemorrhagic infarctions (splinter hemorrhages) which are clinically typical of glaucoma. The functional damage may be a circumscribed scotoma in the visual field.

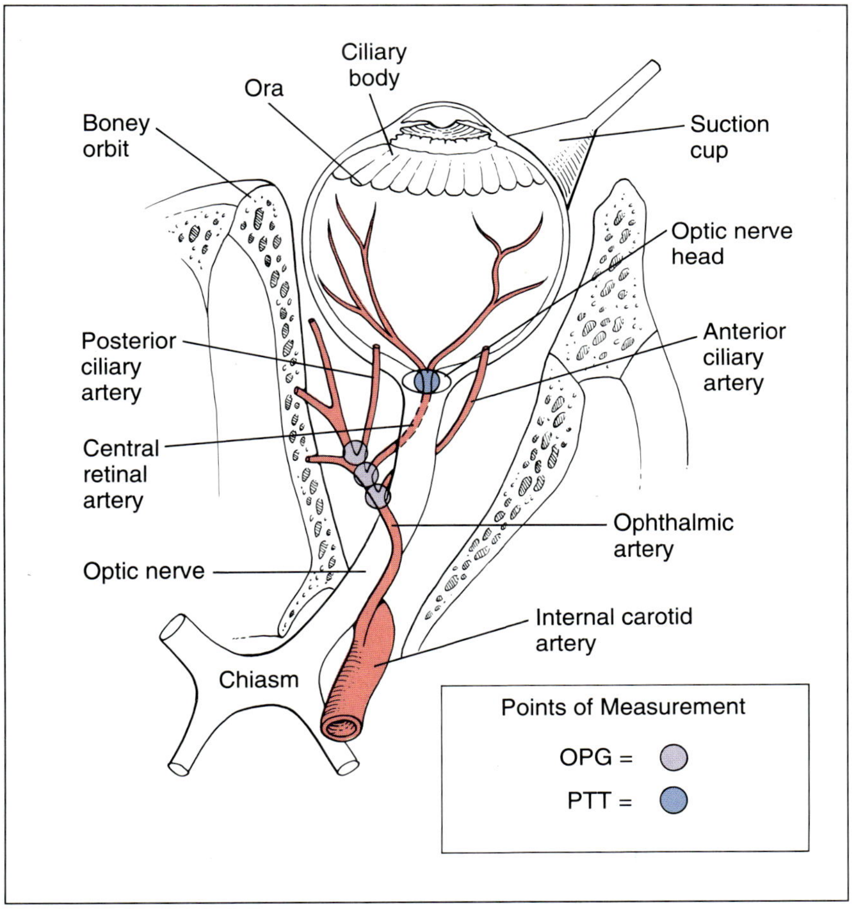

5.16 | Schematic diagram of the blood supply of the eye. By ocular pneumoplethysmography (OPG) and its modifications the blood pressure is measured in the ciliary arteries and in the central retinal artery, i.e., outside the eye and relatively far away from the site of glaucoma damage. In the pressure tolerance test (PTT) the artificial increase of the IOP has its most prominent action in the optic nerve head, i.e., at the site where glaucoma damage occurs.

5.17 | Schematic diagrams showing circulatory autoregulation. *A:* Low recording speed: blood flow plotted versus the perfusion pressure. Curves of this shape may be obtained in animal experiments in kidney, brain or eye. The perfusion pressure is changed by altering systemic blood pressure. *B:* Low recording speed: blood flow plotted versus the intraocular pressure. A curve of this shape can be obtained from the eye in animals and in humans by artificially increasing the IOP. Because an increase in IOP results in a decrease in perfusion pressure, the curve in *B* is essentially the inverse of *A*. Because blood flow and amplitude of the VECP are correlated, the ordinate can represent either. The time required for generating curves *A* and *B* is at least 25 minutes. *C:* High recording speed: amplitude of the VECP (solid line, left ordinate) and IOP (broken line, right ordinate) are plotted versus time. IOP is changed in a step function. The VECP amplitude shows a rapid initial drop and then recovers gradually. *D:* Ordinates and abscissa as in *C*, but IOP is changed in a staircase function. *E:* The amplitudes of the VECP, averaged during each pressure step (ordinate) from *D*, are plotted versus the IOP. (Adapted from Kirchheim H: Kreislaufregulation, in Busse R (ed): *Kreislaufphysiologie*. Stuttgart: Thieme, 1982, 167–210.)

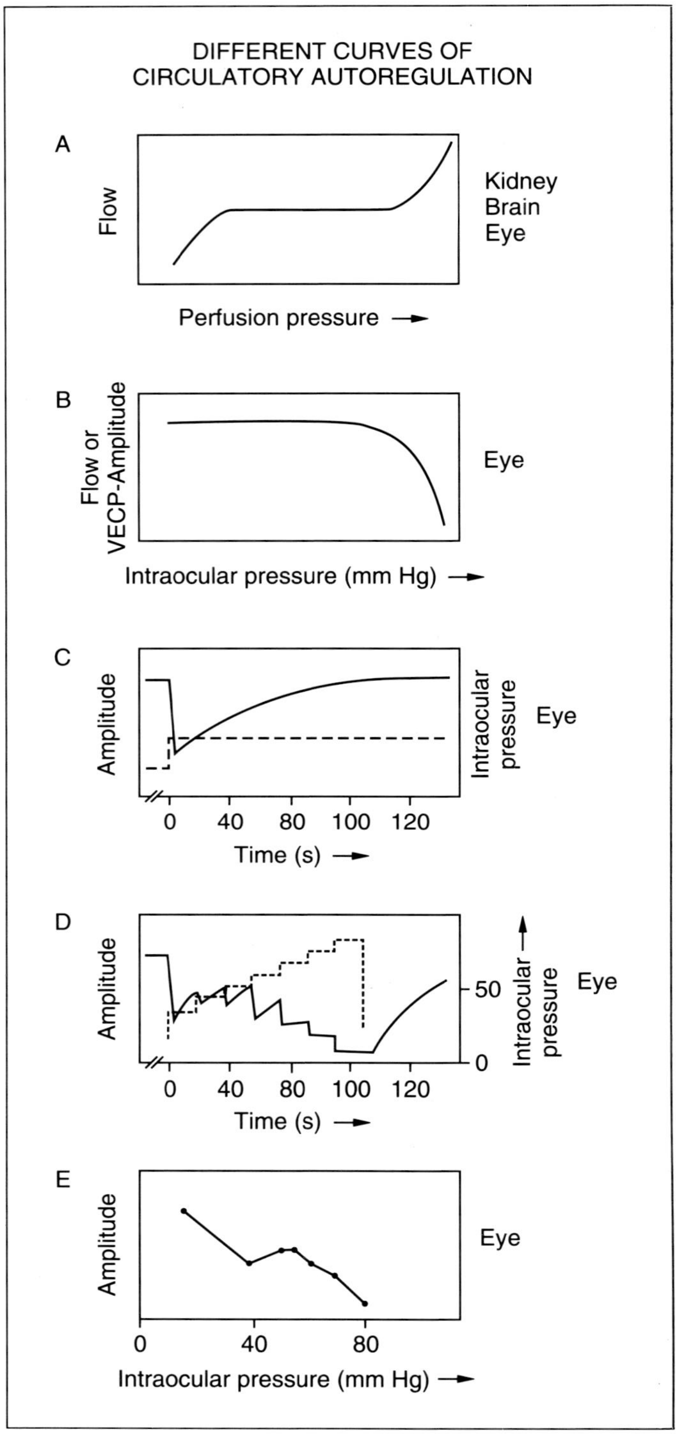

AUTOREGULATION DEMONSTRATED BY DIFFERENT AMPLITUDE/ PRESSURE CURVES

Autoregulation, when present, may maintain the pressure head in the regions in danger. Therefore, as long as autoregulation is present moderate increases in IOP may be tolerated. If autoregulation ceases, damage to the optic nerve may begin.

Healthy eyes maintain their VECP amplitudes despite moderate IOP increases, perhaps because of autoregulation in the vessels of the optic disc, but glaucomatous eyes do not. Autoregulation is a general principle in biology and is seen with regard to blood flow in the kidney or the brain[78] (Fig. 5.17). Curves such as those in Figure 5.17A are derived from experiments in which the blood pressure in the arteries is varied, thus changing the perfusion pressure; blood flow is then measured some minutes later after the system has reached a new steady state. The perfusion pressure in the eye can also be altered by changing the blood pressure, but this is more easily accomplished by increasing the IOP. In this case, a curve such as that in Figure 5.17B results, because an *in*creasing IOP *de*creases the perfusion pressure (see Fig. 5.15).

Immediately after the initial IOP increase, the VECPs decrease and then gradually rise again to a steady-state level (Fig. 5.17C). Such behavior is quite well known in regulated technical and biological systems.[79] The time in which the steady state is reached is about 120 seconds (time constant = 40 seconds). Because the time for each experimental pressure step is 20 seconds, we are always interfering with the recovery process (if it is present) at each pressure step and the recovery process is often stopped by a new pressure step (Fig. 5.17D).

PRESSURE TOLERANCE TEST

In the current technique,[80] the patient sits in front of a TV screen which shows pattern reversal stimuli at a reversal rate of 7.5/second (Fig. 5.18). Steady-state evoked potentials are measured by a vector voltmeter[81] which gives the amplitude and latency of the response at every moment. The evoked potentials are measured first at spontaneous IOP and then at artificially increased intraocular pressure. The IOP is raised in staircase steps at 20-second intervals, using the suction cup method.[73] If certain exclusion criteria are observed, e.g., high myopia or previous intraocular surgery, the suction cup method is safe.[73,74,82,83] When IOP is elevated above the systolic blood pressure, blood is prevented from entering the eye. In the current procedure, total cessation of blood flow to the eye lasts only about 20 *seconds,* while full recovery occurs in healthy eyes even after a cessation of blood flow for *20 minutes.*[84] The most serious unwanted effect may be a subconjunctival hemorrhage. After recording, the amplitudes of the VECP are plotted against IOP, generating amplitude/pressure curves (Figs. 5.17 and 5.18). In healthy subjects, the curve does not decline linearly. Rather, the amplitudes decrease at the first pressure step, but with further increase of the IOP the amplitudes again increase or maintain their value until they decline to the background noise level at quite high IOP. This first inflection of the curve may be described as a kink, and is usually lacking in glaucomatous eyes (see Stodtmeister and Pillunat, Chapter 7).

5.18 | Block diagram of the examination setup for the recording of visually evoked cortical potentials at artificially increased intraocular pressure. The patient is viewing pattern reversal stimuli. The signals are led off by skin electrodes, amplified, and digitally stored. A computer controls the entire examination, including the suction pump. After the end of the examination the computer plots the amplitude of the visually evoked cortical potentials versus the IOP (amplitude/pressure curve).

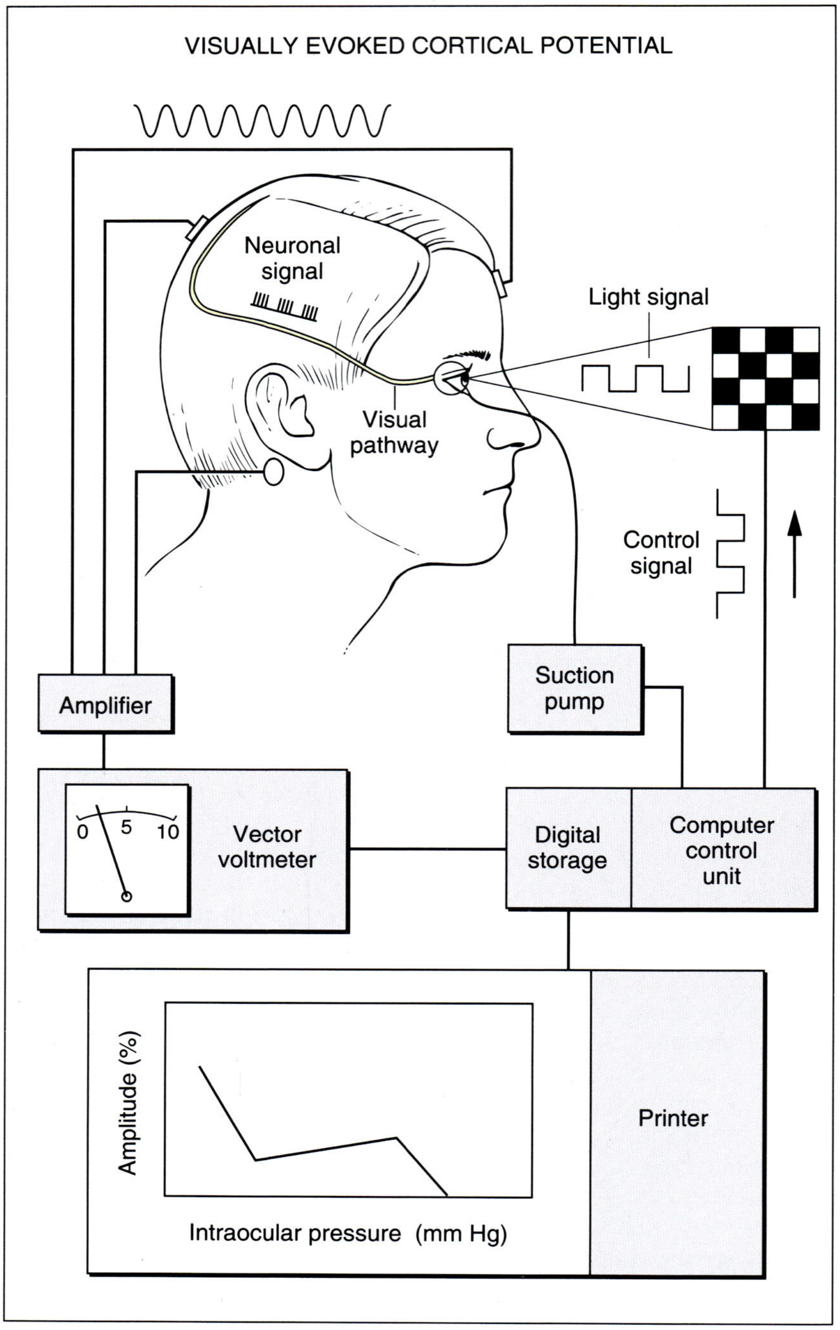

6 | Structure and Appearance of the Optic Nerve Head and Retinal Nerve Fiber Layer in Glaucoma

Section I

Histopathology of the Optic Nerve Head and Retinal Nerve Fiber Layer in Glaucoma

Ronald L. Radius

The principal features of glaucomatous optic neuropathy are irreversible damage to the ganglion cell axon (presumably at the level of the optic nerve head), descending atrophy of the axonal segment within the retina, and death of the ganglion cell of origin.[1–7] Histopathologically, axon loss and ganglion cell drop-out can be recognized in thinning of both the retinal nerve fiber and ganglion cell layers (Fig. 6.1). In most cases, this axon loss is seen throughout the optic nerve cross-section and the inner retinal layers. This pattern is recognized clinically as generalized enlargement of the optic nerve cup with thinning

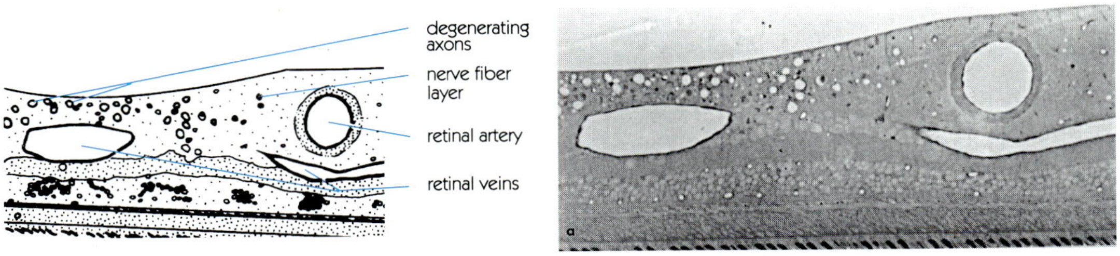

6.1 | Ophthalmoscopic nerve fiber bundle defects are a common finding in eyes with glaucomatous optic neuropathy. Histologically, these defects reflect thinning of the nerve fiber layer (left) in contrast to the thicker axon layer in the more normal adjacent retina (right). (From Radius RL, Anderson DR: The history of retinal nerve fiber layer bundles and bundle defects. *Arch Ophthalmol 1979;97:948.*)

of the neural retinal rim.[2–5] In many cases, however, at some time during the disease process axon damage preferentially involves the superior and inferior poles of the optic nerve head, producing vertical elongation of the enlarging optic cup (Fig. 6.2). Within the retina, there is more localized ganglion cell loss in the region circumscribed by the superior and inferior vascular arcade. The pattern of ganglion cell loss in eyes with experimentally induced glaucoma indicates that axons of larger ganglion cells may be preferentially vulnerable to pressure-induced axon damage.[8–11]

A generalized reduction in tissue volume occurs within the anterior optic nerve head as a result of ongoing axon loss (Fig. 6.3). Remaining columns of glial cells collapse on deeper layers. Within the lamina cribrosa, the laminar sheets are compressed, reduced in number, and begin to bow backward from the horizontal plane of the surrounding retinal layers (Fig. 6.4). In more advanced disease, the region of the lamina scleralis undermines the adjacent choroid, although the size of the optic canal at the level of

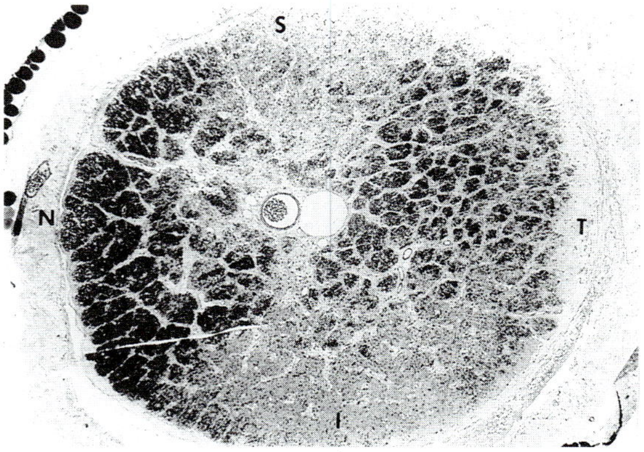

6.2 | In eyes with moderate glaucomatous optic neuropathy, axon loss can be recognized throughout the extent of the nerve section. In many eyes, however, the superior (S) and inferior (I) poles are preferentially involved by the neuron damage. N= nasal; T= temporal. (From Radius RL, Pederson JE: Laser-induced primate glaucoma. *Arch Ophthalmol 1984;102:1693.*)

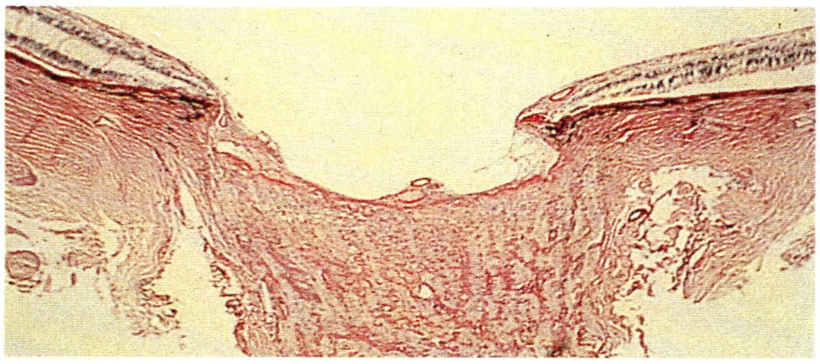

6.3 | Deeply cupped optic nerve head. (From Yanoff M, Fine BS: *Ocular Pathology. A Color Atlas, ed 2.* New York: Gower Medical Publishing, 1992, 16.14.)

Bruch's membrane remains unchanged.[2,4,5,12–16] The number of capillaries is reduced, as is the amount of glial tissue within the anterior optic nerve. With continued retrodisplacement of the lamina cribrosa, the surface area of the lamina increases, leaving the overall amount of glial tissue, both anterior and posterior, slightly increased or little changed (Fig. 6.5).

Remaining axons often demonstrate localized swelling and organelle accumulation similar to that described in experimental models of glaucoma.[16] Axonal columns follow increasingly complex paths through collapsed and misaligned laminar pores. Glial astrocytes fill spaces within these tissue columns as axons die and disappear. More posteriorly, ascending (Wallerian) degeneration of axon segments proceeds along the entire extent of the optic nerve. Myelin loss causes a decrease in the diameter of the retroorbital optic nerve.

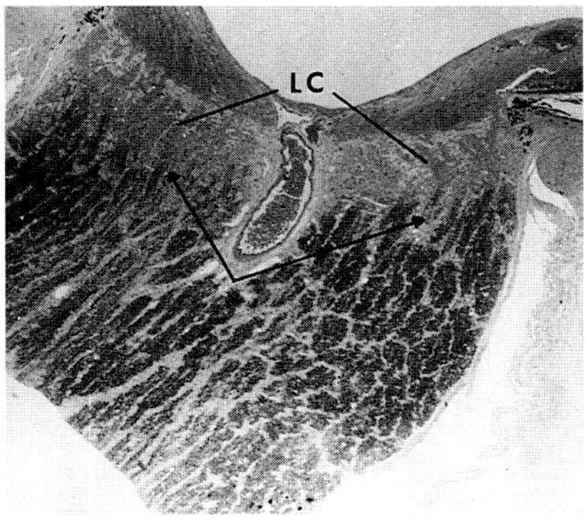

6.4 | In eyes with glaucomatous optic neuropathy, axon loss leads to a reduction in volume of the anterior optic nerve head, and bowing of the posterior lamina cribrosa (LC) can be seen. Loss of myelin (arrows) in the retro-ocular optic nerve is another sign of optic nerve damage in eyes with pressure-induced axon damage (From Radius RL, Pederson JE: Laser-induced primate glaucoma. *Arch Ophthalmol 1984;102:1693.)*

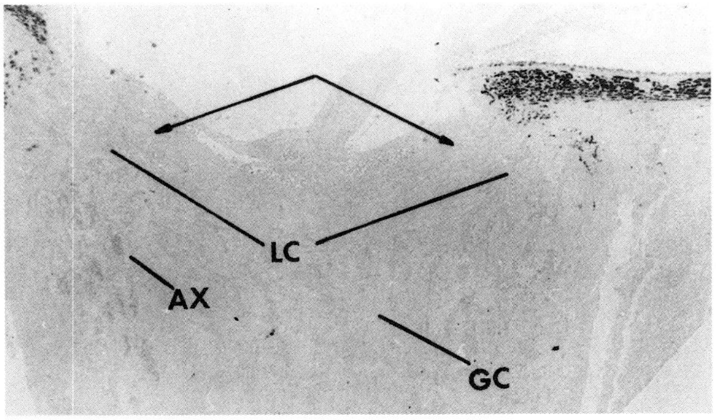

6.5 | In eyes with extensive glaucomatous damage, there may be almost total axon loss. A few neurons (AX) can be identified by the remaining myelin material seen in the intraorbital portion of the nerve behind the globe. The lamina cribrosa (LC) is bowed posteriorly and there is undermining of the scleral rim at the optic nerve head (arrows). Remaining sheets of glial and connective tissue (GC) are collapsed and there is little if any tissue remaining of the anterior optic nerve head. (From Radius RL, Pederson JE: Laser-induced primate glaucoma. *Arch Ophthalmol 1984;102:1693.*)

Section II

Extracellular Matrix of the Human Optic Nerve Head in Glaucoma

M. Rosario Hernandez

When examined by immunofluorescence, the extracellular matrix components of the optic nerve head from human eyes with primary open-angle glaucoma (POAG) differ from those of age-matched normal eyes. Increases in density and in the area occupied by basement membranes in the prelaminar region and in the lamina cribrosa are seen in glaucomatous eyes.[17] A similar observation was recently reported in experimental glaucoma in primates.[18] Histopathologic examination of human eyes in early or moderate stages of glaucoma demonstrated glial hyperplasia in both the laminar and prelaminar regions.[19] These proliferating glial cells are the most likely source of newly synthesized basement membranes and probably represent a response to injury and the loss of axons during the glaucomatous process.

In the cribriform plates of the glaucomatous lamina cribrosa, the extracellular matrix changes markedly and becomes increasingly disorganized with progression of disease. At the ultrastructural level, changes in the elastic fibers are apparent, with loss of the tubular structure of the fibers. Decreases in collagen content as well as thickening and proliferation of basement membrane are evident throughout the lamina cribrosa (Fig. 6.6). In severe primary open-angle glaucoma, there is marked loss of elastin from the cribriform plates immediately bordering the disk surface (Fig. 6.7). The changes in organization and the decreases in density of the elastin fibers in the lamina cribrosa may explain the loss of compliance of the optic nerve head, as measured by laser Doppler velocimetry in primary open-angle glaucoma.[20]

Collagen type VI forms a filamentous network in the extracellular matrix. This form of collagen is present in most tissues, interconnecting fibers of collagen types I and III and near basement membranes.[21] In the normal lamina cribrosa, collagen type VI is localized at the edge of the cribriform plates and as patches of staining in the core. In glaucoma, collagen type VI appears to increase markedly in amount and density, especially in the core of

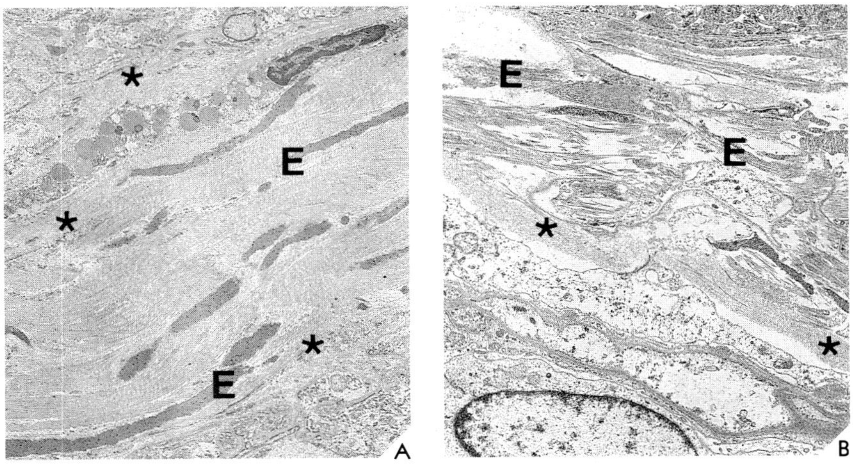

6.6 | Low-magnification electron micrographs of cross-sectional views of cribriform plates. *A:* Normal, 81-year-old subject. Tubular elastic fibers (E) run longitudinally in the core of the cribriform plates. Note the dense collagen matrix surrounding the fibers. Asterisks mark the position of basement membranes not clearly visible at 4,200 magnification. *B:* Mild POAG, 74-year-old patient. The extracellular matrix of the cribriform plates appears disorganized. Fragments of elastic fibers (E) are present in the markedly loose collagen matrix. Asterisks point to thickened basement membranes that serve as reference for the limits of the core of plates. (From Hernandez MR: Ultrastructural immunocytochemical analysis of elastin in the human lamina cribrosa. Changes in elastic fibers in primary open angle glaucoma. *Invest Ophthalmol Vis Sci* 1992; 33:2891-2903.)

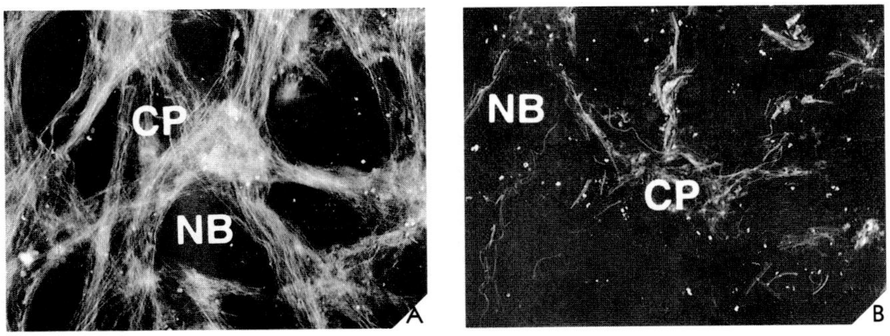

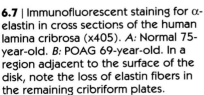

6.7 | Immunofluorescent staining for α-elastin in cross sections of the human lamina cribrosa (x405). *A:* Normal 75-year-old. *B:* POAG 69-year-old. In a region adjacent to the surface of the disk, note the loss of elastin fibers in the remaining cribriform plates. CP=cribriform plate; NB=nerve bundle. (From Hernandez MR, Neufeld AH: The extracellular matrix of the optic nerve, in Drance S, Neufeld AH, Van Buskirk EM (eds): *Pharmacology of the Glaucomas.* Baltimore: Williams and Wilkins, 1992.)

the plates (Fig. 6.8). The increase in collagen type VI is apparent at all stages of the glaucomatous process[17] and throughout the entire lamina cribrosa, suggesting that collagen type VI is a reactional form of collagen in this tissue.

Unfortunately, it is not possible at present to determine whether the changes observed in glaucomatous eyes represent a response to the loss of neural tissue, with subsequent rearrangement of the cribriform plates owing to elevated intraocular pressure (IOP), or whether these changes imply a predisposing weakness in this connective tissue that permits the glaucomatous excavation of the optic nerve head to progress in response to elevated IOP.

Cells grown in tissue culture have helped us to understand better the different responses of the connective tissue in the human lamina cribrosa.[22] These lamina cribrosa cells are broad, flat, and markedly sensitive to the growth factor PDGF, suggesting that they are a form of neuroglial cell.[23] In culture these cells synthesize many of the macromolecular components of the extracellular matrix of the lamina cribrosa, including collagen types I, III, IV, VI, and elastin.

Recently, these lamina cribrosa cells have been grown under hydrostatic pressure 50 mm Hg above atmospheric pressure. Cells grown under high pressure for 7 days become markedly elongated as compared with control cells grown under atmospheric pressure. They also exhibit more mRNA for collagen type I, as determined by dot-blot hybridization and in situ hybridization, and they secrete more collagen type I onto the tissue culture plate, as determined by immunofluorescence[24] (Fig. 6.9). Therefore, in response to hydrostatic pressure in vitro, these cells synthesize and lay down more fibrillar forms of collagen, as though building a more rigid substrate.

The new techniques of molecular biology provide means to study gene expression and regulation of the synthesis of extracellular matrix macromolecules. Cloned human genes, as well as genomic and cDNA probes for collagens, elastin, and attachment factor, are now widely available. Although immunohistochemistry has identified and localized extracellular matrix macromolecules, it does not yield information on the metabolic activity of specific cells, nor does it distinguish newly synthesized from accumulated material. In situ hybridization allows the identification of mRNA within fixed tissue sections of cells in culture by use of radiolabeled cDNA or cRNA probes

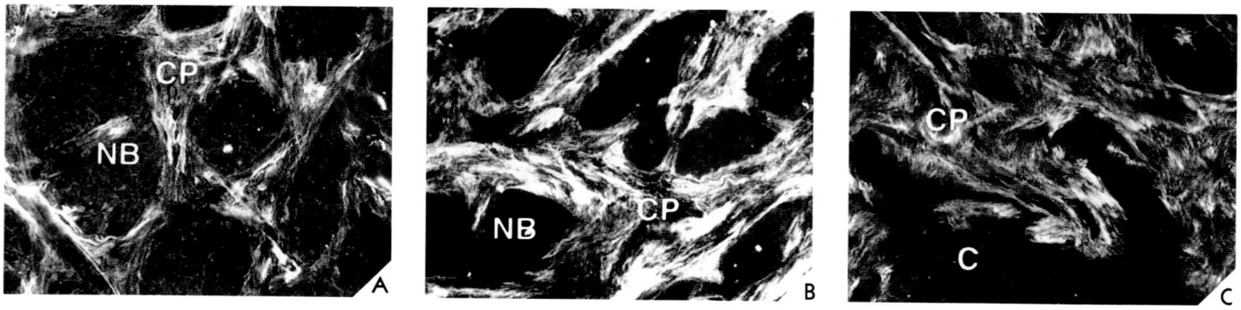

6.8 | Immunofluorescent staining for collagen type VI in cross sections of the human lamina cribrosa (x405). *A:* Normal 75-year-old. Collagen type VI is present at the edges of the cribriform plates (CP) and as patches of staining inside the core. *B:* POAG, 73-year-old. In the region adjacent to the central vessels, note the increase in collagen type VI. *C:* POAG, 69-year-old. In the region adjacent to the surface of the disc, note the increase in collagen type VI in the plates bordering the cup (C). NB=nerve bundles. (From Hernandez MR, Neufeld AH: The extracellular matrix of the optic nerve, in Drance S, Neufeld AH, Van Buskirk EM (eds): *Pharmacology of the Glaucomas.* Baltimore: Williams and Wilkins, 1992.)

followed by autoradiography.[25] Recently, it has been shown with in situ hybridization that cells of the lamina cribrosa express mRNA for both collagen types I and IV in individual human optic nerves throughout life[26] (Fig. 6.10). Future work with the use of this technique will allow the determination of whether the changes observed with age and in glaucoma are due to altered biosynthesis or to degradation of extracellular matrix macromolecules.

Investigations into the extracellular matrix of the human lamina cribrosa are continuing to test the hypothesis that there is a connective tissue component of glaucomatous optic nerve degeneration. Some structural weakness in this tissue, derived from variability of age-related changes, may predispose certain individuals' optic nerves to damage by elevated IOP. Furthermore, inherent defects or weaknesses in the extracellular matrix of the lamina cribrosa of certain individuals, perhaps due to slight changes, errors, or imbalances of key macromolecular components, may produce an optic nerve head that exhibits progressive cupping at normal IOP, causing low-tension glaucoma. Thus, the composition of the extracellular matrix of an individual's lamina cribrosa may provide the optic nerve head with a structure whose biophysical characteristics of rigidity change with age, and are sensitive to IOP. Elucidation of the pathophysiologic role played by connective tissue in the glaucomatous process awaits further investigation.

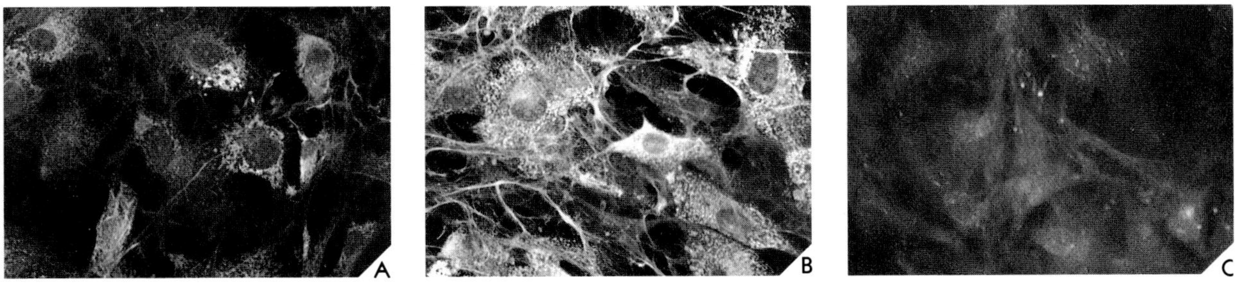

6.9 | Human lamina cribrosa cells in culture. Immunofluorescent staining for collagen type I (x410). *A:* Cells grown under atmospheric pressure show intracellular staining for collagen type I. *B:* Cells grown under elevated hydrostatic pressure show intense intracellular and extracellular staining for collagen type I. *C:* Cells incubated with nonimmune serum instead of the primary antibody show no immunofluorescent staining negative control. (From Hernandez MR, Neufeld AH: The extracellular matrix of the optic nerve, in Drance S, Neufeld AH, Van Buskirk EM (eds): *Pharmacology of the Glaucomas.* Baltimore: Williams and Wilkins, 1992.)

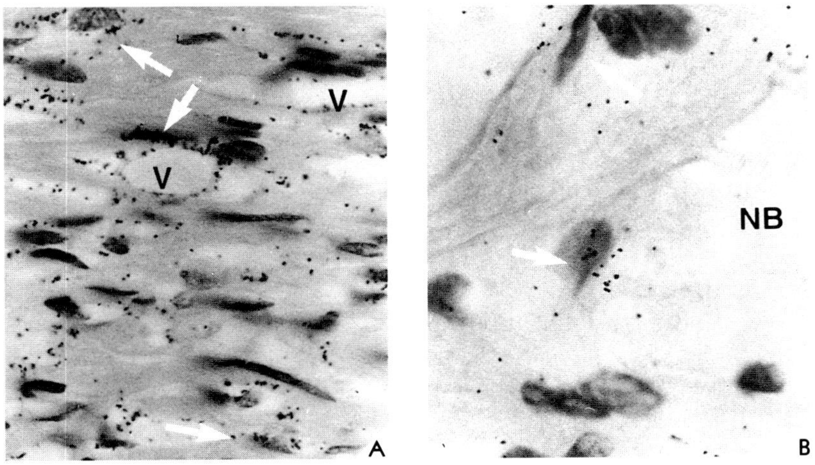

6.10 | Expression of collagen type IV mRNA in human optic nerve heads. In situ hybridization of human lamina cribrosa from normal eyes with ^{35}S-antisense RNA for collagen type IV. *A:* Normal, 56-year-old. Sagittal view of the cribriform plates (x450). Arrows point to labeled cells in the plates and in the blood vessels (V). *B:* Normal, 55-year-old. Cross-sectional view of the cribriform plates (x890). Arrows point to labeled cells lining the plates. NB = nerve bundle. (Adapted from Hernandez MR, Hanley NM, Neufeld AH: Localization of collagen types I and IV mRNAs in human optic nerve head by in situ hybridization. *Invest Ophthalmol Vis Sci 1991;32:2169-2177.*)

Section III

Ophthalmoscopic and Photographic Characteristics of the Optic Nerve Head in Glaucoma

Eve J. Higginbotham

Increased ratio of the optic cup to the disc diameters (C/D ratio) is considered an important risk factor for, and is often a sign of, glaucoma. A C/D ratio below 0.4 occurs in a majority of normal persons, with only 6% having ratios greater than 0.5.[27] Asymmetry of optic nerve head cupping between the eyes is also important (Figs. 6.11–6.13); differences between the C/D ratios of two eyes was noted to be >0.1 in only 8% of Armaly's normal series and >0.2 in less than 1%. A splinter disc hemorrhage (Fig. 6.14) indicates the presence and progression of glaucoma. Prevalence rates of 0%, 0.44%, and 2.44% were found in normal, glaucoma-suspect, and glaucomatous eyes in a prospective study.[28] Therefore, enlarged C/D ratio, C/D asymmetry, and disc hemorrhage are important indicators of optic nerve damage.

Additional glaucomatous changes in the optic nerve include vertical elongation of the cup and saucerization of the nerve head, localized thinning, sloping, or notching of the neuroretinal rim, sharp angulation of vessels crossing the disc margin, baring of the disc vessels (due to loss of surrounding and overlying neural and glial tissue), and peripapillary atrophy (Fig. 6.15). An increase in the vertical diameter of the cup to more than the horizontal diameter, resulting in ovalization of the cup contour, has been considered an early sign of glaucomatous damage.[29] This corresponds well with the postmortem finding of fewer remaining nerve fibers in the superior and inferior poles as compared with other areas in optic nerves of glaucomatous eyes.[30] Localized thinning of the neuroretinal rim[31] (see Fig 6.19) and sharp angulation of vessels exiting the nerve indicate localized nerve loss.[32] Peripapillary atrophy has also been associated with nerve damage.[33] In fact, in cases when glaucomatous optic nerve atrophy occurs in the presence of a small disc, peripapillary atrophy and nerve fiber layer defects may be the only indication of disease on ophthalmoscopic examination.[34] Figure 6.15 summarizes the major ophthalmoscopic findings in glaucoma.

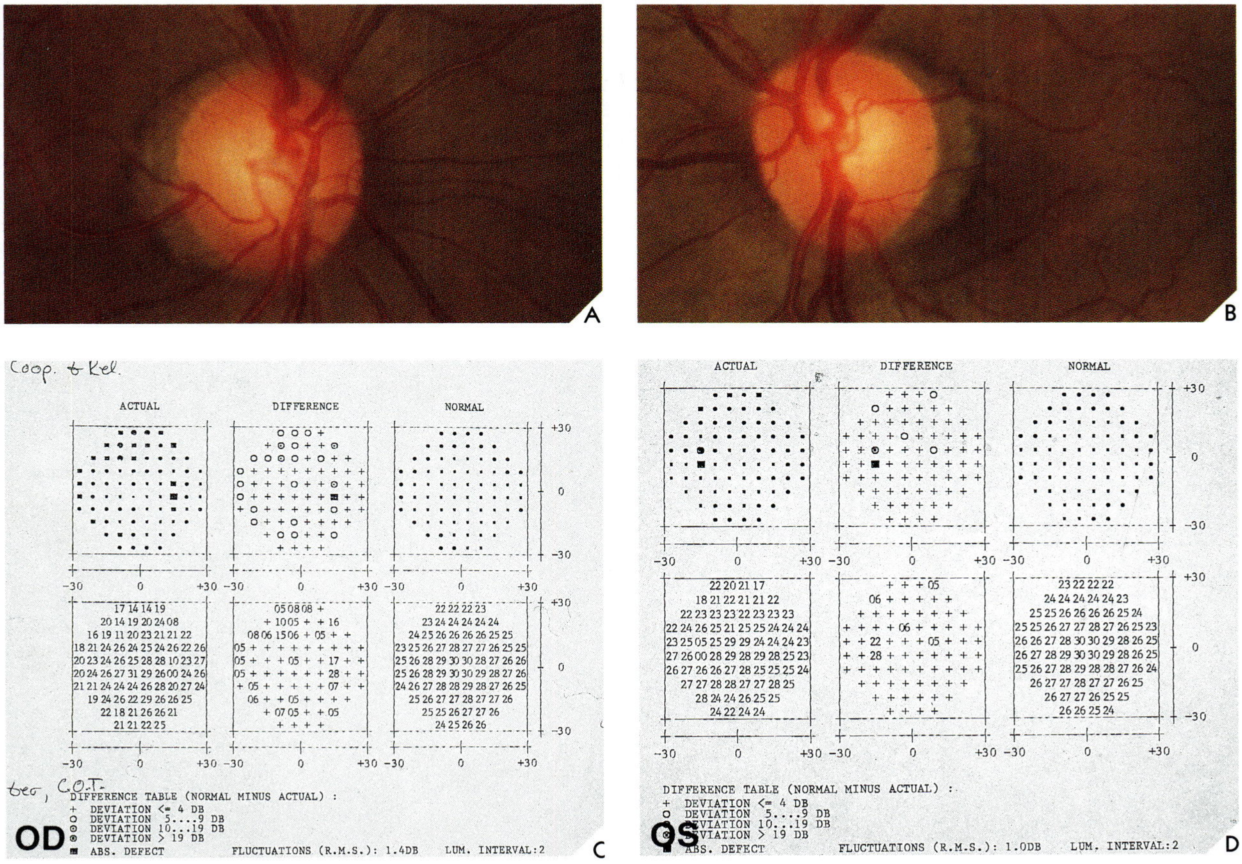

6.11 | The C/D ratio of the right eye (*A*) is 0.7 and the left eye (*B*) 0.5. Note the increased sloping inferotemporally in the right eye as compared with the left eye. This asymmetry corresponded to asymmetric pressures (OD 31 mm Hg; OS 20 mm Hg) and visual fields (*C*, OD and *D*, OS). There are more depressed points (central squares) compared with age-matched normals in the right eye versus the left eye visual field.

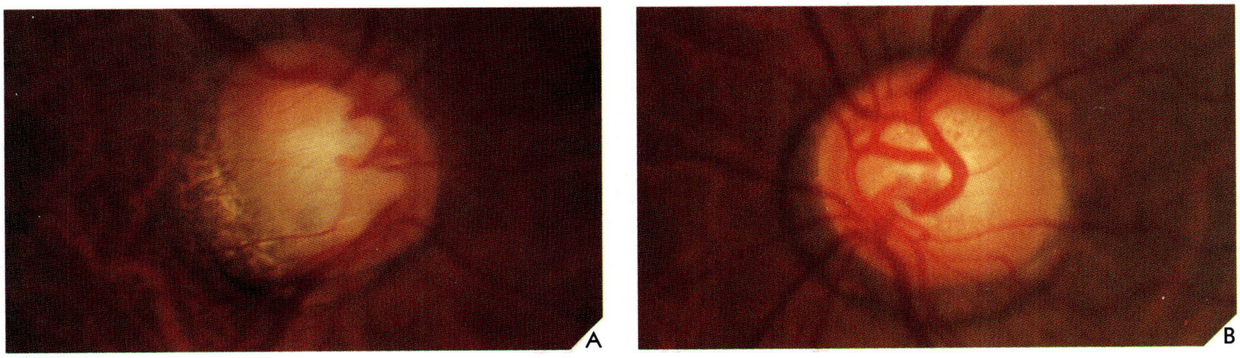

6.12 | Marked asymmetry in cupping and peripapillary changes are noted in this pair of photos (*A*, OD and *B*, OS). Note the extensive loss of the temporal rim in the right eye and the obscuration of the circumlinear vessel.

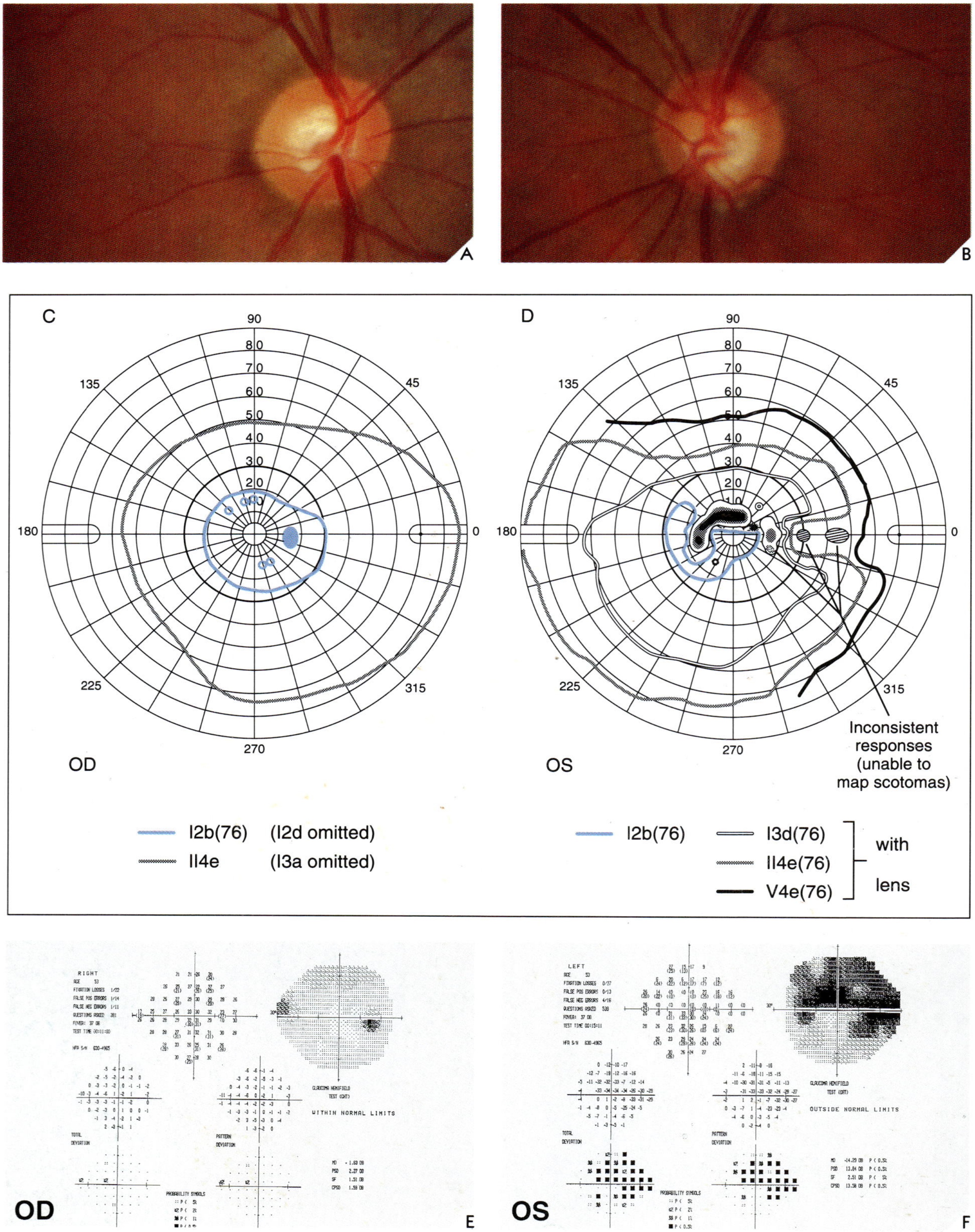

6.13 | Marked asymmetry between nerves, and corresponding asymmetric visual field loss, is illustrated. Note the localized inferior temporal extension of cupping in the left eye (*B*) compared with the right (*A*), and the primarily superior left eye field defect seen with both kinetic (*C* vs. *D*) and static threshold (*E* vs. *F*) perimetry.

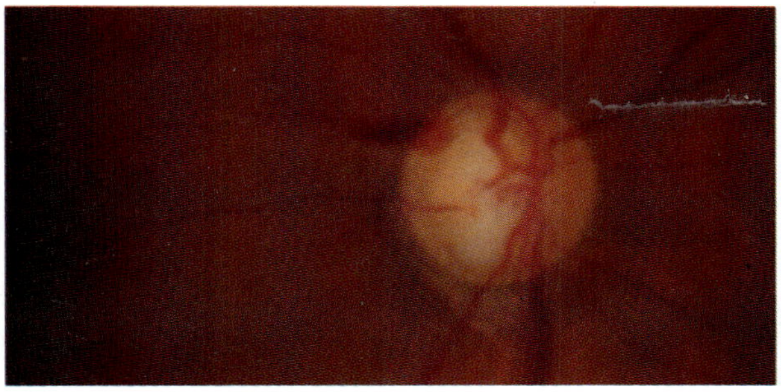

6.14 | A hemorrhage is noted at the margin of the disc in a patient with severe glaucomatous damage.

Figure 6.15. Ophthalmoscopic Indications of Glaucoma

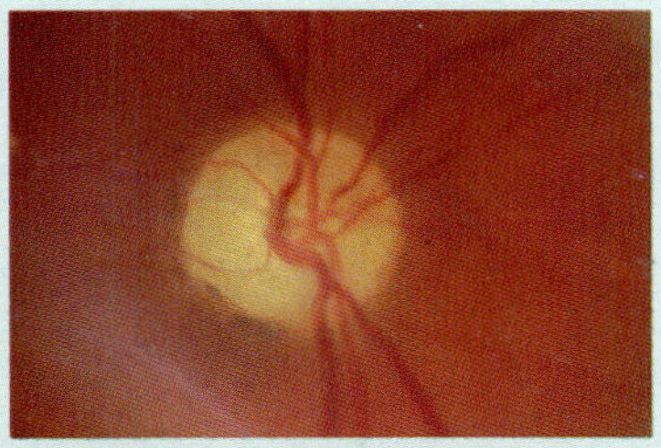

Pallor associated with cupping

Baring of the disc vessels

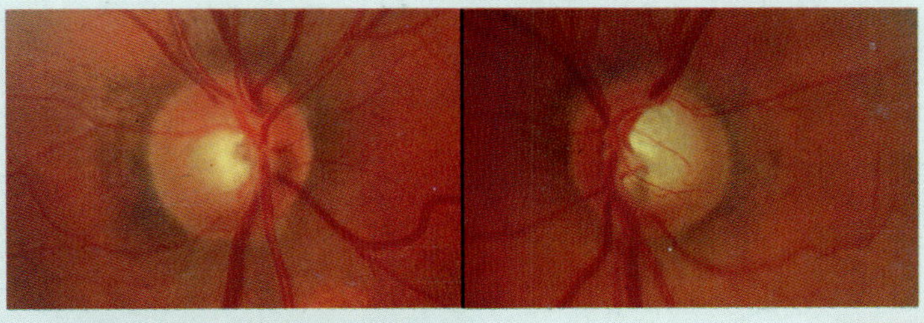

Asymmetry of C/D >0.2 in vertical vs horizontal directions (OS, seen on the right)

Asymmetric extension of cup to margin (notching of rim) (OS)

Exposed lamina cribrosa (OS)

Asymmetry of C/D >0.2 between discs

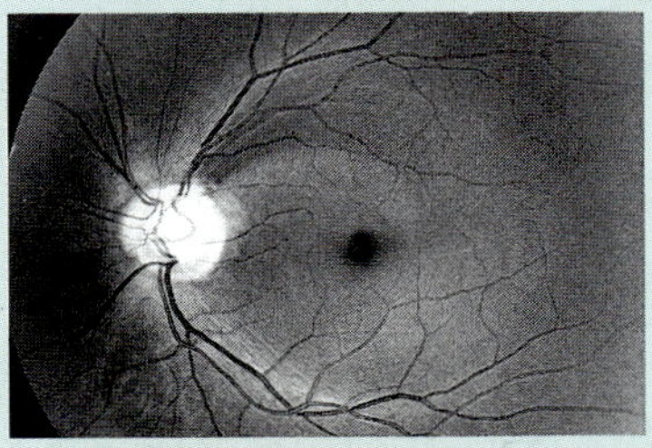

Nerve fiber bundle defects by red free light

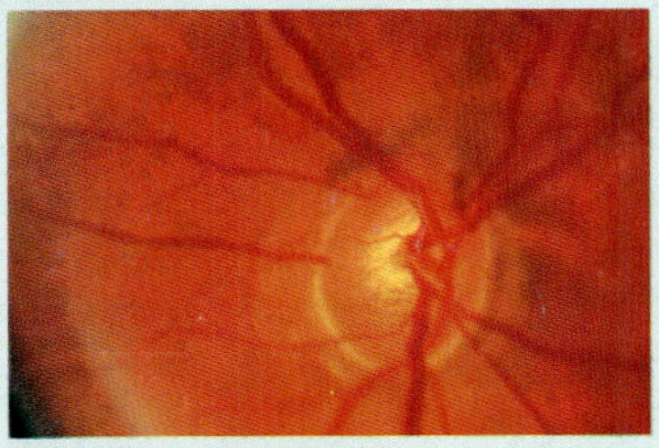

Splinter hemorrhages at the disc margin (11 o'clock)

Asymmetry of cup contour (vertical saucerization)

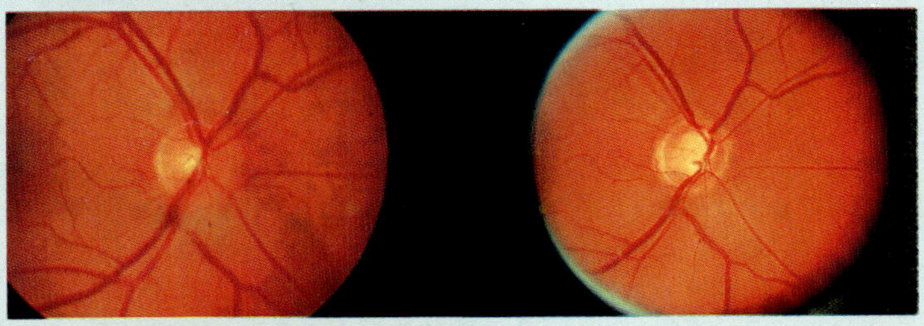

Increased cupping, nasal displacement of vessels, and development of peripapillary atrophy from 1969 (left) to 1977 (right)

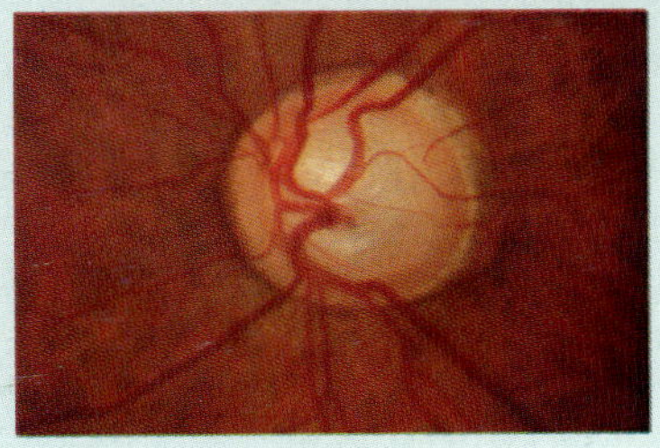

Cupping of the disc margin

Deep cup

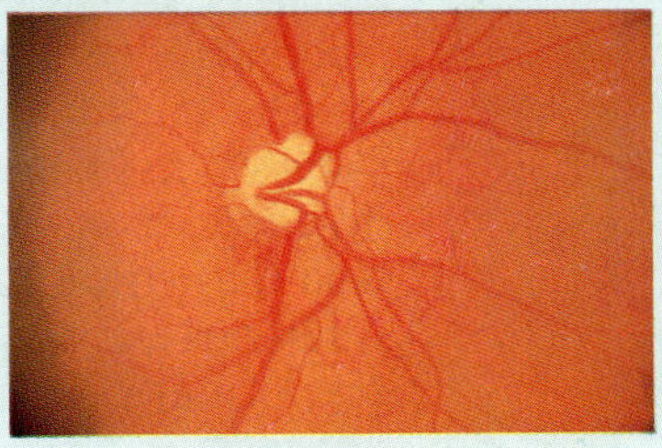

Sharp margins or undermining of large cup

Splinter hemorrhages at the disc margin

Obliteration of the circumlinear vessels

SECTION IV

FUNDUSCOPIC AND PHOTOGRAPHIC CHARACTERISTICS OF THE RETINAL NERVE FIBER LAYER IN GLAUCOMA

Anja Tuulonen
P. Juhani Airaksinen

Glaucoma is a disease of multifactorial causes that produce damage to the ganglion cell axons in the ocular fundus. The loss of nerve fibers gives a typical glaucomatous configuration to the optic nerve head. The structural abnormality leads to functional damage that can be quantified by psychophysical tests, most commonly visual field examination.

In addition to the optic nerve head, the atrophy of ganglion cell axons can also be observed in the retinal nerve fiber layer (RNFL). A defect in the RNFL may, in fact, be the earliest sign of glaucoma, preceding changes in the optic nerve head configuration[35] and the visual field.[36] Therefore, a normal optic disc appearance and a normal visual field do not rule out glaucoma.

PATTERNS OF RNFL ATROPHY

Glaucoma may produce localized or diffuse damage of the RNFL, or a combination of both (Fig. 6.16).[37,38] The beginner's problems with nerve fiber layer evaluation are often based on overestimation of local defects and underestimation of diffuse nerve fiber loss.

In 52% of eyes with developing glaucoma, the first detectable RNFL abnormality is diffuse loss of axons.[39] In early phases this is not always easy to detect. A mottled appearance of the retina (see Fig. 4.21B, Tuulonen and Airaksinen, Chapter 4) is a typical sign of diffuse RNFL damage, in addition to disappearance of the cross-hatched appearance of the small blood vessels and the general darkness and monotony of the image (see Figs. 4.20A, 4.21 Tuulonen and Airaksinen, Chapter 4).

Unlike diffuse damage, localized defects are easier to detect because they are well outlined against the surrounding healthy nerve fiber bundles

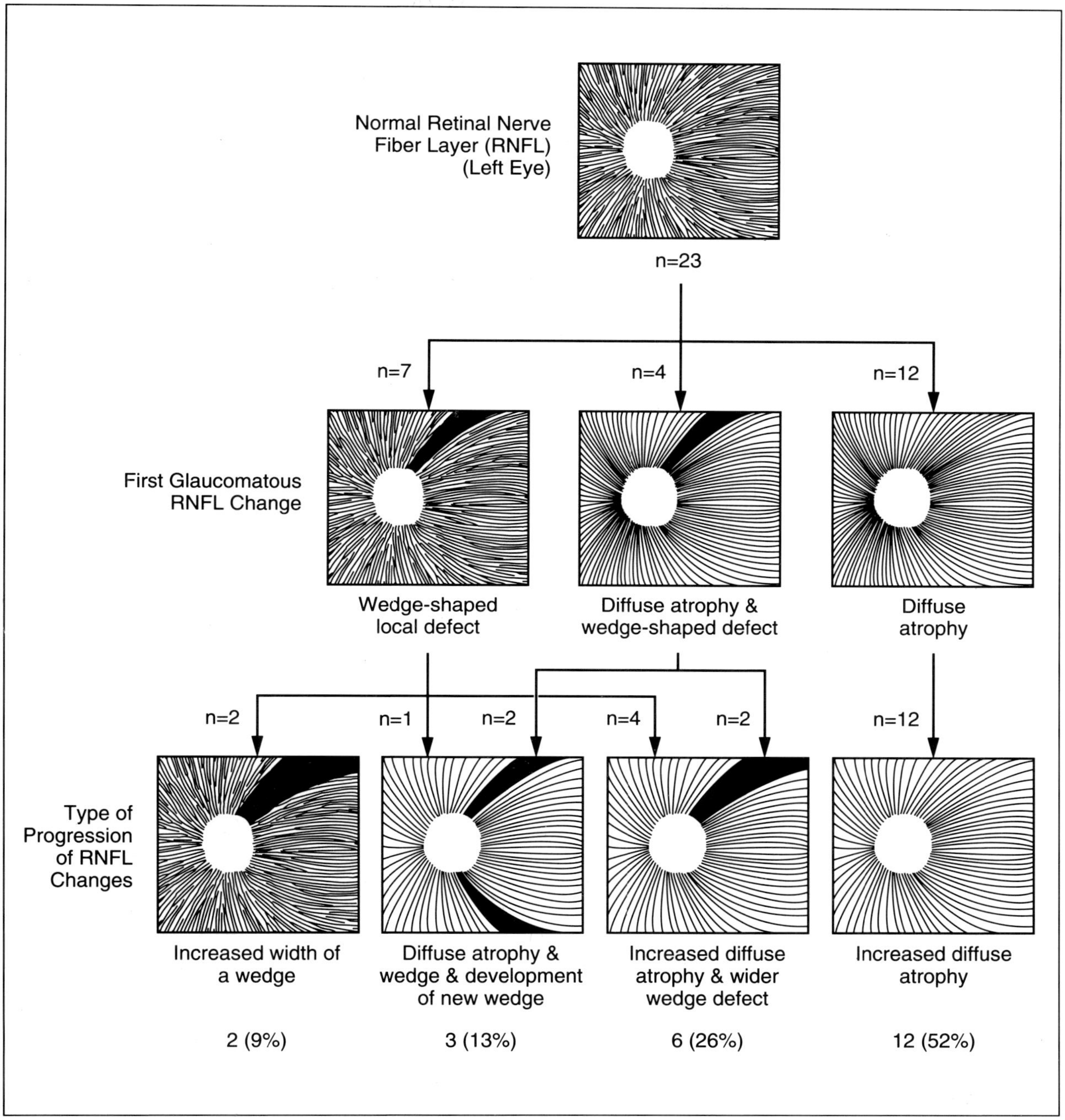

6.16 I The patterns of RNFL atrophy. Localized wedge-shaped defects are found with equal frequency in the upper and lower temporal regions. (Adapted from Tuulonen A, Airaksinen PJ: Initial glaucomatous optic disc and retinal nerve fiber layer abnormalities and their progression. *Am J Ophthalmol 1991;111:485–490.* Published with permission from *The American Journal of Ophthalmology*. Copyright by the Ophthalmic Publishing Company.)

(Fig. 6.17). However, only 30% of eyes with high-tension glaucoma develop a localized RNFL defect as the only initial abnormality. Diffuse atrophy may also be combined with denser localized defects (Fig. 6.18).

RELATIONSHIP OF OPTIC DISC, RNFL, AND VISUAL FIELD ABNORMALITIES

Development and progression of glaucomatous visual field and optic disc abnormalities can be easily understood on the basis of the two- and three-dimensional organization of the RNFL (see Figs. 4.13 and 4.15, Tuulonen and Airaksinen, Chapter 4). For some reason, the first glaucomatous damage affects the upper and lower temporal areas of the optic disc. The affected fibers originate from ganglion cells located about 15–20° from the fovea, close to the temporal raphe (G, Fig. 6.19A). The ganglion cell atrophy cannot be clinically visualized, but the loss of respective axons appears as a wedge-shaped RNFL defect (D) and a small notch (N) at the optic disc margin (see Figs. 6.19A and 6.19B). Corresponding to this localized ganglion cell drop-out, there is an isolated scotoma (VFD, Fig. 6.19A) in the nasal visual field close to the horizontal meridian.

With progression of disease, the RNFL defect becomes wider, the ganglion cell drop-out enlarges along the course of the wedge-shaped RNFL defect, and the visual field defect begins to assume an arcuate shape (see Figs. 6.19C and 6.19D). At this stage the visibility of the RNFL defect is poor near the optic disc because undamaged, more proximally originating axons cover the defect (arrows, Figs. 6.19A and 6.19C).

When the proximally originating axons have also degenerated, the RNFL defect can be visualized all the way to the optic disc. At the same time the notch of the neuroretinal rim reaches the optic disc margin and the arcuate visual field defect connects to the blind spot (see Figs. 6.19E and 6.19F).

Progression of the glaucomatous damage can be seen as further widening of the RNFL defect towards the papillomacular bundles and towards 12

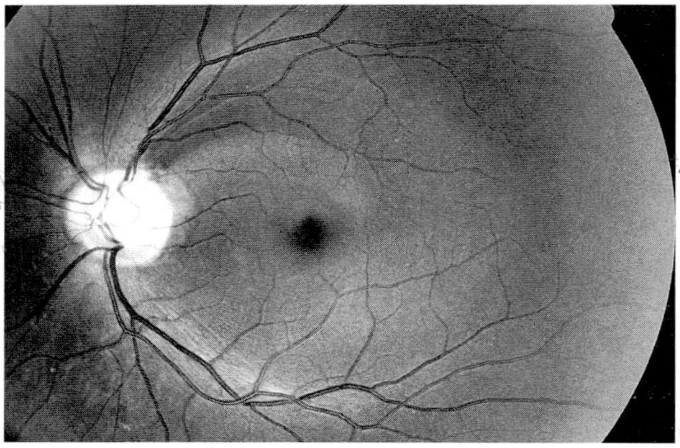

6.17 | Localized RNFL defect in the upper temporal area. A few fibers remain intact within the defect.

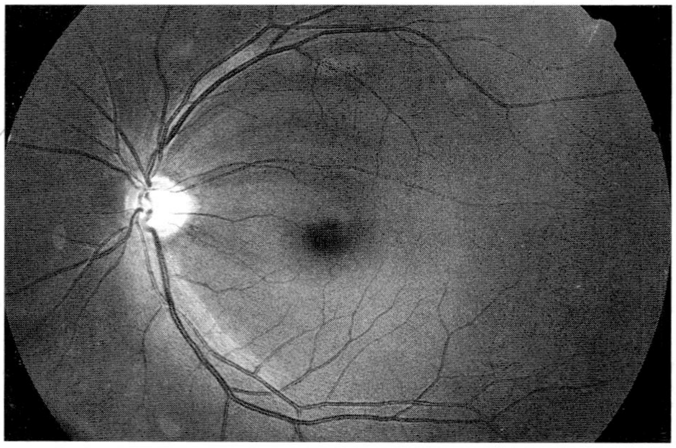

6.18 | Diffuse atrophy in the superior temporal region combined with denser localized defect.

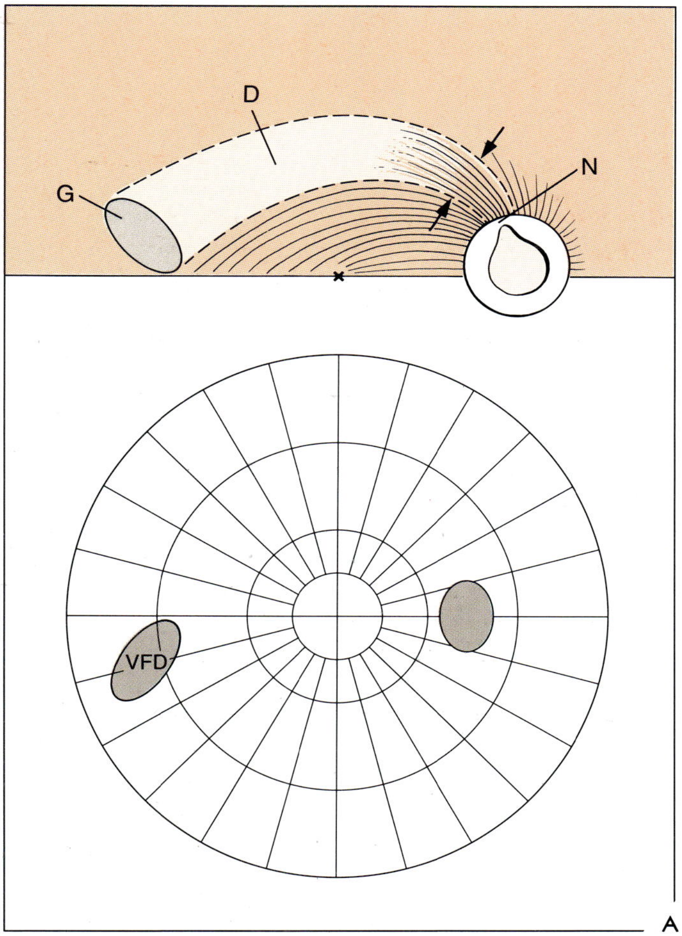

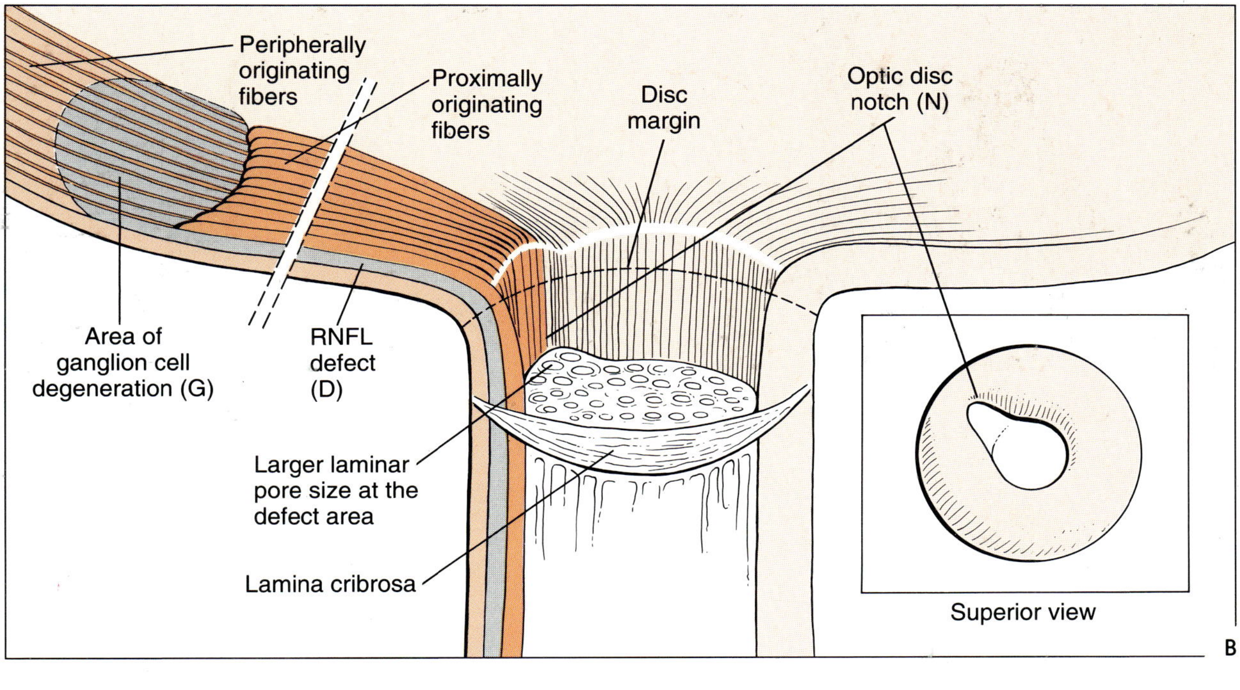

6.19 | Development of classic glaucomatous nerve fiber bundle defect in the visual field. *A:* Isolated scotoma in the nasal visual field. The morphologic changes are depicted at the top and the corresponding visual field defect at the bottom. G=ganglion cell drop-out; D=RNFL defect; N=optic disc notch; VFD=visual field defect. *B:* Three-dimensional illustration of the development of an optic disc notch and a wedge-shaped RNFL defect. (Continued on next page.)

6.19 | (Cont'd.) *C:* The scotoma enlarges and starts to become arcuate in shape. *D:* A clinical example of the previous figure. The patient was a 40-year-old female with low-tension glaucoma seen on August 7, 1989. (Continued on next page.)

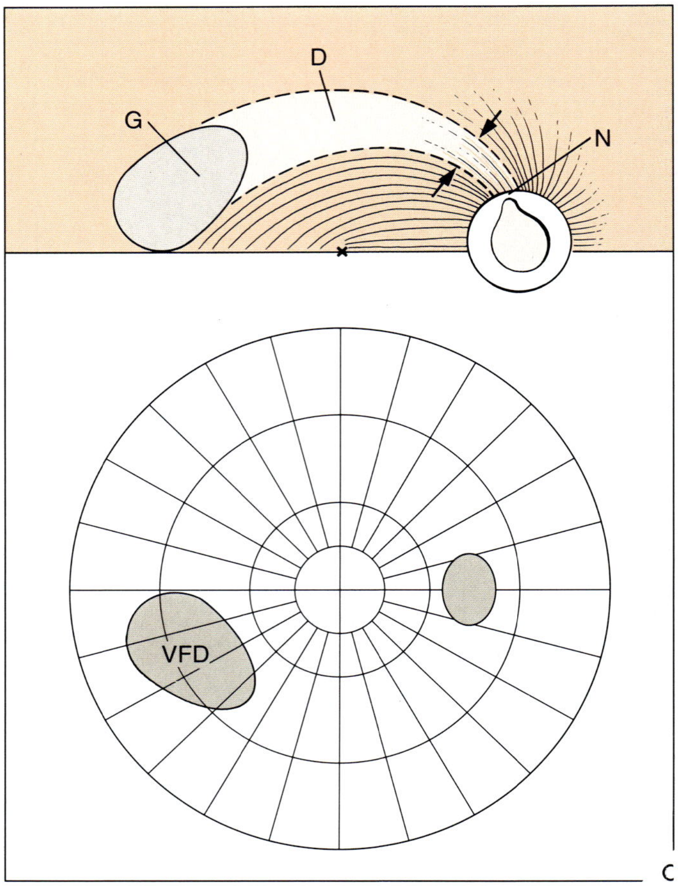

C

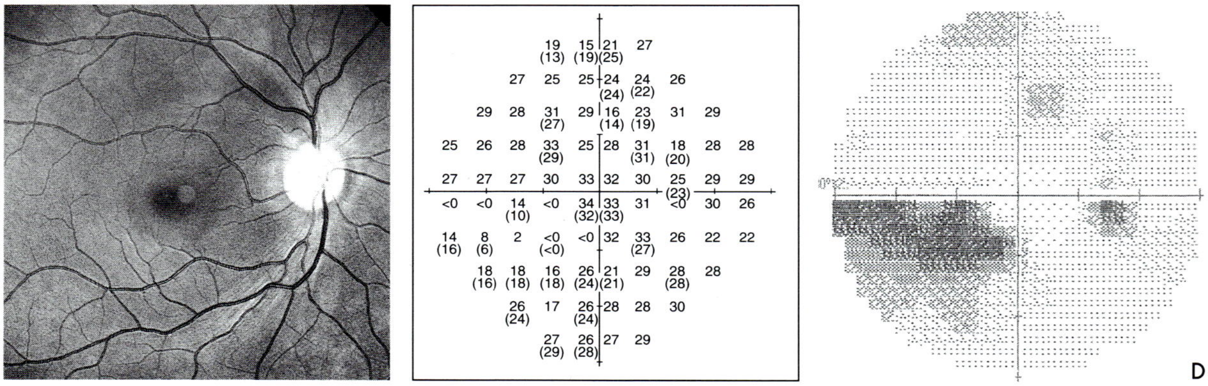

D

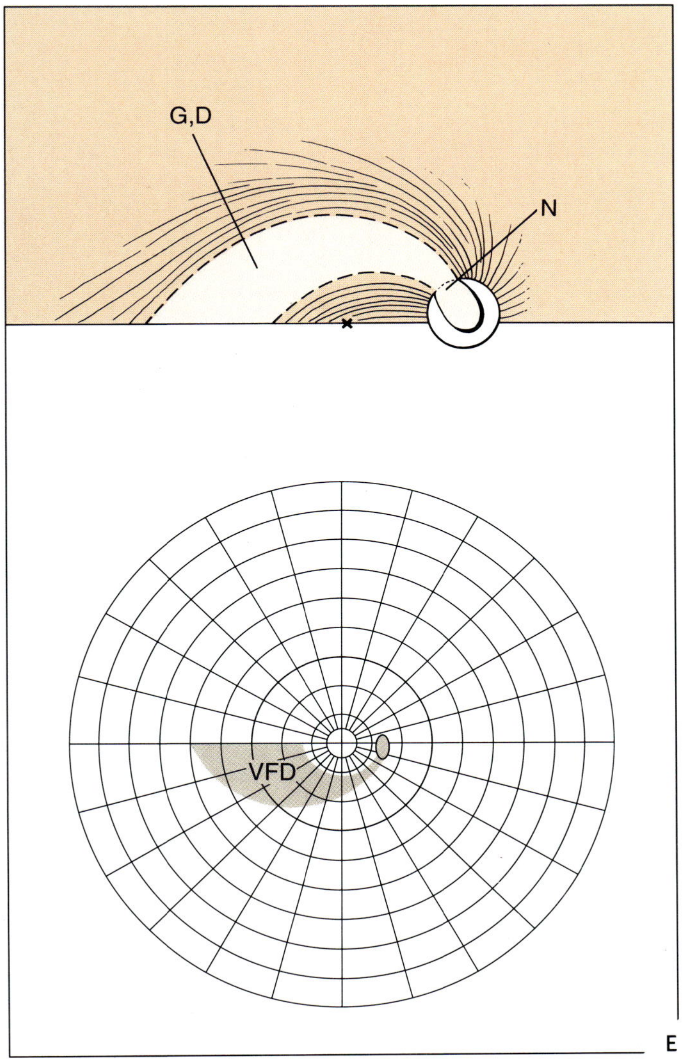

E

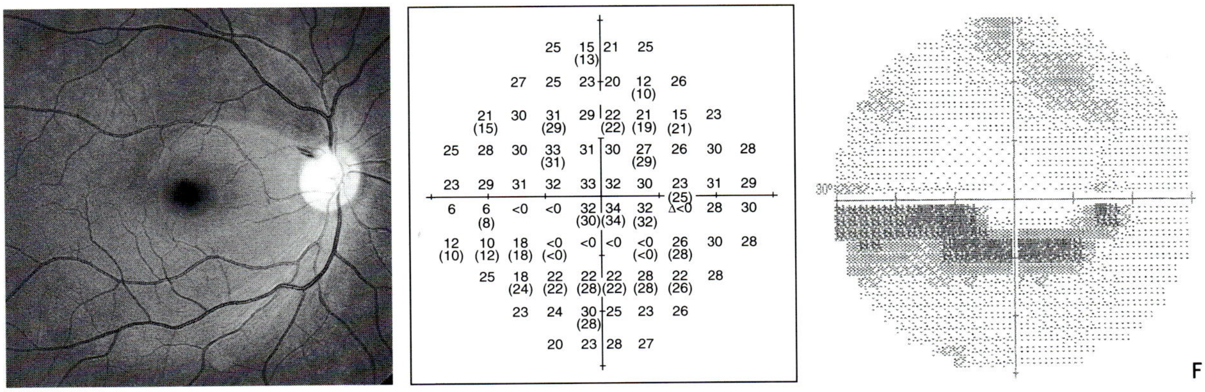

F

6.19 | (Cont'd.) *E:* Connection of arcuate visual field defect into the blind spot. *F:* Clinical example of the previous figure. Same patient as shown in *D,* seen here on August 20, 1991. Note the splinter hemorrhage at disc margin superotemporally. (Continued on next page.)

6.19 | (Cont'd.) *G:* Nasal breakthrough. *H:* Goldmann visual field. Same patient as shown in *D*. Note the breakthrough of arcuate scotoma to the nasal periphery.

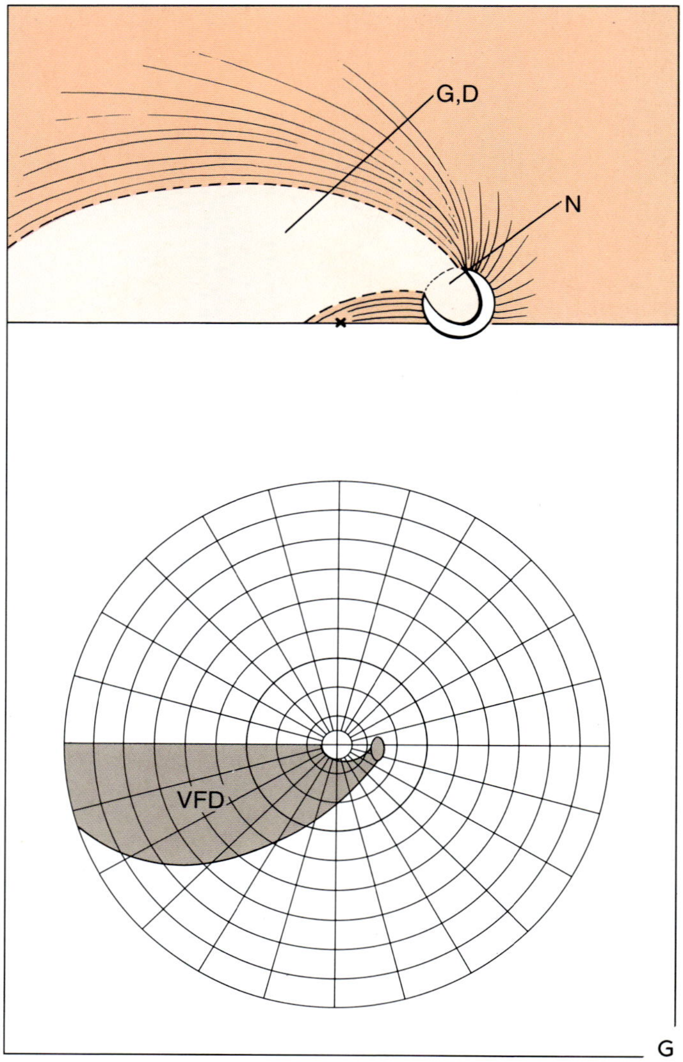

G

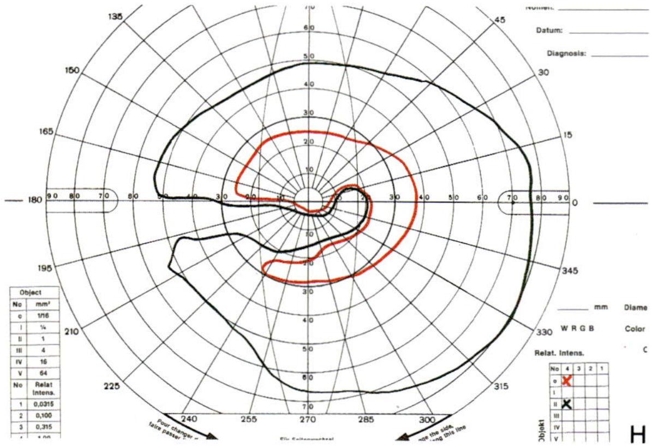

H

o'clock (see Fig. 6.19G). When the papillomacular bundles are threatened, the visual field defect comes closer to fixation. An optic disc hemorrhage at the papillomacular border of the RNFL defect (see Fig. 6.19F) indicates the location of further damage. Progressive loss of axons towards 12 o'clock will gradually produce a nasal breakthrough of the visual field defect (see Figs. 6.19G and 6.19H).

RNFL AS A DIAGNOSTIC TOOL

The diagnosis of glaucoma is always a summary of all the clinical information available. In diagnosing this disease one should not consider the visual fields alone, the optic disc alone, intraocular pressure alone, or RNFL alone. The role and importance of each examination may vary with several patient-related factors such as age, optic media, stage of disease, optic disc size, and other eye diseases.

RNFL observation is helpful when a notch at the disc margin is suspected (Fig. 6.20A–C). If the RNFL is normal, the suspicion was a false alarm. In case of true abnormality, a dark, sharply outlined wedge-shaped defect at a corresponding location on the retina should be seen (Fig. 6.20D). Although

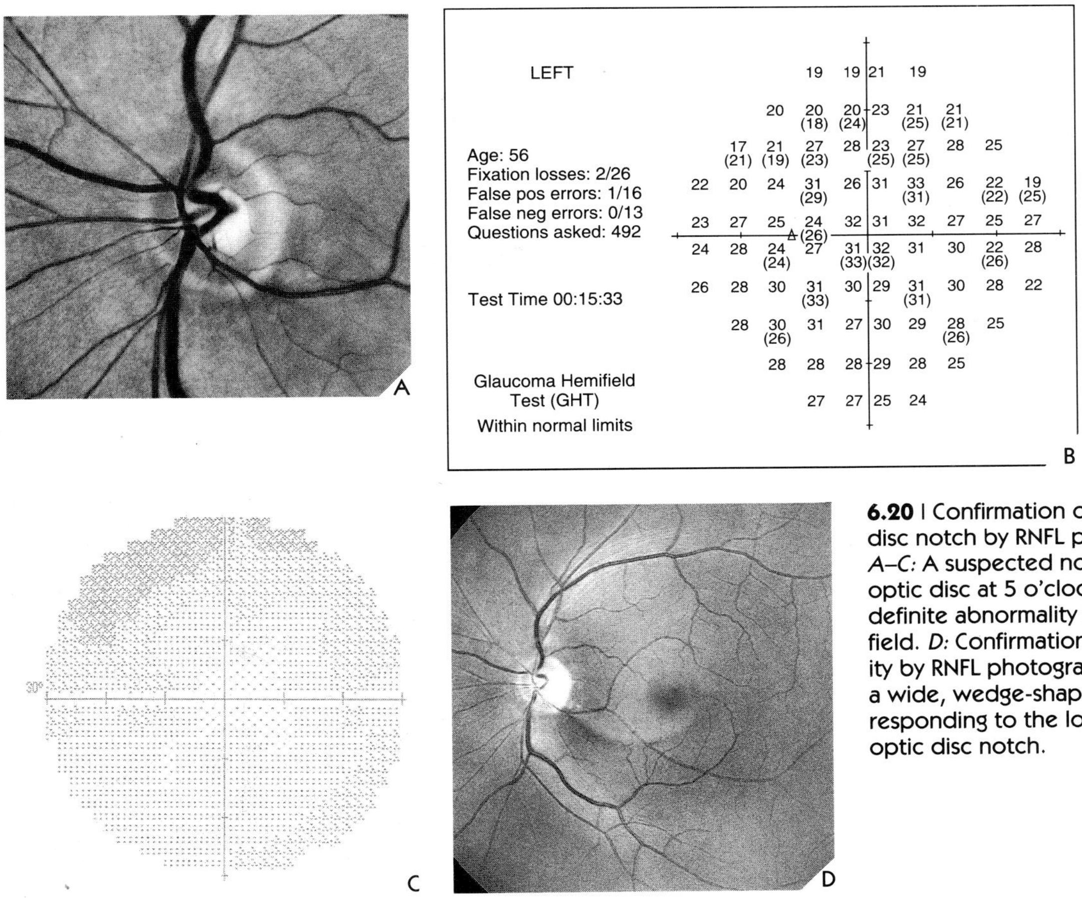

6.20 | Confirmation of an optic disc notch by RNFL photography. *A–C:* A suspected notch of the optic disc at 5 o'clock, with no definite abnormality in the visual field. *D:* Confirmation of abnormality by RNFL photography, showing a wide, wedge-shaped defect corresponding to the location of the optic disc notch.

RNFL analysis is particularly important in the diagnosis and follow-up of early glaucoma, it can also be quite demonstrative in far-advanced cases (Fig. 6.21). In addition, RNFL photography is a useful tool in screening for glaucoma.[40]

Sometimes visual fields exhibit a defect that is hard to anticipate by looking at the optic disc but which can be confirmed by RNFL analysis. A small optic disc may even appear normal despite the presence of an RNFL defect (Fig. 6.22). On the other hand, a large disc with a large cup may look suspicious but the visual field and the RNFL can be normal (Fig. 6.23). If the visual field is abnormal but both optic disc and RNFL appear undamaged, an cause other than glaucoma may produce the field defect.

Although analysis of the RNFL takes some time to learn, it will provide the clinician with much additional information to combine with optic disc and visual field evaluation. One of the drawbacks, however, is that the assessment of RNFL is subjective and qualitative. Recently, new instrumentation has been developed to quantify RNFL abnormalities, by measuring either the RNFL thickness or contour.[41,42] Equipment using a coherent scanning laser beam has the advantage of being relatively insensitive to small pupils and cataracts.[43,44] When they become available to the clinicians, these techniques may greatly improve the diagnosis and follow-up of glaucoma.

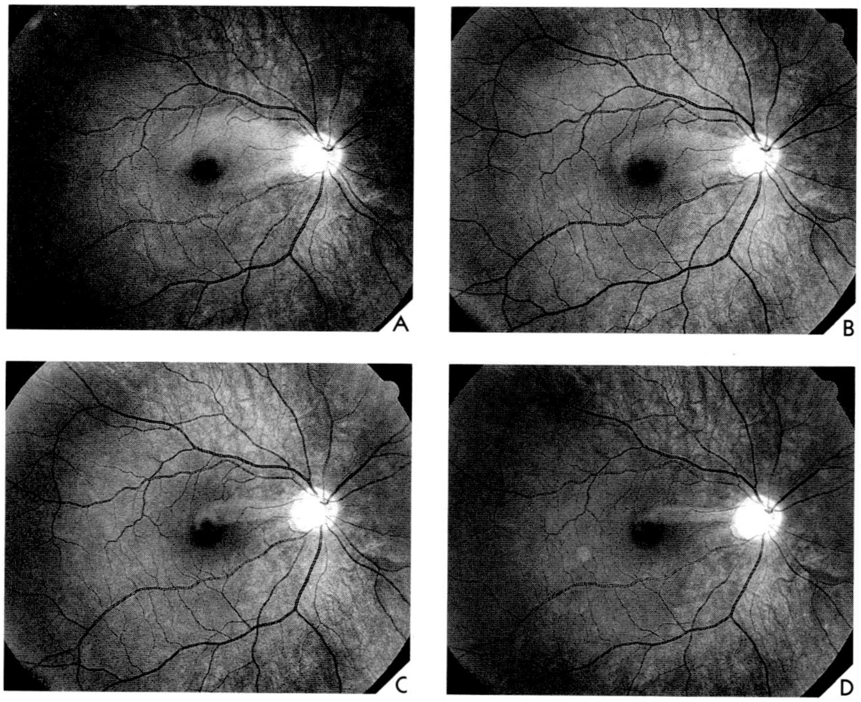

6.21 | Follow-up of end-stage low-tension glaucoma with RNFL photography; 40-year-old female. Only the papillomacular nerve fiber bundles are intact and visible. The photographic series shows progressive damage to the axon bundles. *A:* 1986; *B:* 1988; *C:* 1990; *D:*1991.

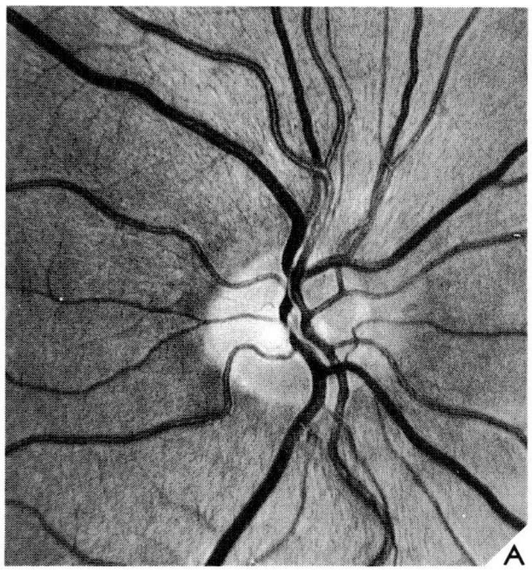

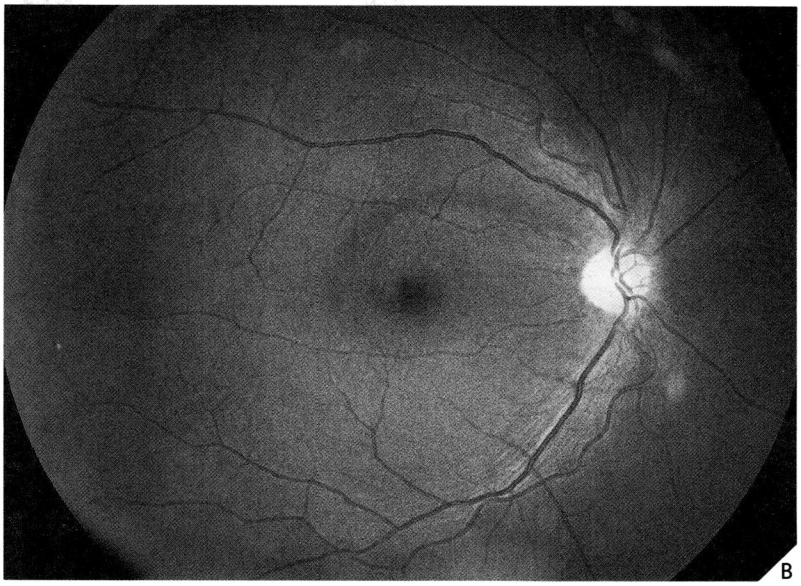

6.22 | *A:* Small optic disc, normal appearance. *B:* RNFL photography reveals a localized defect.

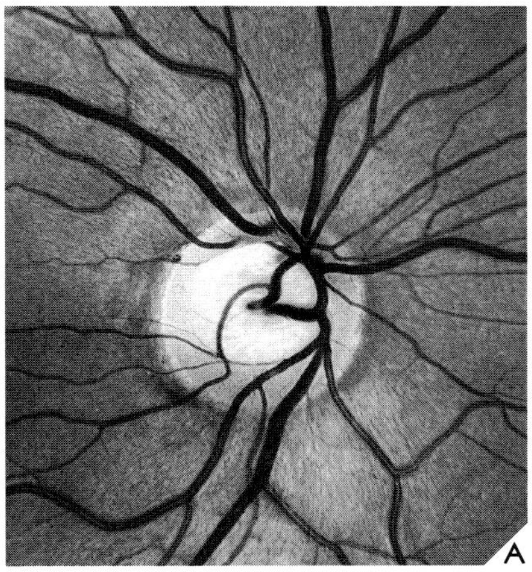

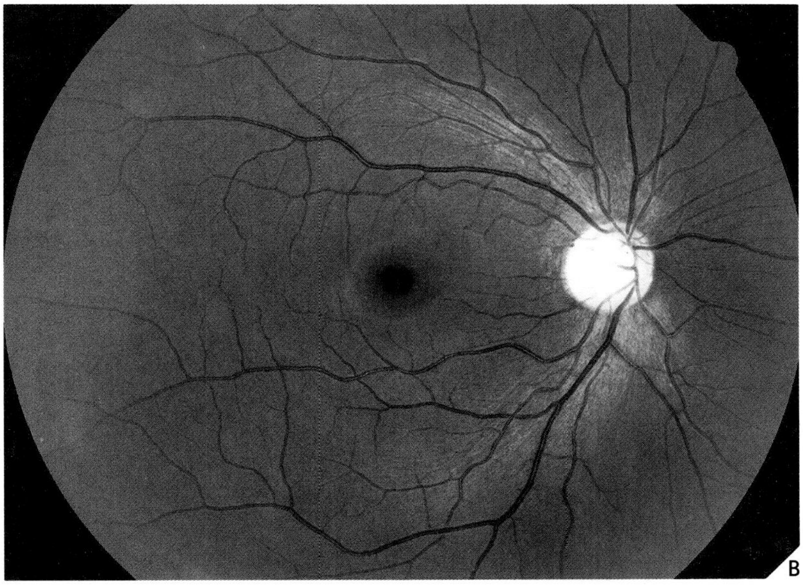

6.23 | *A:* Large, "suspicious" optic disc cupping in a large optic disc. *B:* Normal RNFL and visual fields.

SECTION V

MEASUREMENTS OF THE OPTIC NERVE HEAD AND RETINAL NERVE FIBER LAYER IN GLAUCOMA

Joseph Caprioli
Robert N. Weinreb

Clinical and histologic evidence suggests that glaucomatous eyes lose retinal ganglion cell axons, often manifested by ophthalmoscopically visible changes in the optic nerve head and nerve fiber layer, before loss of visual function can usually be detected.[45–50] An hypothesis about the relationship between clinically detectable structural and functional damage associated with progressive glaucoma is presented in Figure 6.24. Glaucomatous alterations of optic nerve head structure can usually (but not always) be recognized before visual field abnormalities can be measured, even with the most sensitive perimetric techniques. At some later stage of the disease, visual field defects appear; at still more advanced stages of optic nerve damage, significant further loss of visual field may occur with little or no discernible change in the appearance of the optic nerve head. The implications of this are that careful scrutiny of the optic nerve and nerve fiber layer is required in the early stages of the disease and that careful measurements of the visual field are more sensitive indicators of progression in the more advanced stages of the disease.

OPTIC NERVE HEAD

Estimations of C/D ratio poorly describe optic nerve head structure and do not sensitively indicate progressive glaucomatous damage.[51] Figure 6.25 shows two normal optic nerve heads, one with a large disc diameter and the other with a smaller disc diameter. Note that the cup of the large disc is much larger than the cup of the smaller disc. In normal individuals, large discs have large cups and therefore large C/D ratios; the size of the cup depends on the size of the disc. Figure 6.26 shows a series of disc photographs of a patient with progressive glaucomatous damage: there has been narrowing of the disc rim superiorly and inferiorly, with recurrent disc hemorrhages. Estimates of C/D ratio would not be likely to detect this subtle but important change.

Stereoscopic photographs of the optic disc represent the best widely available, standard technique with which to record optic nerve appearance. Subjective comparisons over time of sequential optic nerve photographs can

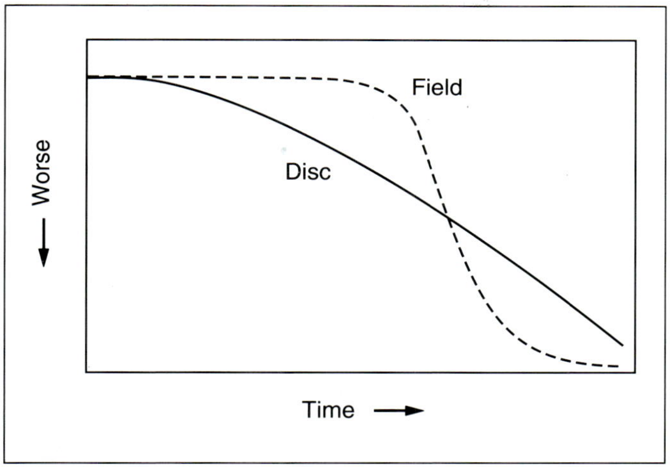

6.24 | A hypothesis about the relationship between clinically detectable structural and functional damage associated with progressive glaucoma. Structural changes in the optic nerve and nerve fiber layer are usually detectable before visual field abnormalities can be measured.

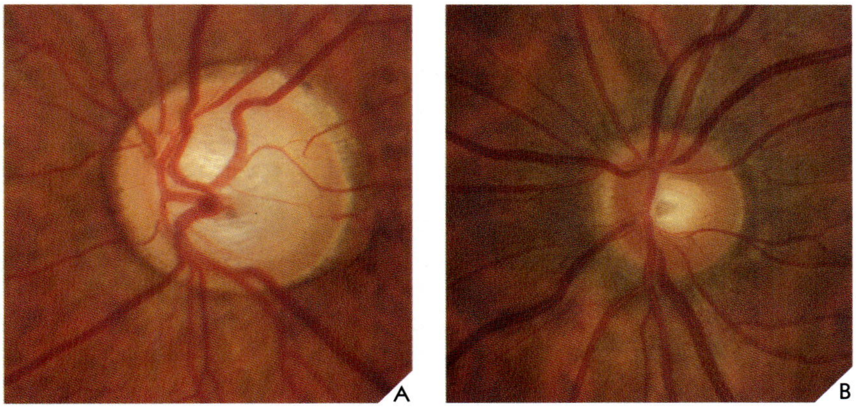

6.25 | The optic nerve in two normal individuals, photographed with the same fundus camera at the same magnification. The area of the optic disc in *A* is approximately four times that of the optic disc in *B*. The size of the cup is highly correlated with the size of the disc.

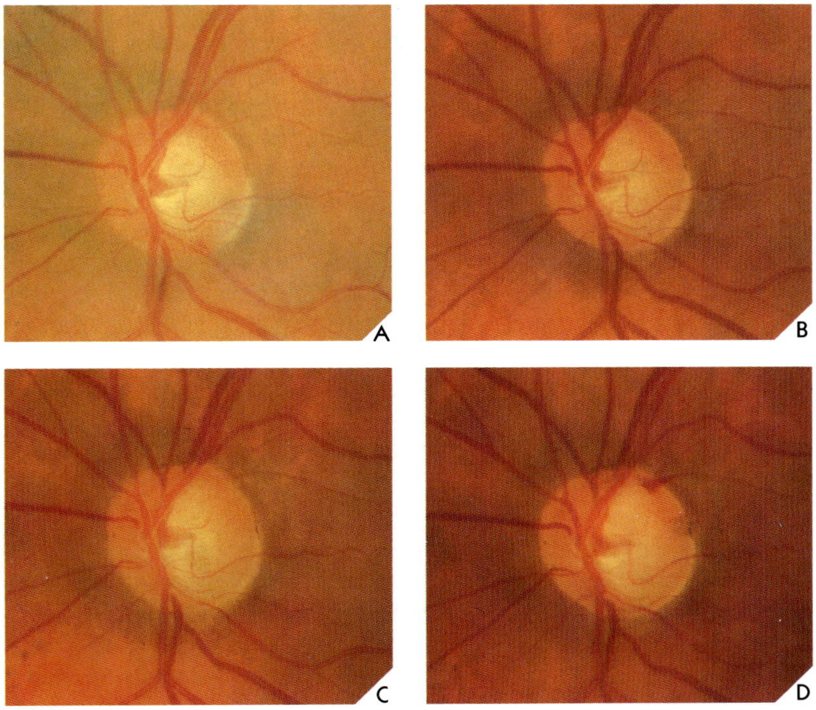

6.26 | *A–D:* Series of disc photographs in a patient with progressive glaucoma. Note progressive thinning at the inferior and superior poles of the disc, and the disc hemorrhages at the same locations. Progressive disc damage such as this often escapes detection when only estimates of C/D ratio are used for evaluation.

often detect small but significant changes that may have important therapeutic implications. Abnormalities of the nerve fiber layer, visible ophthalmoscopically with red-free light and best recorded with monochromatic photography, have been well described[52–54] (see Tuulonen and Airaksinen, Chapters 4 and 6). Evaluation of the optic nerve head and nerve fiber layer are complementary examinations, because both may show the effects of ganglion cell loss. However, a widely held clinical opinion is that the appearance of credible nerve fiber layer defects in the absence of detectable optic disc abnormalities is unusual.

The visual comparison of sequential optic nerve and nerve fiber layer photographs represents the best routine technique with which to detect change with time. The subjective and qualitative nature of these interpretations has stimulated a search for more sensitive and quantitative techniques with which to recognize the earliest structural changes from glaucomatous damage and to detect small changes over follow-up periods. Appropriate markers for glaucomatous damage should be sensitive, specific, objective, and quantitative. Analogue photogrammetry of simultaneous stereoscopic fundus photographs has been used to quantify the topography of the optic nerve head, and computerized image analysis techniques have been used to quantify the area of optic disc pallor.[55,56] In a retrospective study of optic disc pallor in normal subjects and ocular hypertensives, no significant changes were identified in the normal group, whereas the ocular hypertensive group showed significant increases in pallor over a 2-year period.[57]

Planimetric measurements of disc rim area have been reported by Balazsi et al[58] and by Airaksinen and co-workers.[59] Such measurements were initially believed, unlike C/D ratio, to be independent of disc size. Unfortunately, it has been shown that disc rim area also depends on disc size (the larger the disc, the greater the disc rim area), and that this factor must be taken into account when measurements from different eyes are compared. In addition, a great deal of overlap was found between measurements of glaucoma patients and those of normal subjects; this precluded the use of single such measurements to discriminate clearly between normal and glaucomatous eyes. It is not yet known how useful these measurements might be when individual patients are followed over a long period of time.

Computerized image analysis of simultaneous stereoscopic videographic images has been used to study structural parameters of the optic nerve head in normal, glaucoma-suspect, and glaucoma cases.[60] The standard summary parameters first calculated from topographic measurements were C/D ratio, disc rim area, and cup volume (Fig. 6.27). For each of these parameters, the high degree of overlap between diagnostic groups limited its use to detect the earliest glaucomatous changes, but disc rim area provided the best indicator of disease. Correlations between structural parameters and visual field loss in glaucoma were sought and identified (Fig. 6.28).[61,62] Visual field mean defect (an indicator of overall visual field damage) correlated best with disc rim area, but only ≈ 20% of the variation of mean defect could be explained by the variation of rim area.

RETINAL NERVE FIBER LAYER

The limited usefulness of the "standard" disc parameters sparked a search for more specific and sensitive structural markers for early glaucomatous damage. The distillation of a large amount of quantitative topographic information into parameters with which clinicians were previously comfortable, such as C/D ratio, disc rim area, and cup volume, seemed not to be the most efficient way to make use of the new measurements. Computerized image

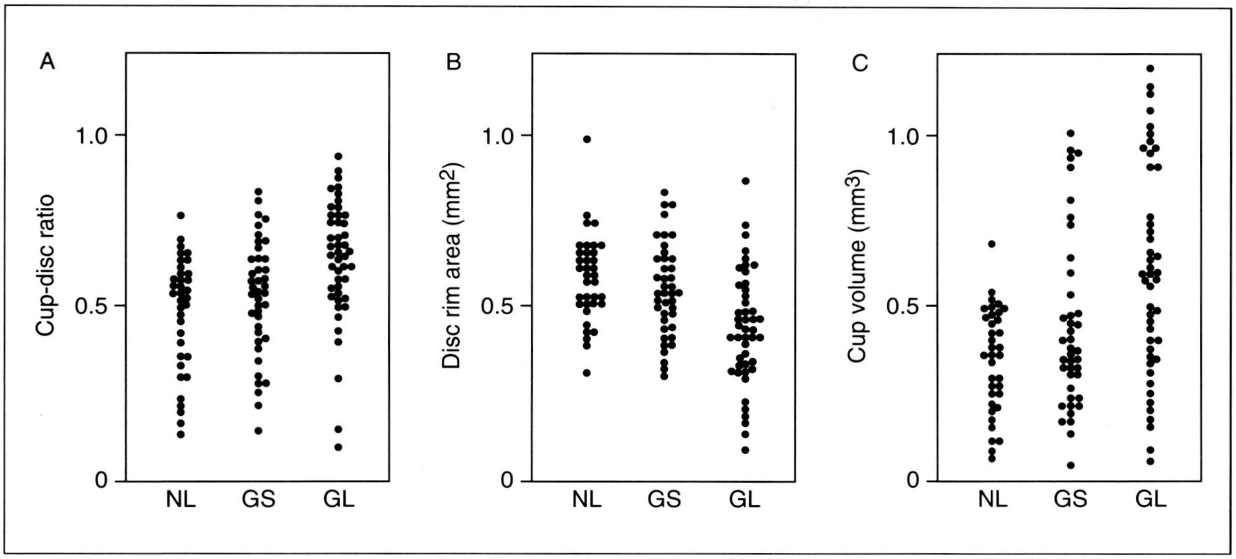

6.27 | Measurements of C/D ratio (*A*), disc rim area (*B*), and cup volume (*C*), made with computerized image analysis of simultaneous stereoscopic photographic images in normal (NL), glaucoma-suspect (GS), and glaucoma (GL) cases. A large degree of overlap for any of these parameters between diagnostic groups makes single measurements of such parameters poor discriminators between normal and glaucomatous eyes.

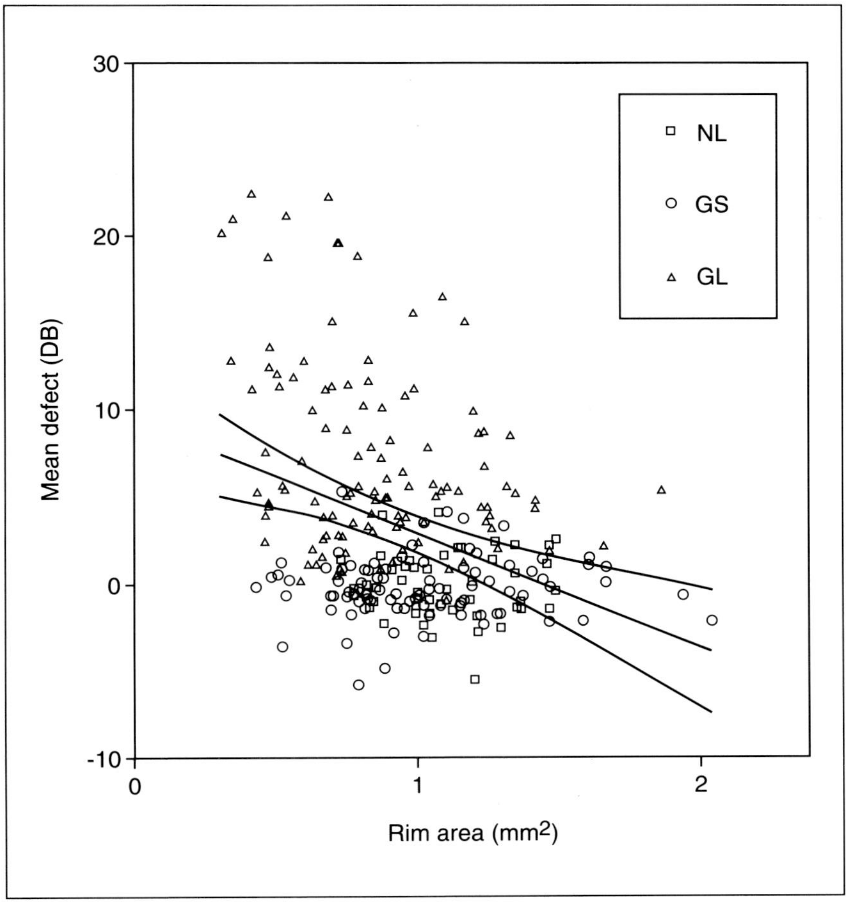

6.28 | Correlation between disc rim area as measured by computerized image analysis and visual field mean defect in glaucoma suspects and glaucoma patients. The correlation is statistically significant (r=-0.36, p=0.001), but variation in rim area accounts for <15% of variation in mean defect (R^2 = 0.13).

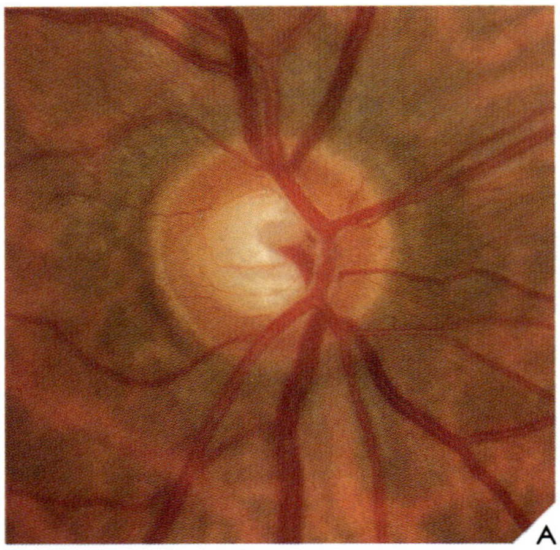

-15	-20	-24	-30	-36	-41	-42	-23	3	7	-14	-35	-57	-78	-95	-60	-9	128	333	295	182	74
-15	-20	-23	-32	-41	-44	-39	-10	26	32	6	-23	-53	-74	-82	-50	-6	123	321	285	175	71
-26	-28	-29	-42	-57	-51	-24	-13	-6	30	92	61	2	-36	-51	-29	3	135	347	306	186	72
-16	-21	-26	-38	-51	-40	-4	22	46	78	113	78	20	-27	-62	-52	-29	48	168	157	105	55
-21	-20	-14	-16	-18	-9	11	45	82	85	52	29	9	-3	-9	-23	-39	-39	-20	-1	18	36
-18	-21	-17	0	17	31	43	67	95	169	279	242	160	107	83	75	72	63	47	43	42	40
-21	-5	18	46	74	113	159	154	132	235	447	405	284	162	50	74	142	166	144	111	74	38
13	28	52	91	132	177	225	255	281	391	568	512	382	241	103	145	244	268	216	146	70	0
9	40	82	127	172	243	342	450	560	641	683	613	508	473	499	395	251	213	276	224	136	53
3	44	97	150	204	354	586	641	643	657	682	650	599	608	668	599	489	376	260	173	95	22
18	52	100	164	229	368	569	621	627	652	690	670	632	653	724	671	581	419	195	111	70	31
32	61	102	166	232	333	466	552	623	680	717	681	622	643	732	640	491	346	213	152	113	76
41	66	103	167	233	299	370	483	610	679	689	666	633	608	585	475	339	230	150	108	76	47
42	61	89	139	191	233	271	410	580	675	690	668	633	549	421	343	280	205	122	85	61	40
31	42	63	111	161	235	334	450	572	648	677	660	629	544	408	318	242	160	78	50	39	29
24	39	60	98	138	179	229	353	501	606	659	616	543	436	299	207	130	63	10	3	10	16
29	39	48	63	79	107	152	253	373	499	616	552	431	331	251	158	61	-17	-72	-61	-29	1
-14	23	30	38	45	75	130	228	339	474	615	528	369	244	152	87	28	-51	-145	-124	-68	-13
-21	-3	17	27	38	56	87	162	250	334	402	335	226	162	141	87	22	-70	-181	-159	-96	-34
-42	-38	-28	-15	-1	23	58	108	161	196	209	172	120	103	118	69	0	-105	-235	-211	-138	-67
-42	-50	-54	-35	-14	10	38	70	104	118	112	90	63	49	48	14	-30	-118	-237	-209	-135	-63
-38	-33	-25	-21	-18	-7	11	33	55	59	44	38	35	30	22	-4	-38	-119	-237	-207	-130	-57
-21	-19	-15	-12	-8	1	19	27	31	31	27	19	9	10	20	6	-15	-118	-288	-254	-156	-63
6	7	1	-9	-20	-7	30	28	12	-1	-11	-17	-22	-8	22	14	-6	-115	-295	-261	-161	-65

B

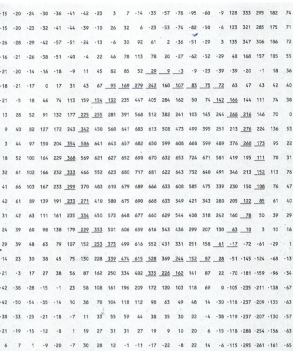

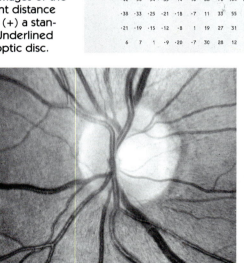

6.29 | A 25 x 25 magnification-corrected data matrix of the fundus (*B*) centered at the optic nerve (*A*). Data were derived from digital image analysis of simultaneously recorded striped video images of the optic nerve. Numbers represent distance in microns above (-) or below (+) a standard retinal reference plane. Underlined values lie on the edge of the optic disc.

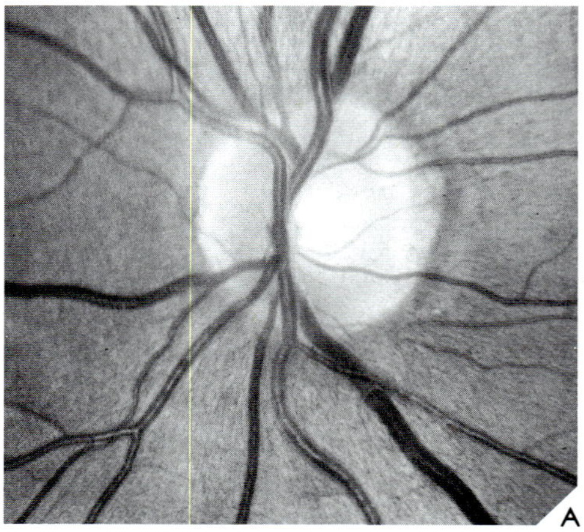

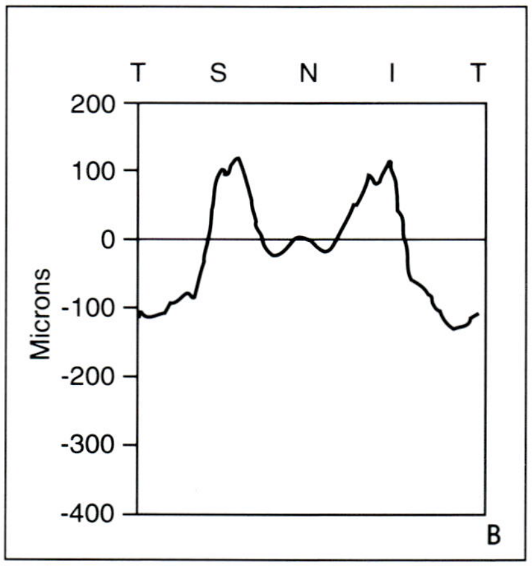

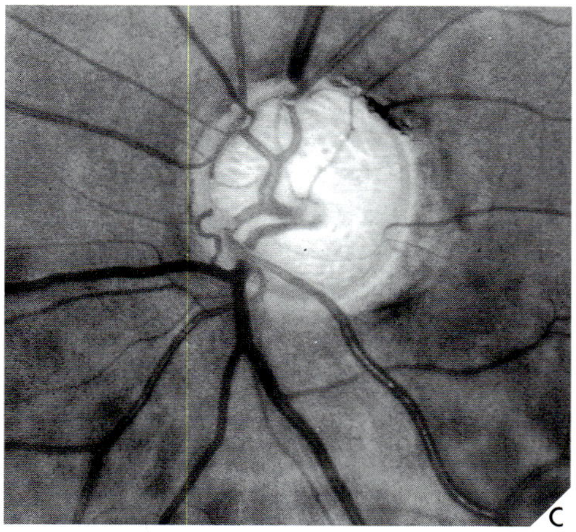

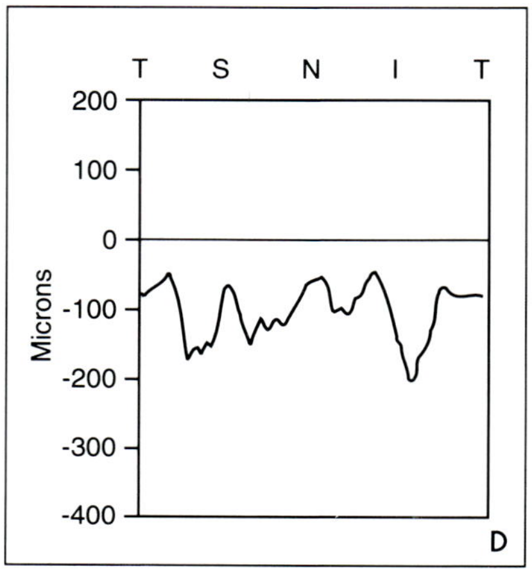

6.30 | Comparisons of optic disc or nerve fiber layer photos with measured profiles of the peripapillary nerve fiber layer surface contour. Temporal, superior, nasal, and inferior locations are indicated by capitals T, S, N, and I, respectively. *A* and *B:* Typical normal eye exhibits a double-hump pattern that reflects thicker fiber bundles at the superior and inferior poles of the disc. *C* and *D:* Patient with advanced glaucomatous visual field loss shows flattening of the profiles with loss of the normal double-hump pattern.

analysis of simultaneous stereoscopic images can produce a depth matrix in absolute measurements of the optic disc and surrounding area as shown in Figure 6.29.[63] Other workers have made preliminary measurements of nerve fiber layer thickness, and systematic studies in glaucoma patients are pending.[64–66] Computerized image analysis can be used to quantify the surface contour of the peripapillary nerve fiber layer[67] (see Weinreb and Caprioli, Chapter 4). Figure 6.30 shows examples of such measurements in normal and glaucomatous eyes. Glaucomatous damage to retinal ganglion cell axons is manifested by a decreased height of the nerve fiber layer and by flattening of the normally thickest portions of this layer at the superior and inferior poles of the disc. The contour of the juxtapapillary nerve fiber layer was measured in glaucoma patients (n = 112), glaucoma suspects (n = 87), and in age-matched normal controls (n = 53).[68] The average relative nerve fiber layer

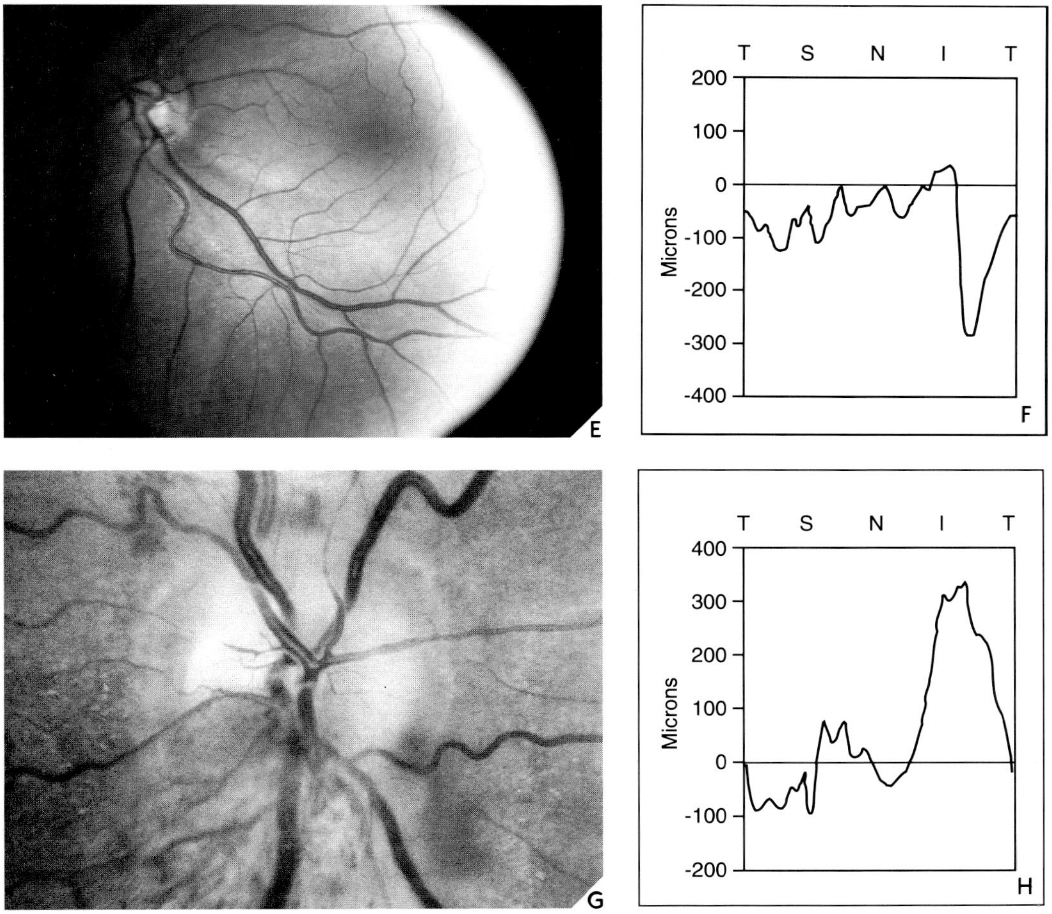

6.30 | (Cont'd.) *E* and *F:* Patient with a localized nerve fiber layer defect from glaucoma shows a wedge-shaped defect of the corresponding area of the profile. *G* and *H:* Eye with acute ischemic optic neuropathy and sector edema of the disc with thickening of the adjacent nerve fiber layer; the profile shows a large elevation of the nerve fiber layer inferiorly. (From Caprioli J, Miller JM: Measurement of relative nerve fiber layer surface height in glaucoma. *Ophthalmology 1989; 96:633–641.*)

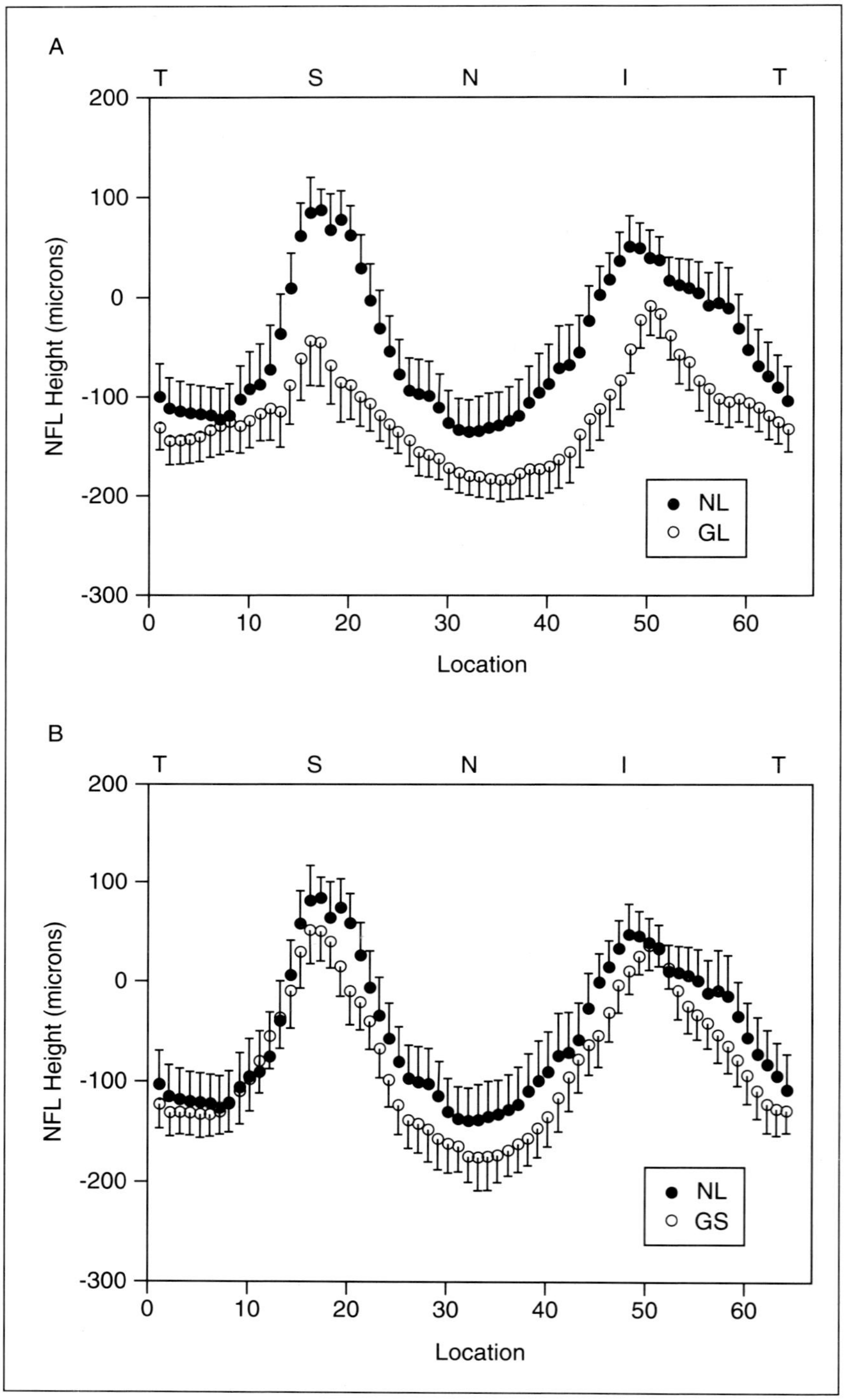

6.31 | Mean relative nerve fiber layer height measurements in (*A*) normal and glaucoma groups and (*B*) normal and glaucoma suspects. The error bars indicate two standard errors of the mean and the locations correspond to those indicated in Figure 6.30. (From Caprioli J: Contour of the juxtapapillary nerve fiber layer in glaucoma. *Ophthalmology 1990;97:358–366.*)

height differed in glaucomas and normals by 70 mm, but differences exceeded 100 mm at the superior and inferior poles of the disc (Fig. 6.31). Mean values for glaucoma suspects were intermediate between those for the normal and glaucoma groups. Measurements of relative nerve fiber layer height correlated better with indices of visual field loss than did any of the standard structural parameters (Fig. 6.32). The ability of nerve fiber layer contour measurements to discriminate between normal and glaucomatous eyes was investigated with receiver operating characteristic curves, and was compared to that of the standard disc parameters. These curves are used to assess a test's diagnostic performance by displaying pairs of sensitivity and specificity values throughout the whole range of a test's measurements. The diagonal of such a plot represents a line of "no information," while curves shifted to the upper left indicate increased specificity and sensitivity; the area

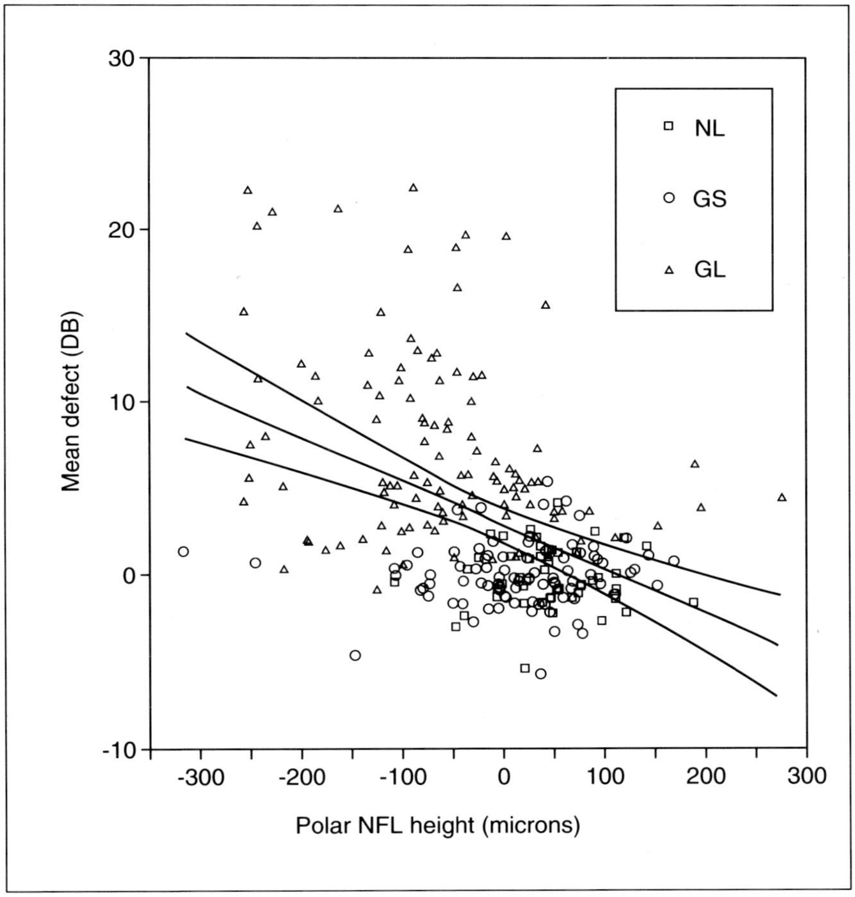

6.32 | Relationship of nerve fiber layer surface contour (as indicated by the height of the nerve fiber layer at the superior and inferior poles of the disc), with visual field mean defect. The correlation was statistically significant (*r*=-0.48, *p*=0.001).

under the curve is therefore proportional to its power to discriminate between two groups. Nerve fiber layer contour was the best discriminator between normal and glaucomatous eyes of all the parameters tested (Fig. 6.33). Measurements of juxtapapillary nerve fiber layer contour or of nerve fiber layer thickness may prove useful to detect glaucomatous optic nerve damage at an early stage and to recognize accurately progressive nerve damage over time.

The goal of having an inexpensive, conveniently performed, sensitive and specific test of early and progressive optic nerve damage has not yet been realized. Much progress has been made in recent years. As technological advances are applied to this area in the near future, significant further progress, which will increase the quality of care generally available to glaucoma patients, will undoubtedly become reality.

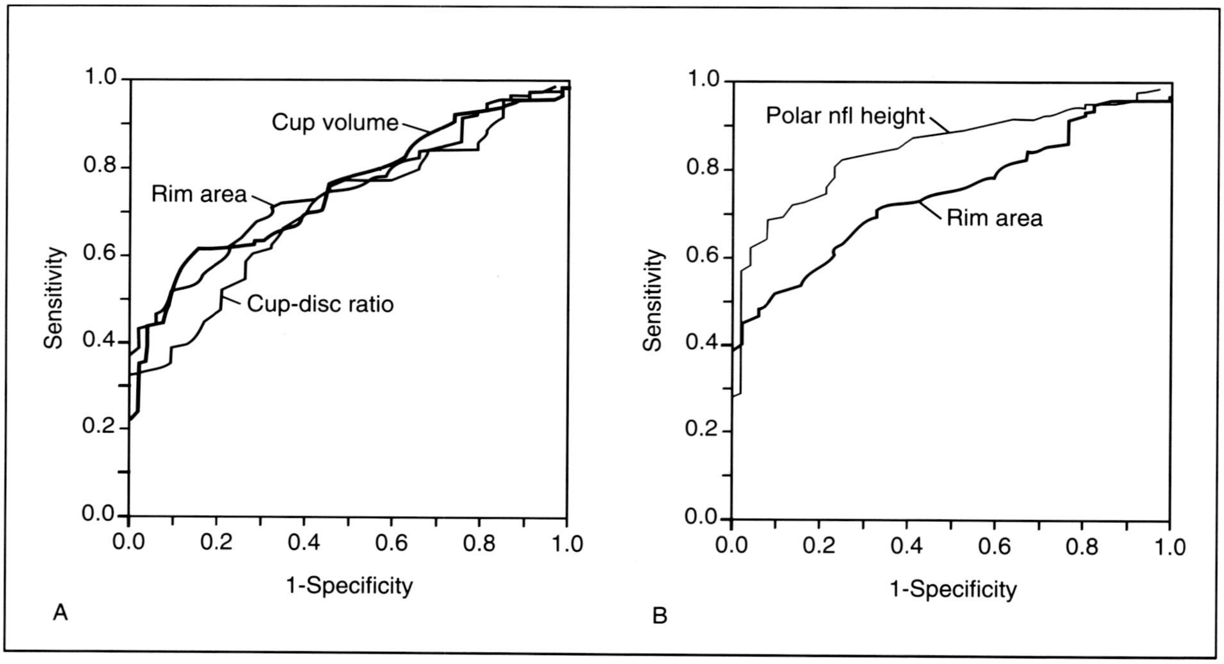

6.33 I Receiver operating characteristic curves for (*A*) the standard disc parameters and for (*B*) a nerve fiber layer contour parameter (polar nerve fiber layer height). Polar nerve fiber layer height was superior to other parameters in its ability to discriminate between normal and glaucomatous eyes. (From Caprioli J: Contour of the juxtapapillary nerve fiber layer in glaucoma. *Ophthalmology 1990;97:358–366.*)

7 Visual Function in Glaucoma

Section I

Psychophysics and Electrophysiology in Glaucoma: An Overview

Stephen M. Drance

It is almost 100 years since it became known that there are characteristic optic nerve head changes, as well as visual field defects, in chronic open-angle glaucoma. Although our knowledge during this time has undergone significant advancement, the pathogenesis of the disease remains a mystery. The recognition of the earliest damage, either to structure or function, may be important for the management of the disease, on the assumed likelihood that an alteration of risk factors and damaging factors at the early stages may arrest the disease before the patient becomes aware of any visual handicaps. This section will provide an overview of the psychophysical and electrophysiologic methods used to evaluate visual function in glaucoma (Fig. 7.1).

Kinetic perimetry, which classically measures the differential increment threshold to light both in the periphery and the center of the visual field, has established the nerve fiber bundle field defect and a generalized contraction of all isopters as the hallmark of the glaucomatous visual field defect. The introduction of the Bjerrum screen for quantitative perimetry by Traquair identified paracentral scotomas, nasal steps, and arcuate scotomas as the classic disturbances of the visual field in open-angle glaucoma. The introduction of quantitative arc perimeters, on the other hand, identified losses of the peripheral nasal visual field as part of glaucomatous damage and a generalized reduction of the entire visual field (a sinking of the island of vision) as a common early field defect. The concept of static perimetry was introduced by Sloan[1] and received further impetus from the work of Harms and Aulhorn[2] and from the introduction of the Goldmann perimeter.[3] This approach emphasized standardization of stimuli and demonstrated that the central and peripheral

FIGURE 7.1. PSYCHOPHYSICAL AND ELECTROPHYSIOLOGIC TECHNIQUES IN GLAUCOMA EVALUATION

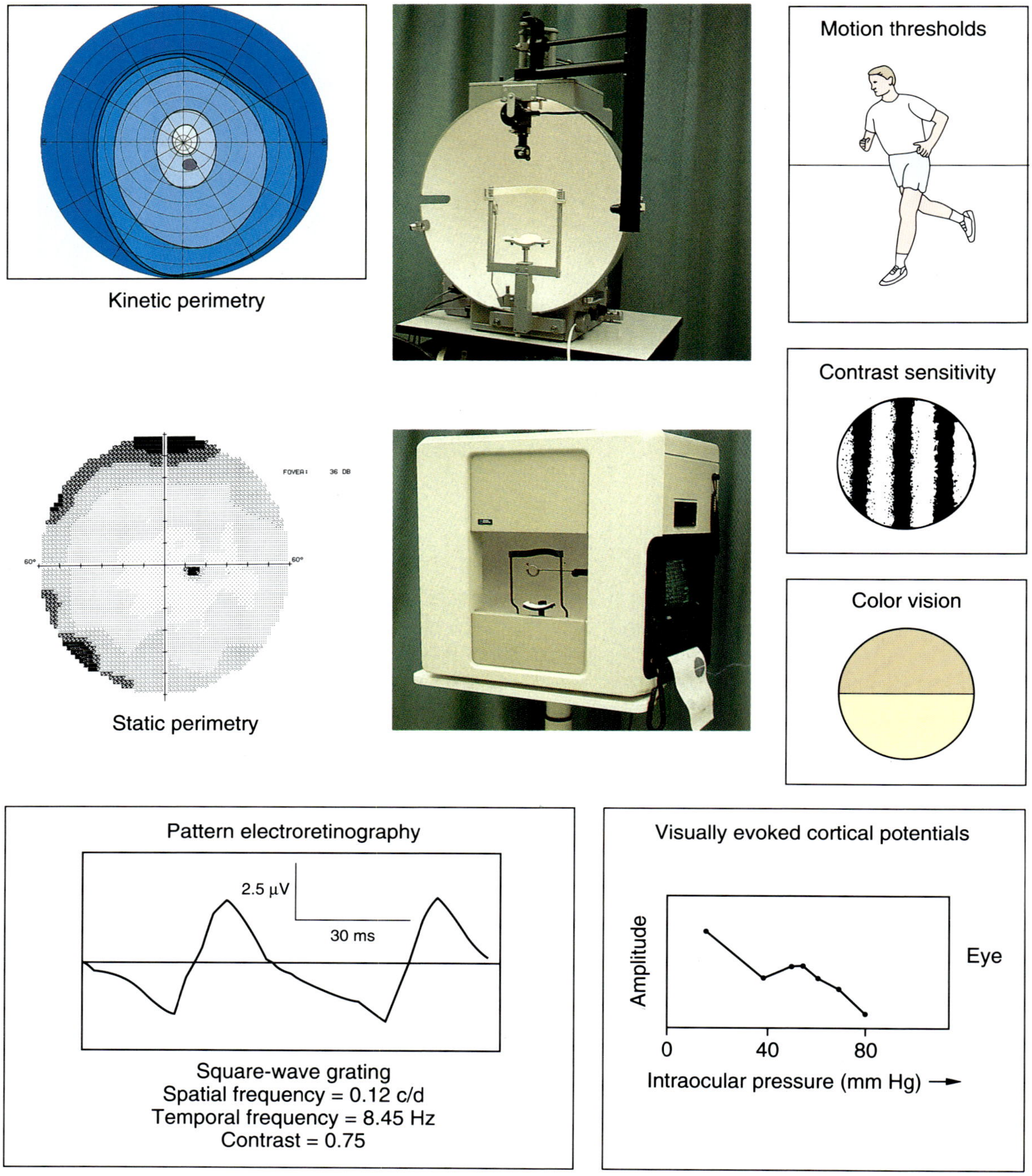

visual field were really part of the same island of vision and could be examined at one sitting. We learned that localized central field defects were quite specific but not pathognomonic for glaucoma, as they also occurred in other optic neuropathies. We also became aware that generalized losses of sensitivity, although common in glaucoma, lack specificity because they are influenced by the clarity of the media,[2] pupil size,[2] refraction, and aging.[4] Instability of thresholds has been shown to precede the development of localized field defects.[5] It has become clear that changes at the optic nerve head can be unaccompanied by localized field defects even with the best perimetry in the world, and that a diffuse loss of retinal nerve fibers can occur without an accompanying localized field defect.[6] The introduction of automatic perimeters not only improved the quality and standardization of perimetry but enabled us to make fairly accurate measurements of thresholds and to analyze this information statistically. The large amount of both short-term and long-term fluctuation became apparent.[7] Structural changes still often precede visual field loss, even when the indices obtained by data reduction are used. However, the gap has narrowed.

Experimental neurobiological studies meanwhile demonstrated differences between small and large ganglion cells of the retina.[8] They generate small and large axons, respectively, and in the lateral geniculate body there is a clear separation of the magnocellular and parvocellular systems.[9] The large ganglion cells constitute about 10% of all retinal ganglion cells and show phasic or transient responses to changes in illumination.[8] They have large overlapping receptive fields[10] that receive input from both rods and cones,[11,12] and are sensitive to high temporal frequencies at relatively low spatial frequencies.[9] The small ganglion cells are part of the midget system.[13] They receive input predominantly from the cones,[14] have very small receptive fields (in many instances from a single cone), and show tonic or sustained responses to luminance contrast.[9] Those with input from cones with shorter wavelength responses are larger and their axons conduct faster than those with cone input sensitive to longer wavelengths.[15] At high stimulation frequencies the tonic cells respond as achromatic cells and are sensitive to high spatial frequencies, whereas at low frequencies they respond as chromatic cells. Important concepts related to these dual response characteristics have been developed.[16,17] Pressure elevation,[18] experimentally obtained in the monkey eye and naturally occurring in human open-angle glaucoma,[19] results in the appearance of cupping of the optic nerve head, diffuse loss of ganglion cells and axons with special predilection for loss of axons at the superior and inferior poles, and a sequential loss of the large ganglion cells followed by the smaller ones.

Because the large axon cells generate the large optic nerve fibers and provide the main input from the retina to the magnocellular visual pathway, which is primarily involved in interpretation of spatial organization based on motion and depth perception,[20–22] it was believed that disturbances in motion might be affected early in open-angle glaucoma. Peripheral displacement thresholds[23] and motion thresholds[24] are significantly elevated in patients with open-angle glaucoma and in glaucoma suspects. In both of those studies there was again overlap between the glaucomatous and normal individuals, which suggests that a number of patients with open-angle glaucoma still have normal motion thresholds. Twenty-one percent of the glaucoma suspects and 42% of the overtly glaucomatous eyes manifested a significant elevation in motion threshold. The findings in the glaucoma suspects suggested that, although most of them fell into the normal motion threshold group, there was a subpopulation with a markedly elevated threshold.

Although color disturbances are nonspecific because they are affected by the clarity of the ocular media and diseases of the retina, many studies have shown that color perception is defective in glaucoma patients.[25–30] While it is difficult to compare the details from different studies because of the differing protocols and conditions of testing, it is generally agreed that the blue–yellow mechanism is disturbed more frequently and earlier in the course of the disease than is the red–green mechanism, that a considerable proportion of glaucoma suspects have such color losses,[31–33] and that blue–yellow disturbances may predict subsequent development of classical localized glaucomatous visual field defects. Diffuse loss of the human retinal nerve fiber layer is related to yellow–blue color losses, whereas localized retinal nerve fiber layer losses do not relate to either yellow–blue or red–green losses.[34]

There are many reports of disturbed spatial and/or temporal contrast sensitivity in the glaucomas. As with color studies, the results are conflicting and are difficult to interpret because of the great variation in the methods and conditions of the testing used and the fact that contrast sensitivity is also affected by media opacities, pupil size, refractive errors, amblyopia, and diseases of the retina.

Earlier work showed that in glaucoma patients and glaucoma suspects contrast sensitivity, primarily to coarse gratings, was reduced.[35–40] Eyes with mild visual field defects, however, exhibited losses of contrast sensitivity primarily to the medium and finer gratings.[41] Such losses could occur before development of localized visual field defects on the Octopus perimeter. Significant reductions in sensitivity with low-contrast Snellen-type charts,[42] rapid flicker of homogeneous field,[43] multiflash campimetry,[44] and temporal modulation[45] of a coarse sinusoidal grating have all been found in established and suspect glaucomatous eyes. In general, eyes with more extensive visual field defects exhibit the largest losses in temporal contrast sensitivity,[37] and with one exception[45] almost all studies favor temporal contrast sensitivity compared with static spatial contrast sensitivity as being more disturbed in open-angle glaucoma.

Flicker has been found to be disturbed before disturbances of the central visual field occur. A reduction in temporal contrast sensitivity in the central part of the visual field, both to diffuse flickering targets and to counterphase targets, was demonstrated in primary open-angle glaucoma and in suspect eyes with elevated IOP. There was considerable overlap between these groups and normal subjects.[46] The best separation between the groups was found to occur when both the diffuse flicker and the counterphase targets were used and the results averaged.[46] By a different methodology, glaucoma patients were shown to have losses to flicker of the midfrequencies of 10–30 Hz.[43] Some 50–70% of glaucoma patients had a decreased temporal contrast sensitivity,[47] but with the exception of one study[48] no significant difference in sensitivity was found between the central 5° of the visual field and the Bjerrum area most commonly involved in glaucoma. A relationship between the amount of flicker loss and the extent of the visual field defect was also established. Testing the entire central field with a computerized flicker perimeter showed that localized flicker defects were larger than with light-sense perimetry and that some flicker defects were present which were undiscovered by light-sense perimetry.[49] Sixty-four percent of glaucoma suspects with normal visual fields had pronounced disturbances on the flicker perimeter.

Studies of visually evoked cortical potentials (VECP) in humans and monkeys have shown evidence of high temporal frequency and low spatial frequency attenuation of visual responses in subjects with open-angle glaucoma and in glaucoma suspects. These abnormalities are usually not pronounced enough to detect glaucomatous damage reliably in individual patients. The latency seems to be a better detector than the amplitude. Newer modifications of VECP testing under the stress of artificially elevated IOP may prove more useful (see Stodtmeister and Pillunat, Chapters 5 and 7).

The pattern electroretinogram (PERG) is believed to come from the ganglion cell layer of the retina,[50] but this hypothesis has been challenged.[51,52] PERG abnormalities precede optic disc damage in monkeys with laser-induced IOP elevations.[53] In glaucoma patients both low and high temporal frequency-stimulated PERGs are abnormal, but, if anything, the higher temporal frequencies are more disturbed.[54] Pressure elevations also produce reductions in the PERG amplitude in individual patients.[55] In groups, however, pressure elevation does not correlate with the PERG amplitude.[56] Increased latency in pattern-evoked visual responses are associated with changes in contrast sensitivity. The PERG as it is presently recorded is small and has great variability. Advances in recording techniques or analysis may make this a more useful objective technique for the evaluation of the glaucomas in the future.

SUMMARY

There is much evidence that psychophysical functions other than merely light increment thresholds are disturbed in patients with open-angle glaucoma. However, a number of patients with marked open-angle glaucoma damage to the light sense do retain some other normal psychophysical functions. There is also evidence that a proportion of glaucoma suspects have abnormal psychophysical functions before the development of recognizable optic nerve head changes and localized disturbances in their visual field. Almost all the psychophysical functions are tested at the fovea, which suggests that the fovea can be disturbed early in glaucoma and can be involved in the diffuse damage to the ganglion cells quite early in the disease. There is evidence that loss in blue–yellow color discrimination is related to diffuse but not localized loss of the retinal nerve fiber layer. Blue–yellow color losses have been related to the light increment threshold at the fovea and also to the pericentral and paracentral parts of the visual field. There is evidence that when suspects with color disturbances are followed longitudinally, the subsequent development of localized visual field defects can be predicted from the color abnormality. There is as yet no longitudinal study to show similar predictive value for the other abnormalities of psychophysical functions, such as spatial and temporal contrast sensitivity, hyperacuity, and motion detection. The electrical functions generated by the ganglion cells and the evoked cortical potentials are disturbed in open-angle glaucoma and, again, a number of patients who are glaucoma suspects have similar disturbances. There are a few longitudinal studies at this time showing that these electrophysiological abnormalities may predict the subsequent development of visual field defects. Structural changes at the optic nerve head usually precede the development of localized visual field defects, but there is as yet no good study that links the development of these early optic nerve head changes to disturbances of the other psychophysical functions. The tools to examine these interrelationships are at hand, and in the coming decade there is a good chance that the pathophysiology of glaucomatous damage and its relationship to elevated IOP will be identified. The possibility of more than one mechanism of damage in the glaucomas and the possible interrelationships of these mechanisms raise some exciting challenges. The various sections comprising this chapter will describe in more detail the present state of our knowledge in these areas.

SECTION II

VISUAL FIELD LOSS AND PERIMETRY IN GLAUCOMA

Anders Heijl

THE NATURE OF GLAUCOMATOUS VISUAL FIELD LOSS

Although consensus does not yet exist on the basic pathophysiologic processes that underlie glaucoma, there does seem to be general agreement that glaucoma is characterized by microscopic lesions at the prelaminar level of the optic disc. These changes, whether due to mechanical stretching of axonal bundles and misalignment vis-à-vis the holes in the lamina or to derangement of small vessel function, lead to axon malfunction and death and, consequently, to visual impairment that manifests as visual field defects. These field defects are, therefore, important signs of disease, which can be used for detection as well as to monitor the effectiveness of therapy.

CONCEPTS OF GLAUCOMATOUS FIELD DEFECTS

Our concept of glaucomatous field loss has changed considerably over time. Albrecht von Graefe was the first to report that glaucomatous eyes showed visual field defects, when he demonstrated typical contractions.[57] The emphasis on peripheral visual field loss in glaucoma continued with the invention of Foerster's perimeter, which was particularly suited for detecting such defects.[58] The arcuate defects now regarded as the hallmark of glaucoma were first demonstrated by Bjerrum.[59] Bjerrum also invented the tangent screen, and was the first to realize the importance of relative field defects and the usefulness of small test targets in kinetic perimetry. Later, Bjerrum and his pupil Rønne demonstrated and emphasized the importance of nasal steps.[59,60]

Although the findings of Bjerrum and Rønne clearly have stood the test of time, other perimetric features once believed to be indicative of glaucomatous field loss have not. Various forms of enlargement of the blind spot were long thought to be important, or even the most important, signs of early glaucoma. These included baring of the blind spot and the Seidel scotoma, a short arcuate scotoma connected to the blind spot. Enlarged blind spots, Seidel scotomas, and baring are not typical of glaucoma, however. The most common location for early defects in glaucoma is nasal to fixation, and baring of the blind spot can also be elicited in most normal eyes.[61]

The idea that enlarged blind spots are indicative of glaucoma may have stemmed from the fact that peripapillary atrophy is particularly common, albeit nonspecific,[62] in glaucoma, and also might be due to artifacts created by nonperfect kinetic isopter perimetry (Fig. 7.2).

Medical understanding of glaucomatous field loss advanced further in the 1960s with the contributions of Aulhorn and Harms,[63] who showed that perimetric defects in early glaucoma occur most commonly in the central 30° field, in the form of paracentral scotomas and nasal steps. They found defects solely involving the periphery to be rare. Paracentral defects can occur anywhere in the central field, but are more common nasally, and tend to be situated closer to fixation in the superior than in the inferior hemifield.[64]

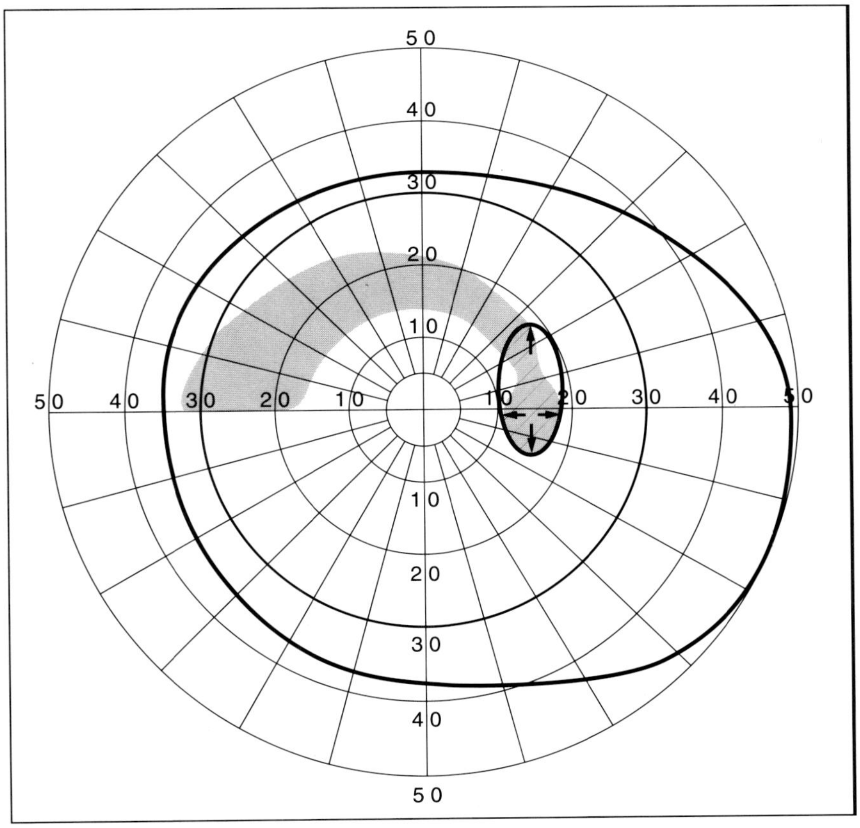

7.2 | Missed arcuate glaucomatous field defect. Kinetic testing has failed to detect complete arcuate defect (stippled), instead only incorrectly indicating enlargement of blind spot.

In progressive glaucoma paracentral scotomas tend to deepen, grow, and merge into more or less arcuate defects (Fig. 7.3), thus reflecting the anatomy of the retinal nerve fiber layer. Static perimetry has been shown to be more suitable for the detection of these typical glaucomatous defects than kinetic perimetry.

Nasal steps are very important signs of glaucoma (see below). When manual perimetry is used they are found as an initial perimetric sign of glaucoma in a large percentage of cases.[65] The importance of peripheral nasal defects outside 30° is still debated. Some studies have indicated that up to 11% of patients may have defects in the nasal periphery while the central field is still normal.[66] Others have found that peripheral nasal steps are virtually nonexistent in glaucoma patients whose central fields are normal as measured with modern computerized perimetry.[67] The most important question, from a practical point of view, is whether any additional time that may be available after assessment of the central visual field with a standard protocol is best spent in further investigation of the central 30° field or in searching for defects outside this area.

VARIABILITY

Even in normal subjects there is considerable intersubject and intrasubject variability in perimetric results; results from different individuals differ somewhat, as do fields from the same eye when plotted at different times. In glaucoma, clear-cut and reproducible field loss is preceded by a long phase characterized by increased local intratest and intertest variability. This has been shown with both manual[68] and computerized methods,[69] but is much more

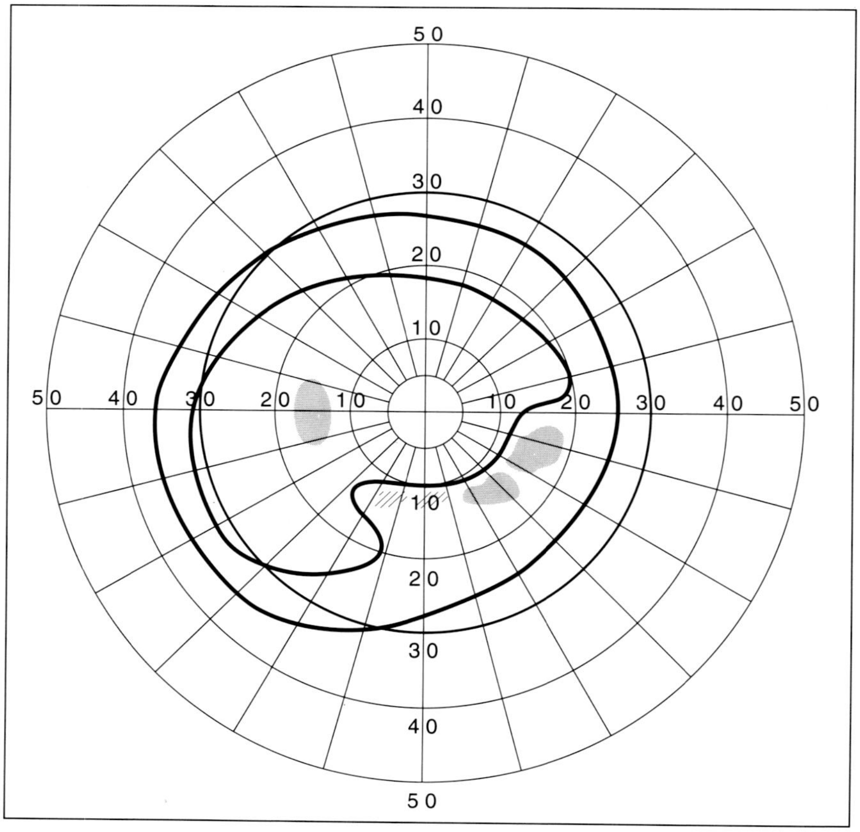

7.3 | Early glaucomatous defects often appear as small paracentral, often poorly delineated defects and as areas with questionable sensitivity (shadowed). Such scotomas, initially unconnected to the blind spot, later merge and grow into full-blown arcuate defects.

obvious when computerized testing is used. Therefore, in eyes converting to glaucoma with field loss, the earliest perimetric changes are typically small, rather nonspecific depressions of sensitivity which seem to come and go in approximately the same area of the field during a long period of time before absolutely clear-cut defects can be registered (Fig. 7.4).

GENERAL REDUCTION OF SENSITIVITY AND FOCAL LOSS

In recent years, diffuse reduction of sensitivity has often been regarded as a sign of glaucoma.[70–73] However, other studies have concluded that entirely diffuse loss is uncommon or nonexistent in glaucoma.[74,75] Even in early cases with widespread loss of sensitivity, some areas always seem to be more affected than others. There are changes in the shape of the hill of vision, not simply an overall lowering. This results in areas of localized loss, i.e., traditional glaucomatous visual field defects.

The concept of diffuse loss of sensitivity in glaucoma may, in part, be a matter of semantics. Mean deviation (MD) has often been regarded as an indicator of diffuse loss, although it is really an index of the total loss, or the sum of diffuse and localized loss[76,77] (see below). In some cases a pathologic MD may have been incorrectly interpreted as an indicator of diffuse, homogeneous depression of the visual field, when it actually may have been caused by localized loss affecting one or more parts of the visual field but not the entire field. Widespread reduction of sensitivity is common in glaucoma, but explanations other than glaucoma (e.g., media opacities or pharmacologically induced miosis) are the rule when test results show only homogeneous and general reduction of sensitivity without any concomitant localized loss.

Although early glaucoma damage, therefore, is usually not diffuse, neither is it usually extremely focal. Even before clear-cut field defects have developed, the area of increased scatter and of variable, nonreproducible

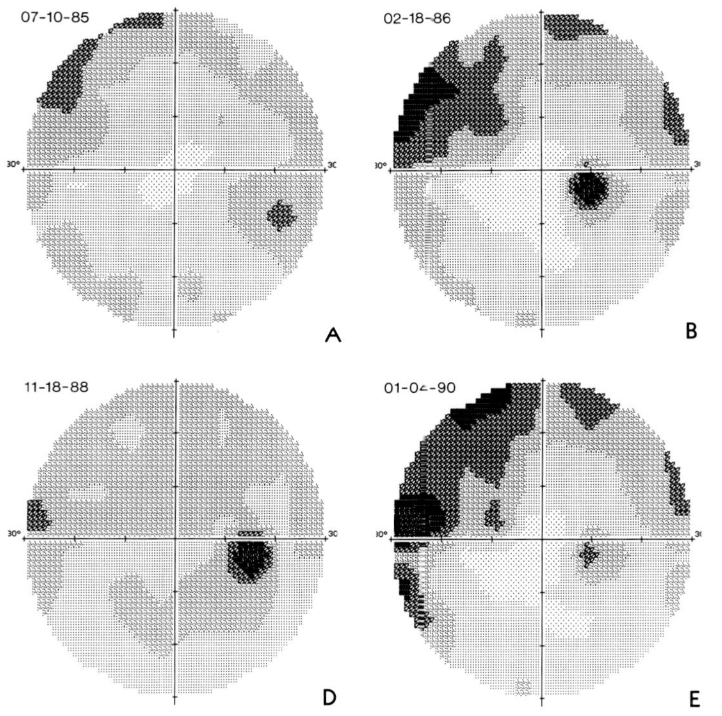

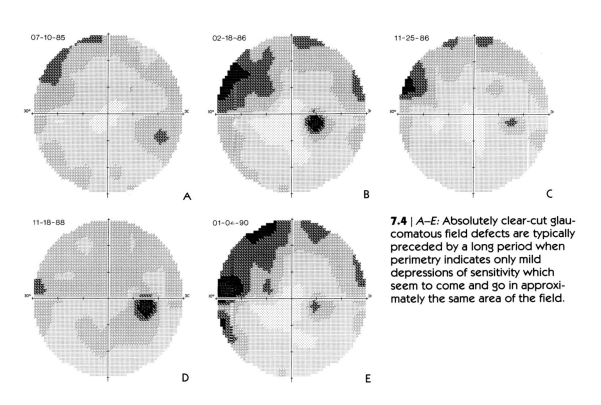

7.4 | *A–E:* Absolutely clear-cut glaucomatous field defects are typically preceded by a long period when perimetry indicates only mild depressions of sensitivity which seem to come and go in approximately the same area of the field.

depressions has been shown to be large enough to encompass several test points in standard computerized central field tests (e.g., the Humphrey 30-2 or 24-2 patterns or the Octopus 32 or G1 programs).[78]

Many reported studies have suggested that diffuse loss is associated with concentric enlargement of the optic cup and high IOP. Localized loss, on the other hand, has frequently been considered typical of low-tension glaucoma and, naturally, with localized abnormalities of the optic disc rim (e.g., notching). It is possible, however, that these observations may turn out to be artifacts of the methods by which new cases are discovered, with high tension more likely to be diagnosed in the absence of definite disc signs, such as notching, through routine tonometry.

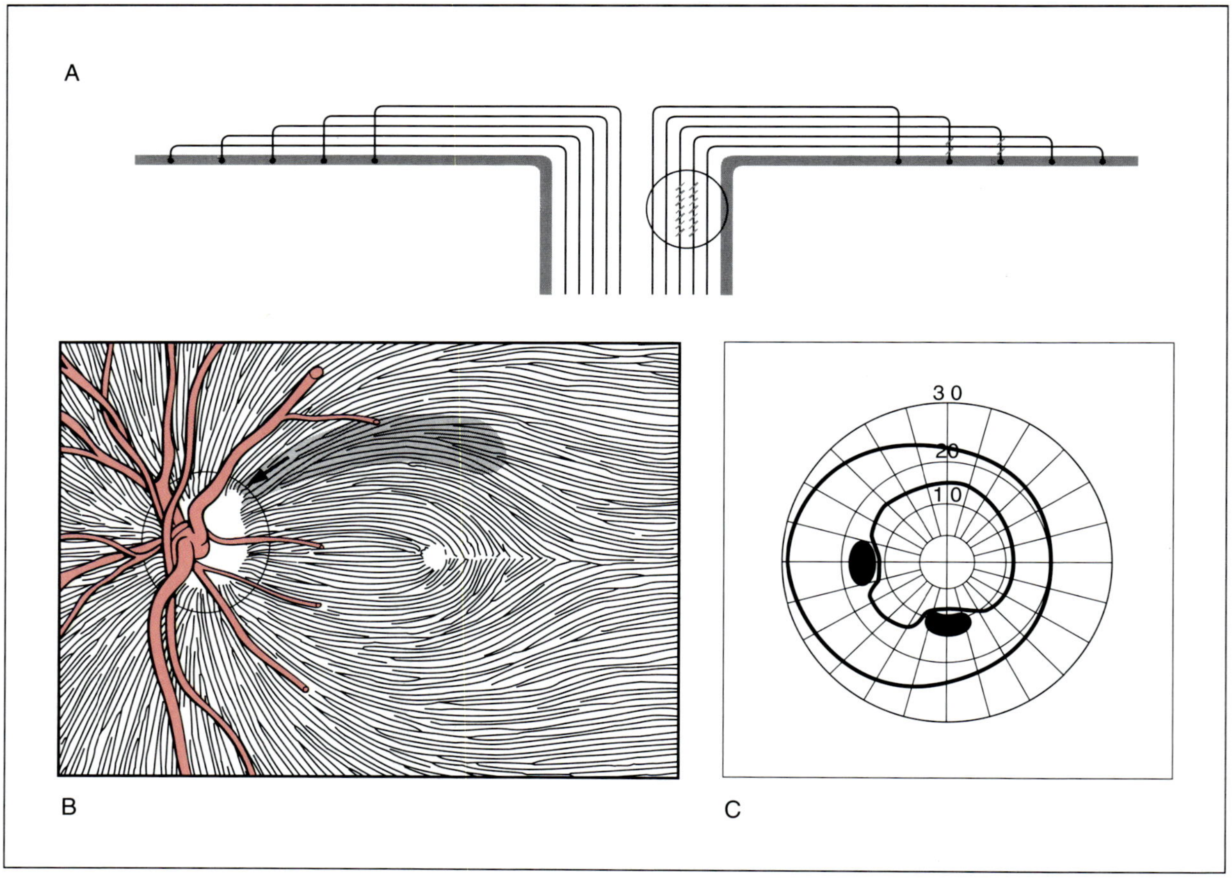

7.5 | Anatomic correlates *(A,B)* to small, arcuate paracentral glaucomatous scotoma *(C)*. Small destruction (circled) in front of lamina cribrosa *(A)* also showing as partial notching (arrow) of disc *(B)* results in loss of axons (stippled) in direction corresponding to lesion. Systematic layering of axons in RNFL with shorter fibers more centrally in disc explains why resulting field defect is not a complete Bjerrum scotoma connected to blind spot.

ANATOMIC CORRELATES

The arcuate arrangement of the retinal nerve fiber layer, and the temporal raphe at the horizontal meridian, naturally explain the full-blown arcuate Bjerrum scotoma and the nasal step. The axonal bundles of the retinal nerve fiber layer are arranged in a systematic way, with the longer axons lying deeper and closer to the neuroretina and the shorter axons lying more superficially and closer to the internal limiting membrane.[79] This organization is retained in the prelaminar region of the optic disc (Fig. 7.5A). A small focal lesion at this level will therefore not result in a complete Bjerrum scotoma, connected to the blind spot and ending at the nasal horizontal meridian, but will only create a paracentral scotoma that tends to respect the arcuate arrangement of the nerve fiber layer (Fig. 7.5B,C). This should not be taken, however, as anatomic support for suggestions that glaucoma frequently produces tiny deep scotomas. On the contrary, it now appears that even very localized lesions at the level of the optic disc cause moderately large areas of ganglion cell death in the retina[79] (Fig. 7.6). This is in agreement with clinical observations that very well-defined, small, and localized glaucomatous scotomas are quite rare. When such small and well-defined field defects occur, they are often located close to the point of fixation, where axonal density is high and receptive fields are small.

Glaucoma often leads to a rather concentric enlargement of the cup. Nevertheless, entirely diffuse loss of sensitivity is also uncommon (see above), presumably because the perfectly homogeneous loss of axon density required to produce it is highly unlikely to occur. Instead, some parts of the disc suffer at least slightly greater damage than others, causing changes in the shape of the hill of vision and thus in localized defects (e.g., nasal steps)

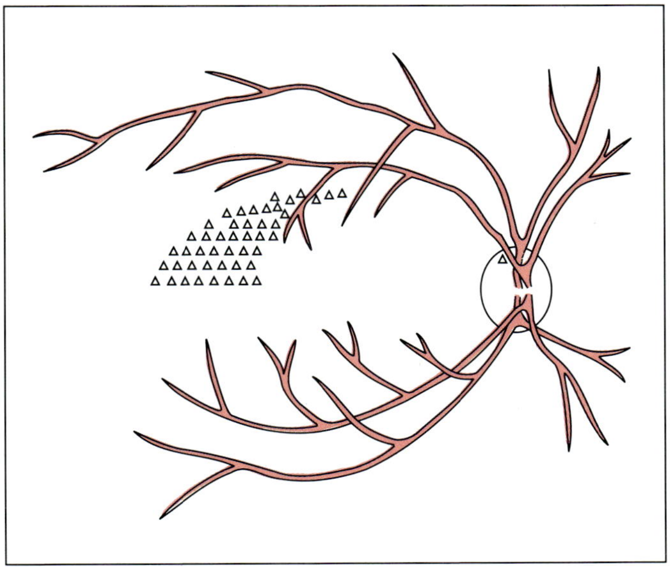

7.6 | Distribution of atrophic ganglion cells in retina after small, focal lesion at the optic disc. Very small disc lesions produce effects over rather large areas of retina. This may help to explain the rarity of extremely focal glaucomatous lesions. (Adapted from Minckler D: The organization of nerve fiber bundles in the primate optic nerve head. *Arch Ophthalmol 1980;98:1630–1636.* Copyright American Medical Association.)

(Fig. 7.7), instead of perfectly homogeneous and diffuse reduction of sensitivity. Therefore, reasonably localized loss and widespread field loss are both common patterns in glaucoma, whereas the extremes (entirely homogeneous and diffuse, or extremely localized loss) are both rare.

SUMMARY

Glaucomatous field defects are the result of lesions at the prelaminar region of the optic disc. They may be widespread, but entirely diffuse loss is uncommon or rare. Extremely small defects are also uncommon. Glaucomatous defects often follow an arcuate pattern, at least in part; this shape is a result of the arcuate course of the normal retinal nerve fiber layer. Early defects usually occur in the central 30° field.

DETECTING GLAUCOMATOUS VISUAL FIELD LOSS

Glaucoma suspects should be subjected to visual field examination at regular intervals. The search for glaucomatous defects should concentrate on the central 30° field, where early changes are most common. Examination of the peripheral field is not nearly as effective and can be omitted (see above). When manual techniques are used, it may be valuable to examine the nasal periphery between 30°–60° (see below).

KINETIC AND STATIC TECHNIQUES

Kinetic perimetry is well suited to detect nasal steps. Several meridians around the nasal horizontal meridian should be examined, at two or three eccentricities. However, kinetic perimetry will miss many scotomas. Scotomas will be detected only if they happen to be situated in the area of plotted isopters, and will then only be visible as a central shifting of the isopter. Therefore, if the examination is carried out only with kinetic stimuli moving towards the point of fixation, scotomas cannot be depicted as such, but only as contractions (see Fig. 5.2, Chapter 5). Static perimetry is a much more effective technique for detecting scotomas, particularly when they are small or are located in relatively flat areas of the hill of vision.

AUTOMATED PERIMETRIC TECHNIQUES FOR GLAUCOMA DETECTION

Automated perimetry is the preferred method of identifying early glaucomatous field defects. It is as sensitive as or even more sensitive than manual perimetry,[80–82] less vulnerable to the inadvertent effects of examiner bias, and may detect defects many years before they can be identified by conventional manual perimetry.[83] The only automated technique that has achieved widespread acceptance and success is static light-sense perimetry. The main emphasis in this chapter will therefore be placed on automated static testing.

Both automated and manual algorithms for visual field testing can be subdivided into two main categories, suprathreshold screening techniques and threshold-measuring programs.[84,85] Suprathreshold screening tests are qualitative tests intended to differentiate between normal and abnormal visual fields. These techniques aim at saving time by presenting the patient with targets at each test location that should be readily perceived by a normal test subject. Suprathreshold tests are therefore quick and can be used to test many locations in the visual field in a short time.

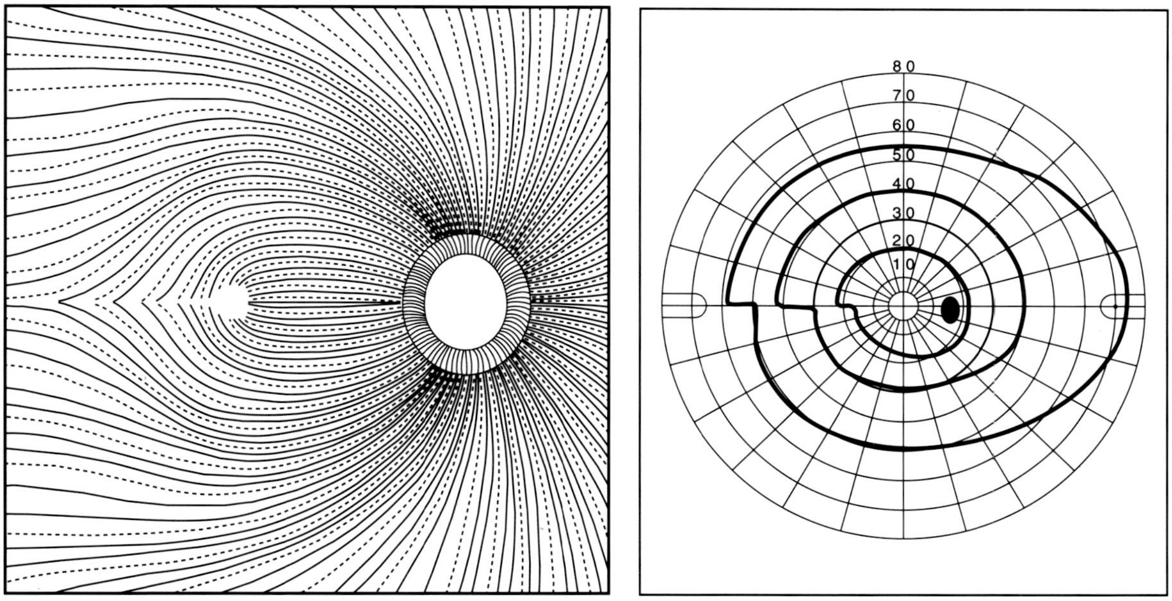

A

B

7.7 I Concentric cupping and field loss. Glaucomatous disc with concentric but somewhat asymmetric increase of disc cupping. Corresponding larger axon loss (interrupted lines) in superior half of retina *(A)*, explains inferior nasal step and contraction of isopters in inferior hemifield *(B)*.

Early automated perimeters often employed one-level screening (Fig. 7.8A), i.e., the same stimulus intensity was used throughout the tested area. This is a nonoptimal approach because stimuli that are bright enough to be seen peripherally will be too bright to detect paracentral losses sensitively, while targets that are suitable for screening of the most central portions of the field will be too dim to be seen peripherally, even by normal subjects.

Eccentricity-compensated testing, in which suprathreshold screening targets increase in intensity with increasing eccentricity (Fig. 7.8B), provides better conditions for efficient detection of field loss. These approaches aim at presenting stimuli at predetermined and constant levels above the anticipated normal threshold of the tested eye (i.e., they are threshold-related). This is usually achieved by actually determining threshold values at a few points in the tested field; an alternative approach is to employ a priori knowledge of normal sensitivities in the form of the age-corrected normal reference field (see below). With this technique sensitivity can be kept more uniform, regardless of point locations, and the risks of false-positive defects in the midperiphery will be reduced.

Threshold-related, eccentricity-compensated, suprathreshold static perimetry can therefore be an efficient way of screening for glaucomatous field defects. In its basic format, this type of algorithm separates screened points into seen points and missed points. Missed points can be submitted to further testing to determine how much sensitivity has been lost at each location. Such quantification may help in interpretation, and adds little time if only a few abnormal points are present.

Threshold-measuring tests (Fig. 7.8C) are more time consuming, because several stimuli, above and below threshold, must be shown at each location. However, they are considerably more efficient detectors of beginning abnormality and can show the highly variable, shallow, nonreproducible defects that appear as the initial perimetric signs of glaucoma (see above and Fig. 7.4). It may be quite helpful to establish a few baseline threshold tests in patients who are considered at high risk to develop field loss in the future.

Threshold tests of the central 30° field are, therefore, well suited for following eyes with suspect glaucoma for the earliest detectable field abnormalities, but threshold-related, eccentricity-compensated tests can also be very effective.

MANUAL PERIMETRY FOR DETECTION

Manual perimetry is also used to search for glaucomatous visual field damage but, again, the examination should be concentrated in the central 30°. Manual perimetry is largely an art, and with a well-trained and motivated perimetrist using suitable and strict techniques it can be a sensitive technique. It is difficult to maintain consistently good results in clinical settings, however, and as a rule computerized perimetry is clearly better in the search for glaucomatous field loss. In manual kinetic perimetry two central isopters, e.g., with Goldmann stimuli I/2 and I/1, could be used. Peripheral testing can be omitted except when nasal steps are sought (see below). When a peripheral isopter is plotted, one should avoid the extremely suprathreshold V/4 target and try I/4 or II/4 instead. Nasal steps (see Fig. 7.7) are easy to discover with manual kinetic techniques, and it is important to search for such steps at two or three eccentricities.

Even very distinct scotomas can easily be missed between isopters unless static spot checking is performed. Such static testing must, therefore, be considered mandatory. The Armaly–Drance glaucoma screening protocol

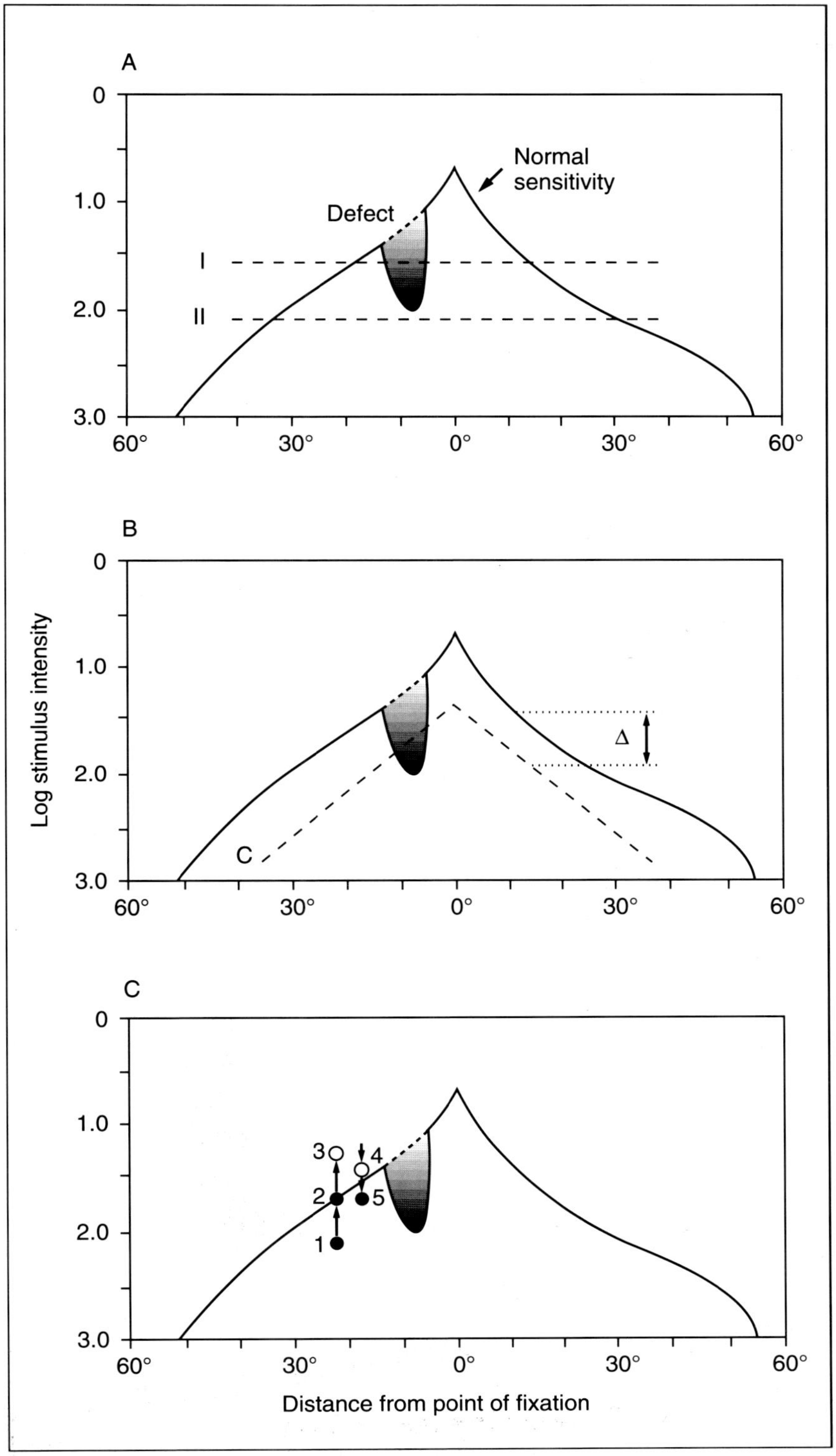

7.8 | Perimetric sensitivity is highest at fovea and decreases with distance from point of fixation. Suprathreshold one-level screening *(A)* may, therefore, easily result in false positive defects in periphery if stimulus is weak (level I) or missing of relative defects centrally if a stronger stimulus is used (level II). Threshold-related eccentricity-compensated screening *(B)* is better. Actual threshold determination *(C)* is best but requires several questions per tested point.

has been specifically designed for detection of early glaucomatous field defects,[86] and has been proven very effective.[87] This technique is still the recommended approach for situations in which manual perimetry must be used for detection of glaucomatous field defects.

FOLLOWING GLAUCOMATOUS VISUAL FIELD LOSS

AUTOMATED PERIMETRY: FULL-THRESHOLD VS. FAST THRESHOLD ALGORITHMS

In follow-up it is important to keep the conditions of testing as constant as possible. Threshold programs should be employed, and the same point pattern, stimulus size, etc., should always be used. In this situation the advantages of computerized perimetry are particularly clear, because differences between examiners, and from day to day in the same examiner, are eliminated.

Glaucomatous field defects progress through extension, through deepening, and by the occurrence of new circumscribed field defects in previously unaffected areas.[88] Recognition of increasing scotoma depth requires threshold measurements.

True threshold-measuring programs, which measure the increment threshold at all point locations, must be differentiated from so-called fast-threshold programs, which are really rather sophisticated screening tests. In one type of fast-threshold test,[89] the perimeter uses a baseline of one or more threshold tests from the same eye to show a supposedly slightly suprathreshold stimulus at all test points. Only missed points are thresholded, and seen points are considered not to have deteriorated. With this technique, random improvements will not be recognized and flagged as such, whereas random deteriorations will be detected. In nonprogressive fields this will result in a number of indications of progression and none of improvement. The clinician may have great difficulties in judging the true clinical meaning of such findings.

Glaucomatous fields are often subject to "visual fatigue," which manifests as a decrease in sensitivity that takes place *during* the test itself.[90] A point that initially shows only slight depression of sensitivity may change into a seriously disturbed point as the test progresses, and the visual field worsens while it is being measured (Fig. 7.9). Therefore, follow-up examinations should always be conducted with tests of approximately the same duration as the baseline test. A fast-threshold test will perform the entire examination while the field is still fairly good and has not started to deteriorate because of visual fatigue. However, a substantial amount of true deterioration may have taken place before this progression can be detected with the fast threshold test. Therefore, full threshold tests are most suitable for follow-up.

VERY SERIOUSLY DISTURBED FIELDS

The basic principle in selecting a test point pattern is to test the same points as those examined when the baseline was established. There is one important exception to this: in very seriously disturbed fields (e.g., where only a central island is preserved), most points in the standard pattern may be in areas of absolute defects; the test then yields only a small number of threshold values better than 0 decibel (DB). In such cases it is advantageous to switch to a test that is concentrated to the remainder of the field, for instance one which covers only the central 10°. This creates a new baseline which will facilitate the detection of any further progression. Similarly, in cases with advanced field loss when the standard test does not give enough data, switching from a standard size III stimulus to a nonstandard size V can change the field drastically and provide a sufficient numerical base for follow-up. Another option in very seriously disturbed glaucomatous fields may be to switch to manual kinetic perimetry (see below).

MANUAL PERIMETRY

Keeping conditions of testing constant is of utmost importance when glaucomatous fields are followed with manual kinetic perimetry. It is important to use the same stimulus sizes and brightnesses as in the baseline field, to check the calibration of the instrument regularly, and to try to use the same stimulus velocity at consecutive examinations.

Manual kinetic perimetry is the examination method of choice in eyes with fields that are so severely disturbed that static automated perimetry indicates mostly absolute defects and therefore does not yield enough data for follow-up. It is also suitable in patients who have great difficulties in conducting standard computerized perimetry. However, it is often difficult to obtain reliable test results in patients who fall into this category, regardless of the technique used.

FREQUENCY AND REPETITION OF TESTS

Ideally, all patients with manifest field loss should be tested twice a year; in seriously affected patients for whom management may critically depend on the outcome of the visual field test, even more frequent examinations may be justified. Test–retest variability is very large in glaucomatous fields, and with results from only two tests it is usually impossible to differentiate between random fluctuations and true progression (see below). Identifying a negative trend becomes much more easy with access to, e.g., four tests.

Glaucoma suspects require less frequent examinations than do patients with confirmed glaucomatous field loss; examination once a year may be perfectly adequate in low-risk ocular hypertension.

When the very first field loss is found in such eyes converting from ocular hypertension to early glaucoma, shallow and variable depressions of sensitivity, usually localized in one area of the field, are characteristic (see above). With access to only one field test these findings are difficult to distinguish from random variability. Only repeated testing can help in the differ-

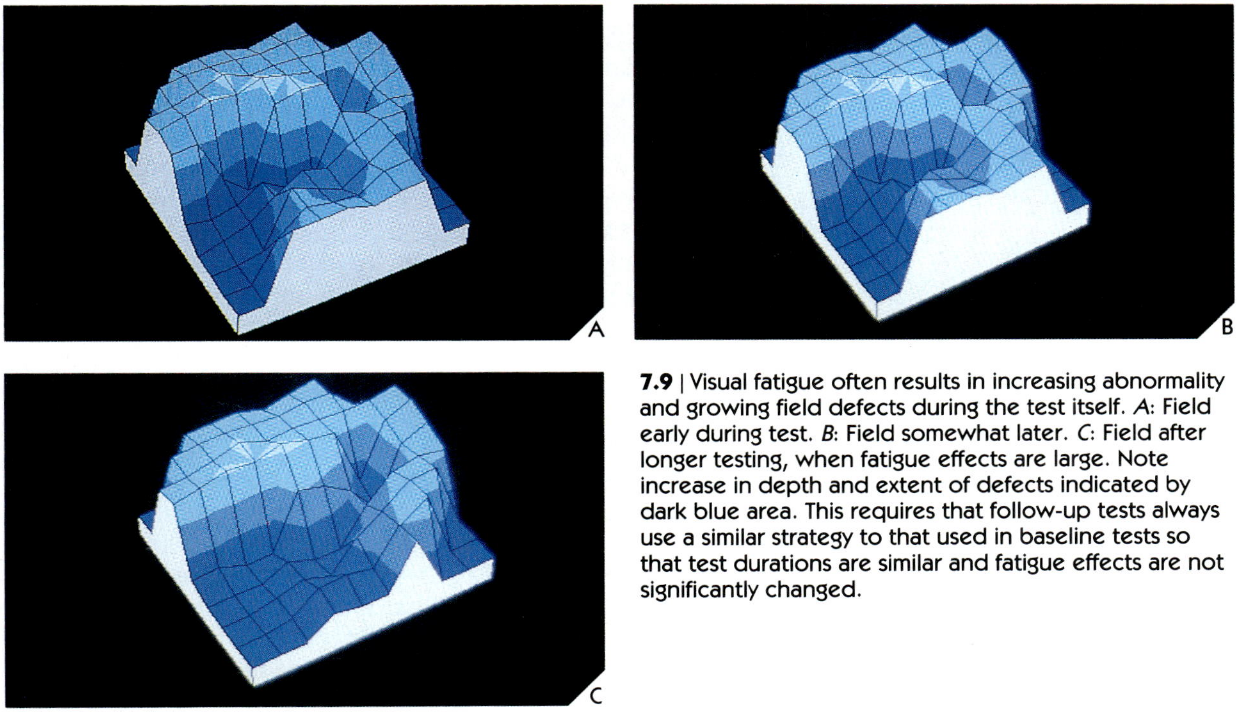

7.9 | Visual fatigue often results in increasing abnormality and growing field defects during the test itself. *A*: Field early during test. *B*: Field somewhat later. *C*: Field after longer testing, when fatigue effects are large. Note increase in depth and extent of defects indicated by dark blue area. This requires that follow-up tests always use a similar strategy to that used in baseline tests so that test durations are similar and fatigue effects are not significantly changed.

entiation. Similarly, if the latest follow-up field indicates progression, it is always wise to repeat the test to confirm the trend before any changes in the therapeutic management are implemented.

ANALYSIS OF INDIVIDUAL VISUAL FIELDS

Interpretation of individual computerized visual fields presents no problem in the majority of cases; often the results are either obviously normal or clearly abnormal. There is a wide gray zone, however, in which classification is more difficult. In a sense, one might say that interpretation of visual fields has become more difficult since the advent of computerized perimetry. Kinetic Goldmann perimetry usually indicated defects only at a stage when these were obvious, credible, and in agreement with optic nerve head topography. The high sensitivity of computerized perimetry makes it possible to identify glaucomatous field loss at a much earlier stage, but it also shows many irregularities and considerable variability in normal fields. Analysis of fields in glaucoma patients and glaucoma suspects has become a question of differentiating between normal and abnormal irregularities. Similarly, recognition of progression has become a question of differentiating between random and significant test–retest variability.

In almost all cases in which true field defects would have been documented with conventional manual methods, the abnormalities will be absolutely clear and more or less impossible to overlook on the gray-scale print-out of a static computerized test. Therefore, it may be defensible to adopt a position of wait-and-see when automated fields are not clearly normal or abnormal. Nevertheless, a systematic approach to interpretation, and some knowledge, will enable the clinician to use the results of the automated perimetric techniques more efficiently. Any such approach should consider the following parameters, among others:

1. Assessment of test reliability parameters and the comments of the perimetrist.
2. Whether the field departs significantly from normality.
3. Whether any departures from normality are artifactual or are due to pathologic processes.
4. If pathologic, whether the field loss is due to glaucoma or to some other pathologic process.

RELIABILITY OF RESULTS

Most automated perimeters present catch trials (false-positive and false-negative checks) and checks of fixation stability during the course of the test. It is important to determine whether the results of these catch trials are within the expected range before any judgments are made about the test itself. False-positive and false-negative answer rates depend somewhat on the perimeter used, but are typically under 20% in normal subjects. Fixation losses tend to be somewhat higher but are often of a similar magnitude.[91] Failure to fall within the given guidelines for catch trials and fixation stability does not necessarily imply that the test must be discarded as unreliable. For example, glaucoma patients commonly produce false-negative catch trial results that fall outside the range found in normal subjects, and a poor fixation score in instruments using the Heijl–Krakau blind-spot method of fixation monitoring is often due to failure of the perimetrist to realize that the instrument has not properly located the blind spot. It is also important to take note of observations made by the perimetrist; often perimetric results make sense only when such comments are taken into account.

DEPARTURE FROM NORMALITY

Many computerized aids are now available to assist in deciding if a visual field result departs from the bounds of normality. These may help by showing the significance of measured departures from normal sensitivity, by pointing out asymmetries across the visual field (especially across the horizontal meridian), and by helping to differentiate between localized field loss and diffuse loss caused by media opacities and miosis. Differences from age-corrected normal values can be displayed on a point-by-point basis as deviation maps, showing the depth of encountered defects[77,89,92] (Fig 7.10). Of course, it is the significance of specific departures from normality rather than their magnitudes which is of interest, and such significances can be shown in probability maps.[77,89,93] (see Fig 7.10). Variability among normal subjects is considerably larger peripherally than paracentrally.[94,95] Therefore, the statistical and clinical significance of a certain depression from the age-corrected normal values is much larger when the depression occurs in the paracentral area than when it

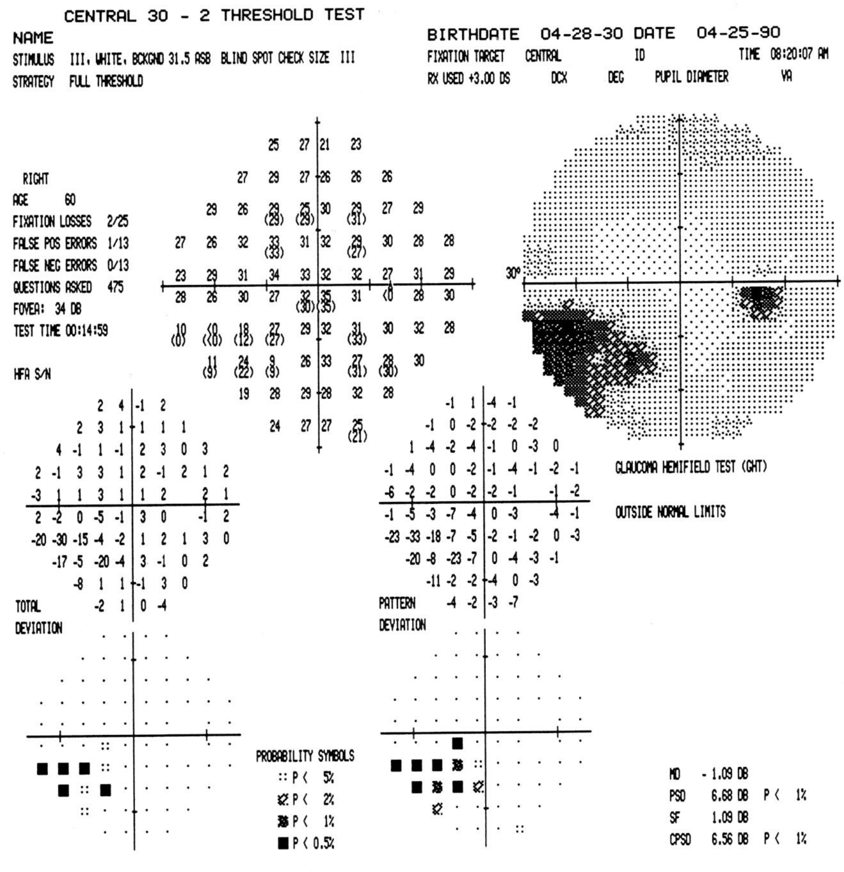

7.10 | Conventional single-field Statpac printout for Humphrey field analyzer. A classic inferior nasal defect is easily seen in all printouts. Numerical total deviation map shows deviations from age-corrected normal threshold value, while probability maps indicate that measured values within defect are highly unusual in normals, and therefore significant. Glaucoma hemifield test identifies field as abnormal; all visual field indexes are also abnormal. Terms and abbreviations are defined in text.

appears farther away from the fixation point (Fig. 7.11). At present, probability maps probably offer the easiest and best tool for differentiating between true field loss and noise, and they often show developing field loss at an early stage when visual field indices are still normal (Fig. 7.12). Departures from age-normal values can be further corrected for the general sensitivity of the patient in question, thus allowing separate consideration of localized and diffuse field loss. Probability maps can again be used to present the significance of localized departures, having removed the effects of diffuse loss due, for example, to cataract or miosis[77,89,93] (Fig. 7.13).

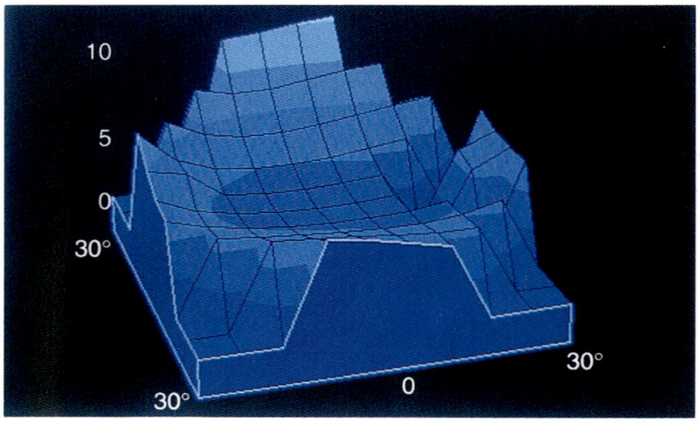

7.11 | Dependence of interindividual threshold variability on point location. Illustration shows central 30° field. Z-axis is measured defect depth (deviation from age-corrected normal threshold values in DB) required to reach significance, at $p<0.05$ level in points with depressed sensitivity. Larger defect depths are required in midperiphery than centrally.

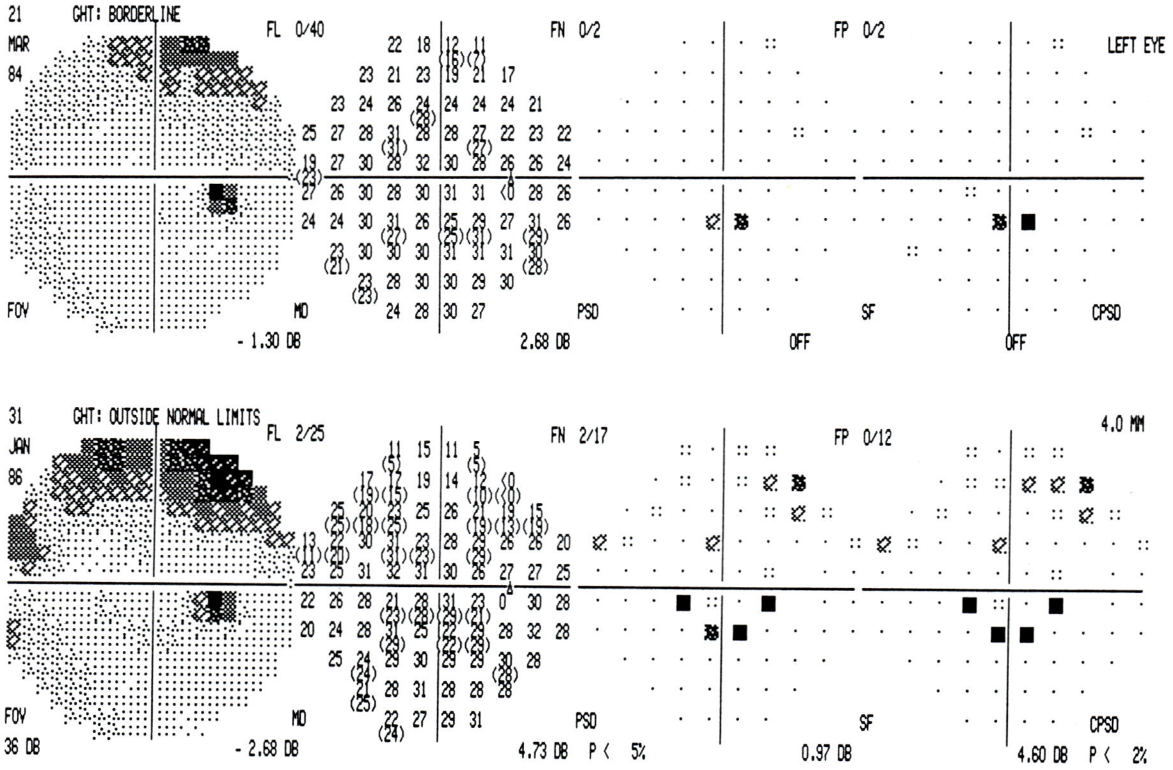

7.12 | Two fields from eye with developing field loss determined with Humphrey field analyzer. Disturbances often appear in probability maps in the paracentral area before they become obvious in conventional gray-scale printouts.

Results of computerized field tests can be condensed into so-called global visual field indices. Such indices can estimate the volume of the measured hill of vision, as in the performance value of the Competer/Digilab perimeter[96] or the mean sensitivity (MS) of the Humphrey and Octopus instruments. MD (mean deviation or mean defect in the Humphrey and Octopus instruments, respectively) is an average total difference, in DB, between the measured field and the age-corrected normal reference field.[76,77] Pattern standard deviation (PSD), corrected pattern standard deviation (CPSD), loss variance (LV), and corrected loss variance (CLV) reflect the difference in shape, but not in height, between the measured field and the age-corrected normal reference field. In some perimeters, normal ranges have been empirically determined for these indices. When MD, PSD, or CPSD is outside these limits, the levels of significance are shown. Visual field indices allow a crude classification of visual fields into normal and pathologic. Present indices are not optimal for diagnosis because, for example, they do not take into account whether points with low sensitivity are grouped into meaningful patterns or whether such points are randomly scattered across the field. Indices do offer a large degree of data reduction, however, and are very convenient in looking for general trends.

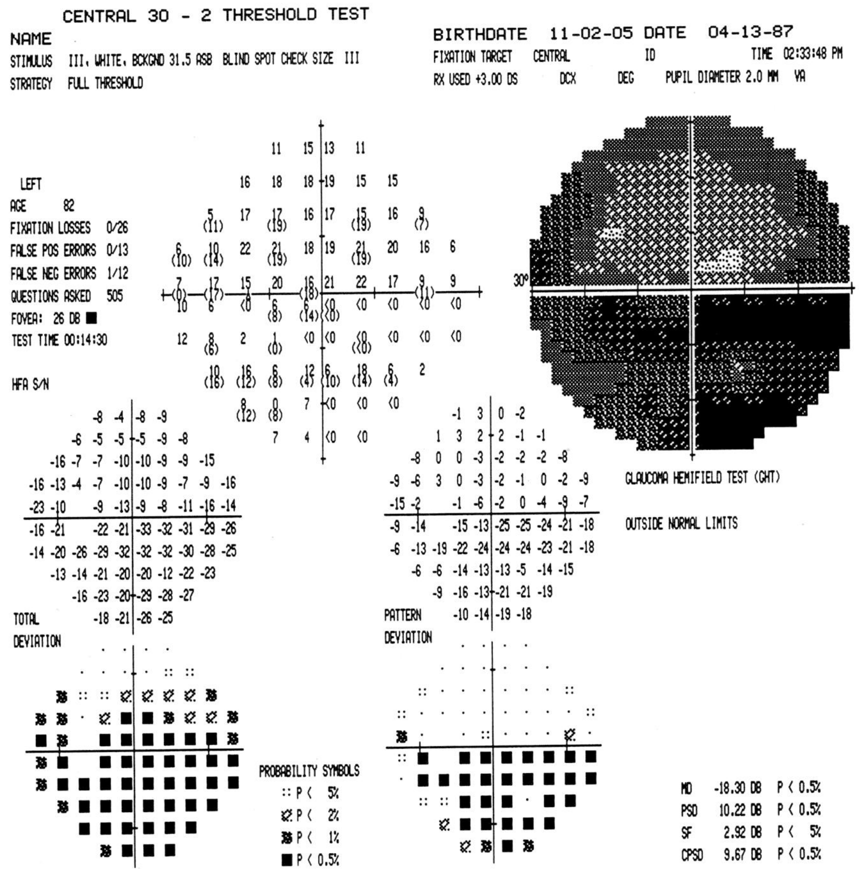

7.13 | Visual field from eye with coexisting glaucoma and cataract. Total deviation probability and numerical maps show that the entire field is depressed. Localized, glaucoma-induced defect is shown in pattern deviation maps. Glaucoma hemifield test indicates abnormal result.

Comparisons of threshold values in the superior and inferior hemifields can help to differentiate between normal and glaucomatous fields,[97] especially when they are based on empirically observed frequencies of deviations from age-corrected normal values rather than on actual sensitivity values.[98] The Glaucoma Hemifield Test of the Humphrey Statpac program is an example of an analysis based on such up–down comparisons plus an estimation of the general level of sensitivity in the best parts of the measured field.[98]

SEPARATION OF ARTIFACTUAL AND PATHOLOGIC FIELD LOSS

False-positive field defects frequently occur outside 20° of eccentricity in all directions, but most often superiorly. In the latter area they are often caused by droopy lids. Rims of corrective lenses or misalignment of such lenses can cause false-positive defects in any direction. Patients who lack previous experience with automated perimetry not uncommonly produce fields that are falsely interpreted as pathologic. Such "untrained" fields typically show concentric contraction, with low sensitivities in the periphery and normal or almost normal values close to the point of fixation[99,100] (Fig. 7.14).

INTERPRETATION OF PATHOLOGIC FIELDS

Nonglaucomatous field defects are quite common, even in supposedly normal subjects (see above). Therefore, when encountered defects do not look typical of glaucoma and when the optic disc appears normal, one should try to exclude other reasons for field loss than glaucoma.

In glaucoma, interpretation of single fields should particularly aim at detection of localized field defects. Homogeneous, diffuse loss is much more commonly caused by media opacities or medically induced miosis than by glaucoma (see above). Naturally, groups of depressed points are more important than isolated or scattered points with somewhat lowered sensitivity, and the patterns of glaucomatous field loss are well documented, as previously discussed. Comparisons of corresponding areas in the two (superior and inferior) hemifields can often be helpful.[97,98] Differences in sensitivity between the superior and inferior hemifields, of course, are the reason for nasal steps. In cases of suspect glaucoma where the most recent test shows questionable abnormalities, it is helpful to look for similar but not identical changes in the preceding tests.

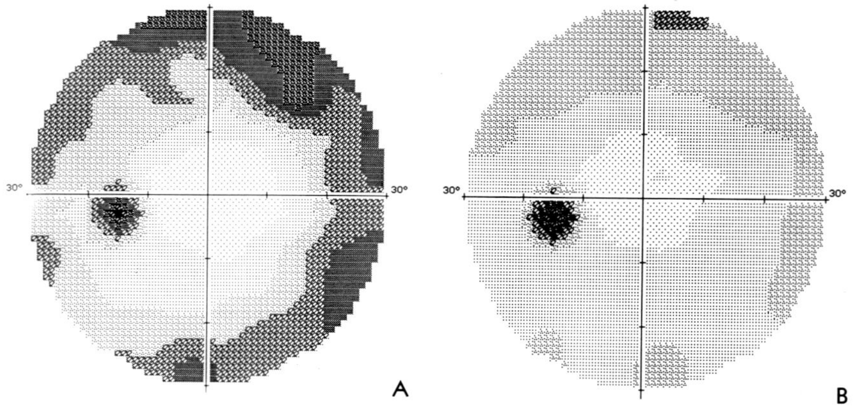

7.14 | Example of perimetric learning in normal subject. *A:* Early field shows typical concentric contraction, with low sensitivities in the periphery and normal or almost normal values close to the point of fixation. *B:* Later field is normal.

INTERPRETATION IN FOLLOW-UP

The advantages of computerized perimetry, as compared with manual techniques, are particularly clear in follow-up, when automation ensures that the examination is performed with exactly the same test strategy every time, and when computer-assisted interpretation routines can help to organize the large amounts of data that accumulate for patients who are followed for many years. Nevertheless, interpretation of series of visual fields in follow-up is considerably more difficult and complicated than is interpretation of single visual fields. There are several reasons for this, the most important being that glaucomatous visual fields are less reproducible than normals and, hence, true differences between tests are more difficult to detect. The large amount of data is a challenge in itself; it should facilitate detection of change, yet it is impossible for the clinician to analyze optimally the massive numbers of threshold values involved in glaucoma patients who have been tested many times with automated perimetry.

Computerized perimeters offer many ways of looking for change over time, and different levels of abstraction can be applied to the data. At the minimal level of abstraction, analysis is made of the raw threshold values of the entire series of tests, an approach that is almost impossible when more than a few fields are available. At the maximal level, analysis is made of a single figure of merit for each test, such as mean deviation. It seems clear, however, that early changes can easily be missed at this level of maximal condensation of data.[101] Many intermediate levels of abstraction exist, and it is at these intermediate levels that the best judgments are to be made.

A number of issues should be kept in mind when series of glaucomatous visual fields are to be analyzed. There are similarities with the analysis of single fields, but the point of view is somewhat different:

1. Suitability, reliability, and sufficiency of available data.
2. Whether observed field changes fall within the limits of normal variability in glaucoma or are likely to indicate significant change.
3. Whether observed changes are artifactual or caused by progressive glaucoma.
4. Treatment implications of observed changes in visual fields.

SUITABILITY, RELIABILITY, AND SUFFICIENCY OF DATA

Field results may not be useful because the test method used was not suitable to the particular situation; incorrect choices of test strategy, pattern, and stimulus size may make it impossible to include certain tests, or to judge the entire series of fields. Reliability parameters should be considered but are of limited value. The rate of false-negative answers is increased in abnormal fields, and false-negative values can hardly be regarded as a reliability indicator in moderately or severely disturbed glaucomatous fields.[91] The same is true for SF, the short-term fluctuation. High percentages of false-positive answers are dependable indicators of inadequate patient performance also in pathologic fields, and are well worth taking into account. A high percentage of false-positive answers tends to increase measured DB threshold values, whereas high numbers of false-negative values have the opposite effect.

It is critical that there be enough baseline and follow-up tests to enable a clinical judgment to be made. Judgments of change can only very rarely be based on only two tests, unless the changes are drastic, such as from a completely normal result to a reasonably well-developed and deep arcuate defect.

This usually happens only with tests which are separated by a very long time interval. Normally, no serious change in treatment regimen should be contemplated on the basis of change seen between only two tests; at least two baseline and two follow-up tests should be available for analysis, and often even this number is insufficient.

NORMAL VARIABILITY VS. SIGNIFICANT CHANGE

Threshold variability in glaucomatous visual fields is much higher than in normal fields. The degree of variability is influenced by the degree of abnormality[102] (Fig 7.15). Therefore, in points that initially show normal threshold values, and therefore a defect depth around 0 DB, the majority will be between +3 and -5 DB from the age-corrected normal value on follow-up. In shallow field defects, however, the variability increases over that found in normality, and when presently available perimeters are used, points having initial defect depths of exceeding 10–15 DB can vary on follow-up from almost normal to absolute defects, by chance alone.

The general status of the field also influences the range of random variation. Fields that are generally more abnormal, as measured by MD, have larger variabilities in individual threshold values than more normal fields. Furthermore, points with the same initial degree of abnormality have a higher chance of showing better sensitivity at follow-up tests when they are situated in reasonably normal fields than when they are part of a more seriously disturbed field.[103] Finally, intertest variability is smaller paracentrally than more peripherally.[102] Therefore, variability in glaucomatous visual fields is substantial and depends on a number of factors. Although it is possible to

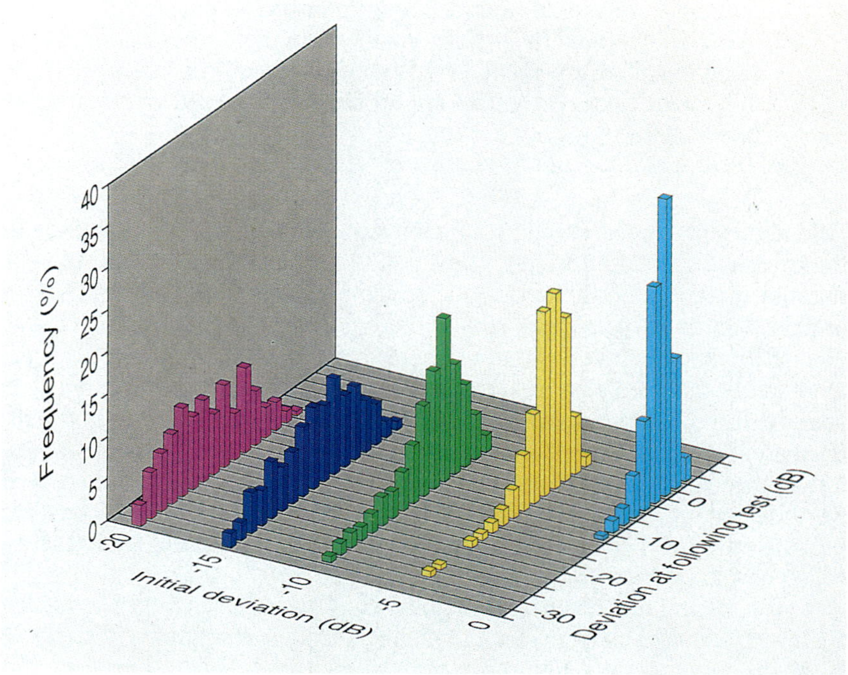

7.15 | Test–retest threshold variability, dependence on defect depth. The five bar diagrams show distributions of measured threshold values at a second test (X-axis) in points stratified according to defect depth at initial test (Y-axis). Initial defect depths vary from normal (turquoise), to 5 DB (yellow), 10 DB (green), 15 DB (blue), and 20 DB (red) below age-corrected normal threshold value. Bar height indicates frequency (in %). Points with normal sensitivity show considerably smaller changes between tests than do abnormal points.

remember a few rules based on these observations, it is much simpler to use analysis programs in which such empirical information has been recorded. At least one statistical package is commercially available which offers analysis of the statistical significance of changes at each point in the visual field, based on empirical data from glaucoma patients[98,104] (Fig. 7.16).

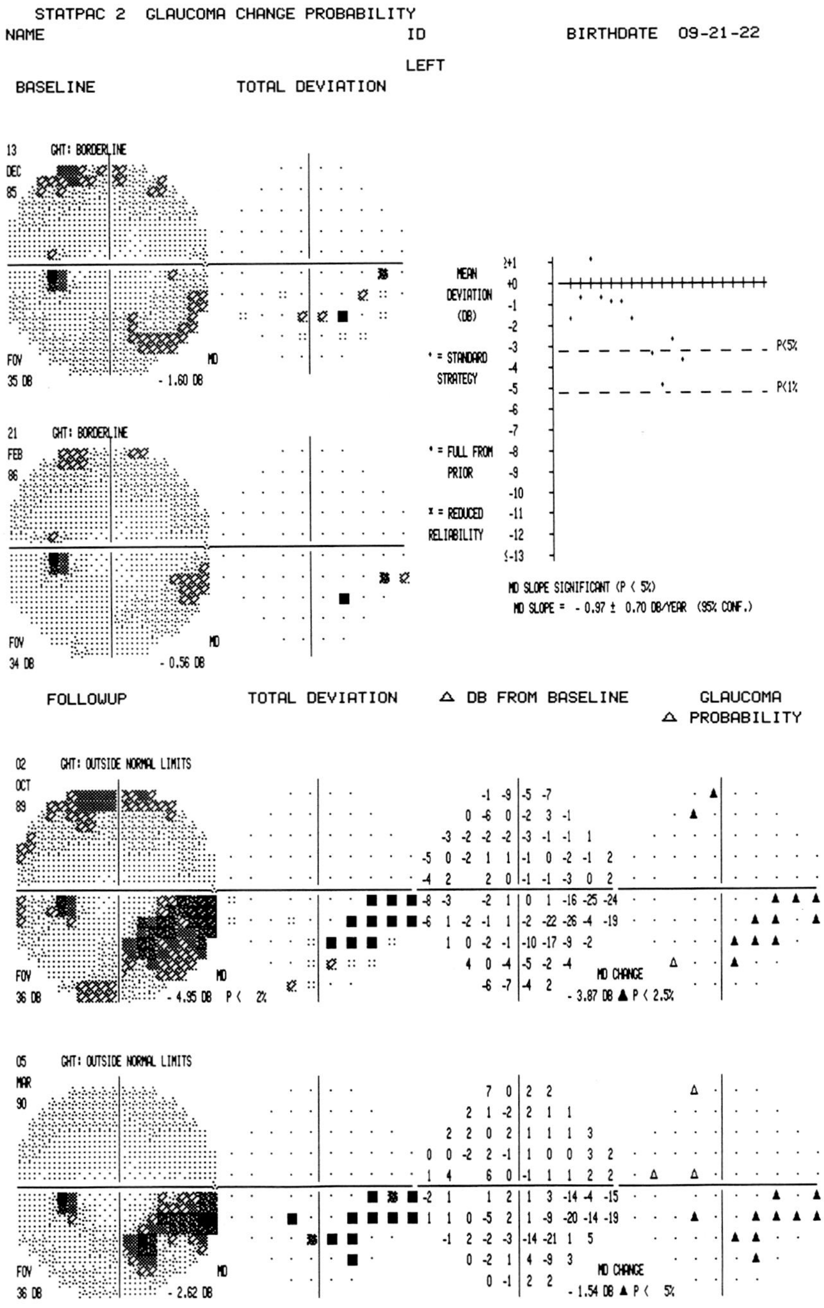

7.16 | Regression analysis and change probability maps, Humphrey field analyzer. Progressive glaucoma with increasing field loss. Scatterplot shows mean deviation worsening significantly over time. Average of first two (upper) fields form baseline. Two late fields in series (below) compared to baseline; numerical deviation maps show differences in DB; probability maps show that deterioration is significant at several points (black triangles).

It is also possible to draw inferences about the significance of apparent visual field changes through the use of regression analysis techniques[77,105] (see Fig. 7.16). Instead of using information about the behavior of glaucomatous visual fields in general, as outlined above, regression analyses consider the consistency of the individual patient's results over time. Comparisons of fields with the help of t-tests[106] are not recommended, however. The threshold values of computer fields are not independent observations, and t-tests often falsely indicate significant deterioration or improvement when no true changes have taken place.[107]

Over long periods of follow-up, defects commonly progress so much that the worsening is obvious just on a rapid glance at the gray-scale printouts of the series of fields. A localized defect that can be seen to engage previously normal areas on several consecutive tests is a good clinical sign of progression.

There is no doubt that computerized interpretation routines will improve in the future and will therefore make it easier to draw correct conclusions about stability and progression. Such programs cannot eliminate the large variations encountered in series of visual fields, however. Even with techniques that use available field data optimally, we can doubt our future ability to detect reliably the very small amount of glaucomatous visual field decay that may take place between two or three patient visits over 6 to 12 months.

GLAUCOMA PROGRESSION OR OTHER REASONS FOR CHANGE

Although glaucomatous fields are characterized by relatively large test–retest variations, the rate of true progression in glaucoma is almost always slow. When really large changes are encountered between two tests, one must consider whether the differences are the result of test artifacts, of some other unexpected disease, or perhaps some inadvertent change in test protocol. Miotic therapy is a common reason for sudden overall deterioration. In particular, when miotics have been added because of suspected visual field progression, one must beware of interpreting the first field test on miotics as confirmation of the questionable negative trend.

In the same way that many normal subjects need previous experience to produce a normal result at automated perimetry, pathologic fields also frequently improve with experience. Some improvement over the first few fields is common, and sometimes such changes are drastic. This is a good reason to disregard the first test in determining the visual field baseline in a particular eye, especially when the first test is generally worse than subsequent ones. Therefore, it is good practice to perform more than one field test early on, to establish an appropriate baseline of at least one "trained" field.

Progressive cataracts are common in patients with glaucoma. It is often difficult to determine whether a worsening of the field in such patients is due to the cataract or to the glaucoma. The important difference is that cataracts influence all parts of the visual field to a similar degree; they lead to a general depression of sensitivity. Glaucoma, on the other hand, produces mainly localized field defects. Therefore, when glaucomatous visual field defects progress, the defects deepen and extend, and new defects appear, while other parts of the field remain unchanged. On the other hand, when worsening is due to progressive lens opacities the deterioration is more widespread, influencing all parts of the visual field.

TREATMENT IMPLICATIONS OF OBSERVED CHANGE

Our ability to detect true change is limited. Small and insignificant changes will pass unrecognized. Therefore, any credible deterioration in visual field status carries with it the obligation to consider seriously a change in treatment. The seriousness of the contemplated intervention must be weighed against the relative certainty that a perimetric change has occurred; minor changes in medications require lower levels of certainty than do decisions to submit the patient to surgery. In situations when there is any uncertainty at all, one should try to confirm suspected deterioration by repeating the test on another day. Poor results are often caused by random variations, and unexpected apparent progression is often followed by improvement without any change in therapy.[108]

SECTION III

CONTRAST SENSITIVITY TESTING IN GLAUCOMA AND OCULAR HYPERTENSION

Ivan Bodis–Wollner

Contrast sensitivity (CS) measurements in glaucoma patients were first reported using printed charts of low- to mid-range spatial frequency sinusoidal gratings which varied lengthwise in contrast[109] (Fig. 7.17). Some follow-up studies using these stimuli have suggested that CS losses also exist in ocular hypertensive (OHT) patients.[110] Other studies revealed little deficit because the overlap between scores of normals and OHT patients was too large.[111] An approach that used stimulus gratings modulated in time and that was produced on an oscilloscopic display appeared to offer diagnostic advantages.[112,113] Instead of static patterns in this stimulus, the dark pattern bands switch place with the bright ones and back several times per second. The result of studies that compared several spatial and temporal frequencies of modulation as stimuli in glaucoma[112–114] suggested that low spatial frequency patterns modulated in time around 8 Hz provide the best statistical discrimination between normal subjects and glaucoma patients (Figs. 7.18 and 7.19). About 50% of OHT patients also showed significant CS losses; this was surprisingly more than the number expected to develop glaucoma proper, i.e., visual field defects. It was suggested that neurons selective for coarse, temporally modulated patterns are especially sensitive to the initial glaucomatous damage.[112,113] Based on the specific visual losses encountered, it appeared (in analogy to the cat retina) that so-called Y-cells are vulnerable. Later work in the primate showed that a better analogy would have been with M-cells of the monkey retina. Several (although not all) histologic studies in humans[115] and in the monkey model of glaucoma[116] are consistent with this suggestion.

Although not negating the fact that slowly modulated patterns also revealed ERG deficits in glaucoma,[117] converging evidence from several subsequent electrophysiologic studies[118–120] are in agreement that, on the whole, so-called steady-state stimuli (above 4 Hz) provide a better discrimination between glaucoma patients and normal subjects than do static or quasistatic patterns. Indeed, in several studies, static or quasistatic (presented for longer than 500 ms) grating stimuli failed to discriminate between glaucoma patients and normal subjects.[121–123] Flickering stimuli without a pattern have been consistently shown to be superior to static targets for detecting visual field defects in glaucoma patients.[124–126] On the basis of an extensive investigation that compared central and paracentral and static and dynamic contrast sensitivity, a recent study[127] therefore suggested that in glaucoma research one should use the more sensitive flickering stimulus.

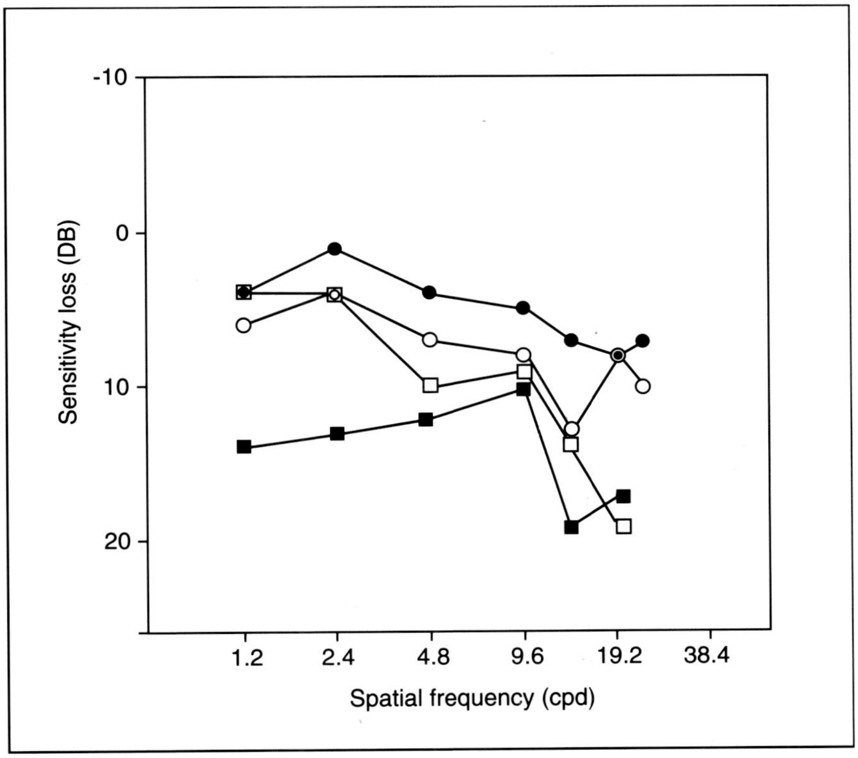

7.17 I Visuograms (ratio of patient to normal contrast sensitivity) at corresponding spatial frequencies for four eyes of two patients. Contrast sensitivity was established with the method of constant stimuli with quasi-stationary (0.5 Hz) presentation. Although all visuograms show high-frequency losses, these are insignificant compared with age-matched controls. Circles represent the data of a patient with low-tension glaucoma, showing little if any deficit at low spatial frequencies. Squares represent the data of a patient with glaucoma who had elevated IOP and arcuate scotoma, showing in one eye a profound low spatial frequency loss. Such a loss is suggestive of advanced glaucoma. Compare this figure with Fig. 5.9 (Bodis–Wollner, Chapter 5) showing high-frequency loss. Temporally modulated patterns are preferred for evaluating visual defects both in OHT and glaucoma. (From Bodis–Wollner I: Differences in low and high spatial frequency vulnerabilities in ocular and cerebral lesions, in Maffei L (ed): *Pathophysiology of the Visual System.* The Hague: Dr. W. Junk Publishers, 1981.)

PREDICTIVE VALUE OF CONTRAST SENSITIVITY IN OHT

One of the most important questions concerning CS is whether or not it predicts the development of glaucoma and, hence, can CS be used as a guide for treatment before the development of field defects? Central CS testing was shown to be superior to automated perimetry[128–132] for revealing defects in a small number of eyes with asymmetric C/D ratios and elevated IOP. However, the converse was reported in at least one study[133] (i.e., there were eyes with normal CS and abnormal fields). This, again, may have resulted from using static targets for CS measurements. The comparative results of using paracentrally presented static gratings and routine perimetry[122] have been only moderately encouraging, whereas paracentral dynamic CS has been shown to be more sensitive than static perimetry to field losses.[127] At this point, the predictive value of dynamic (temporally modulated) CS testing in OHT has to be further pursued.

In summary, the screening value of CS in glaucoma and OHT is well proven. Several but not all studies suggest that low spatial frequency-modulat-

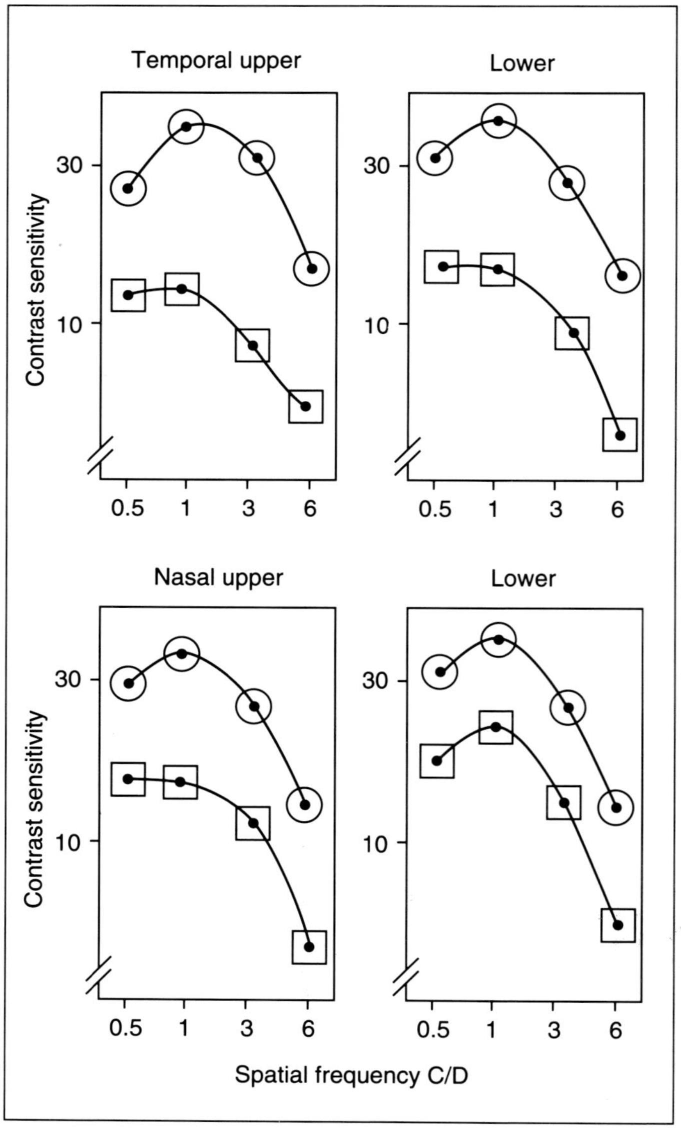

7.18 | Average spatiotemporal (ST) CS near the peak of the normal curve (10 Hz between 0.5 and 6 cpd) determined in four quadrants of the visual field in age-matched controls (circles) and glaucoma patients (squares), all above 50 years of age. Note major loss involving low and medium spatial frequencies in all four quadrants. The patterns were centered on 11.3 degrees from the fovea and subtended 5.5 degrees x 4.4 degrees.

ed patterns are needed for optimal discrimination, although precise statistics are not available because large-scale studies have not been reported. The question of whether or not CS abnormalities predict the development of glaucoma in high-risk OHT patients is being addressed by studies using dynamic (modulated) sinusoidal gratings[112,134] and/or peripheral CS testing.[127,135]

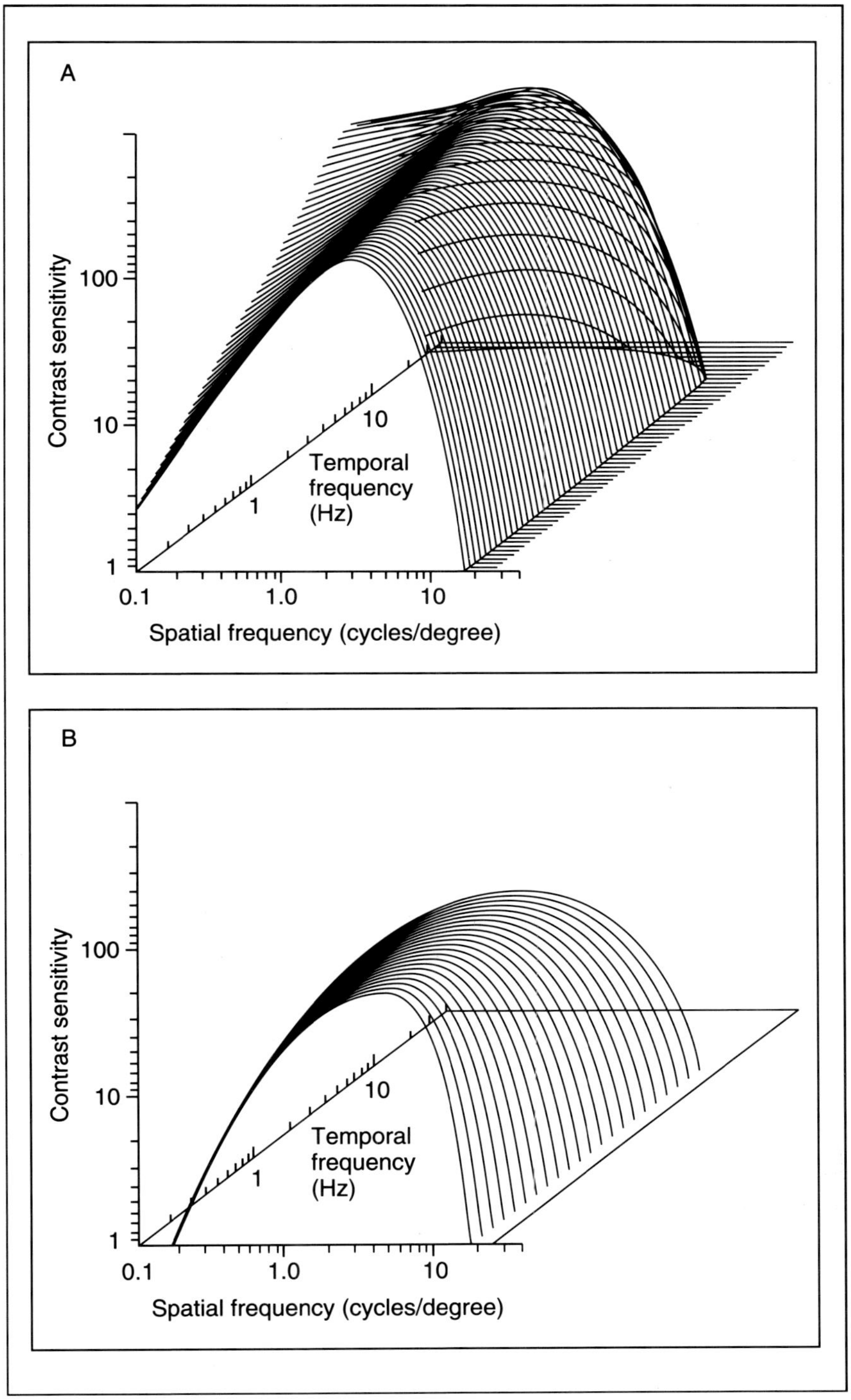

7.19 | The hypothetical three-dimensional spatiotemporal (ST) contrast sensitivity surface of a normal subject *(A)* and a glaucoma patient *(B)*. The glaucomatous ST surface is based on studies of several investigators referred to in the text. Notice how in *A* the surface peaks at 2–3 cycles/degree, with higher sensitivity increasing toward low spatial frequencies. Compare this normal ST surface with Fig. 5.7 (Bodis–Wollner, Chapter 5) of contrast sensitivity at various temporal frequencies. Note the lack of high temporal–low spatial frequency peak in *B* for the glaucomatous ST surface.

SECTION IV

COLOR PERCEPTION IN GLAUCOMA

Stephen M. Drance
Ruth D. Williams
Robert L. Stamper

Color perception is largely a foveal function.[136–138] Color vision pathways are distinct from light perception pathways,[139,140] but both are transmitted by the ganglion cell layer. Although the ganglion cell axons in the superior and inferior poles of the optic nerve head are most susceptible to glaucomatous damage, diffuse nerve fiber loss occurs even in patients with normal Goldmann visual fields (see Airaksinen, Chapter 6). Color perception is usually defective in glaucoma patients,[141–146] often occurring so early as to precede visual field defects. It is the diffuse type of nerve fiber layer defect that correlates with color vision loss in glaucoma.

Although it is difficult to compare the details because of the differing protocols and testing conditions, most studies report a correlation between the extent of visual field loss and the color vision disturbance. However, up to 25% of patients with open-angle glaucoma and severe visual field defects retain statistically normal color perception.[141,143,144] This does not mean that in these individual patients there has not been a change in color perception over time, but it does mean that color perception tested at the macula remains within normal statistical bounds for an age-matched normal population. It also almost certainly means that in the presence of advanced field defects to light-sense perimetry, color vision in these individuals is either normal or only slightly disturbed.

It appears that blue–yellow color vision is more often and more severely affected than red–green color vision. Most of the color tests stimulate only the central 2° of the visual field, but significant correlations between color vision loss and decrease in light sensitivity at the fovea and in the paracentral and midperipheral parts of the visual field have been found.[147] Heron et al[148] were the first to demonstrate that glaucoma patients had generalized losses of blue sensitivity, with confirmed cases exhibiting a 0.6–0.8 log unit generalized loss of blue sensitivity and suspect cases a 0.2–0.3 log unit loss.

These authors also showed a generalized reduction in achromatic sensitivity, which was confirmed by Drum et al,[149] who found that in glaucoma for every log unit loss of photopic sensitivity there was a diffuse 1.4 log unit loss of scotopic sensitivity, and that the earlier losses were photopic and the later ones scotopic. Lakowski et al[150] confirmed Heron's findings of the losses of blue and achromatic sensitivity at the fovea and found that they did not occur in all glaucoma patients, but instead predominated in those who had diffuse loss of the retinal nerve fiber layer as opposed to those with purely localized retinal nerve fiber layer defects. This was manifested by a progressive shift to higher error scores in the 100 Hue test with increased visual field loss. In subjects with localized retinal nerve fiber loss, the prevalence of error scores above the 95th percentile for the normal population was only 7% (almost identical to the normals), while 32% of the subjects with diffuse retinal nerve fiber loss showed color loss scores above the 95th percentile for normals. Determination of green–blue matching ratios with the anomaloscope yielded similar findings. Patients with diffuse retinal nerve fiber loss again showed shifts to the blue, similar to those with glaucomatous field defects, whereas those with localized retinal nerve fiber layer defects behaved like their normal counterparts. The percentage of patients with extreme green–blue losses increased with the extent of the visual field defect, and the number with green–blue loss was greater in those with diffuse retinal nerve fiber layer loss than in those with localized retinal nerve fiber loss.

Patients with low-tension glaucoma, for yet unknown reasons, have much less diffuse field loss by light sense perimetry than their counterparts with elevated IOP,[151] and they also have far less blue cone loss than glaucoma patients with elevated pressure.[152] There is a possibility that some of these differences may be due to "referral bias," because patients with low-tension glaucoma are usually identified as a result of localized disc anomalies, less often because of uniformly large cups, and certainly not because of pressure elevations. Such referral bias would detract from the implication of a fundamental difference between the high- and low-tension glaucoma groups but would reinforce the relationship between localized disc and retinal nerve fiber layer losses and loss of color and achromatic sensitivity.

It, therefore, appears that the disturbance of the blue–yellow color mechanism at the fovea can occur before the development of localized visual field defects and is related to diffuse loss of retinal nerve fibers. Although color disturbances are nonspecific because they are affected by the clarity of the ocular media and diseases of the retina, in the absence of such diseases they can predict the occurrence of subsequent localized visual field defects.[139] Thus, in the absence of other causes, a considerable proportion of glaucoma suspects have blue–yellow disturbances[153–155] that are predictive of subsequent development of classic localized glaucomatous visual field defects. Prospectively, 77% of eyes with color defects developed localized field defects, whereas only 19% of eyes with normal color vision developed field defects over the same period of time.[139] In a population of 14 glaucoma suspects with only an asymmetry of optic nerve heads, 29% showed blue–yellow loss on the 100 Hue test, whereas 93% showed such an abnormality when measured on the anomaloscope.[155] In another ocular hypertensive group, color vision abnormalities were found but there was no correlation between color deficits and optic nerve cupping.[156]

Hart et al[157] suggested that using blue-on-yellow perimetry is more sensitive than standard white light-sense perimetry for detecting moderate glaucoma damage, but appears to have no advantage for defects deeper than 1 log unit. Hart[158] also pointed out that red–green sensitivity is homogeneous in the central 2° of the visual field, whereas sensitivity to blue–yellow is greatly reduced in the central 30 minutes of the fovea and is maximal 2° from fixation. Hart suggested that diseases that destroy the afferents from the fovea result in red–green dyschromatopsia, whereas diseases that are mainly extrafoveal produce primarily blue–yellow dyschromatopsia. In fully developed glaucoma there is a dissociation between the development of localized field defects and color disturbances. Chromatic and luminance flicker deficits have been shown in both glaucoma patients and suspects. Although both groups showed abnormalities in the blue–yellow and luminance flicker, a mild attenuation to red–green flicker was found only in the glaucoma suspects.[159]

The color vision tests used in the above studies are considered too cumbersome for routine clinical use, while the clinically practical tests are not as sensitive for blue–yellow deficits. The sensitivity for three clinically practical tests, the AO-HRR plates, the Farnsworth D15 panel, and a desaturated Farnsworth D15 panel, can be enhanced by changing the definition of a test failure.[160] A modified scoring technique for the Farnsworth D15 panels increases the sensitivity of the tests for evaluation of patients with early open-angle glaucoma, ocular hypertension, and age-matched controls. Color vision defects are significantly increased in the early glaucoma and ocular hypertensive groups for all three tests, but the increased sensitivity brought about by the modified scoring decreases the specificity. The AO-HRR plate test is helpful clinically to detect retinal and optic nerve disease. About 50% of glaucoma eyes show a blue–yellow defect with this test, but it does not discriminate between glaucoma suspects and normal subjects.[160] Therefore, AO-HRR plates are useful for screening but have limited diagnostic value.

Recently, a video tangent screen for color perimetry has been devised.[161] This device utilizes colored test objects which are matched in luminance to a white surround, thus solving the problem of luminance and saturation. Even with such careful control, this color perimetry was no more sensitive in detecting the presence of defects than white light perimetry. However, in 30% of subjects the defects were larger and deeper with color perimetry.

At present, there is great interest in identifying tests of visual function that allow detection of nerve fiber damage before visual field loss. Color vision testing offers this potential and may also provide an additional method of monitoring the progression or stability of damage over time (see also Drance, this Chapter). However, the evaluation of color vision deficits is complex, and the sensitivity and specificity of color vision tests are not yet established. For color vision testing to become clinically valuable, it must be easy to use, quickly administered, and diagnostically specific. Each of the tests presently available has advantages and disadvantages, and further research is necessary to establish their role in the diagnosis and monitoring of glaucoma.

SECTION V

ELECTRORETINOGRAPHY IN GLAUCOMA

Scott E. Brodie
Stephen M. Drance

Selected variants of the electroretinogram (ERG), i.e., the pattern ERG (PERG) and the oscillatory potentials (OPs), elicited by modifications of basic ERG techniques, have shown promise in distinguishing the glaucomatous from the normal state. The nature of the PERG and OPs, and the methods of eliciting and recording them, have been covered in Chapter 5.

It has been demonstrated in cats, monkeys, and human patients that the PERG is selectively extinguished after optic nerve section, although the ERG response to pure luminance modulation (flicker) is preserved.[162–164] The suggestive parallel with the optic atrophy of glaucoma has subsequently been pursued by many investigators.

PERG abnormalities precede optic disc damage in monkeys with laser-induced pressure elevations.[165] In glaucoma patients, both low and high temporal frequency-stimulated PERGs are abnormal, but the higher temporal frequencies are, if anything, more disturbed.[166] Pressure elevations also produce reductions in the PERG amplitude in individual patients,[167] and the PERG is reduced in most glaucoma patients and in many ocular hypertensives[167–169] (Fig. 7.20). In groups of patients, however, pressure elevation does not correlate with the PERG amplitude.[167] Increased latency in pattern-evoked visual responses is associated with changes in contrast sensitivity,[170] and preliminary studies have suggested that reduction of the PERG does indicate a higher risk for subsequent visual field loss.[171,172] However, assessment of the value of the PERG as a prognostic indicator in glaucoma suspects awaits longitudinal clinical trials. In addition, the PERG as it is presently recorded is small and has great variability. Advances in recording techniques or analysis may make this a more useful objective technique for evaluation of the glaucomas in the future.

The oscillatory potentials (OPs) are sensitive to many sorts of damage to the inner retina, including inflammatory disease and ischemia resulting from diabetic retinopathy.[173] Recent reports have demonstrated reductions in the OPs in patients with glaucoma (Fig. 7.21) and lesser reductions in glaucoma suspects[174,175] (Fig. 7.22). Longitudinal follow-up is not as yet available.

It must be emphasized that these ERG techniques remain research tools at present. The value of these tests as prognostic indicators of glaucomatous visual field loss has not been demonstrated in adequate longitudinal clinical trials. There is likewise scant evidence comparing the predictive value of these electrophysiologic procedures with the various psychophysical tests such as contrast sensitivity, coherence perimetry, motion sensitivity, and color vision, which have also been proposed as possible early indicators of the glaucomatous process and are discussed elsewhere in this volume.

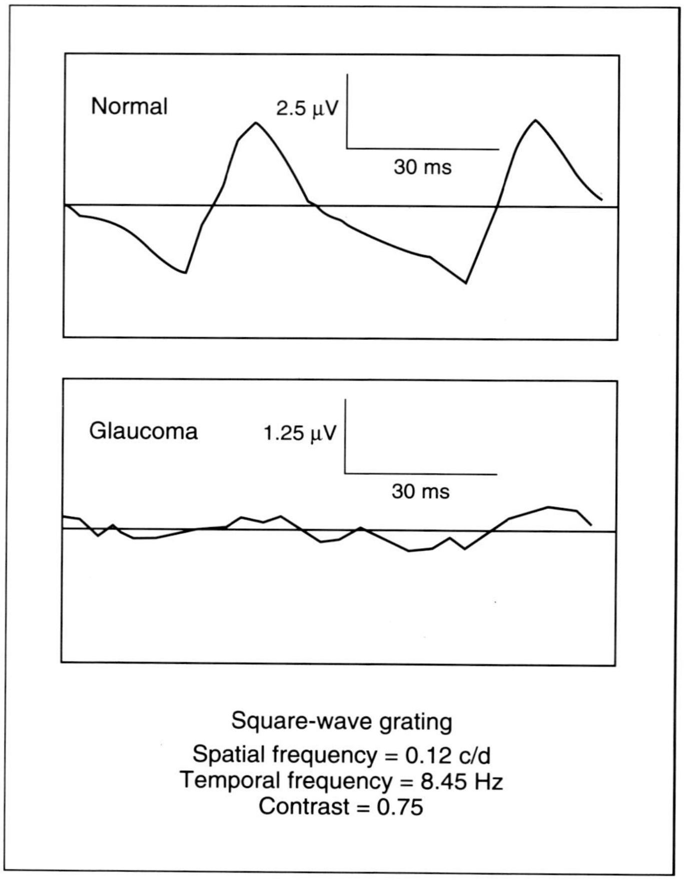

7.20 | Steady-state PERGs from a normal (top) and a glaucomatous eye (bottom).

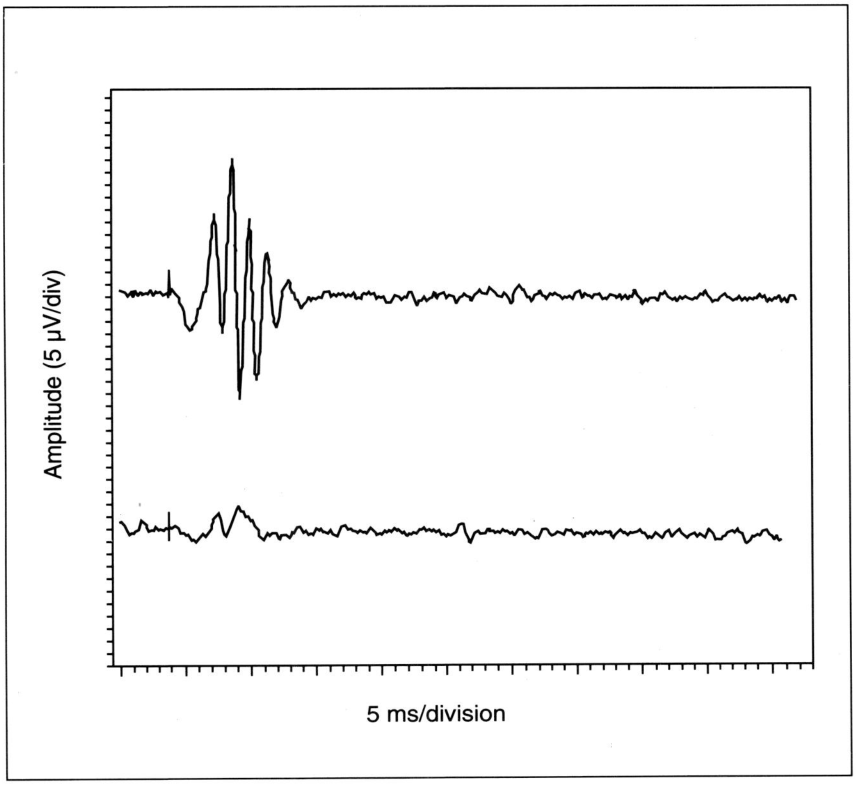

7.21 | Oscillatory potentials from a normal eye (top) and a glaucomatous eye (bottom).

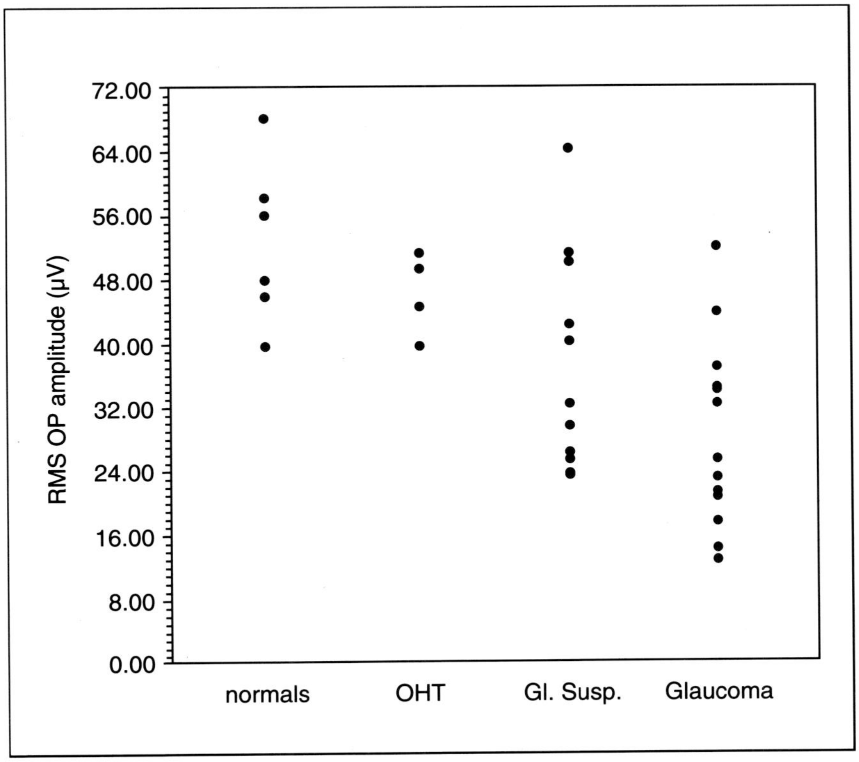

7.22 | Distribution of oscillatory potential root-mean-square amplitudes for normal eyes, low-risk ocular hypertensives, glaucoma suspects (most with elevated IOP), and patients with confirmed glaucomatous field loss.

SECTION VI

VISUALLY EVOKED CORTICAL POTENTIALS IN GLAUCOMA

Richard Stodtmeister
Lutz E. Pillunat

Recordings at spontaneous IOP of the mean latencies and amplitudes of visually evoked cortical potentials (VECP) differ significantly between glaucoma patients and normal subjects,[176–178] but the distributions overlap widely. The VECP recorded at artificially increased IOP also differ in normals and in glaucoma patients.[179] More important, the amplitude/pressure curves generated from the "pressure tolerance test" (see Stodtmeister and Pillunat, Chapter 5) are quasi-linear in glaucomatous eyes but not in healthy ones, i.e., the glaucomatous eyes lack the initial inflection, or "autoregulatory kink" in the curve (Fig. 7.23). In a series of 81 healthy subjects and 56 glaucoma patients, 86% of the healthy eyes and 86% of the glaucomatous eyes were correctly diagnosed on this basis alone. The ultimate diagnostic and prognostic role of this test awaits further study.

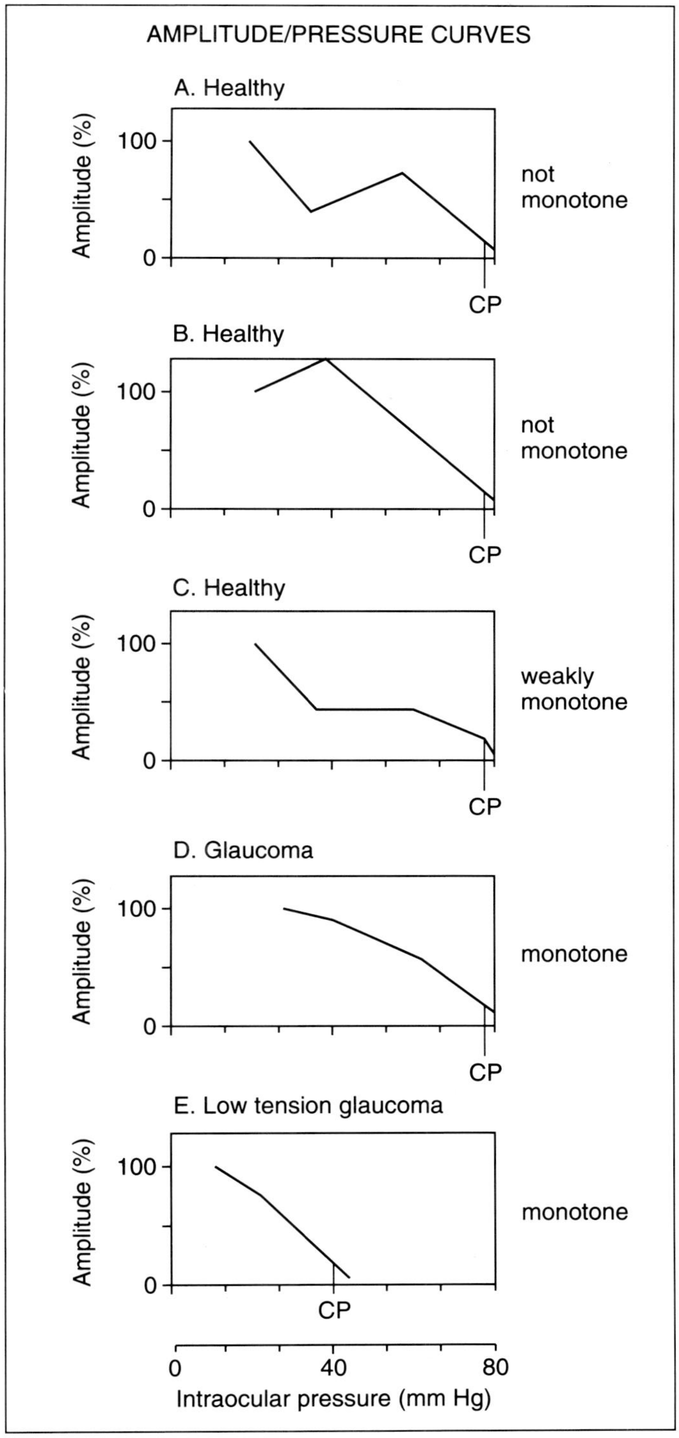

7.23 | Amplitude/pressure curves obtained by recording VECP at stepwise increases of intraocular pressure. The mathematical classification is given at the right of the curves. CP=critical pressure, i.e., that intraocular pressure at which the amplitude of the VECP decreases to 20% of the initial value.

8 SPECIFIC TYPES OF GLAUCOMA

SECTION I

GONIOSCOPIC FINDINGS IN GLAUCOMA

Alan H. Zalta

The changes in optic nerve structure and appearance and in visual function are essentially the same regardless of the type of glaucoma producing them. In contrast, the clinical and histologic appearance of the anterior ocular segment, and the pathophysiology of the obstruction to aqueous outflow, vary markedly in the different glaucomas. This section will provide a brief overview of the different types of gonioscopic abnormalities associated with various glaucomas.

From a gonioscopic viewpoint, angle abnormalities can be classified according to the type of pathology visualized. The most common abnormalities that occur in the anterior-chamber angle are peripheral anterior synechiae, neovascularization, excessive pigmentation, and structural defects.

PERIPHERAL ANTERIOR SYNECHIAE

Peripheral anterior synechiae (PAS) are variable-sized adhesions of the peripheral iris which abut angle structures and occlude the angle as high as Schwalbe's line. The appearance, extent, and location of PAS vary depending on their etiology. The more common mechanisms that may lead to the formation of PAS include a primary pupillary block, a fibrovascular or endothelial membrane, trauma, inflammation, a secondary pupillary block due to iris bombé or pseudophakia, and an intumescent or subluxed lens. Configuration parameters are also important in the differentiation of PAS from iris processes that are a variant of normal anatomy. Although PAS are commonly thought of as small tent-shaped extensions of the peripheral iris, they may be difficult to recognize in extensive areas of angle closure or when they are low lying, extending only to the scleral spur.

Primary-angle closure occurs as the result of a posterior mechanism in which the peripheral iris is pushed into the angle. In this process, a functional block between the pupillary iris and anterior lens surface traps aqueous humor in the posterior chamber, shifts the peripheral iris forward, and closes the anterior chamber angle (Fig. 8.1) (see Skuta, this chapter). There may be a subtle transition from open to closed angle with a gradual increase in area of the iris and trabecular meshwork contact. The PAS usually occlude the trabecular meshwork to a variable degree, depending on the severity of the process, and do not extend above Schwalbe's line. Often a Sampaolesi line (see Zalta, Chapter 3; Ritch and Liebmann, this chapter) seen above a closed angle is mistaken for the trabecular meshwork band.

Peripheral anterior synechiae in iridocorneal endothelial (ICE) syndrome occur as the result of an anterior mechanism in which the peripheral iris is pulled into the angle (see Skuta, this chapter). In this spectrum of diseases, a membrane grows from abnormal corneal endothelium across the anterior chamber angle onto the iris surface and contracts, causing the formation of PAS and iris abnormalities. All three disorders in the ICE syndrome, essential iris atrophy, Chandler syndrome, and Cogan–Reese syndrome, are characterized by a unilateral corneal endothelial abnormality, PAS that extend up to or beyond Schwalbe's line, and abnormalities of the iris. In Chandler syndrome, a progressive iridocorneal membrane causes corneal edema, broad loops of PAS to the peripheral cornea (Fig. 8.2), stromal iris atrophy, corectopia, and ectropion uvea.

Inflammatory PAS can be finger-like or broad-based, conical or cylindrical, and may insert as high as Schwalbe's line (Fig. 8.3).

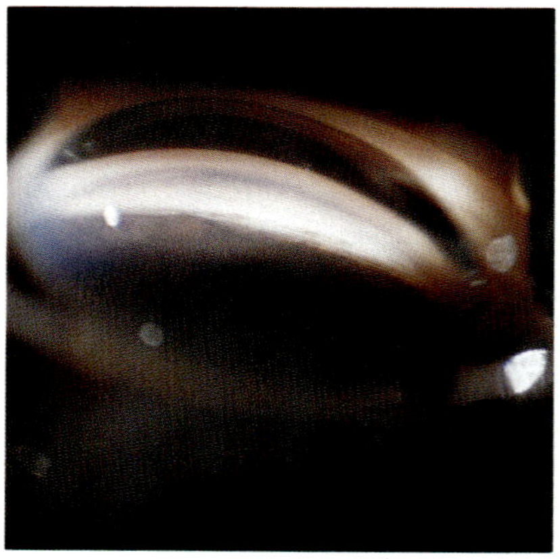

8.1 | Peripheral anterior synechiae in primary angle-closure glaucoma occludes the left half of the anterior chamber angle. The Sampaolesi line may be mistaken for the trabecular meshwork on the left but can be clearly identified by the presence of trabecular meshwork and scleral spur on the right.

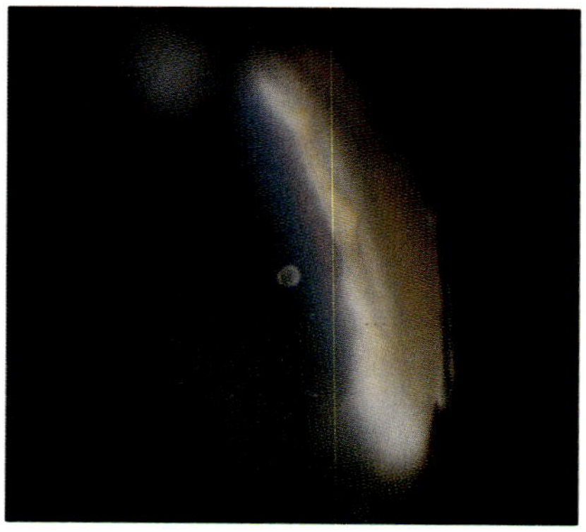

8.2 | Peripheral anterior synechiae in Chandler syndrome, seen through corneal edema, extend in broad loops anterior to Schwalbe's line onto the posterior cornea.

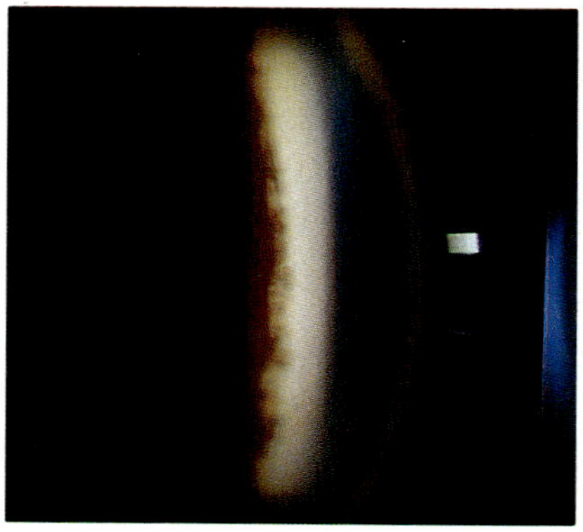

8.3 | PAS in chronic uveitis with variable shape, extent, and height.

ANGLE NEOVASCULARIZATION

Angle neovascularization occurs most commonly as a result of proliferative diabetic retinopathy, retinal vascular occlusion, carotid artery disease, and chronic uveitis (see Skuta, this chapter). In its early stages (Fig. 8.4), subtle vascular stalks cross the ciliary body and scleral spur to arborize in the trabecular meshwork. During gonioscopy, early angle neovascularization can be easily overlooked or mistaken for pigment or iris processes when bright illumination is used or when excessive pressure from the goniolens occludes the vessels. As the neovascular process progresses (Fig. 8.5), arborizations in the trabecular meshwork from different feeding vessels join and a fibrovascular membrane develops along the larger vessels. This fibrovascular membrane contracts the peripheral iris stroma into the angle and slowly "zippers" closed all angle structures.

EXCESSIVE PIGMENTATION

Dense trabecular meshwork pigmentation affecting the entire circumference of the angle is present in pigmentary dispersion syndrome and glaucoma (see Ritch and Liebmann, this chapter), exfoliation syndrome and glaucoma (see Ritch and Liebmann, this chapter), and sometimes in melanomas of the uveal tract (see Van Buskirk, this chapter). Occasionally, excessive trabecular pigmentation is seen in the inferior angle after severe angle closure, after intraocular surgery, with uveitis, or as a normal aging phenomenon. A Sampaolesi line of variable density always accompanies these conditions. Pigmentary glaucoma, a bilateral disorder of the iris pigment epithelium which predominantly affects young adult myopic men, characteristically accumulates dense, homogeneous pigmentation on the trabecular meshwork throughout the entire circumference of the angle (Fig. 8.6). In contrast, the

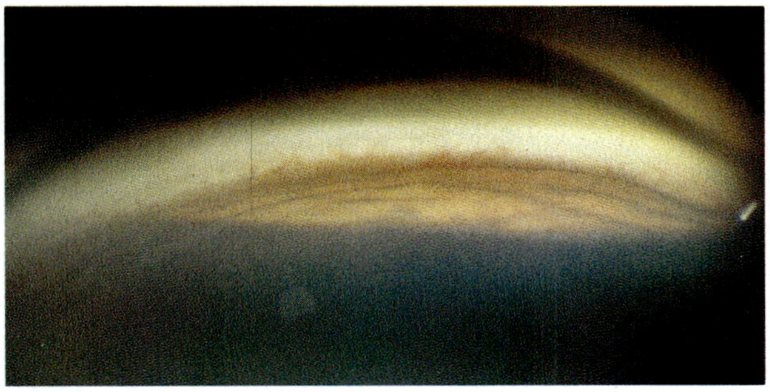

8.4 | Early angle neovascularization in which many subtle vascular stalks cross the scleral spur to join or arborize in the trabecular meshwork.

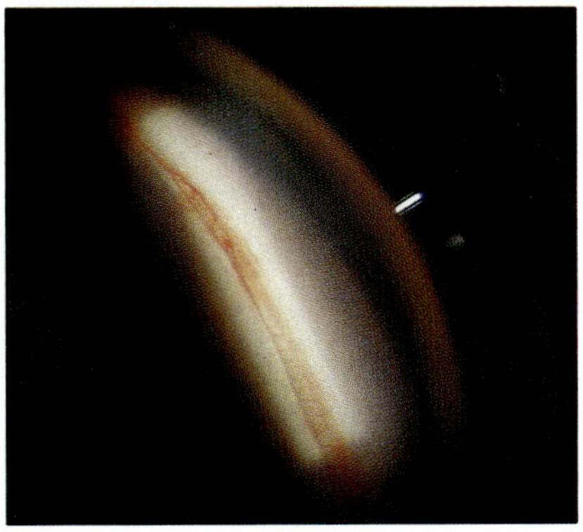

8.5 | Florid angle neovascularization with synechial closure adjacent to peripheral rubeosis iridis superiorly.

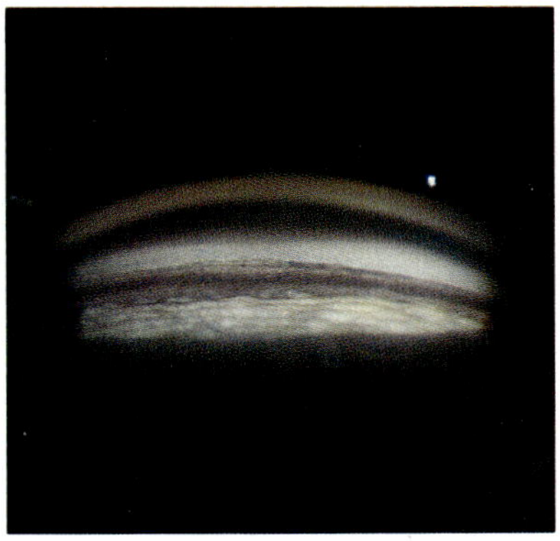

8.6 | Dense, homogeneous pigmentation of the trabecular meshwork and a Sampaolesi line in pigmentary glaucoma.

dense trabecular pigmentation in exfoliation glaucoma, an anterior segment basement membrane disease that affects the elderly, is characteristically patchy and segmental in nature. With iris or iris–ciliary body melanomas, increased angle pigmentation is due to phagocytosis of melanin by macrophages or to direct seeding of tumor cells in the angle (Fig. 8.7). Iris and ciliary body nevi in the angle are rare and may present as discrete pigmented lesions of the iris root and ciliary body band (Fig. 8.8).

STRUCTURAL DEFECTS
ANGLE RECESSION

Angle recession (Fig. 8.9) occurs as the result of a traumatic tear in the anterior face of the ciliary body (see Van Buskirk, this chapter). Typically, the ciliary body band and angle recess are of variable width and there is an irregular, posterior insertion of the iris. Occasionally there is a whitish scar in the recessed areas (Fig. 8.10). Distinguishing extensive traumatic angle recession from a normal, deep angle recess is often difficult and is usually accomplished

8.7 | Increased pigmentation of the trabecular meshwork and tiny pigmented mass lesions in angle due to an iris melanoma.

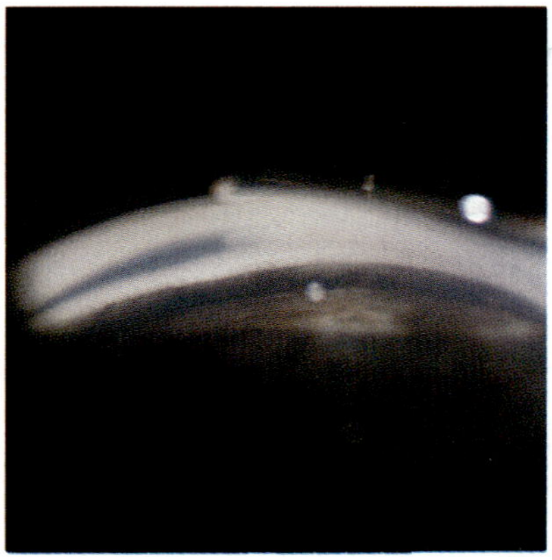

8.8 | Nevi on iris and ciliary body band. The gonioscopic appearance of these lesions has not changed in five years.

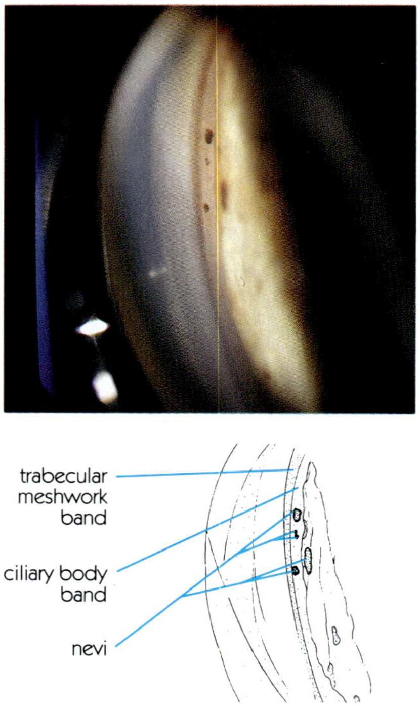

8.9 | Traumatic angle recession with gradual transition from normal iris insertion inferiorly to irregular, posterior iris insertion superiorly, with increasing width of the ciliary body band.

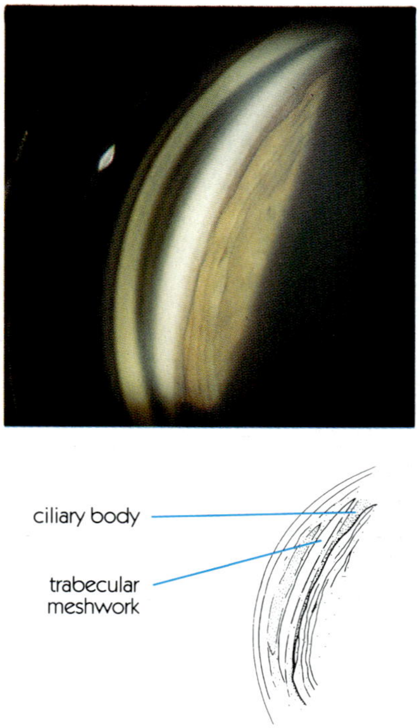

by comparative gonioscopy of the unaffected eye. In an extremely deep angle recess, which is a variant of the normal open angle, the iris inserts posteriorly and exposes a broad ciliary body band symmetrically for 360° in both eyes.

CLEFTS

An iridodialysis cleft (Fig. 8.11), resulting from a traumatic tear and disinsertion of the peripheral iris, exposes the ciliary body and the ciliary processes at the iris root (see Van Buskirk, this chapter). Because iridodialysis clefts are usually caused by severe blunt trauma, angle recession and PAS are often present. Trabeculectomy clefts (Fig. 8.12) are iatrogenic fistulas created through the sclera and trabecular meshwork during glaucoma filtration surgery to allow an open communication between the anterior chamber and the subconjunctival space (see Smythe and Herschler, Chapter 9). A cyclodialysis

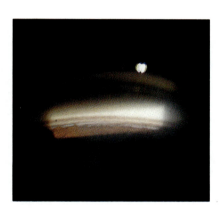

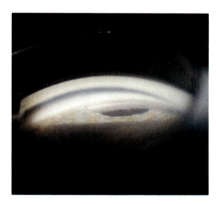

8.10 | Traumatic angle recession with two white fibrotic scars, one in the angle recess on the right and the other crossing the ciliary body band to the scleral spur on the left.

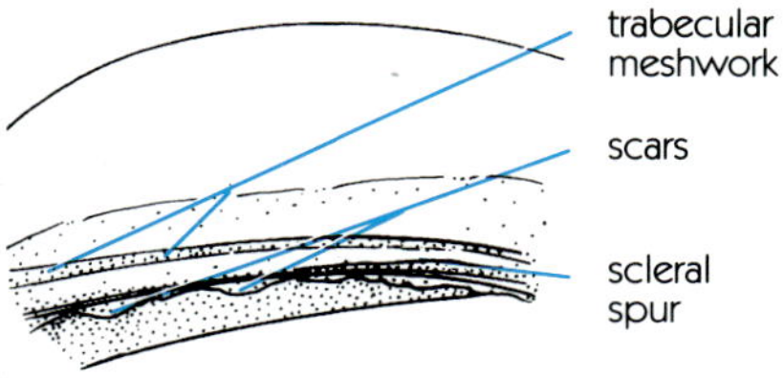

8.11 | Traumatic iridodialysis which exposes the ciliary body is bordered on the right by angle recession and on the left by peripheral anterior synechiae.

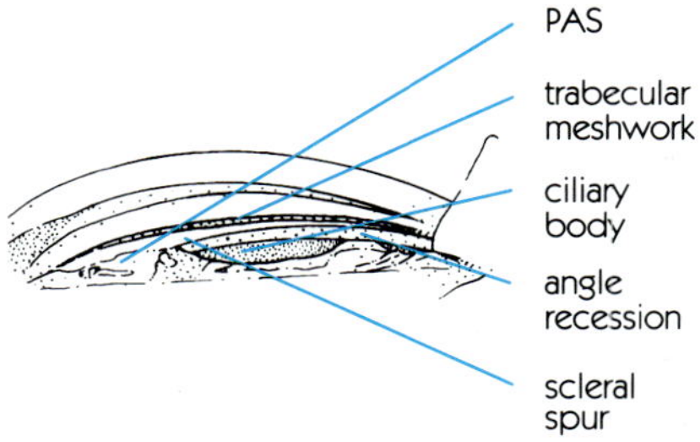

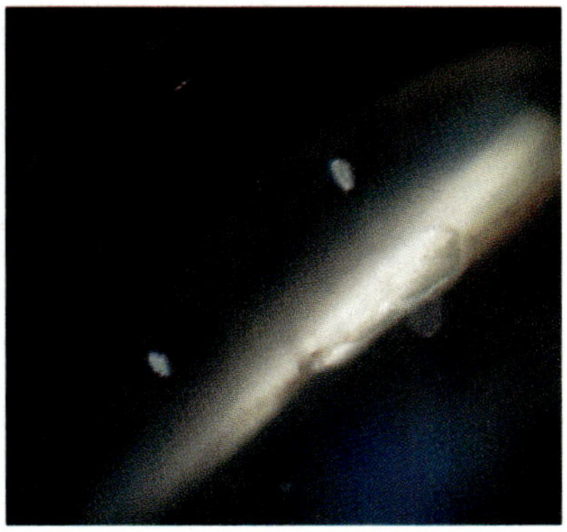

8.12 | Trabeculectomy cleft allows communication between the anterior chamber and subconjunctival space.

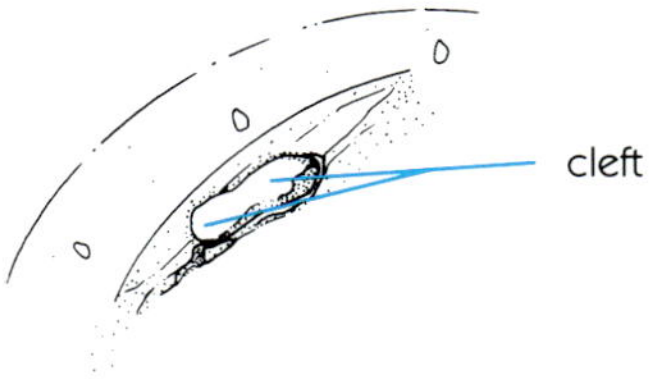

cleft (Fig. 8.13) separates the ciliary body from the scleral spur and allows communication between the anterior chamber and the suprachoroidal space. It may be due to trauma or to a cyclodialysis procedure, a form of glaucoma-filtering surgery that has lost popularity in recent years.

FOREIGN BODIES

Sharp foreign bodies traveling at high velocity may penetrate the cornea and lodge in the inferior anterior chamber angle. If they are of a biologically inert material, such as glass, they may evoke little or no inflammatory reaction, and the only external sign of their presence may be the corneal entry wound or scar, as well as localized corneal edema inferiorly. In such cases, gonioscopy is diagnostic (Fig. 8.14).

ACKNOWLEDGMENT

Earl Choromokos, FOPS, provided expert photographic assistance during the preparation of this chapter.

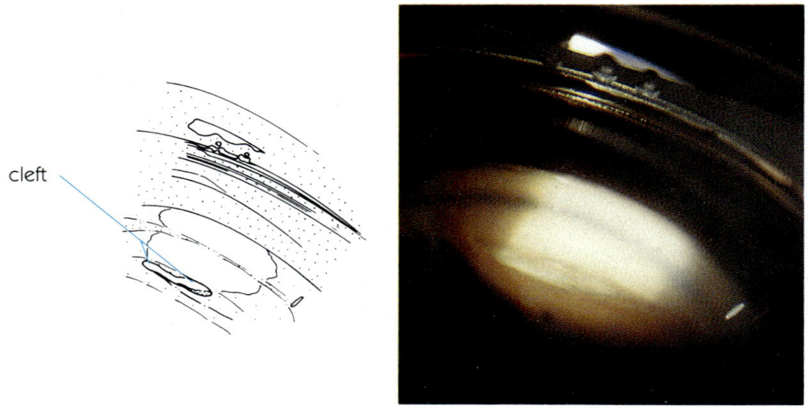

8.13 | Cyclodialysis cleft allows communication between the anterior chamber and supra-choroidal space.

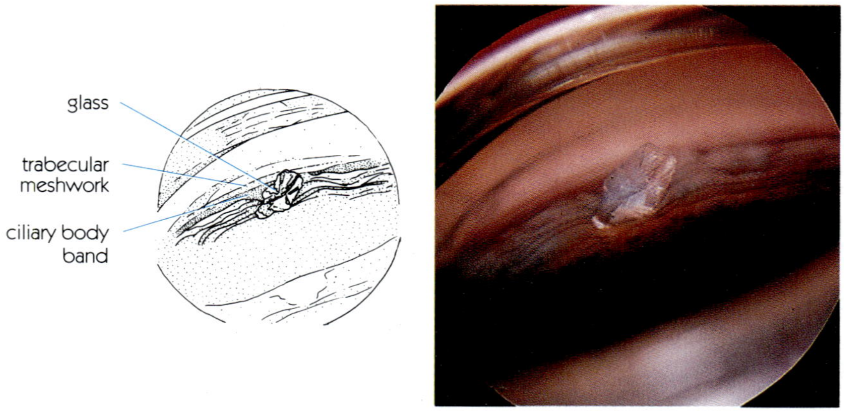

8.14 | Glass foreign body in the inferior angle. (Courtesy of Drs. Harry Roth and Paul L. Kaufman.)

SECTION II

THE ANGLE-CLOSURE GLAUCOMAS

Gregory L. Skuta

The angle-closure glaucomas include a variety of acute and chronic conditions in which temporary and/or permanent obstruction of the trabecular meshwork by the iris results in decreased aqueous outflow and elevated intraocular pressure. This section reviews the diagnosis and treatment of the primary and secondary angle-closure glaucomas, including acute primary angle-closure glaucoma, subacute angle-closure glaucoma, chronic angle-closure glaucoma, plateau iris syndrome, neovascular glaucoma, and ciliary-block glaucoma, as well as other secondary angle-closure glaucomas.

ACUTE PRIMARY ANGLE-CLOSURE GLAUCOMA

Primary angle-closure glaucoma is less common than primary open-angle glaucoma. Although the incidence is not well defined,[1] some studies have suggested ratios of 1:4 to 1:10 (primary-angle closure glaucoma: primary open-angle glaucoma) for white patients.[2] There appears to be a hereditary influence on the depth of the anterior chamber angle and, consequently, on the risk of developing primary angle-closure glaucoma.[3] However, a family history of angle closure may not be particularly useful in predicting the development of this condition in an individual situation.[1] Indeed, most cases appear to be sporadic.[2]

Among whites, primary angle-closure glaucoma appears to be more common in women as compared to men.[1,2,4] It is less common among blacks and Native Americans.[5] However, among Eskimos, an estimated 2–3% of individuals over age 40 develop primary angle-closure glaucoma, presumably due to smaller corneal diameters and anterior chamber depths in addition to thicker, more anterior lenses.[1,6]

Eyes with small anterior segments are predisposed to pupillary block and attacks of angle closure. Although myopic eyes may develop primary angle-closure glaucoma,[7] hyperopic eyes are more likely to be affected because they have smaller anterior chamber volumes and shallower anterior chambers.[4] Thickening and anterior displacement of the lens associated with aging[8] may themselves produce narrowing of the anterior chamber angle and further compromise an already narrow angle to increase the likelihood of an angle closure attack. In addition, the pupil becomes smaller with age, thus increasing the amount of relative pupillary block.[1,2] Not surprisingly, primary angle-closure glaucoma occurs more commonly in the elderly, although it may be seen in younger adults and even in children.[9]

PATHOPHYSIOLOGY

Exposure to dim light, emotional upset with associated sympathetic stimulation, and use of pharmacologic agents with anticholinergic or sympathomimetic properties all result in pupillary dilatation and potential closure of the anterior chamber angle.[1,2,10] Under normal conditions, contact between the iris and lens results in a relative obstruction to the flow of aqueous from the posterior to the anterior chamber, causing higher pressure to be exerted by aqueous posterior to the iris. This phenomenon can be referred to as *relative pupillary block*.[1,2,11] In predisposed eyes, a mid-dilated pupil, caused by the factors described above, appears to maximize the forces that increase pupillary block, anterior bowing of the iris (iris bombé), and secondary obstruction of the anterior chamber angle as seen in primary angle-closure glaucoma (Fig. 8.15).

Although agents that produce pupillary dilatation are most commonly implicated, cholinergic agents can also potentially exacerbate pupillary-block and angle-closure glaucoma.[1,2,10] Increased contact between the iris and lens can potentiate the posterior forces that produce pupillary block. In addition, anterior displacement of the lens–iris diaphragm by cholinergic agents can also increase pupillary block.

8.15 | Contact between lens and iris *(A)* with pupil in mid-dilated position maximizes pupillary block, causing peripheral iris to bow forward *(B)* and block outflow channels.

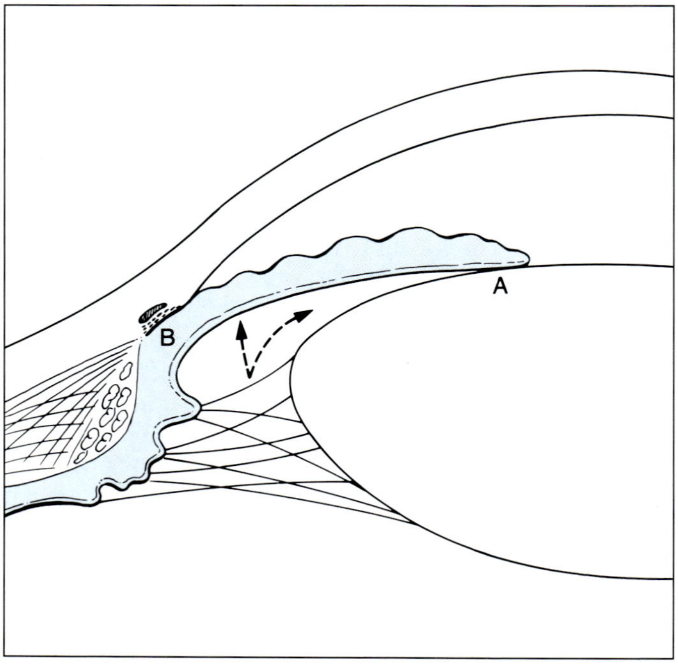

DIAGNOSIS

Patients with acute primary angle-closure glaucoma typically present with sudden unilateral onset of pain, decreased vision, halos around lights, and injection of the eye.[1,2] The abrupt rise in intraocular pressure (IOP) may produce autonomic stimulation and associated nausea, vomiting, bradycardia, and diaphoresis. On examination, the eye typically shows marked conjunctival injection and ciliary flush (Fig. 8.16). The cornea usually displays epithelial edema and sometimes exhibits stromal swelling and folds in Descemet's membrane. The anterior chamber is usually shallow centrally but is particularly shallow peripherally, where anterior bowing of the iris may lead to apposition of the iris and cornea. Anterior chamber inflammation, particularly aqueous flare, is common. The pupil, which is usually in a mid-dilated position with a pupillary diameter of 3.5–6 mm, may be irregular and, because of associated ischemia, is usually sluggish or nonreactive.[1,2,12] Sector atrophy of the iris, usually greater superiorly, often results from pressure-related ischemia (Fig. 8.17). Dispersion of pigment may also be seen.[1,2] The lens may exhibit

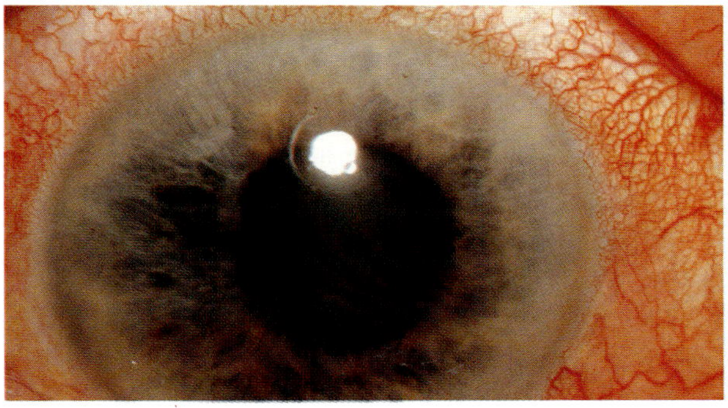

8.16 | Eye in attack of acute primary angle-closure glaucoma. Note conjunctival injection and ciliary flush, mid-dilated pupil, and probable iris atrophy (left side). (Courtesy of Dr. Terry J. Bergstrom.)

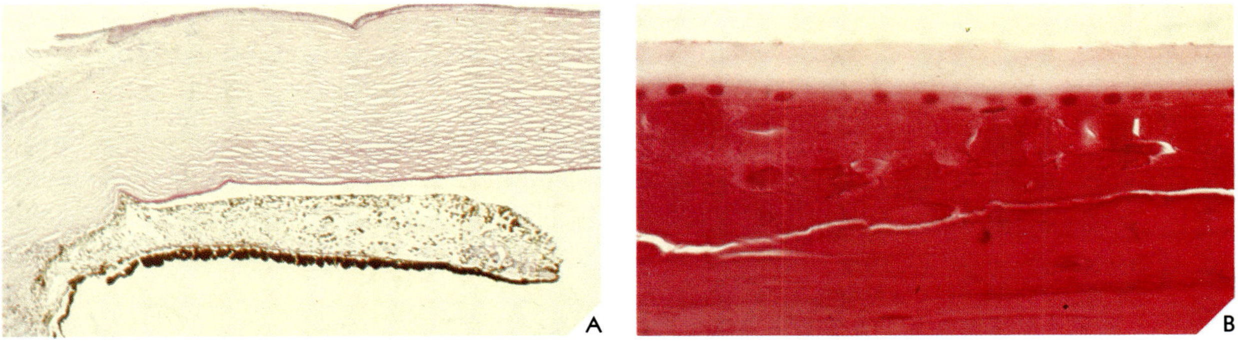

8.17 | Primary angle-closure glaucoma. *A:* The anterior chamber angle is completely occluded by a peripheral anterior synechia. The iris shows segmental necrosis consisting of stromal atrophy, loss of the dilator muscle, and necrosis of the sphincter muscle. Segmental iris necrosis can be mimicked clinically by herpes zoster. *B:* This histologic section shows small areas of epithelial necrosis in the lens, and tiny adjacent areas of subcapsular cortical degeneration. (*A*, PAS stain.) (From Yanoff M, Fine BS: *Ocular Pathology. A Color Atlas*, ed 2. New York: Gower Medical Publishing, 1992, 16.4.)

glaukomflecken (Fig. 8.18), anterior subcapsular lens opacities[1,2] that are represented histopathologically by focal necrosis of the anterior subcapsular lens epithelium[13] (see Fig. 8.17). IOP is usually highly elevated, typically greater than 40 mm Hg and often greater than 50 mm Hg. Gonioscopically, the angle is closed, although it may be possible to open the angle with compression if no permanent peripheral anterior synechiae are present. (Because of corneal edema, it may be necessary to apply topical glycerin to clear the cornea, or to delay gonioscopy until the IOP is lowered by medical therapy with subsequent improvement of the edema.) The optic nerve may be normal in appearance, although hyperemia and edema of the nerve are often present during the initial period of an attack.[1,2,14] Optic nerve pallor without cupping may be seen after an attack, although glaucomatous cupping has been described in eyes that had had previous episodes of angle closure.[15] Visual fields most often show generalized or nonspecific constriction, more often of the superior hemifield,[16] although arcuate defects and other nerve fiber bundle defects have been documented.[15]

Examination of the fellow eye may assist in making a diagnosis of acute angle-closure glaucoma in the eye of concern, since the anterior chamber angle of the fellow eye will, in general, also exhibit a narrow angle. If the angle is deep, another process must be considered.

DIFFERENTIAL DIAGNOSIS

The clinical presentation of acute primary angle-closure glaucoma is usually easy to recognize. The differential diagnosis (Fig. 8.19) includes a variety of disorders with and without pupillary block: uveitic glaucoma, glaucomatocyclitic crisis, open-angle glaucomas with markedly elevated intraocular pressures (e.g., exfoliative glaucoma, angle-recession glaucoma, primary open-angle glaucoma, or POAG), iridocorneal endothelial syndrome (ICE), lens-induced glaucoma, aphakic and pseudophakic pupillary block, angle closure secondary to scleral buckling surgery or after panretinal photocoagulation, angle-closure glaucoma in nanophthalmos, glaucoma secondary to intraocular tumors or cysts, suprachoroidal hemorrhage or other intraocular hemorrhage, central retinal vein occlusion, retinopathy of prematurity, epithelial or fibrous ingrowth, neovascular glaucoma, and ciliary-block glaucoma. These disorders are discussed elsewhere in this chapter and text. In particular, the differentiation between ciliary-block glaucoma and primary angle-closure glaucoma with pupillary block is discussed elsewhere in this volume.

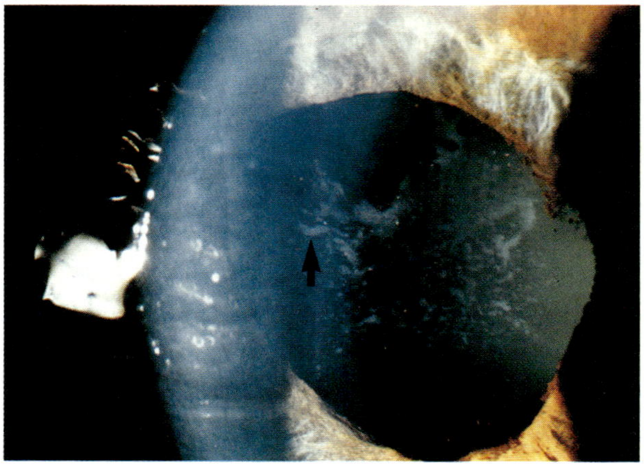

8.18 | Glaukomflecken (arrows) of lens and superior iris atrophy after attack of primary angle-closure glaucoma. (Courtesy of Dr. Paul R. Lichter.)

MANAGEMENT

Management of acute primary angle-closure glaucoma consists of medical therapy to break the acute attack, more definitive surgical intervention (usually laser iridotomy) to permanently relieve pupillary block, medical and/or surgical treatment of any residual glaucoma, and prophylactic iridotomy in the fellow eye to eliminate the risk of an attack in that eye.

MEDICAL THERAPY

Initial medical therapy of acute primary angle-closure glaucoma includes administration of (1) 1–4 drops of pilocarpine (1–2%) over 30 minutes to produce miosis and break the attack; (2) a topical beta-blocker and apraclonidine to reduce aqueous production and help lower IOP; and (3) oral or intravenous acetazolamide (250–500 mg), also to reduce aqueous production. If the attack is not quickly broken with this approach and the patient is able to tolerate oral agents, an osmotic agent (50% glycerin or 45% isosorbide, 1–2 g/kg) may be given. Otherwise, 20% mannitol may be administered intravenously. If the pupillary sphincter has become ischemic as a result of the attack, the pupil may remain in the mid-dilated position despite the pilocarpine therapy.[1,2,12] In some cases, reduced IOP caused by aqueous suppressants[17] and/or hyperosmotic agents may make the sphincter more responsive to miotic agents. However, prolonged administration of additional pilo-

Figure 8.19. Differential Diagnosis of Primary Angle-Closure Glaucoma

Angle-Closure Glaucomas Associated with Pupillary Block

- Acute primary angle-closure glaucoma
- Subacute angle-closure glaucoma
- Chronic angle-closure glaucoma
- Uveitic glaucoma with posterior synechiae and pupillary block
- Lens-induced angle-closure glaucomas
  - Phacomorphic
  - Dislocated lens
  - Microspherophakia
- Aphakic and pseudophakic pupillary block
- Drug-induced secondary angle-closure glaucoma

Open-Angle Glaucomas Associated with Highly Elevated Intraocular Pressures

- Uveitic glaucoma with open angle
- Glaucomatocyclitic crisis
- Primary open-angle glaucoma
- Secondary open-angle glaucoma (e.g., exfoliative glaucoma, pigmentary glaucoma, angle-recession glaucoma)

Angle-Closure Glaucomas Not Associated with Pupillary Block

- Plateau-iris syndrome
- Ciliary-block glaucoma
- Neovascular glaucoma
- Uveitic glaucoma with synechial closure but no pupillary block
- Iridocorneal endothelial syndrome
- Lens-induced glaucomas without pupillary block (phacomorphic glaucoma)
- Angle-closure glaucoma secondary to scleral buckling surgery
- Angle-closure glaucoma secondary to panretinal photocoagulation
- Angle-closure glaucoma in nanophthalmos
- Angle-closure glaucoma secondary to intraocular tumors or cysts
- Angle closure secondary to suprachoroidal hemorrhage
- Angle-closure glaucoma secondary to central retinal vein occlusion
- Angle-closure glaucoma secondary to retinopathy of prematurity
- Angle-closure glaucoma secondary to epithelial or fibrous ingrowth

carpine or the use of echothiophate is unlikely to be beneficial; it may only induce further ocular congestion and inflammation and, possibly, systemic toxicity (nausea, vomiting, diarrhea, bradycardia, and hypotension).[2] Frequent application of a potent topical corticosteroid may reduce the ocular inflammation associated with an angle closure attack.

Although not currently available in the United States, thymoxamine, an alpha-adrenergic antagonist,[18] may be useful, at least in theory, in the treatment of acute angle-closure glaucoma. Dapiprazole, another alpha-adrenergic antagonist which is now commercially available in the United States,[19] may also have a role in treatment. By relaxing the pupillary dilator muscle, these agents produce miosis without affecting the lens–iris diaphragm and increasing the likelihood of pupillary block.

In eyes in which medical therapy does not break an acute attack, corneal compression with a tonometer tip, a cotton-tip applicator (Fig. 8.20), a muscle hook, or a four-mirror goniolens may help to break the attack by mechanically pushing aqueous into the peripheral anterior chamber to open the angle.[1,2,20] Other alternatives in resistant eyes include laser iridoplasty and peaking of the pupil with the argon laser.[21]

Surgical Therapy

After initiation of medical therapy, laser iridotomy should be performed to provide more definitive treatment of the underlying disease process (Fig. 8.21). Laser iridotomy is most easily accomplished after the attack has been

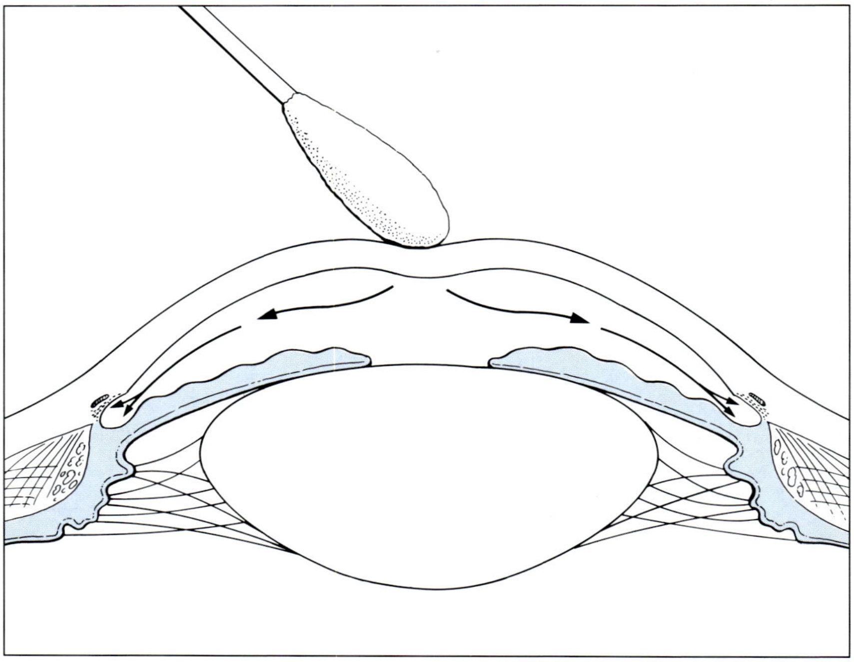

8.20 | Corneal compression with cotton-tip applicator may help break attack of angle-closure glaucoma by pushing aqueous into peripheral anterior chamber. Compression may also be performed with tonometer tip, muscle hook, or four-mirror goniolens.

broken by the methods described above. However, in cases resistant to medical therapy, laser iridotomy may be necessary to break the attack itself. Specific techniques for laser iridotomy are described by Skuta in Chapter 9.

In eyes in which laser iridotomy cannot be successfully completed for technical reasons or because of inadequate patient cooperation, surgical peripheral iridectomy may be necessary.

In the past, determination of the extent of peripheral anterior synechiae was often believed to be important in planning appropriate surgical therapy. Because the degree of permanent angle closure was felt to be related to ultimate control of the glaucoma, some surgeons chose to perform filtering surgery rather than peripheral iridectomy alone if 50–75% of the angle was closed by peripheral anterior synechiae.[2] Others still recommended peripheral iridectomy alone, followed by medical therapy and later by filtering surgery if medical therapy was inadequate in controlling the glaucoma.

With the advent of laser iridotomy, the decision-making process is simplified by first performing laser surgery. If necessary, chronic medical therapy can be utilized. If this is inadequate in controlling IOP, further options include filtering surgery and argon laser trabeculoplasty (if enough open angle remains for adequate treatment).[1,2] Goniosynechialysis is another surgical alternative in which peripheral anterior synechiae are stripped away

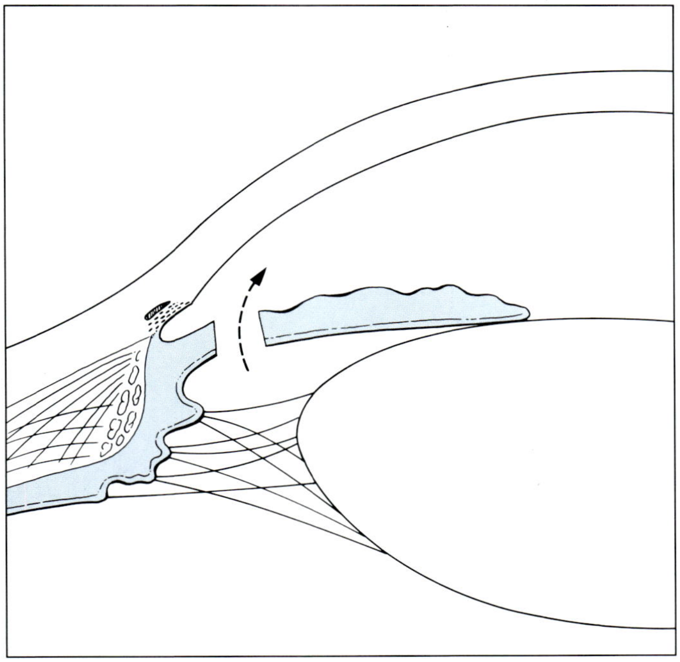

8.21 | Opening in peripheral iris has relieved relative pupillary block and closure of the anterior chamber angle.

to reopen the trabecular meshwork[22] (Fig. 8.22). This treatment has been reported to be most effective in eyes in which the angle closure occurred within 12 months of surgical intervention.

FELLOW EYE

In a patient with a history of primary acute angle-closure glaucoma in one eye, the fellow eye is also at risk for developing an acute attack. It is estimated that 50–75% of such patients develop an acute event in their fellow unoperated eye within 5–10 years, even with the use of chronic miotic therapy.[1,23] Prompt prophylactic laser iridotomy in the fellow eye, therefore, is appropriate.

OTHER PRIMARY ANGLE-CLOSURE GLAUCOMAS

SUBACUTE ANGLE-CLOSURE GLAUCOMA

Some patients may describe intermittent episodes of blurred vision and ocular discomfort, which, in the presence of a narrow angle, are suggestive of subacute angle-closure glaucoma.[1,2,24] These episodes may be relieved by light-induced or sleep-induced miosis. In some cases, repeated subacute attacks may result in the development of permanent peripheral anterior synechiae. Treatment consists of laser iridotomy. If IOPs remain elevated after laser iridotomy in the presence of optic nerve and/or visual field damage, then long-term medical therapy, laser trabeculoplasty, or filtering surgery may be required.

CHRONIC ANGLE-CLOSURE GLAUCOMA

As noted above, recurrent subacute attacks of angle closure may lead to the development of permanent peripheral anterior synechiae. In another form of chronic angle-closure glaucoma, also sometimes known as creeping angle-closure glaucoma,[1,2,25] appositional angle closure with or without the presence of permanent peripheral anterior synechiae may result in elevated IOPs. When peripheral anterior synechiae develop, they tend to begin superiorly, where the angle is usually narrowest.

Chronic angle-closure glaucoma is the most common type of angle closure in black individuals. The Baltimore Eye Survey has reported a higher rate of primary angle-closure glaucoma in blacks as compared with whites.[26] Clinical experience at the Bascom Palmer Eye Institute suggests that chronic

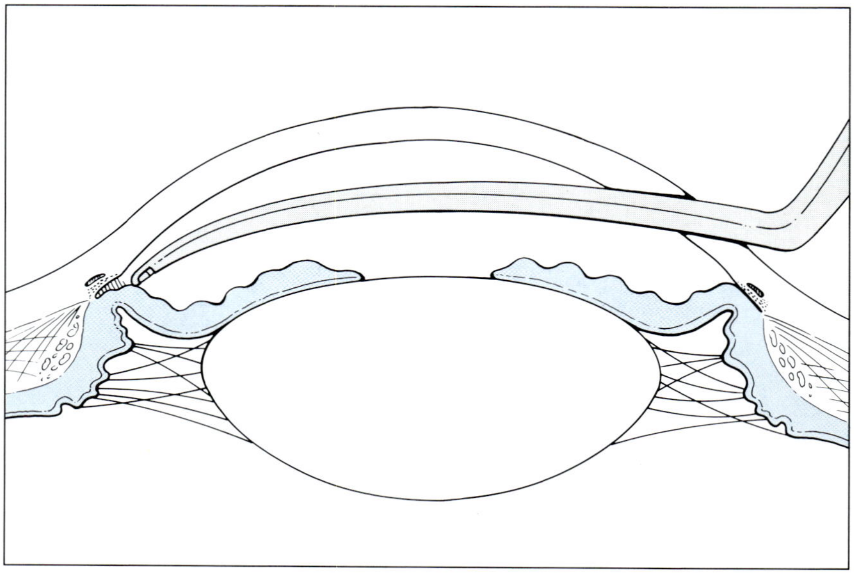

8.22 | In goniosynechialysis, peripheral anterior synechiae are separated from trabecular meshwork with a smooth-tipped irrigating cyclodialysis spatula. (Adapted from Campbell DG, Vela A: Modern goniosynechialysis for the treatment of synechial angle-closure glaucoma. *Ophthalmology 1984;91:1054.*)

angle-closure glaucoma is also relatively more common among Hispanic patients.

Chronic angle-closure glaucoma is usually asymptomatic and may resemble primary open-angle glaucoma in its presentation. Diagnosis depends on careful initial gonioscopy, which should be repeated periodically in all patients with glaucoma because progressive narrowing of the angle can occur over time, especially in patients on cholinergic therapy. Compression or indentation gonioscopy is particularly helpful in distinguishing between appositional closure and synechial closure.[27]

Treatment consists of laser iridotomy, although trabecular damage often requires long-term medical therapy and sometimes laser trabeculoplasty or glaucoma filtering surgery for control of IOP.

PLATEAU IRIS SYNDROME

In some eyes with relative pupillary block, the iris configuration is relatively flat, with an abrupt posterior turn near the iris insertion. Many of these eyes with a so-called "plateau iris configuration" respond to laser iridotomy.[28] However, in a small number of eyes with "plateau iris syndrome," angle closure may occur after dilatation as the peripheral iris bunches up to occlude the angle even in the presence of a patent iridotomy (Fig. 8.23).

In some cases, elevated IOP persists and progressive peripheral anterior synechiae may develop. Progressive permanent angle closure can be prevented by treatment with chronic miotic therapy or peripheral iridoplasty to pull the peripheral iris away from the angle.[1,2]

PROVOCATIVE TESTING

In patients with narrow anterior chamber angles on gonioscopy, some clinicians base their decision regarding the need for laser iridotomy on provocative testing, in which patients are subjected to mydriasis, a dark room, or a prone position to assess the effect on the angle appearance and the IOP.[1,2,29] Test results are regarded as positive when IOP rises 8 mm Hg or more in the presence of a closed angle. The value of such provocative testing has not been proven, however, and many others rely on the patient's history (e.g., symptoms of subacute angle closure or strong family history of angle closure) or physical findings (signs of previous episodes of angle closure, or appositional angle closure with or without an elevated IOP) in arriving at a clinical decision.[2, 29A]

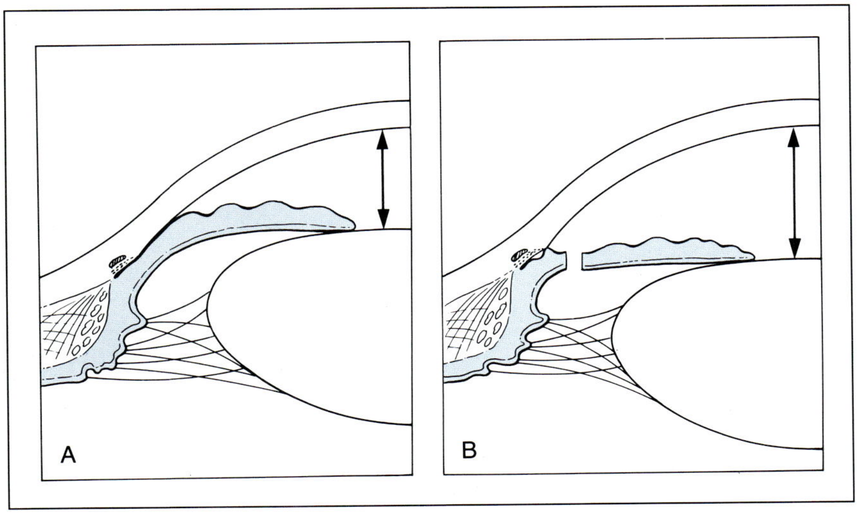

8.23 | In contrast to typical angle closure secondary to pupillary block *(A)*, peripheral iris may still occlude the anterior chamber angle even after laser iridotomy in plateau iris syndrome *(B)*.

NEOVASCULAR GLAUCOMA

Neovascular glaucoma was first described in 1866 after a central retinal vein occlusion.[30] The condition is characterized by anterior segment neovascularization which may lead to closure of the anterior chamber angle and a severe secondary glaucoma.

PATHOPHYSIOLOGY

Neovascular glaucoma is usually associated with an underlying ischemic process involving the retina.[31,32] The most common predisposing conditions include diabetic retinopathy and retinal vascular occlusions (Fig. 8.24).

Diabetes mellitus accounts for approximately one third of cases of neovascular glaucoma.[30–32] In general, anterior segment neovascularization and neovascular glaucoma are associated with proliferative diabetic retinopathy, although neovascular glaucoma may occur even in the absence of posterior segment neovascularization.[33] In diabetic patients, anterior segment neovascularization is not invariably followed by neovascular glaucoma.[33] However, it is well known that vitrectomy and lensectomy may be associated with rapid progression of iris neovascularization and subsequent development of neovascular glaucoma.[34,35]

Central retinal vein occlusion is the second most common cause of neovascular glaucoma, accounting for nearly one third of cases.[36] According

Figure 8.24. Associations With Anterior Segment Neovascularization

Diabetic Retinopathy

Retinal Vascular Occlusions
- Central retinal vein occlusion
- Central retinal artery occlusion
- Branch retinal vein occlusion

Carotid Artery Obstructive Disease

Associated Chorioretinal Disorders
- Chronic retinal detachment
- Choroidal melanoma
- Retinoblastoma
- Metastatic carcinoma
- Reticular cell sarcoma
- Coats' exudative retinopathy
- Sickle cell retinopathy
- Eales' disease
- Retinopathy of prematurity
- Persistent hyperplastic primary vitreous
- Syphilitic retinal vasculitis
- Retinoschisis
- Stickler syndrome
- Radiation retinopathy

Other Ocular and Systemic Disorders
- Chronic uveitis
- Endophthalmitis
- Carotid–cavernous fistula
- Giant cell arteritis
- Takayasu's pulseless disease
- Trauma

(Modified from *Glaucoma, Lens, and Anterior Segment Trauma,* Section 8, Basic and Clinical Science Course. San Francisco: American Academy of Ophthalmology, 1989–90, 75.)

to Hayreh et al,[36] approximately 75–80% of central retinal vein occlusions are nonischemic, and 20–25% are ischemic. Among the ischemic central retinal vein occlusions, approximately 60% develop iris neovascularization and 33% develop neovascular glaucoma. Therefore, the degree of retinal ischemia is strongly correlated with the development of iris neovascularization. Signs of retinal ischemia include extensive retinal capillary nonperfusion on fluorescein angiography, a marked decline in vision, 10 or more cotton-wool spots, a reduced b/a wave ratio (<1.2) on electroretinography, and a significant relative afferent pupillary defect.[37]

Neovascular glaucoma after central retinal vein occlusion may progress more rapidly than in diabetes. Although the secondary glaucoma after central retinal vein occlusion is often referred to as "90-day glaucoma" or "100-day glaucoma," neovascularization may develop within 2 weeks or many months after the vascular event.[38] However, approximately 80% of cases develop within 6 months.[36]

Although central retinal vein occlusion is associated with the vast majority of neovascular glaucoma cases related to vascular occlusions, neovascular glaucoma may also be seen after central retinal artery occlusion[39] and branch retinal vein occlusion.[40]

A variety of other disorders may be associated with neovascular glaucoma. Other chorioretinal disorders include chronic retinal detachment, choroidal melanoma, retinoblastoma, Coats' exudative retinopathy, retinopathy of prematurity, sickle cell retinopathy, syphilitic retinal vasculitis, retinoschisis, and Stickler syndrome.[30–32] Carotid artery obstructive disease, which may also cause ocular ischemia, is probably the third most common cause of neovascular glaucoma. In one series it accounted for 13% of neovascular glaucomas.[41] Carotid–cavernous fistula, which is often associated with increased episcleral venous pressure, also shunts arterial blood away from the eye, resulting in ocular ischemia and secondary neovascularization.[42] Uveitis may also be associated with anterior segment neovascularization and glaucoma.[36,41]

In the above disorders, it is widely theorized that hypoxic retinal tissue releases angiogenic factors which diffuse forward and cause new vessel formation.[30–32,43] The vitreous and lens may act as barriers to these angiogenic factors,[34,35,44] and may themselves exhibit some vasoinhibitory abilities.[45,46] Therefore, removal of these barriers by cataract extraction or vitrectomy in conditions such as diabetes may be associated with rapid progression of anterior segment neovascularization.[34,35] It also appears that extracapsular cataract extraction with maintenance of an intact posterior capsule is less likely than intracapsular extraction to be associated with neovascularization, since an intact posterior capsule may still serve as a barrier to angiogenic factors.[47,48]

DIAGNOSIS (CLINICAL FINDINGS)

Most glaucomatologists classify iris neovascularization into three clinical categories: iris neovascularization without glaucoma; open-angle glaucoma; and angle-closure glaucoma.[31] In iris neovascularization without glaucoma, the first subclinical sign is increased permeability of blood vessels at the pupil margin, as demonstrated by fluorescein angiography.[49] Clinically, dilated tufts of vessels are seen at the pupil margin, typically progress towards the iris root[31] (Fig. 8.25), and may begin to involve the anterior-chamber angle[18] (Fig. 8.26). Neovascular iris vessels are irregular in size and course, branch frequently, and lie on the iris surface. They differ in appearance from engorged iris vessels such as those seen in an inflamed eye, where the vessels are more uniform in size, have a radial course, do not branch within the iris, and lie in the iris stroma.[30]

In open-angle glaucoma, more extensive iris and angle neovascularization is present, although the normal angle structures can still be identified.[31] Although the angle appears "open," it and the iris are, in fact, often covered by a fibrovascular membrane. At this stage, anterior-segment inflammation and hyphema are often seen.

Eventually, the fibrovascular membrane described above causes progressive secondary angle closure (Fig. 8.27) and may give the iris stroma a smooth, flattened appearance[30,31,50] (Fig. 8.28). Further contraction of this membrane, which consists of a superficial layer of myofibroblasts overlying the new vessels[50] (Fig. 8.29), results in ectropion iridis, a dilated pupil, and extensive synechial closure of the angle[30,31] (Fig. 8.30). The secondary angle-closure glaucoma which results from this process is usually very severe.

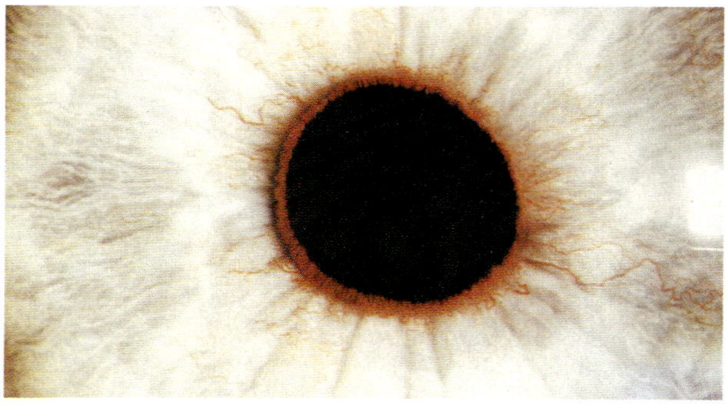

8.25 | Peripupillary iris neovascularization in diabetic patient with vessels progressing towards iris root on right. (Courtesy of Dr. Scott R. Sneed.)

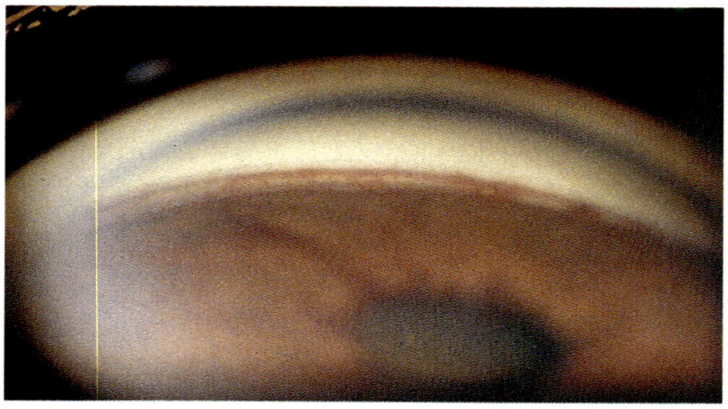

8.26 | Fine abnormal anterior chamber angle vessels (arrow) in early neovascular glaucoma. (Courtesy of Martin Wand.)

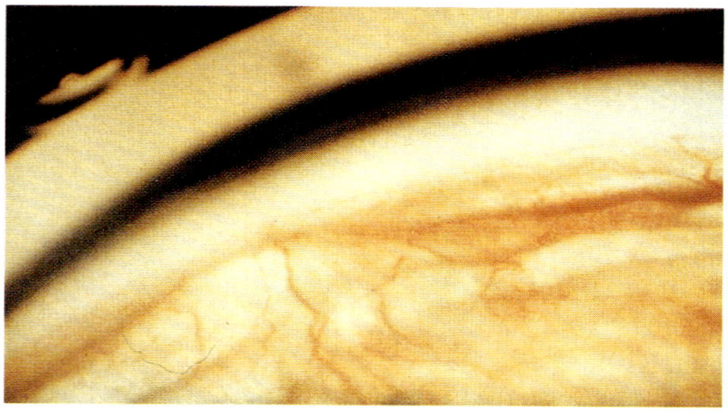

8.27 | Iris and anterior chamber angle neovascularization with early secondary angle closure in neovascular glaucoma. (From Van Buskirk EM: *Clinical Atlas of Glaucoma.* Philadelphia: WB Saunders, 1986, 75.)

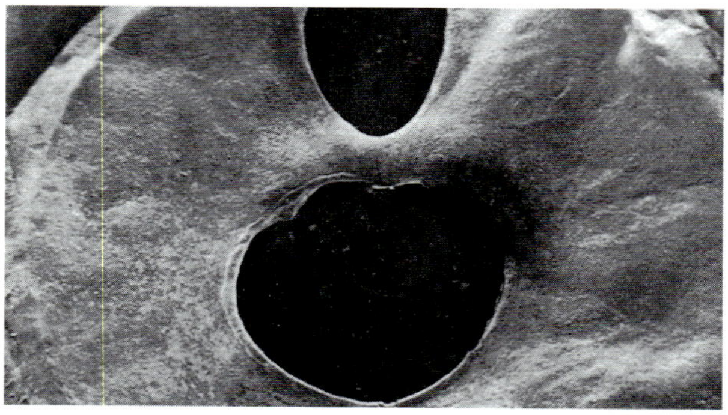

8.28 | Scanning electron micrograph shows smooth iris surface secondary to proliferation of fibrovascular membrane in neovascular glaucoma. (From John T, Sassani JW, Eagle RC Jr: The myofibroblastic component of rubeosis iridis. *Ophthalmology 1983;90:722.*)

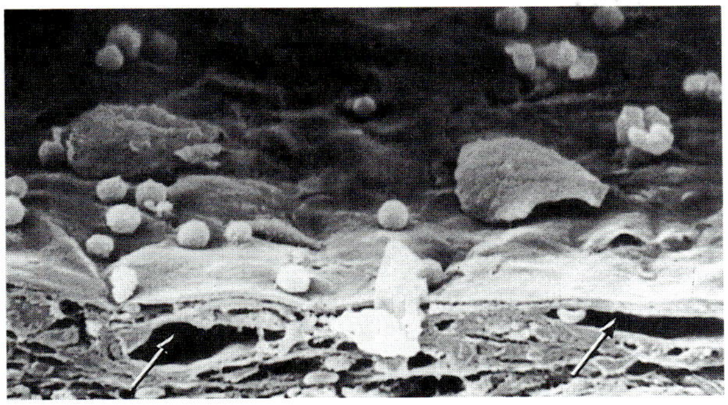

8.29 | Scanning electron micrograph reveals superficial layer of myofibroblasts which overlies new iris vessels (arrows). (From John T, Sassani JW, Eagle RC Jr: The myofibroblastic component of rubeosis iridis. *Ophthalmology 1983;90:724.*)

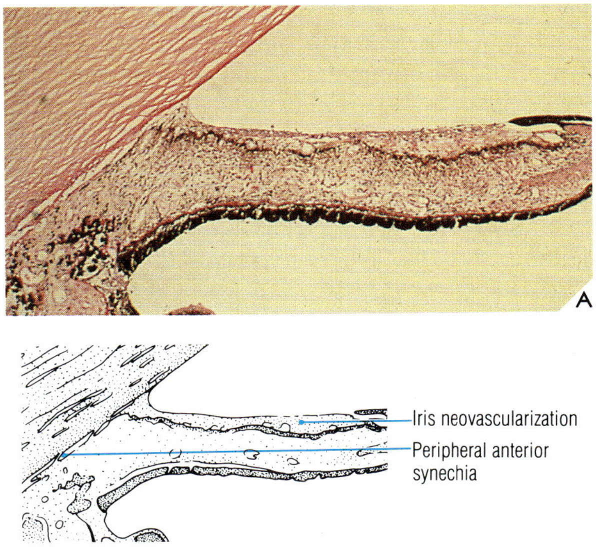

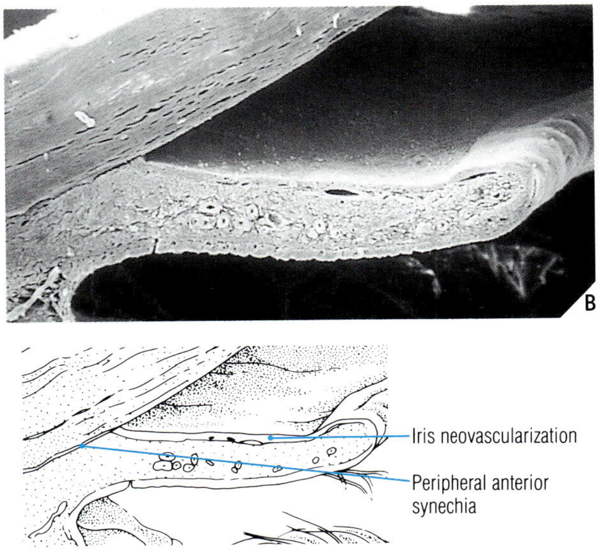

8.30 | *A:* Histologic section shows vascular channels and fibrous tissue present above the anterior border layer of the iris in the form of iris neovascularization. The membrane has caused a peripheral anterior synechia. Shrinkage of the membrane has produced an ectropion uvea. *B:* In a scanning electron microscope view, the anterior chamber angle and peripheral iris are covered by a fibrovascular membrane, and the angle is closed by a peripheral anterior synechia. (*A:* PAS stain. *B:* Courtesy of Drs. RC Eagle Jr and JW Sassani.) (From Yanoff M, Fine BS: *Ocular Pathology. A Color Atlas,* ed 2. New York: Gower Medical Publishing, 1992, 16.9.)

DIFFERENTIAL DIAGNOSIS

The differential diagnosis of neovascular glaucoma includes the uveitic glaucomas, Fuchs' heterochromic iridocyclitis, acute angle-closure glaucoma, and some of the secondary angle-closure glaucomas described elsewhere in this section and text.

MANAGEMENT

Medical therapy in neovascular glaucoma usually consists of aqueous suppressants, including topical ß-blockers and apraclonidine, and systemic carbonic anhydrase inhibitors.[31] Cholinergic agents, which tend to increase inflammation and cause further breakdown of the blood–aqueous barrier, should be avoided in the presence of active neovascularization.[51] After retinal ablation, if regression of the neovascularization occurs and the angle remains open, cholinergic therapy may later become an option in medical management.[52] Because acute neovascular glaucoma is usually associated with significant anterior segment inflammation, topical corticosteroids and cycloplegic agents are often helpful.[52] There is some evidence to suggest that corticosteroids play a role in causing regression of the neovascularization.[53]

When the presenting IOP is extremely high, some clinicians choose to administer a systemic hyperosmotic agent,[30–32] especially when the cornea is edematous. However, these agents may be less effective in neovascular glaucoma than in other conditions, since the abnormal permeability of the new vessels may decrease the osmotic gradient between the eye and the systemic circulation. Because patients with neovascular glaucoma are often medically compromised, particular care should be taken in administering hyperosmotic agents. In diabetic patients, isosorbide is the oral agent of choice since, in contrast to glycerin, it is not metabolized.

Because of the underlying retinal ischemia, panretinal photocoagulation is critical to the initial management of iris neovascularization and neovascular glaucoma to reduce or eliminate the anterior-segment neovascularization and to limit progressive closure of the angle.[54] After an ischemic central retinal vein occlusion with extensive capillary nonperfusion, many surgeons recommend prophylactic treatment in the absence of new vessels, since the risk of rapidly progressive anterior-segment neovascularization is high.[55] However, others wait until new vessels are actually seen clinically. In diabetes, where progression of iris neovascularization is usually less rapid, treatment is indicated for anterior-segment neovascularization even in the absence of posterior-segment proliferative changes.[31] When panretinal photocoagulation is not possible because of media opacities, peripheral panretinal cryoablation can be performed.[56]

In goniophotocoagulation, the new angle vessels are directly treated with the argon laser.[57] Typical treatment parameters include 0.2-second duration, 100–200-µm spot size, and 200–400-mW power, settings that usually result in closure of the new vessels. Although goniophotocoagulation may serve as an adjunct in treatment, it does not eliminate the more critical need for retinal ablation.

Historically, the prognosis of filtering surgery in neovascular glaucoma has been poor owing to intraoperative bleeding and postoperative fibrovascular proliferation, resulting in closure of the filtering site.[31] With successful preoperative retinal ablation and careful intraoperative hemostasis, Allen et al[58] have reported a 67% success rate for filtering surgery in neovascular glaucoma. Many surgeons advocate the use of the antifibrotic agents 5-fluorouracil[59] or mitomycin[60] to increase the likelihood of surgical success, whereas others recommend the placement of aqueous shunting devices such as the Molteno implant for the primary surgical treatment of neovascular glaucoma.[61]

In cases with limited visual potential or failure of other surgical modalities, cyclodestructive procedures can be considered.[30–32] Cyclocryotherapy has been the most widely utilized cyclodestructive procedure. Other alternatives include Nd:YAG laser transscleral cyclophotocoagulation, endophotocoagulation, and therapeutic ultrasound. These modalities and their advantages and disadvantages are discussed by Shields in Chapter 9.

CILIARY-BLOCK (MALIGNANT) GLAUCOMA

Ciliary-block glaucoma refers to a relatively rare form of angle-closure glaucoma in which aqueous is misdirected into the vitreous cavity in predisposed eyes. It most commonly occurs after intraocular surgery. Because of a historically poor response to standard treatment of angle-closure glaucoma, it has also been commonly called malignant glaucoma.[30,62,63] Other terms include direct-lens block, aqueous misdirection syndrome, and cilio–vitreo–lenticular block.[30]

PATHOPHYSIOLOGY

In phakic hyperopic eyes with small anterior segments, (1) uveal congestion and/or anterior rotation of the ciliary processes related to intraocular surgery, and ocular decompression in combination with (2) a thickened anterior hyaloid appear to predispose to posterior misdirection of aqueous into the vitreous cavity. This, in turn, results in forward displacement of the lens–iris diaphragm, closure of the angle, and increased IOP[64] (Fig. 8.31). A relatively large lens with close apposition to the ciliary body, laxity of the lens zonules,[65] or ciliary spasm from any variety of causes (including miotic therapy)[66] may also predispose to the development of this condition.

In aphakic eyes, iridovitreal synechiae, a dense or thickened vitreous face, and/or adherence of the vitreous to the ciliary body[30,62,64] may predis-

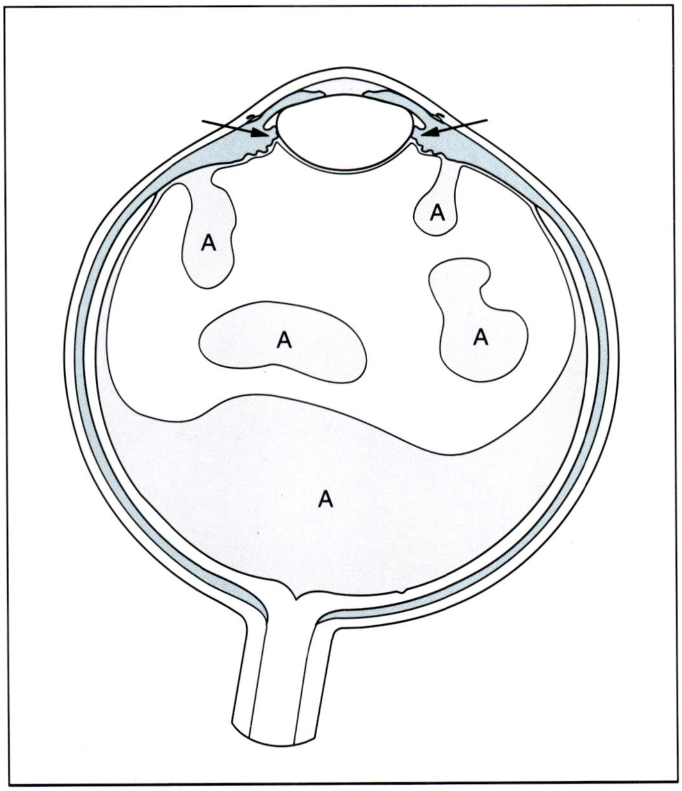

8.31 I In phakic eye, apposition of anteriorly rotated ciliary processes (arrows) and thickened anterior hyaloid predisposes to posterior misdirection of aqueous (A) into vitreous cavity, with forward displacement of the lens–iris diaphragm, closure of the angle, and increased intraocular pressure.

pose to the posterior misdirection of aqueous (Fig. 8.32). In the presence of a posterior vitreous detachment, the fluid may accumulate behind the vitreous.[67] Ciliary block may also occur in pseudophakic eyes.

DIAGNOSIS (CLINICAL FINDINGS)

Ciliary-block glaucoma has been most commonly observed after surgical peripheral iridectomy, filtering surgery, or cyclodialysis for the treatment of chronic and acute angle-closure glaucoma.[68] The presence of a partially or completely closed anterior-chamber angle appears to predispose to the development of this condition.[69] It has also been described after intracapsular and extracapsular cataract extraction[69,70] and may be induced by miotic agents,[71] trauma, and ocular inflammation.[66] Spontaneous ciliary-block glaucoma[69,72] and ciliary block in association with retinopathy of prematurity[73] have also been reported.

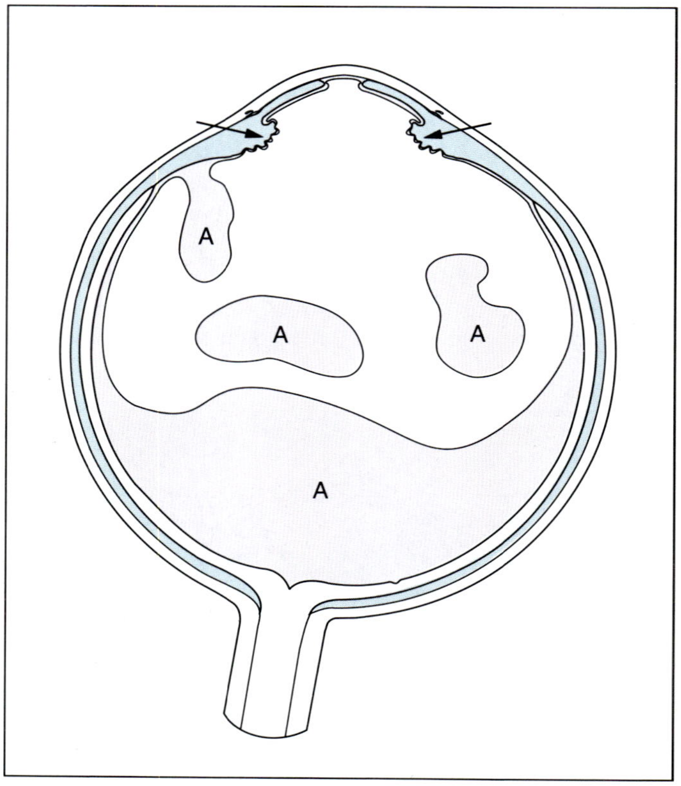

8.32 | In the aphakic eye, iridovitreal synechiae, dense or thickened vitreous face, and/or adherence of vitreous to ciliary processes (arrows) may predispose to posterior misdirection of aqueous (A).

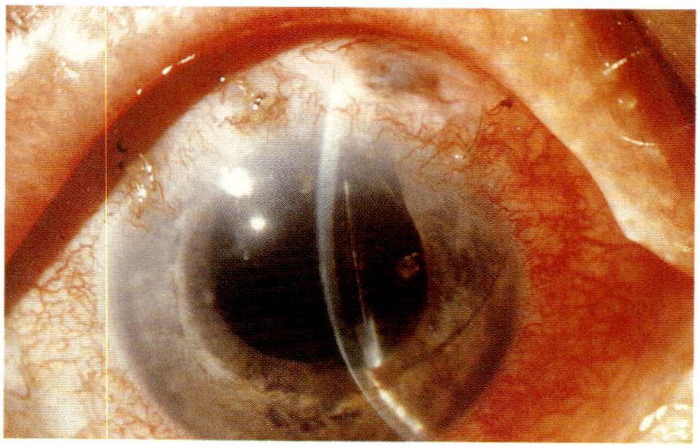

8.33 | Completely flat anterior chamber with apposition of posterior chamber intraocular lens and iris to cornea in presence of patent superior sector iridectomy. (Courtesy of Dr. Elizabeth Hodapp.)

In ciliary-block glaucoma, the anterior chamber is typically shallow or flat and the IOP is elevated even in the presence of a patent iridectomy (Fig. 8.33). In their initial descriptions of ciliary-block glaucoma, Chandler and Grant noted that cholinergic therapy worsened the condition, and cycloplegic therapy lessened the ciliary block.[65]

DIFFERENTIAL DIAGNOSIS

A shallow or flat anterior chamber in the presence of an elevated IOP, especially in a postoperative eye, must be differentiated from pupillary block and angle closure glaucoma or suprachoroidal hemorrhage. Wound leaks and serous choroidal detachments may also result in a shallow anterior chamber; however, the IOP is usually low.[30,62,68]

In pupillary block, iris bombé is typically present, with a shallow anterior chamber peripherally and a deeper chamber centrally. This differs from ciliary block, in which the anterior chamber is uniformly shallow, even in the presence of a patent iridectomy[30,62] (Fig. 8.34). In pupillary

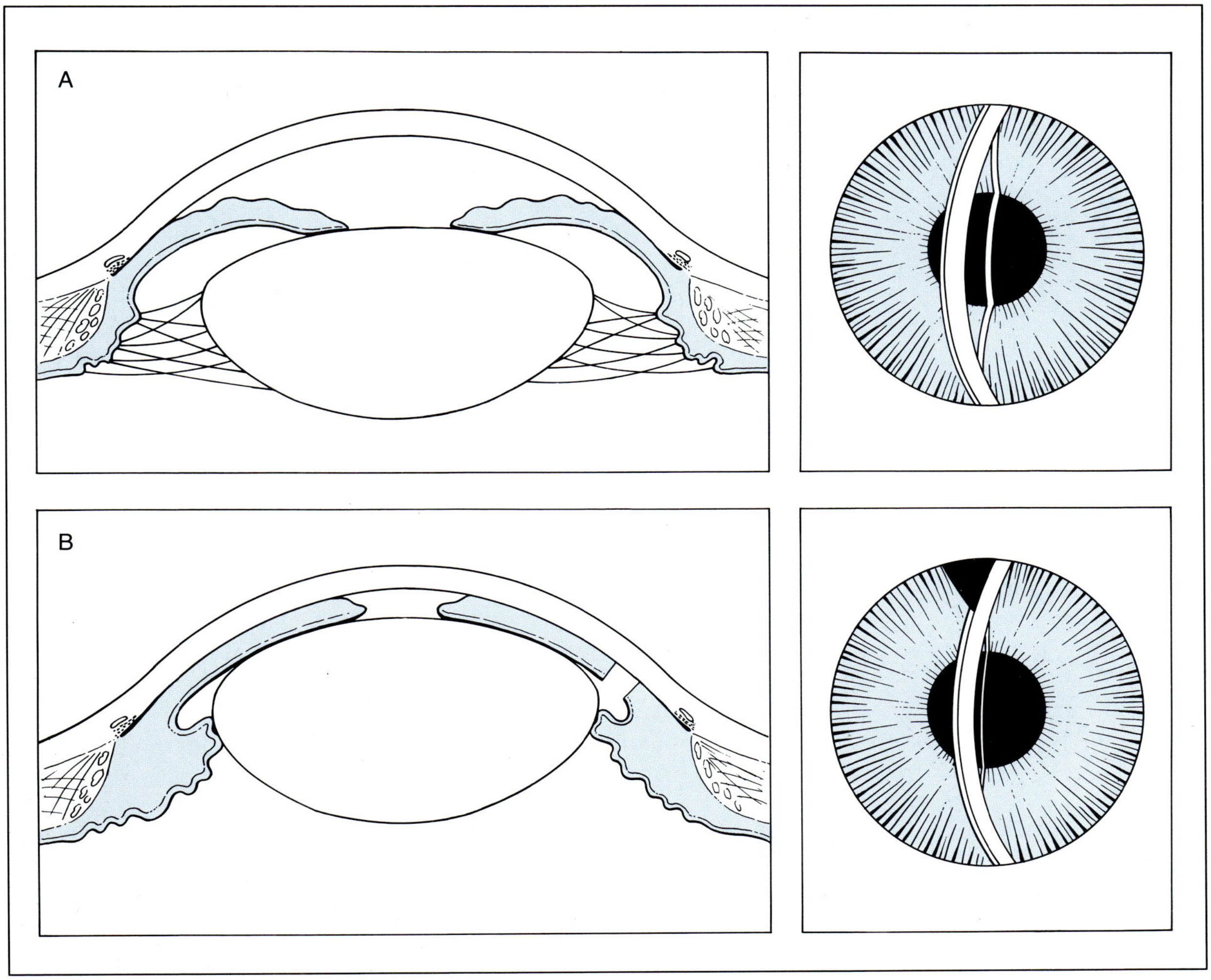

8.34 | Differentiation of pupillary block (A) from ciliary block (B). In *A* the anterior chamber is more shallow peripherally than centrally due to iris bombé, whereas in *B* the anterior chamber is more uniformly shallow, even in presence of patent iridectomy.

block, laser iridotomy can be performed to release the aqueous trapped behind the iris.

Postoperative suprachoroidal hemorrhage is often associated with sudden onset of pain, a shallow or flat anterior chamber, and frequently with an elevated IOP. Fundus examination usually reveals large dark choroidal elevations.[30,62,68]

MANAGEMENT

Medical Therapy

When no iridectomy is present, then laser iridotomy should be performed to eliminate the possibility of pupillary block.[30] If the presumed ciliary block persists, then medical therapy is initiated. Medical therapy consists of discontinuation of any cholinergic agents, since these drugs increase ciliary body tone, relax the zonules, result in anterior displacement and an increased anterior-to-posterior diameter of the lens, and increase relative pupillary block.[65,68,69] Instead, cycloplegic agents such as atropine (1% four times daily) are administered, since they decrease ciliary body tone, increase tension on the zonules, and produce axial thinning and retrodisplacement of the lens. Because sympathomimetic agents may cause further relaxation of the ciliary musculature, phenylephrine 2.5% or 10% is often used in conjunction with topical atropine.

Aqueous suppressants, including topical beta-blockers the α_2-adrenergic agonist apraclonidine, and oral carbonic anhydrase inhibitors, reduce the amount of aqueous being directed posteriorly and also act to lower IOP, which is often 40 mm Hg or higher.[30,62,68,69] Hyperosmotic agents, which include oral glycerin or isosorbide or intravenous mannitol, cause shrinkage of the vitreous and may help to reestablish normal anterior aqueous flow.[64,68,69] The usual dose is 1–2 g/kg every 6–8 hours. To reduce inflammation and any associated uveal congestion, intensive topical corticosteroids should be administered.

Within 4 to 5 days, intensive medical therapy leads to resolution of the ciliary block in approximately 50% of cases.[68,69] In eyes that respond medically, therapy can be slowly tapered with discontinuation of the hyperosmotic agent(s), discontinuation of the carbonic anhydrase inhibitor and apraclonidine and later, if possible, the beta-blocker, discontinuation of phenylephrine, and tapering of the atropine. Many eyes require continuation of atropine indefinitely to prevent recurrences of ciliary-block glaucoma.

Surgical Therapy

As previously noted, even in conjunction with initial medical therapy, laser iridotomy can be performed in the absence of a patent iridectomy to eliminate any possible element of pupillary-block glaucoma. In eyes that do not respond to laser iridotomy and medical therapy, surgical intervention becomes necessary. Argon laser treatment of the ciliary processes through a patent iridectomy has also been described in the treatment of ciliary-block glaucoma in phakic eyes.[74] This treatment presumably produces shrinkage of the ciliary processes and reduces ciliolenticular block, although it has been proposed that this treatment may also be effective in disrupting a portion of the anterior hyaloid.[30] In eyes unresponsive to these modalities, vitrectomy and anterior chamber reformation are indicated. Reported methods include needle aspiration of vitreous through the pars plana in conjunction with anterior chamber re-formation using balanced salt solution, a viscoelastic substance, or air.[64,68] With current technical capabilities, conventional pars plana vitrectomy with aspiration of as much anterior vitreous as possible may be more controlled than needle vitreous aspiration[75] (Fig. 8.35).

In eyes unresponsive even to vitrectomy, lens extraction may be necessary.[30,62] If extracapsular surgery is performed, a primary posterior capsulotomy should be completed to increase the likelihood of reestablishing normal aqueous direction.

In aphakic or pseudophakic ciliary block, photodisruption of the anterior vitreous face (and, in some cases, the posterior lens capsule) with the neodymium:YAG laser has led to resolution of ciliary-block glaucoma[76] (Fig. 8.36).

Because the fellow eye usually has a narrow anterior-chamber angle and is at risk for developing ciliary block after future intraocular surgery, prophylactic laser iridotomy should be performed.[62] However, it should be noted that cases of ciliary-block glaucoma after laser iridotomy have been recently described.[77]

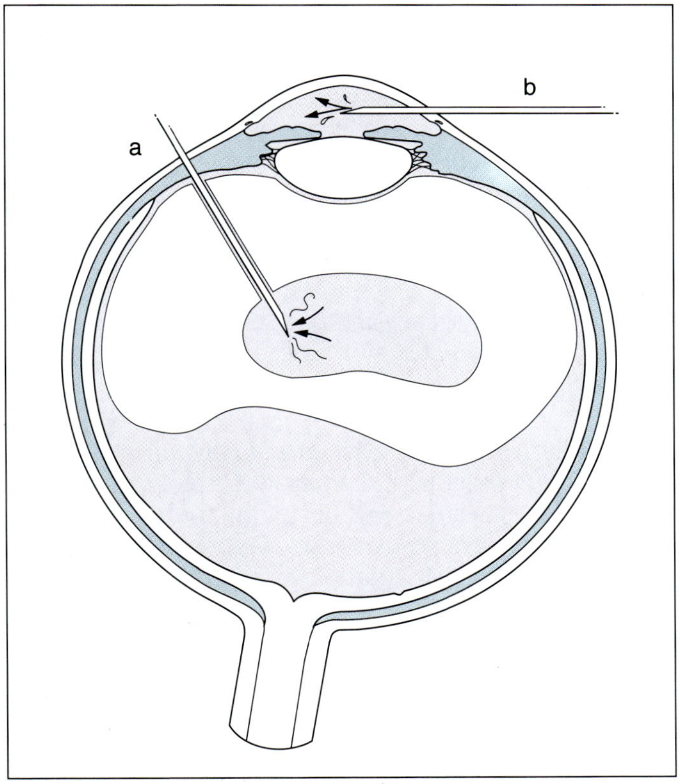

8.35 | Surgical management of medically unresponsive ciliary-block glaucoma may require drainage of fluid and/or aspiration of vitreous using needle *(A)* or standard vitrectomy instruments in conjunction with anterior chamber reformation *(B)* with air, balanced salt solution, or viscoelastic substances.

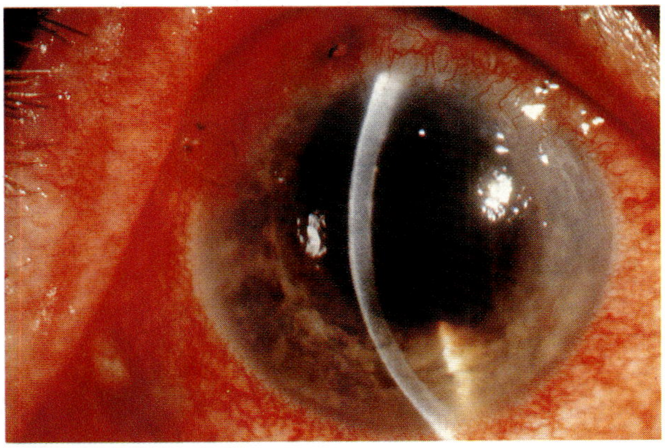

8.36 | Eye shown in Figure 8.33 after photodisruption of posterior capsule and anterior vitreous face with Nd:YAG laser. (Courtesy of Dr. Elizabeth Hodapp.)

OTHER SECONDARY ANGLE-CLOSURE GLAUCOMAS

UVEITIC GLAUCOMA

A variety of conditions not described elsewhere in this section can be associated with secondary angle closure.

Although uveitic glaucoma is often a secondary open-angle glaucoma, the development of dense posterior synechiae may predispose to the development of iris bombé and severe pupillary block, which can be treated with laser iridotomy.[2,78] In some patients with chronic inflammation, peripheral anterior synechiae may develop even in the absence of pupillary block.

LENS-INDUCED GLAUCOMA

In phacomorphic glaucoma, increasing lens thickness with age results in progressive closure of the anterior-chamber angle through anterior displacement of the lens–iris diaphragm and increased pupillary block.[79] Pupillary block can be relieved by laser iridotomy, although the angle may remain narrow until lens extraction is performed.

Angle-closure glaucoma may also occur in such conditions as microspherophakia (seen most commonly in association with Weill–Marchesani syndrome), in which the small, thickened lens sometimes migrates anteriorly to block the pupil.[2,79] Miotic therapy may worsen this condition, which is relieved by laser iridotomy and cycloplegic therapy.

APHAKIC AND PSEUDOPHAKIC PUPILLARY BLOCK

In aphakic and pseudophakic patients, vitreous may fill the pupillary space and/or plug iridectomies and cause pupillary block[2,80] (Fig. 8.37). Alternatively, iris adhesions to the intraocular lens implant, posterior capsule, or vitreous face may also produce pupillary block, which can be relieved by medical therapy (including cycloplegic agents) and laser iridotomy. Some authors have suggested that postoperative posterior synechiae are more likely to occur in diabetic patients after extracapsular cataract surgery.[81]

IRIDOCORNEAL ENDOTHELIAL SYNDROME

Iridocorneal endothelial (ICE) syndrome refers to a usually unilateral condition characterized by corneal endothelial abnormalities, progressive formation of peripheral anterior synechiae without pupillary block, and iris defects.[82] Corneal edema and secondary glaucoma are common. The clinical findings are secondary to endothelialization of the anterior-chamber angle

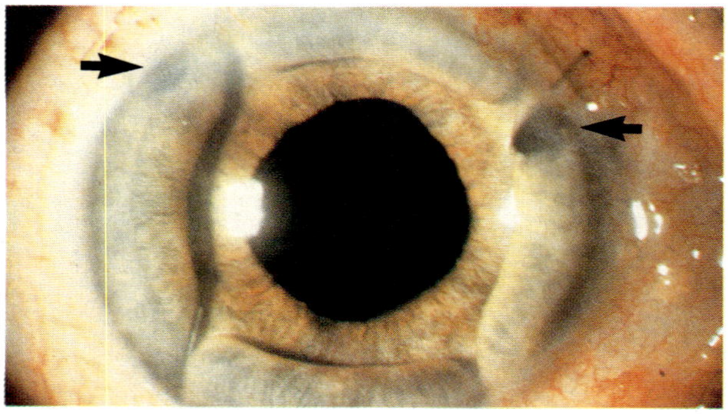

8.37 | Eye with anterior-chamber intraocular lens and iris bombé around implant despite presence of peripheral iridectomies (arrows), which have become blocked by vitreous. (Courtesy of Dr. Eve J. Higginbotham.)

with corneal endothelium and Descemet's membrane extending across the trabecular meshwork onto the anterior iris surface (Fig. 8.38).

Clinical variants include progressive essential iris atrophy (iris changes predominate), Chandler syndrome (corneal changes predominate), and iris–nevus or Cogan–Reese syndromes (nevi or nodules on iris surface predominate). See Van Buskirk, this chapter, for a more complete description of the ICE syndrome and its variants. Treatment consists of medical and/or surgical control of the secondary glaucoma and corneal edema.

ANGLE CLOSURE AFTER SCLERAL BUCKLING SURGERY AND PANRETINAL PHOTOCOAGULATION

Inflammation, uveal congestion with anterior rotation of the ciliary processes, and mechanical anterior displacement of the lens–iris diaphragm may result in angle closure glaucoma after scleral buckling surgery.[83] This usually responds to medical therapy, including topical corticosteroids, cycloplegic agents, and aqueous suppressants. Occasionally, peripheral iridoplasty may be necessary to pull the peripheral iris away from the angle structures.[84] Other alternatives include drainage of any accumulated suprachoroidal fluid or adjustment of the scleral buckle.[30]

After panretinal photocoagulation, ciliary body swelling may produce angle closure.[83] Typically, this responds to topical corticosteroids, cycloplegics, and aqueous suppressants, although unresponsive eyes may require peripheral iridoplasty.[30] When any element of pupillary block is suspected (e.g., narrow angle in fellow eye), laser iridotomy can be performed.

CENTRAL RETINAL VEIN OCCLUSION

Rarely, uveal congestion and anterior rotation of the ciliary processes secondary to central retinal vein occlusion produces a shallow anterior chamber and closure of the angle.[30,85] Treatment is similar to that described above after scleral buckling surgery and panretinal photocoagulation.

ANGLE CLOSURE DUE TO TUMORS AND CYSTS

Intraocular tumors, most commonly malignant melanoma, may cause secondary glaucoma through a variety of mechanisms (see Van Buskirk, this chapter), including anterior displacement of the lens–iris diaphragm and angle-closure glaucoma.[30] Such glaucoma is managed medically.

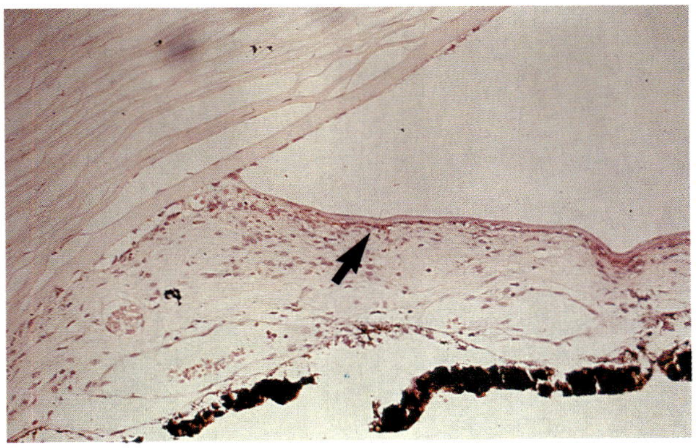

8.38 | Histopathology of iridocorneal endothelial syndrome, showing abnormal endothelium and Descemet's membrane extending onto anterior iris surface (arrow) with associated peripheral anterior synechia formation. (Courtesy of Dr. Morton Smith.)

Epithelial cysts of the iris and ciliary body, if large enough, can also produce an anterior shift of the iris with significant angle closure.[86] Treatment alternatives include puncture of the cysts with argon or Nd:YAG lasers if the cysts are visible at the pupillary margin. Otherwise, laser iridotomy can be performed over the site of the cyst. Glaucoma due to residual peripheral anterior synechiae after cyst puncture may require medical therapy and, in some cases, filtering surgery.[30]

NANOPHTHALMOS

Very small hyperopic eyes with nanophthalmos may often have narrow anterior-chamber angles and angle closure due to (1) a relatively large lens in the presence of a short axial length (high lens/eye volume ratio) and small cornea[87] and (2) spontaneous choroidal effusion with a forward shift of the iris and lens.[88,89] If the angle is occludable or closed, laser iridotomy should be performed, although peripheral iridoplasty may also be necessary.[87,88] Residual glaucoma may require medical therapy. Because of thickened sclera and possible obstruction of drainage from the vortex veins, uveal congestion may be present.[90] As already noted, this congestion appears to contribute to angle-closure glaucoma in some eyes.[88,89] This is also of great importance if intraocular surgery should be necessary, because prophylactic sclerotomies should be performed to reduce the risk of massive choroidal effusions, nonrhegmatogenous retinal detachment, and flat anterior chamber.[30]

EPITHELIAL AND FIBROVASCULAR DOWNGROWTH

As the result of inadequate postoperative wound apposition or after trauma, epithelial or fibrovascular ingrowth may occur and produce a severe secondary angle-closure glaucoma.[30] Treatment of the downgrowth may require extensive surgery, often with a poor prognosis.

SECTION III

EPIDEMIOLOGY OF OPEN-ANGLE GLAUCOMA

Jacob T. Wilensky

It is estimated that approximately two million people in the United States have glaucoma. A large majority of them have primary open-angle glaucoma (POAG), and approximately half are not aware of their disease. Moreover, there obviously was a period when some of the people who now know they have glaucoma had not yet been diagnosed. Many patients are first diagnosed at a stage when significant damage has already occurred. Therefore, identification and treatment of patients who will develop glaucoma is a highly desired goal if visual loss due to this disease is to be minimized.

RISK FACTORS

ELEVATED INTRAOCULAR PRESSURES

A number of risk factors are associated with the development of POAG. The one which has the highest predictive value is the level of intraocular pressure (IOP).[91,92] In general, the higher the IOP, the greater the likelihood of progressive optic nerve damage (Fig. 8.39). The relationship, however, is far from

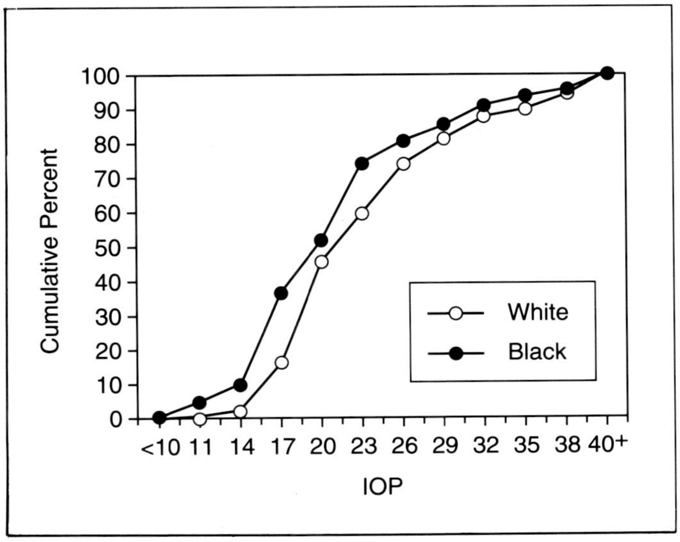

8.39 | Distribution of primary open-angle glaucoma by IOP. (Adapted from Tielsch J: Epidemiology of blindness and glaucoma: racial variations, in Cowan CL Jr (ed): *The Third Caribbean Glaucoma Symposium*. New York: Della Corte, 1991, 4. Copyright © 1991, Lawrence Della Corte Publications, Inc.)

direct, and there are many eyes with IOPs above the normal range that have been followed for a number of years without any signs of glaucomatous cupping or visual field loss. Conversely, many eyes that never experienced IOPs above the normal range develop what appears to be glaucomatous damage.

"Normal" IOP is difficult to define. If one assumes that IOP has a normal distribution in the statistical sense, then the average IOP is approximately 16 mm Hg. Two standard deviations from this mean will encompass a range from 10 to 22 mm Hg. By statistical definition, two standard deviations from the mean indicates that the value outside this range has less than a 5% chance of being a normal value. When studies have been performed in large populations over 40 years of age, it has been found that the number of individuals with an IOP above 22 mm Hg approximates 5–10%, which is considerably greater than the 2.5% that would be expected on a purely statistical basis.[93–95] On the other hand, a large majority of individuals with an IOP above 22 mm Hg do not have either glaucomatous cupping or visual field loss. Therefore, it is now generally accepted that IOP does not have a normal distribution but is skewed to the high side.

Another problem in assessing the role of IOP is that IOP is not a constant value, but instead fluctuates throughout the day. These fairly regular diurnal variations seem related to the body's biological rhythm.[96] In addition, there are shorter-term variations that may be related to environmental influences, including food and fluid consumption. The diurnal variation in normal eyes ranges from 3.5–5 mm Hg, but is greater in untreated POAG.[97] Some authors have stated that a diurnal fluctuation range above a selected value is diagnostic of glaucoma, but no prospective studies have attempted to correlate the range of diurnal IOP fluctuation with subsequent development of visual field loss and cupping.

These confounding IOP variables have led to the finding in several large population surveys that about 50% of the eyes diagnosed as having open-angle glaucoma did not have elevated IOP on initial examination. In these and other studies, some of the patients with elevated IOP but normal visual fields ("ocular hypertensives") were followed prospectively. In general, only a small percentage (0.5–2.0% per year) of patients developed glaucomatous visual field loss during the follow-up period.[98]

LARGE OPTIC DISK CUPS

Another risk factor associated with the development of glaucomatous damage is the presence of a large cup in the optic nerve head. Because progressive enlargement of the cup is one of the signs of glaucomatous damage, when a patient presents with a large cup there is always the suspicion that this represents an early sign of the disease. On the other hand, there is a normal range to the distribution of cup sizes, so that individuals with larger than average cups do not necessarily have glaucoma.

However, one may ask whether eyes with larger cups, even though they are physiologic, have a greater risk of developing glaucomatous damage at a given IOP than do eyes with smaller cups. A growing body of evidence supports the contention that larger cups acquired as the result of glaucomatous damage are more susceptible to damage at a given IOP level.[92,99] There has not been much work trying to correlate the presence of a physiologic large cup with the subsequent development of glaucomatous damage. Two groups of patients known to have a higher incidence of open-angle glaucoma, namely high myopes and blacks,[100] tend to have cups that are larger than average. Whether these larger cups contribute to the greater prevalence of glaucoma damage in these two populations is not certain at this point.

RACE

A third risk factor in open-angle glaucoma is race. There is a higher prevalence of open-angle glaucoma in blacks as compared to whites and Orientals (Fig. 8.40). In the United States this relative prevalence appears to be of the order of 2 to 1, but there are suggestions that it may even be greater in some populations.[101,102] In two recent glaucoma surveys conducted on Caribbean islands, the prevalence of POAG in black populations over 40 years of age was around 14%, which is considerably higher than the approximately 1–2% prevalence for whites reported in other studies.[103,104]

There are also data suggesting that POAG is a more severe disease in blacks than in whites. Age-adjusted data show that the incidence of blindness from glaucoma is approximately eight times greater in blacks than in whites in the United States.[105] Blacks also appear to require higher doses of medication to achieve comparable drug effects, and the success rate for surgery in blacks has been reported to be lower than that in whites.

AGE

Another risk factor is increasing age (see Fig. 8.40). POAG is an uncommon disease in young individuals. In the Framingham Study the prevalence of glaucoma was 0.7% in individuals 52–64 years of age, increased to 1.6% in individuals of 65–74 years of age, and to 4.2% in individuals 75–85 years of age.[106] A similar increase with age was seen in the Ferndale Glaucoma Study.[103]

FAMILY HISTORY

POAG appears to be a familial disease. There have been several surveys of the incidence of glaucoma in relatives of patients with POAG.[107,108] The studies are somewhat limited because of incomplete data capture and because many children have not yet reached the age at which manifest glaucoma might be expected. Nevertheless, these studies have been fairly similar in indicating an approximately 1 in 10 risk that an individual who has a first-degree relative (parent, sibling, or offspring) with POAG will develop the disease. This seems to be at least a tenfold increased risk compared with that of the general population.

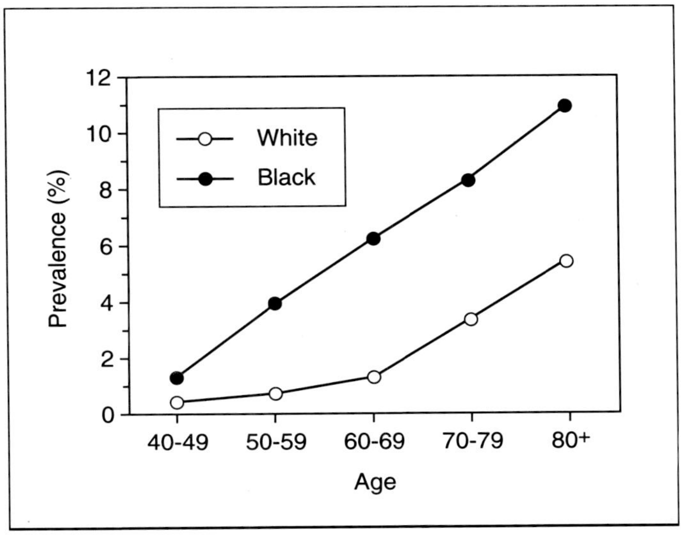

8.40 | Prevalence of primary open-angle glaucoma by age and race. (Adapted from Tielsch J: Epidemiology of blindness and glaucoma: racial variations, in Cowan CL Jr (ed): *The Third Caribbean Glaucoma Symposium.* New York: Della Corte, 1991, 4. Copyright © 1991, Lawrence Della Corte Publications, Inc.)

SYSTEMIC DISEASES

An increased incidence of open-angle glaucoma has been associated with two systemic disease conditions, diabetes mellitus and arterial hypertension. There are several reports indicating that POAG is up to three times more prevalent in diabetics than in nondiabetics.[109] In a case control study of risk factors in POAG, systemic hypertension stood out,[110] and there was considerable difference in relative risk between untreated and treated hypertension.

ASSOCIATED OCULAR CONDITIONS

Two ocular findings have been associated with an increased risk of specific secondary forms of open-angle glaucoma, which must be distinguished from POAG. One is the presence of exfoliative material on the anterior lens capsule. Studies have shown that approximately 5–15% of individuals over 60 years of age have exfoliation of the lens capsule. In one large study, it was found that 5.3% of eyes presenting with exfoliation and normal IOP developed elevated IOP within 5 years and 15.4% within 10 years[111] (see Ritch and Liebmann, this chapter).

Another ocular risk factor for a secondary open-angle glaucoma is the presence of pigmentary dispersion syndrome as manifested by Krukenberg spindles and/or peripheral wedge-shaped transillumination defects in the iris. In one long-term follow-up study of patients with pigmentary dispersion syndrome and elevated IOP but normal visual fields, almost a third of the eyes subsequently developed visual field defects[112] (see Ritch and Liebmann, this chapter).

The presence of myopia appears to be a risk factor for POAG itself. A higher percentage of POAG eyes are myopic than would be found in a nonglaucomatous population.[113] Some glaucoma specialists feel that there is a significant incidence of POAG in eyes with high myopia, but this has not been clearly documented in the literature.[114] A large percentage of patients with pigmentary glaucoma have mild to moderate myopia, but pigmentary glaucoma accounts for only a small fraction of all open-angle glaucoma.

SUSCEPTIBILITY FACTORS

It is fairly clear that no individual risk factor is very predictive, in and of itself, of the future development of glaucomatous damage in an eye. Even when we combine a number of factors, we still are unable to predict accu-

Figure 8.41. Major Risk Factors for Primary Open-Angle Glaucoma

"Elevated" IOP	Family history of glaucoma
"Large" optic disk cup	Diabetes mellitus
Black race	Systemic hypertension
Age	Myopia

rately the majority of eyes that will go on to develop glaucomatous damage.[115] This is probably because these are susceptibility factors as well as risk factors, and we have not yet defined the nature of these susceptibility factors. There might be differences in the vasculature, collagen, or anatomic structure of the optic nerve head, among many possibilities.

From patients with secondary glaucoma, we know that if the IOP is elevated high enough for long enough, the eye will develop glaucomatous damage. However, there are eyes with no elevations of IOP that develop what appear to be glaucomatous cupping and field loss. It is assumed that these eyes have such severe susceptibility factors that they develop damage even in the presence of what would otherwise be considered a normal IOP.

Most eyes fall somewhere between these extremes. They have some degree of susceptibility and, therefore, in the face of moderate stress (e.g., in the form of elevated IOP), they may develop glaucomatous cupping and field loss. If they have a greater degree of susceptibility, it will occur sooner. If they have a lesser degree of susceptibility, it will take longer. Therefore, time becomes another element of the equation that ultimately determines whether a patient will develop glaucomatous damage during his/her lifetime. If one has two patients with similar risk factors, including similar IOPs, but one individual is in his 40s and the other in his 70s, the younger patient has a greater possibility of developing damage during his/her lifetime because he/she will be exposed to these factors for a 30-year period, whereas the patient in his/her 70s, who has a life expectancy of less than 10 years, will be exposed to them for a much shorter time. Of course, although this may be true statistically, there will be 40-year-old individuals who will die of a heart attack or other cause in a year or two and 70-year-old individuals who will live well into their 90s. For a list of risk factors, see Figure 8.41.

SUMMARY

To date, we have identified one major risk or causative factor for primary open angle glaucoma, i.e., elevated IOP. We have further identified at least two factors, exfoliation of the lens capsule and pigmentary dispersion, that dispose towards elevation of IOP. We have also identified a number of associated factors that seem to place an eye at greater risk for developing glaucomatous damage. These include large cups, diabetes mellitus, systemic hypertension, family history of glaucoma, age, black race, and possibly high myopia. It is not yet clear whether they constitute causative factors, susceptibility factors, or possibly both. In the interaction, it is clear that eyes with both causative and susceptibility factors have a substantially increased risk of developing glaucomatous damage, but as yet we still cannot identify with a high degree of sensitivity or specificity a significant proportion of those eyes that will develop glaucomatous damage.

Section IV

Clinical Presentation of Primary Open-Angle Glaucoma

Eve J. Higginbotham

Primary open-angle glaucoma (POAG) can be defined as an optic neuropathy which is accompanied by characteristic visual field defects and is sometimes associated with an elevation of intraocular pressure (IOP). By definition, there is no apparent obstruction of the trabecular meshwork by structures such as the iris on gonioscopic examination.

The evaluation of the patient suspected of having glaucoma begins with recording a thorough history. Because of the insidious and painless nature of POAG, patients often do not report symptoms. Nevertheless, the patient should be questioned regarding decreased or blurred vision, pain, redness, observations of halos around lights, trauma, surgery, previous ocular disease, and systemic medications. In general, however, an affirmative response to most of these inquiries points to an alternative mechanism, such as angle-closure glaucoma. The examiner should also keep in mind the nonocular risk factors for POAG such as age, race, family history, diabetes mellitus, and systemic vascular disease (see Wilensky, this chapter).

As the physician examines the patient, POAG-associated ocular risk factors and findings should be kept in mind. Myopia has been linked to POAG, but IOP is usually considered to be the primary causal factor. Difficulty arises, however, when one considers patients with high IOP and no ocular damage (glaucoma suspect) and patients with normal pressures and glaucomatous damage (low-tension or normotensive glaucoma). A mean IOP measuring 16 ± 2.5 mm Hg (range 10–21 mm Hg) is seen in nonglaucomatous eyes. An IOP measuring 21 mm Hg was formerly thought to be the cut-off between a glaucomatous and nonglaucomatous level. However, the distribution of IOP in the general population is not Gaussian, being skewed to the right (i.e., there are more individuals with pressures in the low twenties than would have been predicted by Gaussian statistics).[116] Rather, the chance of discovering a glaucomatous field defect on examination increases with IOP across the entire range, and is present even at pressures in the low "normal" range. The examiner must also keep in mind the diurnal variation of IOP. Therefore, on the basis of IOP, a diagnosis of POAG can be difficult to make, especially depending on the time of day of the evaluation.

Evaluation of the optic nerve is critical in determining the presence of glaucomatous disease. In fact, changes in the optic nerve will often precede any changes in perimetry. The clinical characteristics of glaucomatous optic neuropathy are described and illustrated by Schwartz, Chapter 4, and in this author's section in Chapter 6. When changes in the optic nerve are evaluated, it is important to consider nonglaucomatous entities such as ischemic optic neuropathy, compressive lesions of the chiasm and optic nerve, and congenital anomalies of the optic nerve such as tilted discs and optic pits. When the usefulness of four disc characteristics (pallor of the neuroretinal rim tissue, thinning of the rim tissue, diffuse obliteration of the neuroretinal rim, and laminar dots) in distinguishing between nonglaucomatous and glaucomatous excavation of the optic disc was analyzed, pallor proved to be 94% specific for nonglaucomatous atrophy and focal or diffuse loss of neuroretinal tissue was 87% specific for glaucoma; the presence of laminar dots was nonspecific.[117] Attention is presently concentrated on developing techniques to detect early glaucomatous atrophy of the optic disc and retinal nerve fiber layer (see Airaksinen and Weinreb/Caprioli, Chapter 6).

Additional ocular signs are important in making the diagnosis of POAG. Depending on the asymmetry and the severity of the field defect, there may be an afferent pupillary defect in the more severely affected eye. Because the increase in IOP in POAG is usually only moderate and insidious, the cornea will be clear unless there is a concomitant corneal problem. If there is any evidence of keratic precipitates or a Krukenberg spindle, a secondary mechanism is implicated. The anterior chamber is deep, with at least one quarter corneal thickness separating the corneal endothelium and the anterior surface of the iris at the peripheral cornea. By definition, the anterior chamber angle will be free of any peripheral anterior synechiae, new vessels, recession, exfoliation material, excessive pigmentation, or foreign body, all of which would indicate a secondary rather than a primary mechanism. For a more detailed description of the technique of gonioscopy and findings related to glaucoma, see Zalta, Chapter 6, and Ritch and Liebmann, Van Buskirk, and Sakamoto and Hetherington, this chapter.

There are two basic types of perimetry: kinetic and static threshold. Kinetic perimetry essentially plots the circumference of the hill of vision at a particular height, whereas static threshold perimetry quantitates the height at a particular location (see Heijl, Chapter 5). The goal of perimetry is to detect changes in visual function that may occur secondary to glaucoma and, whenever possible, to quantitate those changes. The earlier in the course of the disease these changes can be detected, the sooner appropriate treatment can be instituted. Nonspecific early changes include generalized constriction or decrease in sensitivity and baring of the blind spot. More specific changes caused by glaucoma include paracentral scotoma, arcuate scotomas, nasal steps, and temporal wedges. Along with optic nerve head cupping, visual field defects are currently the sine qua non for the definitive diagnosis of glaucoma. For a more detailed description of techniques and visual field findings in glaucoma see Heijl, Chapters 5 and 7.

Although outflow facility is almost invariably reduced in POAG (and even in low- or normal tension glaucoma), tonography is no longer an integral part of the standard clinical evaluation. Tonography provides no information about optic nerve structure or function, and the parameter that may be compromising the optic nerve, intraocular pressure, is obtainable by simple applanation tonometry.

Finally, POAG is typically a bilateral disease. Although asymmetry of IOP and optic nerve damage can certainly exist, advanced abnormalities in one eye in the company of an entirely normal fellow eye suggest another diagnosis. Entities such as previous ocular trauma, ocular or periocular use of glucocorticoids, exfoliation syndrome, and glaucomatocyclitic crisis should be considered, as they can present in a quiet eye with no or only very subtle signs of their presence. Meticulous history and clinical examination are especially called for in such unilateral cases (see Ritch and Liebmann, as well as Van Buskirk, this chapter).

In summary, the clinical evaluation of a patient with POAG begins with a thorough history. The examiner should keep in mind the nonocular and ocular risk factors such as age, race, family history, diabetes mellitus, hypertension, intraocular pressure, large cup-to-disc ratio, and myopia. Accurate measurement of IOP, careful biomicroscopy, gonioscopy, ophthalmoscopy, and perimetry are essential. The therapy of POAG is discussed in the last portion of this volume (Chapter 9).

Section V

Pathology of the Trabecular Meshwork in Primary Open-Angle Glaucoma

Elke Lütjen-Drecoll
Johannes W. Rohen

In trabeculectomy specimens from primary open-angle glaucoma eyes, clusters of extracellular material are found predominantly within the cribriform layer of the trabecular meshwork.[118,119] These so-called "plaques" derive mainly from the sheath of the elastic-like fibers located within the cribriform layer or they develop around the connecting fibrils which then thicken and merge (Figs. 8.42, 8.43, and 8.44). The amount of this "sheath-derived" plaque material (SD plaques) increases with age but is significantly greater in glaucomatous than in normal eyes.[120] Recently, trabeculectomy specimens from 30 glaucoma patients with no medication before surgery were studied [unpublished]. In these cases, too, the amount of plaque material was significantly greater than in normal eyes, indicating that the disease and not iatrogenic effects was responsible. Plaque formation seems to be a continuous, age-dependent process. Therefore, the morphologic changes of the trabecular meshwork in glaucomatous eyes cannot be considered simply as an age-dependent phenomenon. Deposits of the SD plaque material have also been found in the outer wall of Schlemm's canal and in the ciliary muscle between the anterior muscle tips[121] (see Fig. 8.44). This indicates that plaque formation is a more generalized process in the anterior segment, which becomes deleterious only when the aqueous pathways situated in the inner wall of Schlemm's canal or in the cribriform layer are already narrowed or obstructed.

Blockage of these channels can also occur when extracellular material other than SD plaques is deposited within or around the cribriform pathways. Therefore, if clusters of pseudoexfoliation material, pigment granules, or lens material accumulate within the cribriform layer underneath the inner wall endothelium, outflow resistance and consequently intraocular pressure can rise. This explains why in cases of exfoliation glaucoma the amount of SD plaque material is not significantly different from that present in normal eyes of the same age group.[120]

In primary open-angle glaucoma, loss of trabecular endothelial cells is greater than in normal eyes of the same age group. It has been assumed that in glaucomatous eyes a smaller number of trabecular cells exist at birth, so that there may be a genetic disposition for this disease.[122,123]

Loss of trabecular cells is often accompanied by thickening of the uveal and corneoscleral lamellae, due to an increase in the basement membranes, and by augmentation of deposits of long-spacing collagen and SD plaque material (see Fig. 8.42). Thickening of trabecular lamellae will lead to narrowing of the intertrabecular spaces. Finally, complete adhesion or fusion of trabecular beams might develop so that the uveal and corneoscleral pathways become obstructed, resulting in elevation of outflow resistance in these regions. The related areas of the cribriform layer are then underperfused, leading to increased plaque formation. Thus, a vicious circle might develop which could finally lead to a complete obstruction of the trabecular meshwork. However, there are great regional differences in such pathology over the circumference of the trabecular meshwork.

ACKNOWLEDGMENTS

This work was supported by the Academy of Science and Literature, Mainz/Rh.,Germany and by the Deutsche Forschungsgemeinschaft, Bonn-Bad Godesberg (Dre 124/6-1).

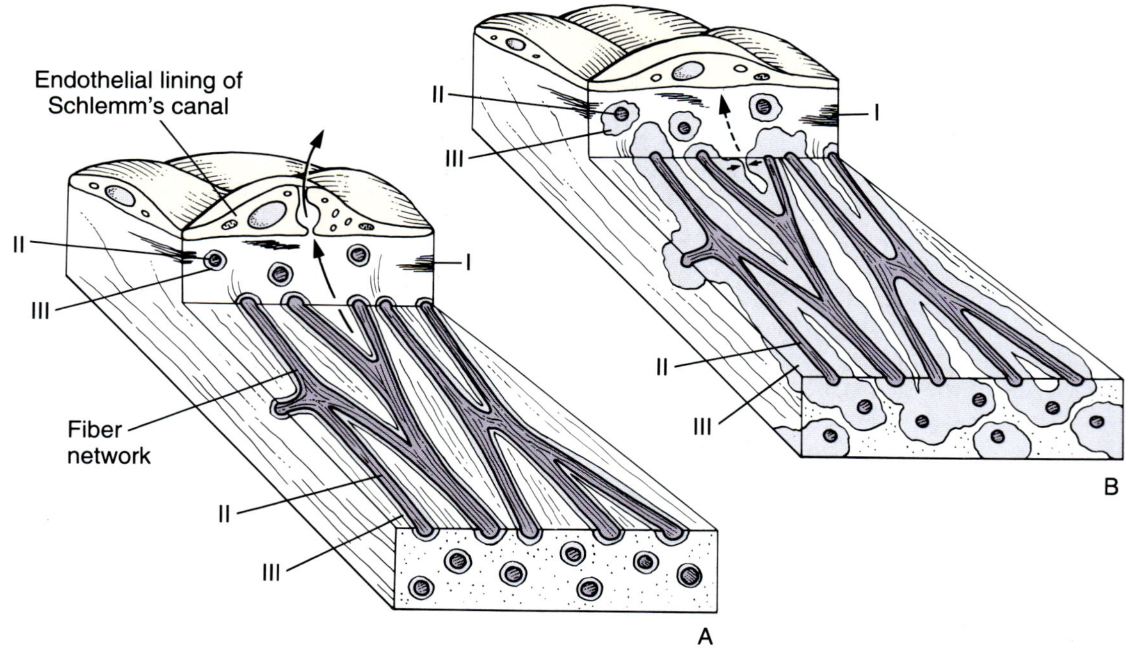

8.42 | Inner wall of Schlemm's canal and the subendothelially located elastic-like fiber network in normal (*A*) and primary open-angle glaucoma (*B*). The thickening of the sheaths by so-called sheath-derived plaques (type III is shown in *B*. I, II, and III indicate type I, II, or III plaques. The long arrows show the direction of aqueous outflow through a giant vacuole. In primary open-angle glaucoma the outflow pathways are narrowed by SD plaque material (small arrows), so that the giant vacuole disappears.

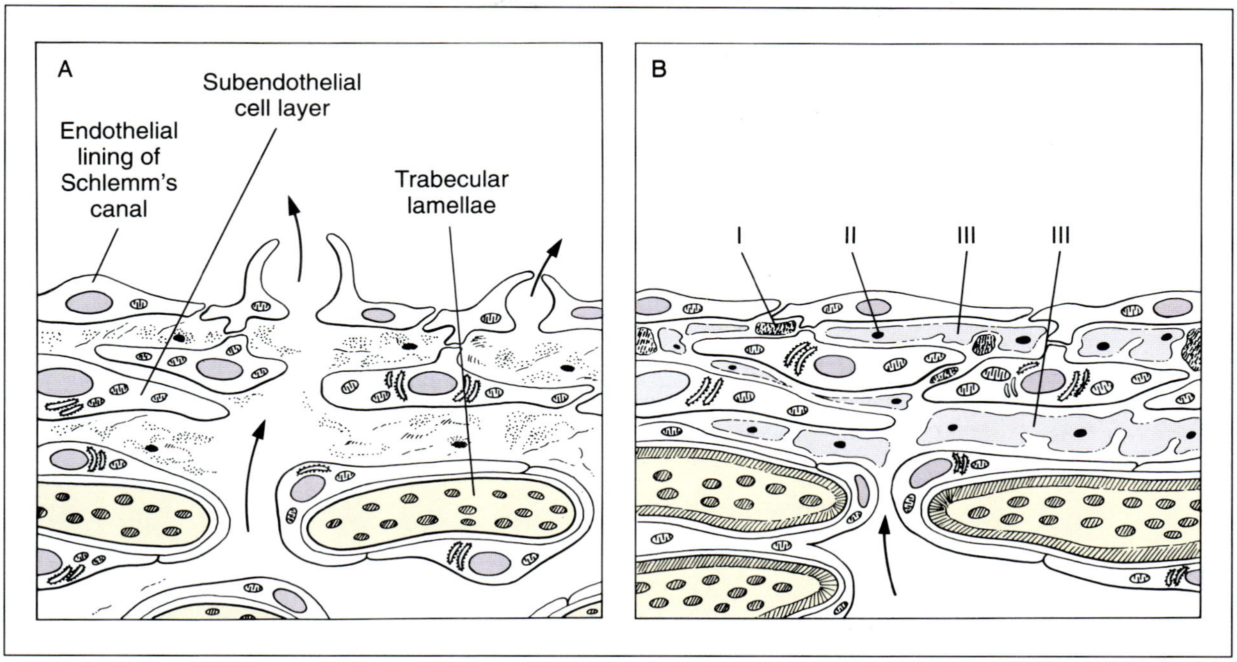

8.43 | Ultrastructure of the cribriform layer and inner wall endothelium in normal (*A*) and glaucomatous (*B*) eyes. Arrows = direction of aqueous outflow. I, II, III = type I, II or III plaques.

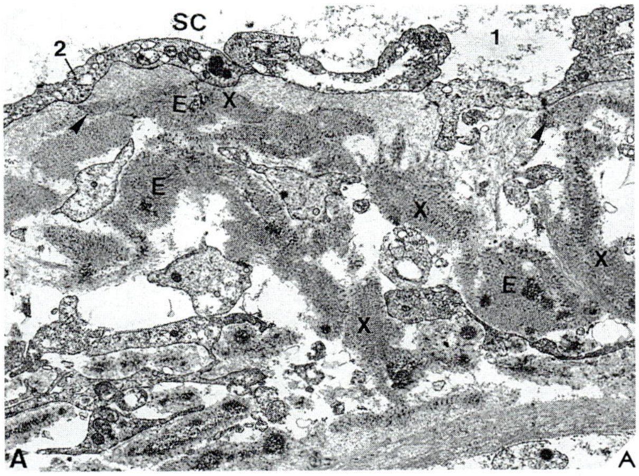

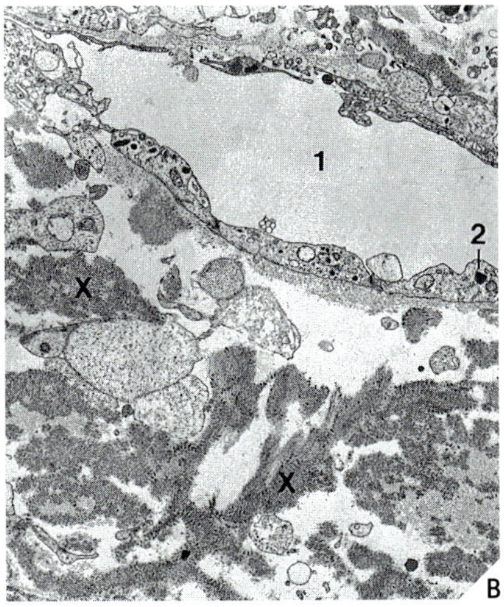

8.44 | Electron micrographs show plaque formation within the inner (*A*) and outer wall (*B*) of Schlemm's canal in a case of primary open-angle glaucoma. 1 = lumen of Schlemm's canal (SC). 2 = endothelial lining of the canal. E = central core of elastic-like fibers. X = sheath material of elastic-like fibers. SC = Schlemm's canal.

Section VI

Pigment Dispersion Syndrome

Robert Ritch
Jeffrey Liebmann

CLINICAL FEATURES

The pigment dispersion syndrome (PDS) is a bilateral disorder characterized by liberation of pigment from the iris pigment epithelium and its deposition throughout the anterior segment. This process produces the classic clinical findings of a Krukenberg spindle (Fig. 8.45); a homogeneous, dense band of pigment on the trabecular meshwork (Fig. 8.46); and slit-like radial transillumination defects in the midperipheral iris (Figs. 8.47 and 8.48). In addition, dispersed iris pigment may be deposited on Schwalbe's line, the anterior iris surface (Fig. 8.49), the lens surface, zonules, and the ciliary body. Blockage of or damage to the aqueous outflow pathways by pigment is believed to be the cause of glaucoma.

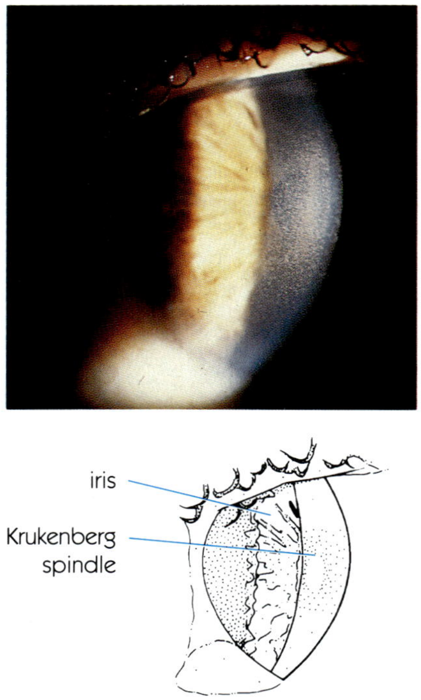

8.45 | Krukenberg spindle.

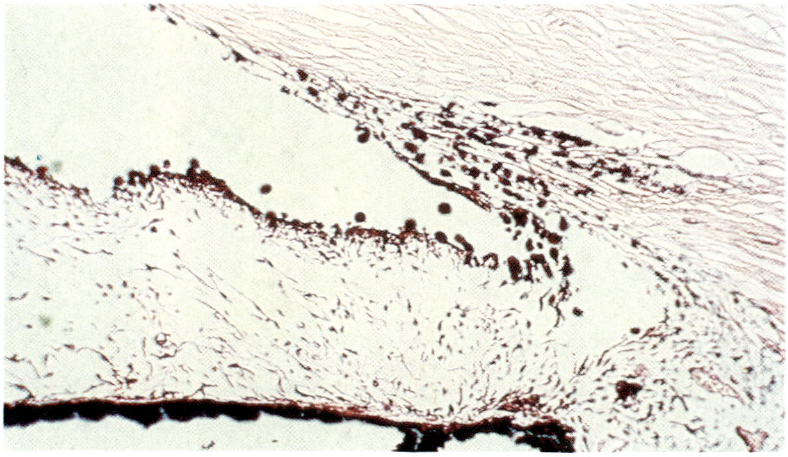

8.46 | Goniophotograph of the anterior chamber angle from a patient with pigmentary glaucoma, showing a dense band of pigment on the trabecular meshwork. (From Yanoff M, Fine BS: *Ocular Pathology. A Color Atlas,* ed 2. New York: Gower Medical Publishing, 1992, 16.10.)

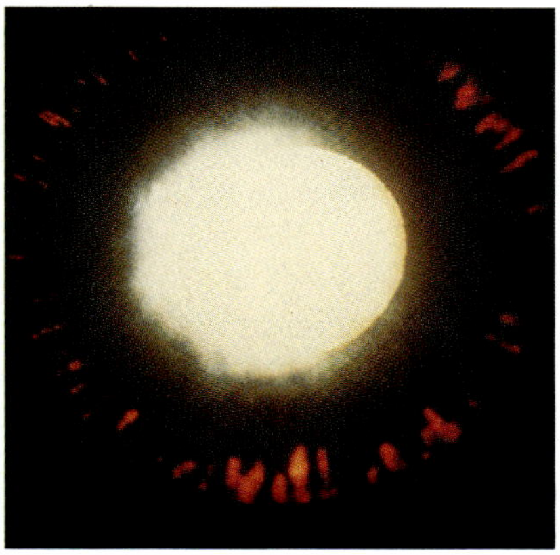

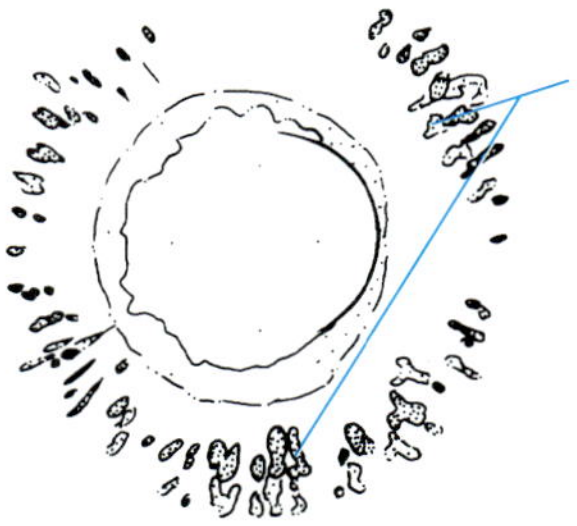

8.47 | Iris transillumination in a patient with pigmentary glaucoma shows radial, slit-like, midperipheral defects resulting from the loss of pigment epithelium.

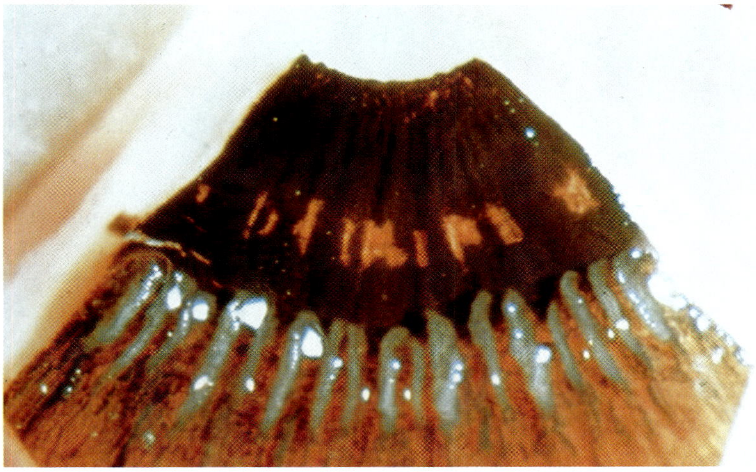

8.48 | Gross specimen reveals loss of pigment epithelium from the back of the iris. (From Yanoff M, Fine BS: *Ocular Pathology. A Color Atlas*, ed 2. New York: Gower Medical Publishing, 1992, 16.12.)

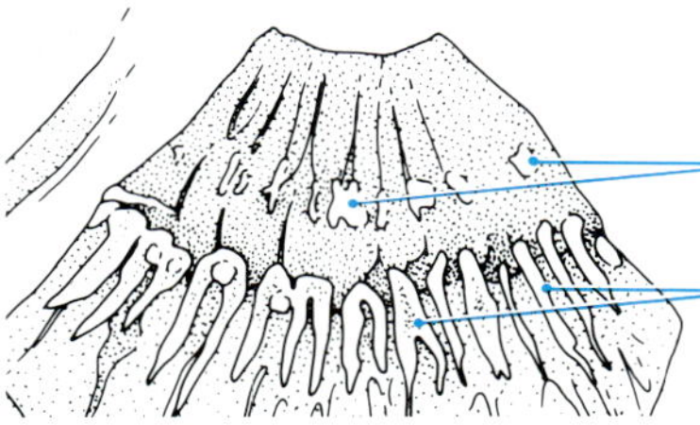

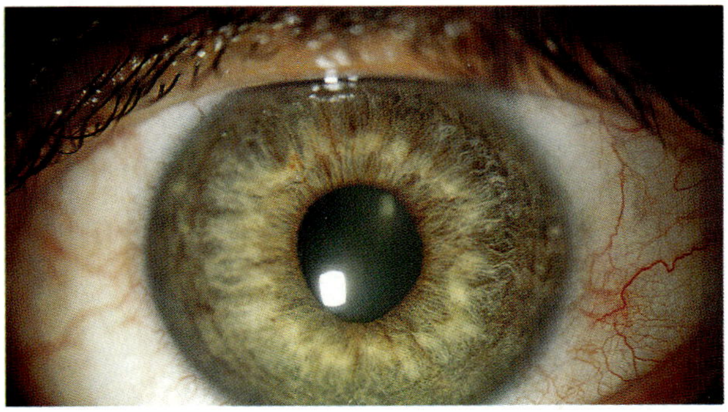

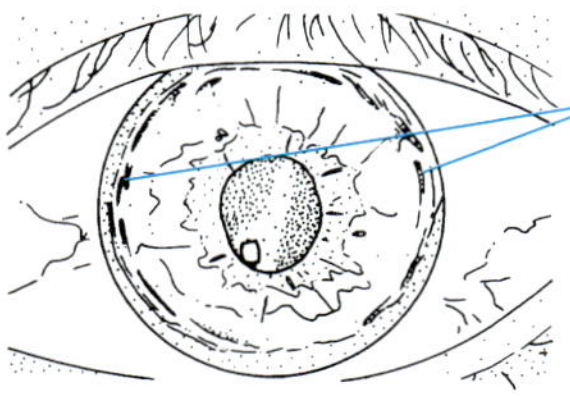

8.49 | Pigment deposition in concentric furrows on the anterior surface of the peripheral iris.

CORNEA

Pigment deposited on the corneal endothelium usually appears as a central, vertical brown band 1–6 mm long and up to 3 mm wide. Its shape is believed due to aqueous convection currents. Pigment deposits become phagocytosed by endothelial cells and remain for many years (Fig. 8.50). With time, the spindle becomes smaller and lighter and often requires more than cursory examination to identify it.

IRIS

The areas from which iris pigment has been lost appear as radial, slit-like, midperipheral transillumination defects most easily detected by careful transillumination. The defects can best be observed by a dark-adapted examiner using a fiberoptic transilluminator placed directly against the sclera so as to achieve a bright red reflex through the pupil. Pigment may also be deposited on the anterior iris surface, where it appears as concentric rings of fine pigment, densest in furrows peripherally.

ANTERIOR CHAMBER AND ANGLE

The anterior chamber is characteristically deep and the iris assumes a concave configuration, most prominent in the midperiphery. The angles are widely open and the iris insertion is usually markedly posterior, with a wide, sometimes ill-defined scleral spur. Pigment deposition on the trabecular meshwork classically appears as a homogeneous, dense band covering the filtering meshwork and a ring of pigment along Schwalbe's line (Sampaolesi line). In extreme cases, the entire angle from Schwalbe's line to the scleral spur may be covered with pigment. Glaucoma appears to be more severe in

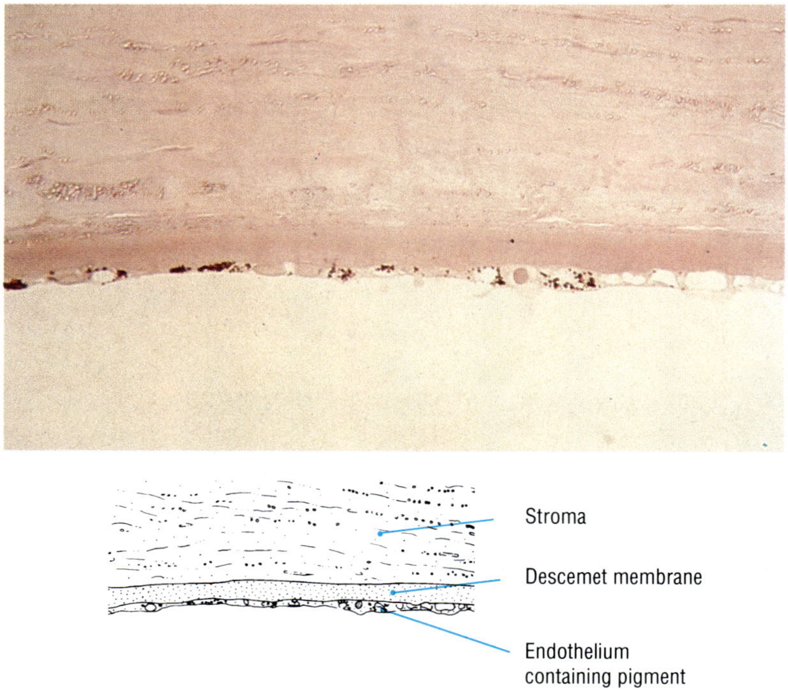

8.50 | Pigment dispersion syndrome. Granules of melanin pigment are present within corneal endothelial cells. (From Yanoff M, Fine BS: *Ocular Pathology. A Color Atlas*, ed 2. New York: Gower Medical Publishing, 1992, 16.11.)

the eye with the more heavily pigmented angle.[124] Pigment is deposited on the zonular fibers as well as on the lens surface, where it is usually found on the posterior capsule at the insertion of the posterior zonular fibers.

RETINA

Retinal detachments occur commonly in patients with PDS. The incidence does not appear to be related to the presence of glaucoma or treatment with miotics. In one series, the incidence of retinal detachments was 6.6% of patients with PDS and normal intraocular pressure (IOP) and 7.6% of those with glaucoma.[124] Most detachments occurred in males who were phakic and not highly myopic.

EPIDEMIOLOGY

PREVALENCE

The actual prevalence of PDS in the population is unknown, and many cases, perhaps most, go undiagnosed. Pigmentary glaucoma has been estimated to comprise approximately 5% of glaucoma patients, but this figure may include persons with PDS and normal IOP. In a series of 9,200 patients in a glaucoma referral practice, PDS was present in 407, of whom 259 had normal IOP, 47 had ocular hypertension, and 104 had glaucoma.[124]

Although some patients develop pigment dispersion in their early teens, most probably develop it in the third decade. PDS appears to be inherited as an autosomal dominant trait.[125,126] The mean age at diagnosis for patients with pigmentary glaucoma in most series is about 35–45 years for men and 40–50 years for women. The mean age at the time of diagnosis of patients with PDS with normal IOPs is younger at the time of diagnosis than those with glaucoma.

Most patients with PDS are white, and the disease is rare in blacks and Asians. There is an approximately equal sex distribution in patients with PDS and normal IOPs. Of patients with pigmentary glaucoma, however, male:female ratios between 1.7:1 and 4.4:1 have been reported.[124,127–129] The onset of glaucoma appears to occur earlier in males. The reason for this difference is unknown.

PATHOLOGY AND PATHOPHYSIOLOGY

REFRACTIVE ERROR

In most series, about 80% of patients with pigmentary glaucoma are myopic. The majority of reported patients with PDS without glaucoma are also myopic. The diagnosis of PDS is probably less likely to be made in emmetropes, who would be examined with lower frequency. It is also possible that myopia may enhance the phenotypic expression of the gene. The higher the myopia, the younger the age at which glaucomatous damage develops.[129] Patients with PDS and glaucoma are significantly more myopic than those without glaucoma.[130] Myopia appears to be a strong risk factor for the development of glaucoma.[131]

MECHANISM OF PIGMENT LIBERATION

At the present time, it is felt that accumulation of melanin pigment in the trabecular meshwork blocks the flow of aqueous humor through the outflow channels. Pigment particles perfused into enucleated eyes increase the resistance to outflow.[132,133] In individuals with normal IOP or primary open-angle glaucoma, phenylephrine either reduces or has no effect on IOP.

Patients with either pigmentary glaucoma or exfoliation syndrome may develop an acute rise in IOP associated with pigment release after exercise or pupillary dilatation, suggesting that these eyes are more susceptible to temporary obstruction of the aqueous outflow system by pigment particles.[134–136] There is a concomitant decrease in the facility of outflow.[137]

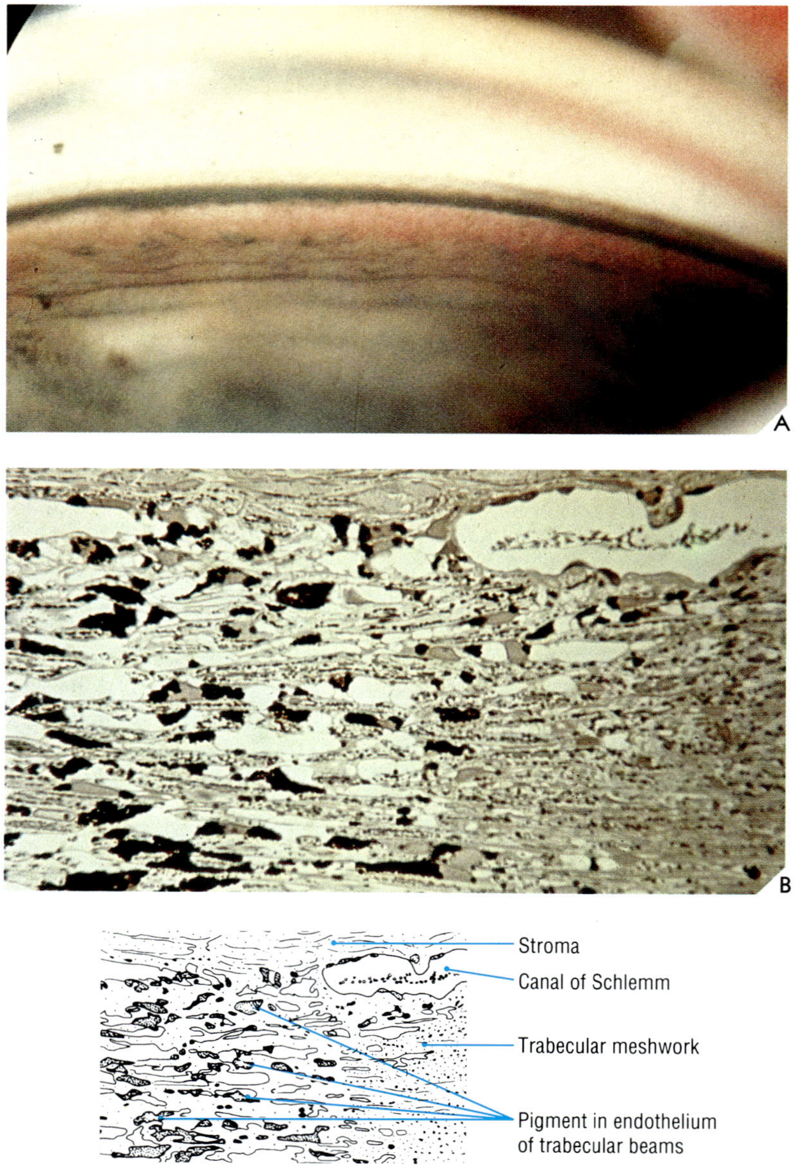

8.51 | Pigment dispersion syndrome. *A:* The anterior chamber angle is deeply pigmented. *B:* Melanin pigment is present within the endothelial cells lining the beams of the trabecular meshwork. (From Yanoff M, Fine BS: *Ocular Pathology. A Color Atlas*, ed 2. New York: Gower Medical Publishing, 1992, 16.11.)

In 1979, Campbell proposed that physiologic movement of the pupil in the presence of a posteriorly concave iris results in rubbing of the pigment epithelium against the zonular bundles, dislodging pigment granules.[128] The loss of pigment and of cells that overlie the zonules corresponds well with the midperipheral radial pattern of iris transillumination defects. This has been confirmed by scanning electron microscopy.[139] Campbell felt that young male myopes are most typically affected because an increase in the size of the myopic globe may be associated with an enlargement of the ciliary body ring in relation to the lens. This enlargement causes the peripheral iris to sag and establish contact with the zonules. Male predominance may occur because men have eyes of greater size. Richardson has hypothesized that the relative rarity of PDS in blacks and Asians might be related to heavy pigmentation and iris stromal compactness, which might prevent peripheral iris sagging.[140]

DEVELOPMENT OF GLAUCOMA

The time between diagnosis of pigment dispersion and the onset of glaucoma varies considerably. Other patients may never develop glaucoma. A recent long-term retrospective analysis involving 65 patients reported development of glaucoma in 36% of male and 33% of female patients with PDS after a mean follow-up of 17 years.[128]

The pigment particles are located both within and outside the cells that line the trabeculum.[141–143] There is degeneration of endothelial cells of the trabecular meshwork, trapping of cell debris or breakdown products of pigment-containing cells, which is different from melanomalytic glaucoma, and sclerosis of the trabecular beams (Figs. 8.51 and 8.52)(see Van Buskirk, this chapter). The trabeculae are left denuded and there is breakdown and collapse of the intertrabecular spaces with degeneration and sclerosis of the trabeculae.

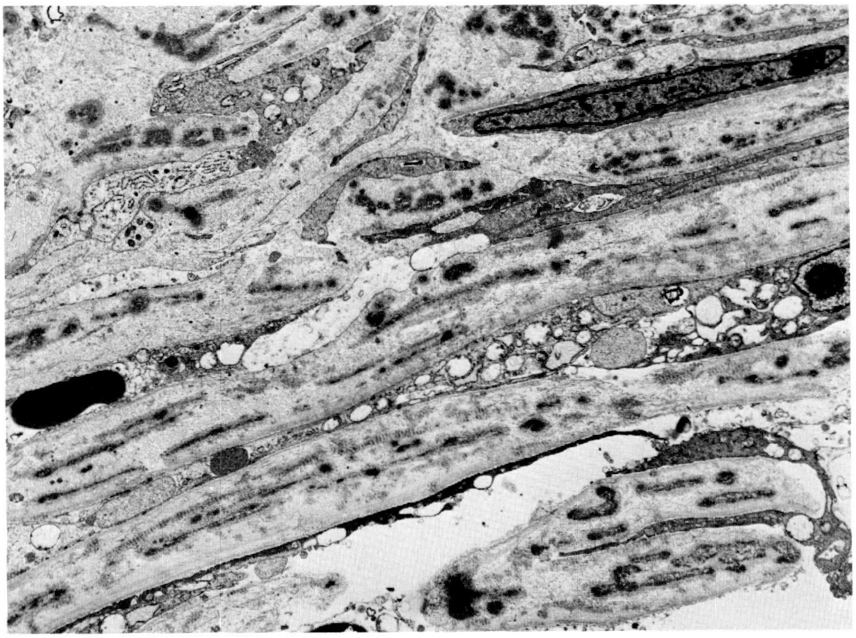

8.52 | Electron micrograph of the trabecular meshwork in pigmentary glaucoma. Trabecular sheets have collapsed and fused, leading to obliteration of the aqueous pathway. (From Ritch R, Shields MB, Krupin T (eds): *The Glaucomas.* St. Louis: CV Mosby, 1989, 988.)

Richardson postulated that obstruction of the aqueous outflow system and the development of glaucoma occur in two stages (Fig. 8.53). Accumulation of pigment in moderate amounts over a short period may acutely obstruct the intertrabecular space and result in transient elevation of IOP. With migration of the trabecular cells away from the beams and cell autolysis, the remaining attached cells spread over the denuded portions of the meshwork. When the meshwork loses the capacity to undergo self-repair, the trabecular beams degenerate and the second stage is entered.

NATURAL HISTORY

Although pigmentary glaucoma is usually a progressive disease that requires medical or surgical management to prevent damage to the optic nerve and glaucomatous visual field loss, it sometimes pursues a mild course and occasionally becomes less severe, particularly with increasing age. Trabecular pigmentation, Krukenberg spindles, and iris transillumination defects may also regress.[138,144] In a few patients, the IOP has been noted to return toward normal after several years of treatment, permitting reduction of medications.[145] Others may develop glaucomatous damage but remain undiagnosed and later ameliorate spontaneously, so that when the damage is finally detected an erroneous diagnosis of low-tension glaucoma is made.[146] Cases of so-

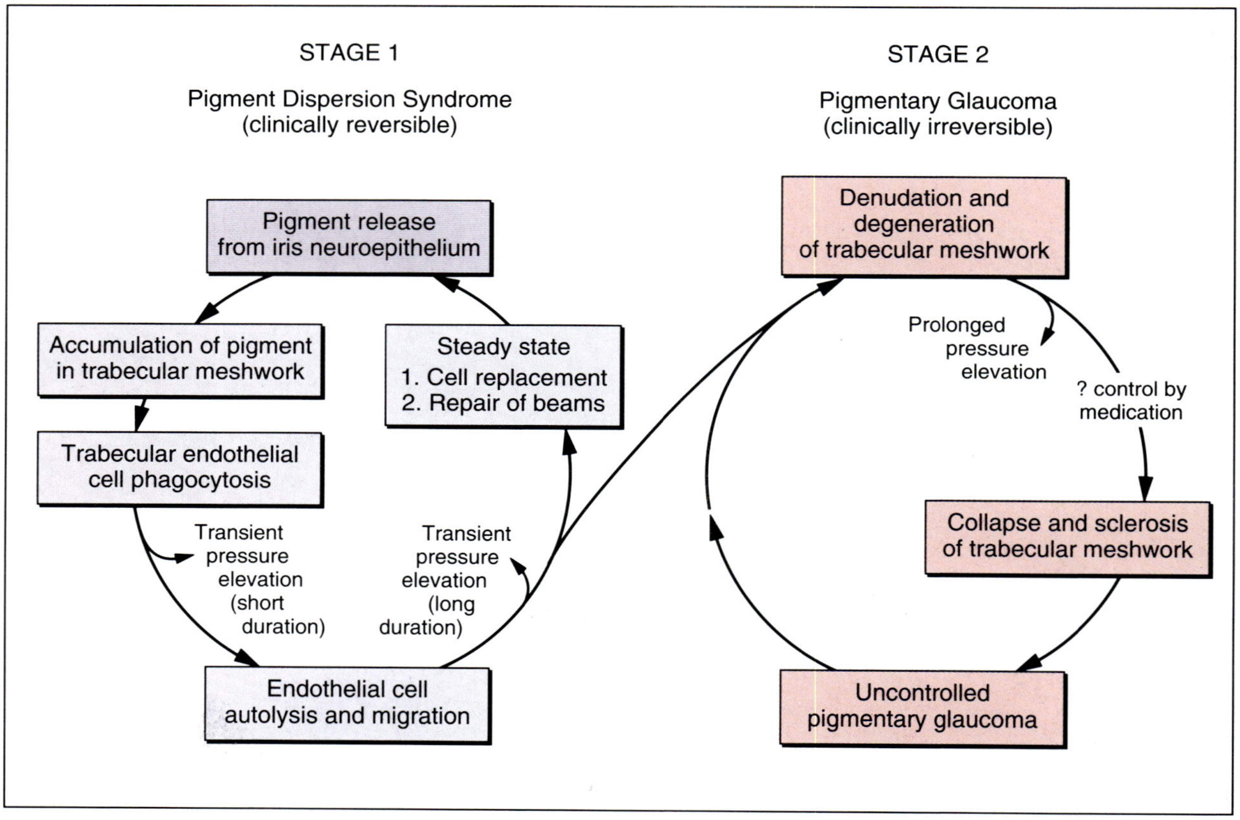

8.53 | Hypothetical mechanism that may explain the pathophysiology of pigmentary glaucoma. The first stage of the disease is clinically reversible and gives rise to transient rises in IOP. The second stage, characterized by irreparable damage to the trabecular meshwork, is irreversible and is accompanied by uncontrolled glaucoma. (Adapted from Ritch R, Shields MB, Krupin T (eds): *The Glaucomas.* St. Louis: CV Mosby, 1989, 990.)

called "burned out" glaucoma in the older literature may well have included patients with pigmentary glaucoma that remitted spontaneously after cessation of pigment liberation.

Speakman[145] has hypothesized that pigment liberation occurs only for a limited number of years and eventually ceases. As the patient ages, the lens continues to grow slowly and the average size of the pupil decreases. The combination of increasing lens diameter and decreasing pupil size creates a relative pupillary block, which causes an anterior shift in the peripheral iris away from the zonules.[138] Pigmentary glaucoma has also been noted to remit after lens subluxation.[147]

MANAGEMENT

MEDICAL THERAPY

Although patients with elevated IOP are usually begun on a beta-blocking agent, miotics may be the treatment of choice for pigmentary glaucoma. Stabilization of pigment liberation or regression of deposited pigment should be a goal of therapy. The beneficial effects of miotics are potentially twofold. First, they reduce pupillary movement with lighting conditions, thereby reducing movement of the iris against the zonules. Second, they increase iridolenticular contact, producing a relative pupillary block and flattening of the peripheral iris, which reduces or eliminates iridozonular apposition. Pilocarpine Ocuserts® are well tolerated by younger patients with pigment dispersion. Because of the increased incidence of retinal detachment in patients with pigment dispersion syndrome, a careful retinal examination should be peformed before and after initiating treatment with cholinergic agents.

An alpha-adrenergic blocking agent, such as thymoxamine hydrochloride or dapiprazole, which constricts the pupil but does not affect accommodation or aqueous humor dynamics, could prove beneficial. Their potential therapeutic use in patients with pigmentary glaucoma or prophylactically in patients with pigment dispersion syndrome and pressure fluctuations is quite intriguing. Epinephrine compounds, beta-adrenergic blocking agents, and carbonic anhydrase inhibitors appear to be effective in patients with pigmentary glaucoma.

LASER AND SURGICAL TREATMENT

In contradistinction to all other forms of open-angle glaucoma, younger patients with pigmentary glaucoma have better results with argon laser trabeculoplasty than older ones.[148–154] In the series with longest follow-up to date, the cumulative success rate at 6 years was 72% for patients under age 42 and 18% for those over.[150] This may relate to the distribution of pigment in the trabecular meshwork. Examination of specimens removed at the time of trabeculectomy in younger patients showed the pigment to be primarily in the uveoscleral and corneoscleral meshwork, whereas in older patients it was localized to the juxtacanalicular meshwork and external wall of Schlemm's canal (Ritch R, Gennaro J, unpublished observations). Argon laser trabeculoplasty, therefore, might lead to collapse and sclerosis of Schlemm's canal in older patients.

The surgical management of patients with pigmentary glaucoma follows the same principles and considerations used in the management of primary open-angle glaucoma. The appearance and change in the optic nerve, along with visual field defects, should be the principal guidelines used in deciding whether surgery is needed. Most patients respond well to standard filtration operations. Adjunctive 5-fluorouracil injections may be helpful in younger patients.

Section VII

Exfoliation Syndrome

Robert Ritch
Jeffrey Liebmann

Exfoliation syndrome is the single most common identifiable cause of open-angle glaucoma in the world. In many countries it comprises the majority of open-angle glaucoma patients. In addition, many patients with exfoliation syndrome develop angle-closure glaucoma. As with pigmentary glaucoma, exfoliation syndrome is vastly underdiagnosed, particularly in its early stages, as it often requires a high index of suspicion on the part of the examiner and a second slit-lamp examination, after pupillary dilatation, to make the diagnosis.

Many terms have been used to describe this syndrome over the years. The most common has been *pseudoexfoliation*, coined to differentiate it from true exfoliation of the lens capsule seen in glass blowers and others exposed to intense heat sources. Because the latter is extremely rare, we have elected to use the simpler term *exfoliation syndrome* (XFS). The term *glaucoma capsulare* is common in the Scandinavian literature. *Ocular elastosis* has recently been suggested as being more appropriate in light of recent advances in our knowledge of the underlying cause of the disorder.[151]

EPIDEMIOLOGY

First described in 1917 by Lindberg, XFS was thought for many years to be peculiar to Scandinavia and northern Europe, a misconception still common among many ophthalmologists. The prevalence of XFS increases with age. In Norway, it was found to range from 0.4% for ages 50–59 to 7.9% for ages 80–89.[152] In Finland, rates of 14.2% for ages 60–69 to 34.7% for patients over 80 were noted.[153] In the Framingham Eye Study, age-specific prevalence rates in patients not identified specifically as having glaucoma rose from 0.6% for ages 52–64 to 5% for ages 75–85.[154] In the southeastern United States, XFS was found in 1.6% over age 30 and 3.2% older than 60.[155]

Observer bias is reduced when the same clinician examines patients in different locations. Aasved found a 4% prevalence of XFS in the general population in England, 4.7% in Germany, and 6.3% in Norway.[156] Forsius found 0% in Eskimos, 12% in Russians, and 29% in Icelanders.[157] It is common in Japan, India, among Navajo Indians, Australian aborigines, and South African blacks, but not among American blacks.

The reasons for variation among populations are unknown. No clear pattern of inheritance has been discerned, nor has any environmental factor been proven to predispose to the disorder. Intraocular pressure (IOP) response to topical corticosteroid testing is similar to that found in the normal population. It usually presents unilaterally (really asymmetrically), but tends eventually to affect both eyes. Henry et al found that the probability of developing XFS in the fellow eye was 6.8% at 5 years and 16.8% at 10 years.[158]

The reported prevalence of XFS in patients with open-angle glaucoma also varies widely, for example: Iceland 72%, England 0–14%, Scotland 16–62%, Germany 0–11%, USA 3–28%, Italy 15–60%, India 18–24%, and Japan 11–26%.[159]

Glaucoma occurs more frequently among persons with XFS. When both glaucoma and XFS are unilateral, they virtually always are ipsilateral. In 100 consecutive patients with XFS, 78% had normal IOP, 15% had ocular hypertension, and 7% had glaucoma.[160] XFS was unilateral in 76% and bilateral in 24%. Men comprised 21% and women 79% of eyes with XFS without glaucoma, whereas there was no sex predilection for those with glaucoma. In a well-defined study, the 5- and 10-year cumulative probabilities of initially nonglaucomatous eyes with XFS developing glaucoma were 5.3% and 15.4%, respectively, a significantly higher rate than would be expected in a similar group of patients without the disease.[158]

Glaucoma in XFS has a poorer prognosis than primary open-angle glaucoma, presents with higher IOP and more severe disc and visual field damage than primary open-angle glaucoma, has a more serious clinical course, and has been considered more difficult to control.

Although XFS is usually considered an ocular disease, recent electron micrographic studies have revealed typical exfoliation material in the skin, heart, lungs, liver, kidney, gallbladder, and meninges of patients with XFS.[158A, 158B] This indicates that XFS may be a systemic disease involving abnormal connective tissue metabolism throughout the body.

CLINICAL FINDINGS

XFS is characterized clinically by the presence of small, grayish deposits of fibrillar–granular exfoliation material within the anterior segment of the eye. These are most commonly seen on the pupillary border and anterior lens capsule, but are also found on the cornea, trabecular meshwork, zonules, and ciliary body.

LENS

Exfoliation material on the anterior lens capsule is the sine qua non of XFS. It is distributed in a classic pattern: a central zone or disc, an intermediate clear zone, and a peripheral granular zone.

The central zone is a homogeneous light-gray or white sheet lying on the anterior surface of the lens capsule (Fig. 8.54). Its diameter varies from 1.5–3.0

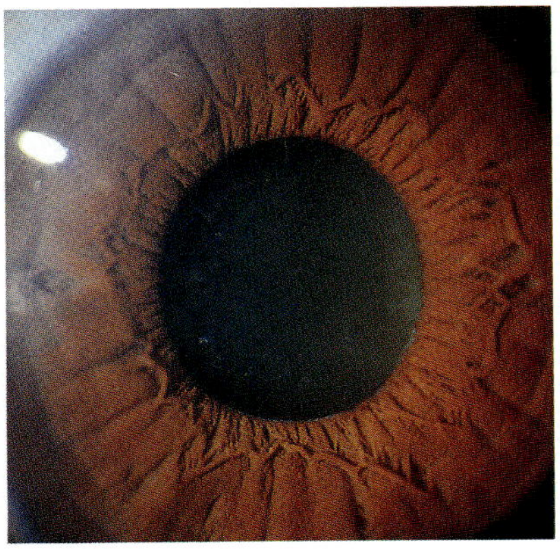

8.54 | The central zone is flat, homogeneous, white to gray, and often difficult to visualize in the undilated state.

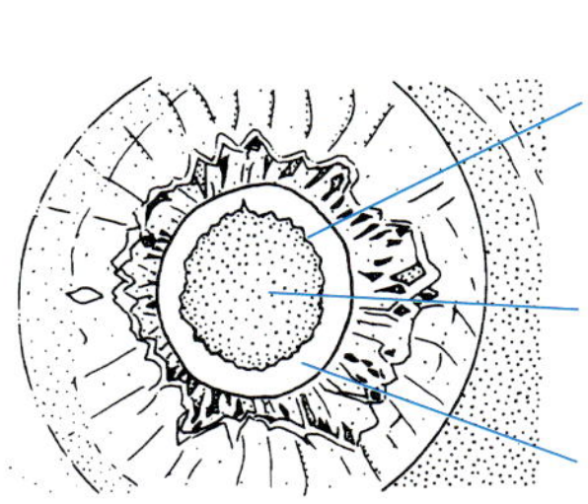

mm and it is usually slightly smaller than the physiologic pupil. In some cases the exfoliation material at the peripheral edge of the zone is rolled up, possibly due to physiologic movement of the iris sphincter butting against it.

The intermediate clear zone, extending from the pupillary border 1–2 mm peripherally, is an area of anterior lens capsule that is usually free of visible exfoliation material. Pupillary constriction and dilatation causes the exfoliation material to be brushed free of the lens capsule in this region.

The peripheral zone is a grayish-white granular ring which becomes visible when the pupil is dilated and is typically granular in the periphery and frosty white centrally (Fig. 8.55). Radial striations are often seen, and layers may be present. Equatorially it extends as granular tongue-shaped projections which merge into the normal capsule before reaching the anterior zone of insertion of the zonular fibers.

Many patients do not have this classic appearance, particularly in the early stages of the disease. Our present concept of the development of the appearance of exfoliation material on the lens surface is that it is first deposited as a fine, homogeneous layer, at which stage it cannot be recognized clinically. Clefts then appear in the region of the future intermediate zone as the iris sphincter rubs against the material. When most of the intermediate zone has been cleared, the remaining exfoliation material appears as bridges between the central and peripheral zones. In visualizing the earlier stages at the slit-lamp, placing the slit beam at 45° to the axis of observation, reducing the light source, and focusing temporally may help to highlight the deposits on the lens surface.

Lens subluxation or dislocation may occur spontaneously or with minimal history of trauma.

IRIS

Changes in the appearance of the iris occur in virtually all patients with XFS and involve the pupillary ruff, sphincter, crypts, vessels, and pigment epithelium.

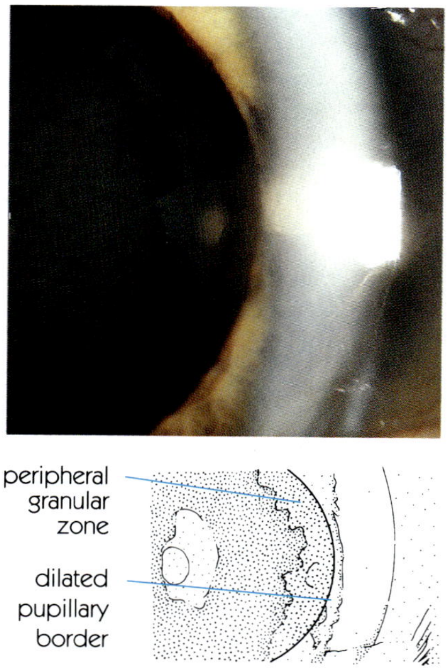

8.55 | Exfoliation material present in the peripheral granular zone on the anterior surface of the lens capsule.

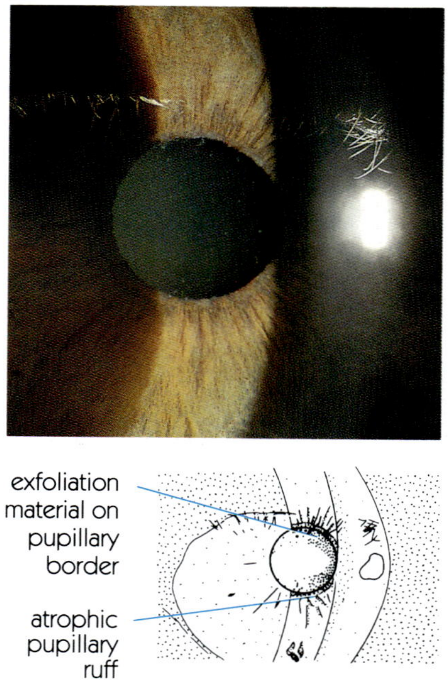

8.56 | Exfoliation material present on the pupillary border. Atrophy of the pupillary ruff is an important secondary clinical sign of the disease and may be present before the development of visible exfoliation material on the iris or lens.

Deposits of exfoliation material on the iris sphincter and pupillary margin are a hallmark of the diagnosis (Fig. 8.56). Only recently appreciated are the findings associated with more subtle signs related to loss of pigment from the epithelium in the iris sphincter region. We believe at present that the pigment is lost secondary to the iris rubbing against the exfoliation material on the lens surface, so that, while the iris dislodges the exfoliation material, the exfoliation material acts like sandpaper, rubbing off iris pigment and leading to its dispersion throughout the anterior segment. It is this aspect which makes us regard XFS as a pigment dispersion syndrome of the elderly.

The most prominent of these signs involves defects in the pupillary ruff.[161-163] Ruff atrophy is often accompanied by a moth-eaten appearance of iris sphincter transillumination. When pigment loss is severe the entire sphincter region may transilluminate. There may be a patchy, punctate pattern of transillumination over the iris peripheral to the sphincter. Deposition of pigment granules on the iris surface is more commonly seen in blue irides and may be difficult to detect in darkly pigmented ones (Fig. 8.57). Particulate pigment deposition on the sphincter is characteristic of XFS and may assume a whorl-like pattern.[163]

On angiography, iris vessels are characterized by a reduced number, lack of normal radial pattern, neovascular clumps, and leakage of fluorescein.[164,165]

ZONULES AND CILIARY BODY

Exfoliation material is often prominent on the zonules and ciliary body, where it may be detected before visualization on the anterior lens surface. The zonules may be weakened and broken, and this presumably leads to the phakodonesis and partial lens subluxation commonly seen with extensive exfoliation (Fig. 8.58).

CORNEA

Scattered flakes or clumps of exfoliation material may be deposited on the endothelium and may adhere to it. A more consistent finding is a diffuse, nonspecific pigmentation on the central corneal endothelium, occasionally

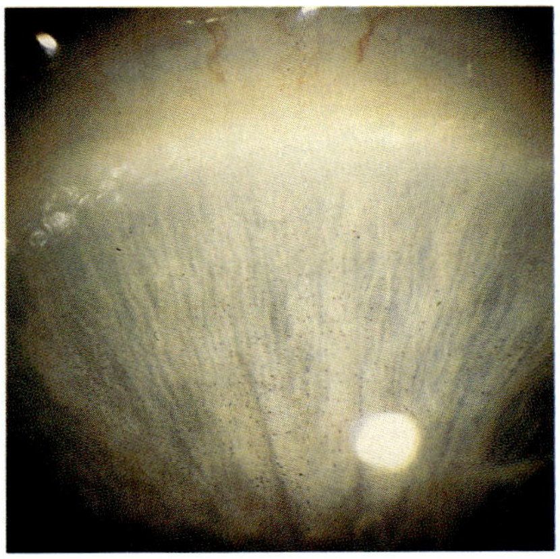

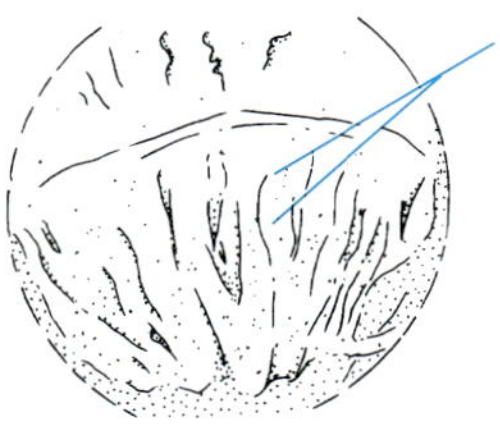

8.57 | Particulate pigment deposited diffusely on the anterior surface of the iris. Compare this to the pattern often found in pigment dispersion syndrome (Fig. 8.49).

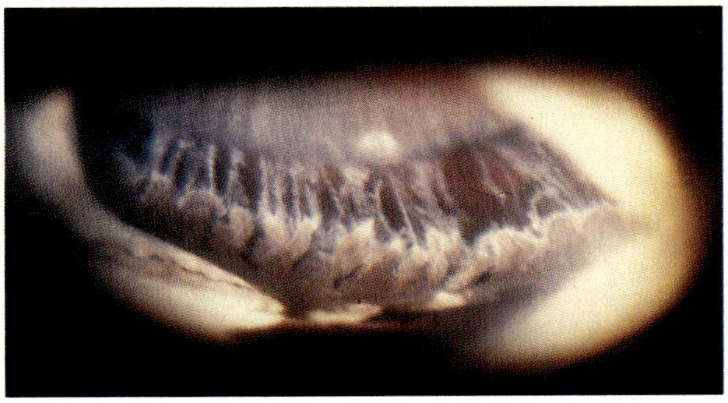

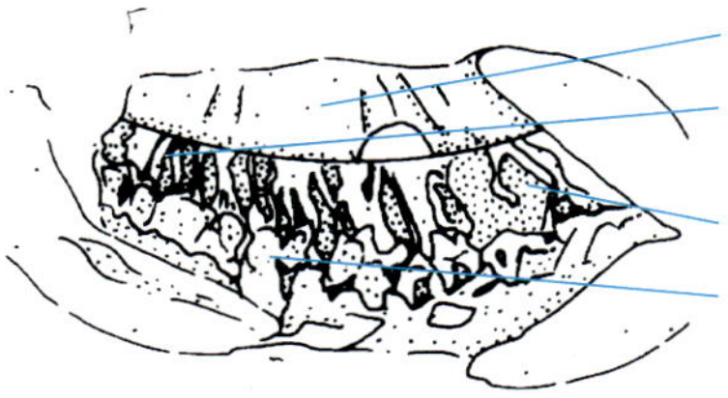

8.58 | Zonules covered with exfoliation material. Many of the zonules are broken, leading to lens subluxation.

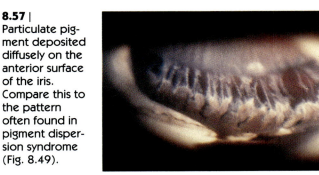

in the form of a Krukenberg spindle. A decreased cell count has been noted in unilateral XFS with[166] and without glaucoma.[167] Polymegathism and polymorphism have been found in both the affected and unaffected eyes of patients with unilateral XFS, suggesting that changes in the corneal endothelium may provide evidence for early diagnosis.[168]

ANTERIOR CHAMBER AND ANGLE

Pigment dispersion in the anterior chamber and deposition on the anterior segment structures are a hallmark of the XFS. After mydriasis, extensive pigment dispersion is often present. This pigment is released from the posterior pigment epithelium of the iris as the pupil dilates.

Increased meshwork pigmentation is a prominent sign of XFS. Unlike pigment dispersion syndrome, the distribution tends to be uneven or splotchy, and less well defined. Pigment is often deposited on Schwalbe's line or on the corneal endothelium anterior to it. Increased meshwork pigmentation may be an early diagnostic finding before the appearance of deposits of exfoliation material on the pupillary margin or anterior lens capsule.[169] However, the extent of pigmentation and severity of glaucoma do not always correlate.[170] Finally, flecks of exfoliation material may also be seen adherent to the trabecular meshwork.

Although most patients have open angles, narrow angles occur in approximately 23–32% of patients,[170,171] with peripheral anterior synechiae present in 14%.[171] Pupillary block may be caused by posterior synechiae, anterior lens movement secondary to zonular weakness or dialysis, or increased iris thickness or rigidity.

HISTOPATHOLOGY

Exfoliation material appears to be produced by the equatorial lens epithelium, iris pigment epithelium, and nonpigmented ciliary epithelium. At these locations it is commonly found within epithelial cells in association with abnormal basement membrane.[172] The lens capsule itself appears normal, although it may contain amorphous material. The exfoliation material on the surface of the lens is believed to result partially from deposition of material produced by the iris and ciliary body and partially from material produced by the lens epithelium which passively diffuses through the anterior lens capsule (Fig. 8.59).

Exfoliation material is found in the conjunctiva of eyes both with XFS and in fellow eyes without clinical evidence of disease.[173] More recently, it has been shown that XFS can be diagnosed before the appearance of exfoliation material on the anterior lens surface by conjunctival biopsy.[169] The conjunctiva appears to be an independent source of exfoliation material that precedes clinical recognition of exfoliation material on anterior segment structures.

Exfoliation material is deposited on the iris surface and is found in close proximity to stromal fibroblasts. Pigment epithelial degeneration leads to pigment liberation and dispersion in the anterior chamber. Iris vessel lumens are often narrowed and may become obliterated, leading to vessel dropout, patchy iris neovascularization, and leakage of dye during fluorescein angiography.

In the trabecular meshwork, exfoliation material is present on and between the trabecular beams, beneath the trabecular endothelial cells, and beneath the endothelium of both inner and outer walls of Schlemm's canal, but not in the canal itself.[172,174–176] Extensive deposits of exfoliation material may be present in the meshwork of normotensive eyes.[177] It is unclear whether the exfoliation material is merely deposited on the angle structures and later phagocytosed or is produced in the meshwork itelf.

Exfoliation material is often deposited on the zonules and ciliary body early in the course of the disease (Fig. 8.60). It may be deposited on the vitreous face long after cataract extraction. Eagle et al found exfoliation material in the wall of a short posterior ciliary artery.[178] These authors suggested it to be an abnormal basement membrane synthesized at multiple sites by aging cells. Streeten et al suggested that exfoliation fibers can derive from cells which do not normally form basement membrane.[151] Biopsies of the skin and oral mucosa for extraocular involvement have not revealed any conclusive information.

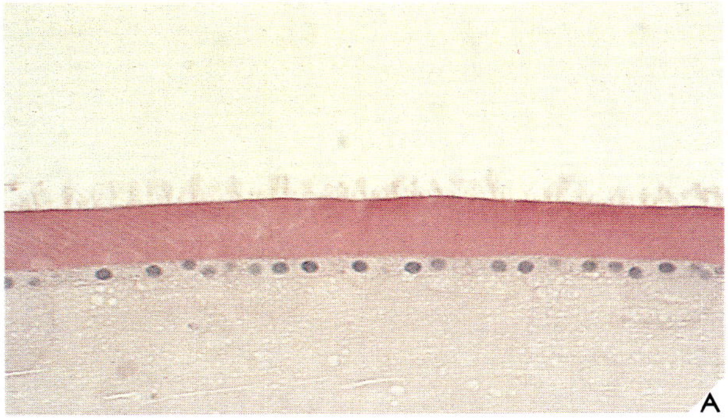

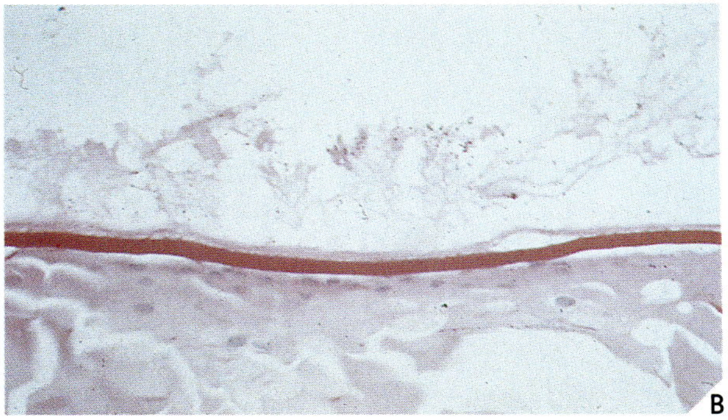

8.59 | Exfoliation material peeling off the anterior lens capsule. *A:* In the central disc area, the exfoliation material is deposited in small slivers that line up parallel to each other. *B:* In the peripheral granular area, the material is in great abundance and has a thick, dendritic appearance (*A* and *B*, PAS stain.) (From Yanoff M, Fine BS: *Ocular Pathology. A Color Atlas*, ed 2. New York: Gower Medical Publishing, 1992, 10.5.)

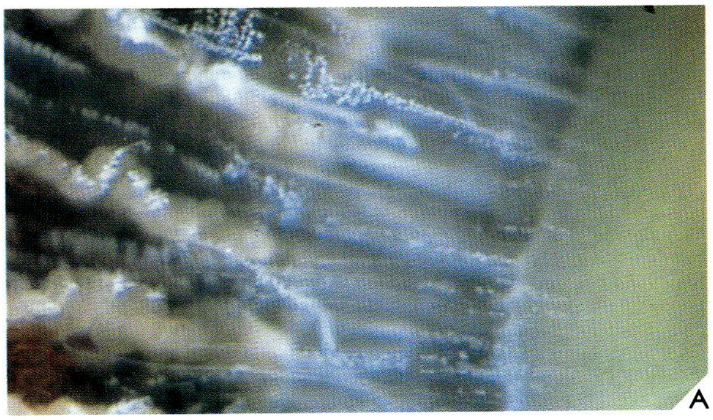

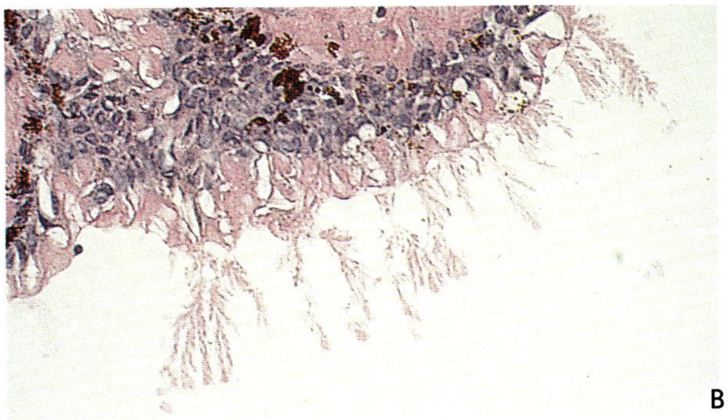

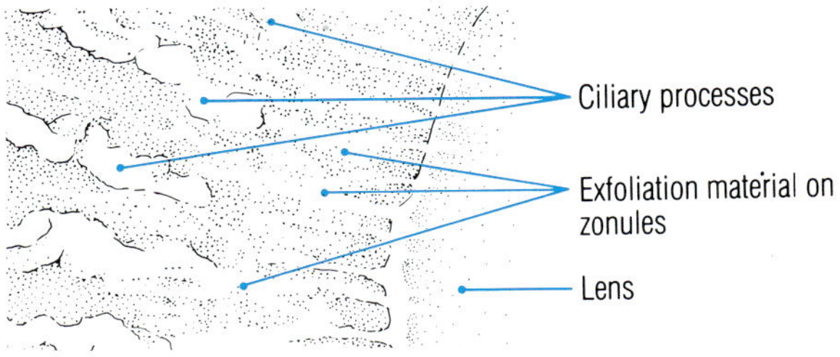

8.60 | *A* and *B:* Exfoliation material near the zonular insertion. (*A*, courtesy of Dr. RC Eagle Jr. *B*, PAS stain.) (From Yanoff M, Fine BS: *Ocular Pathology. A Color Atlas*, ed 2. New York: Gower Medical Publishing, 1992, 10.6.)

NATURE OF THE EXFOLIATION MATERIAL

Electron microscopy of exfoliation material reveals characteristic cross-banded fibrils and filamentous subunits associated with an amorphous ground substance.[172,179] The fibrils, each about 30 nm in diameter, form an irregular meshwork within a loose fibrogranular matrix containing 6–10-nm microfibrils.[151,179] The biochemical composition is consistent with a glycosaminoglycan or glycoprotein.[180,189] Lectin staining suggests a complex carbohydrate composition, with both *O*-linked sialomucin-type and *N*-linked oligosaccharide chains.[182] There are histochemical and antigenic similarities between zonular elastic microfibrils and exfoliation material.[183–186] Streeten et al[151] found typical fibrils of exfoliation material in close proximity to oxytalan fibers, leading them to suggest that XFS might be a form of elastosis. Li et al recently reported the presence of binding sites to amyloid P protein on exfoliation fibrils, similar to the binding sites found on normal elastic fibers.[187]

MECHANISM OF GLAUCOMA

OPEN-ANGLE GLAUCOMA

Potential mechanisms of glaucoma in XFS include alterations of the trabecular cell surface, blockage of the meshwork by exogenous exfoliation material, blockage of the meshwork by liberated iris pigment, and concomitant primary open-angle glaucoma. Obstruction of the aqueous outflow system directly by or consequent to interaction of the trabecular cells with pigment is usually considered to be the predominant cause of glaucoma in XFS.

ANGLE-CLOSURE GLAUCOMA

Angle-closure glaucoma occurring with XFS is much more common than previously realized. The weakened zonules appear to allow the lens to move slightly more anteriorly than normal, while the pupil does not dilate as well as in eyes without XFS. The iris may also be thicker than normal, but this remains conjectural. These factors tend to promote the development of relative pupillary block.

DIFFERENTIAL DIAGNOSIS

The differential diagnosis of XFS includes diseases associated with pigment dispersion in the anterior segment and true exfoliation of the lens capsule. The trabecular meshwork in patients with uveitis tends to have splotchy pigment, with peripheral anterior synechiae (PAS). In chronic angle-closure glaucoma, after iridectomy, the widened angle may have areas of increased pigmentation. True exfoliation of the lens capsule is a rare clinical entity associated with exposure to high temperatures, and is associated with cataract but not with glaucoma. A traumatic exoliation or peeling of the lens capsule can occur, but appears to be extremely rare. Other conditions characterized by pigment changes, such as Fuchs' heterochromic iridocyclitis, pigmentation of the chamber angle with aging or after surgery, and pigmentation secondary to intraocular tumors can usually be readily distinguished.

MANAGEMENT

The approach to the management of XFS has been considered to be no different from that for primary open-angle glaucoma. However, the response to intervention differs in comparison with primary open-angle glaucoma. Glaucoma in XFS responds less well to ß-blockers, and ß-blockers alone are often insufficient to control IOP. Patients with glaucoma and XFS are more likely to require laser or surgical treatment than those with primary open-angle glaucoma.

Cholinergic agents are effective and have been reported to have a greater additive effect with ß-blockers than in primary open-angle glaucoma.[188] Miotics may prove to be the drugs of choice for open-angle glaucoma in XFS, just as in pigmentary glaucoma. Certainly, they should be considered in patients not controlled on ß-blockers alone, and if the combination suffices the ß-blocker should be discontinued to see if the miotics alone can control the pressure. The effectiveness of epinephrine compounds is variable. Carbonic anhydrase inhibitors are often effective.

Argon laser trabeculoplasty (ALT) is particularly effective, at least early on, in eyes with XFS. The baseline IOP is usually higher than in eyes with primary open-angle glaucoma undergoing ALT, and the initial drop in IOP is greater. About 20% of eyes treated with ALT develop sudden, late rises in IOP, possibly due to continued pigment liberation into the anterior chamber and further blockage of the trabecular meshwork.[189,190]

If surgery is required, the procedure of choice is trabeculectomy. Surgical complications are more common in eyes with XFS. Zonular support is typically weak, and marked intraoperative anterior lens movement or subluxation may occur, leading to inadvertent lens damage during iridectomy, vitreous loss, or late incarceration of vitreous into the internal ostium. Previously undetected iris neovascularization may lead to intraoperative or delayed hyphema from the surgical iridectomy.

Patients with XFS are elderly and often have coexisting cataract. Eyes with XFS are more prone to complications at the time of cataract surgery than eyes without XFS. These complications include insufficient mydriasis, zonular dialyses, lens dislocation, rupture of the posterior capsule, and vitreous loss.[191–193] Patients may require one or more sphincterotomies to enlarge the pupil. Spontaneous lens displacement, which may not be visible preoperatively, may worsen considerably on entering the eye or beginning anterior capsulectomy. The presence of subtle iridodonesis or phakodonesis indicates loose or ruptured zonules. Postoperatively, these patients are at greater risk for developing an immediate elevation of intraocular pressure.[194]

Section VIII

Other Secondary Glaucomas

E. Michael Van Buskirk

OCULAR TRAUMA

Any form of eye trauma can disrupt the aqueous humor outflow pathways and cause glaucoma. Blunt trauma distorts the spherical configuration of the multilaminate ocular globe.[195] Sudden shearing of one layer against another during blunt injury produces separation of the uveal tract at the chamber angle. In some cases, the disruption tears the root of the iris away from the ciliary body, manifesting as iridodialysis[196] (Fig. 8.61). In other cases, the ciliary body and iris together are separated away from the sclera, leaving a gap or a cyclodialysis[196] (Fig. 8.62). In most cases, however, the attachments between the iridociliary body and the chamber angle are partially disrupted, leading to a configuration of the chamber angle known as anterior chamber

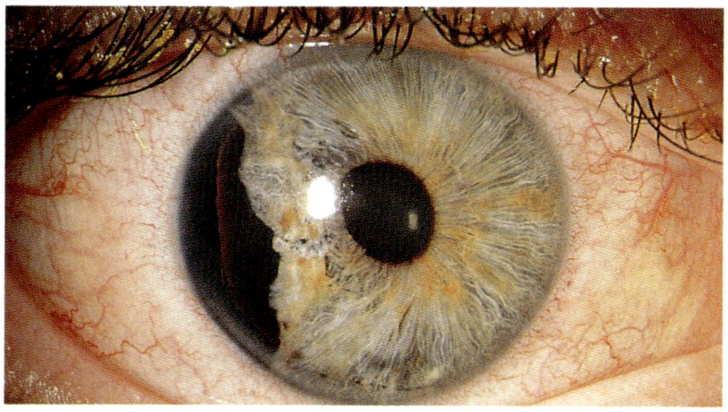

8.61 | Iridodialysis. Separation of the iris root from its attachment to the ciliary body after blunt trauma.

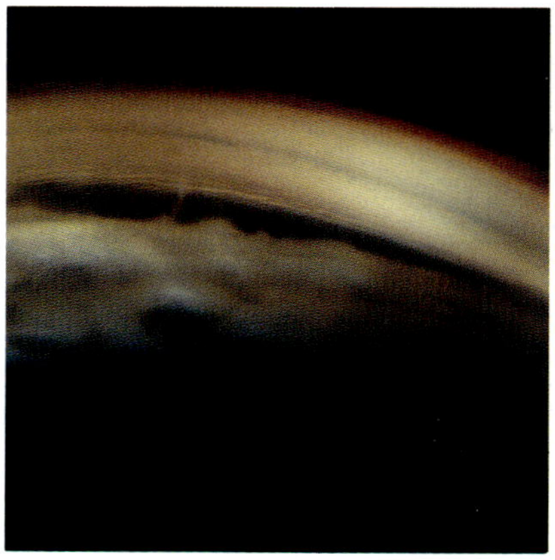

8.62 | Cyclodialysis. Separation of the ciliary body and iris from its attachment to the scleral spur, creating a cleft between the uvea and the inner wall of the sclera after blunt trauma.

angle recession, where the ciliary band becomes many times wider than normal[197] (Figs. 8.63 and 8.64). Tearing away of the uveal meshwork and ciliary muscle fibers causes the scleral spur to stand out brightly as a sharply demarcated white line. The ciliary band develops a slate gray appearance; in some cases, the bare white sclera can be seen (see Fig. 8.63). With this disruption of tissue there is often showering of pigment into the chamber angle that tends to accumulate inferiorly, appearing spattered over the surface of the trabecular meshwork (Fig. 8.65). There may be enough associated inflammation to create peripheral anterior synechia within areas of recessed or even nonrecessed angle. Balls or clumps of pigment commonly rest in the inferior angle after blunt trauma (see Fig. 8.65), even when angle recession is not clinically manifest.

Because the ciliary muscle is an important modulator of trabecular outflow, damage to it may cause increased resistance to aqueous humor outflow, diminished outflow reserve, and elevated intraocular pressure (IOP), depending

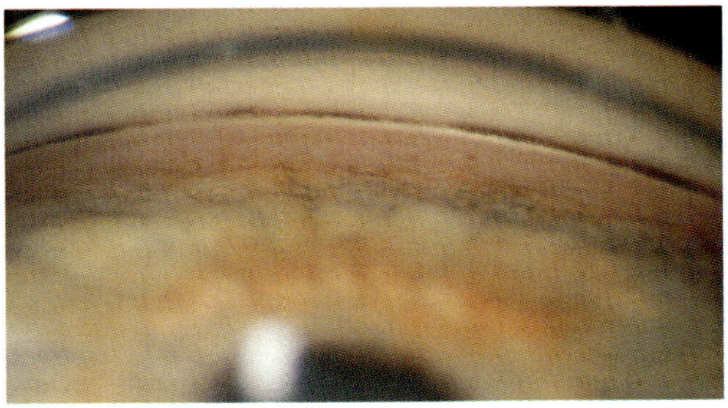

8.63 | Recessed anterior chamber angle after blunt trauma shows a slate-gray, widened ciliary band and a prominent scleral spur below the pigmented trabecular meshwork.

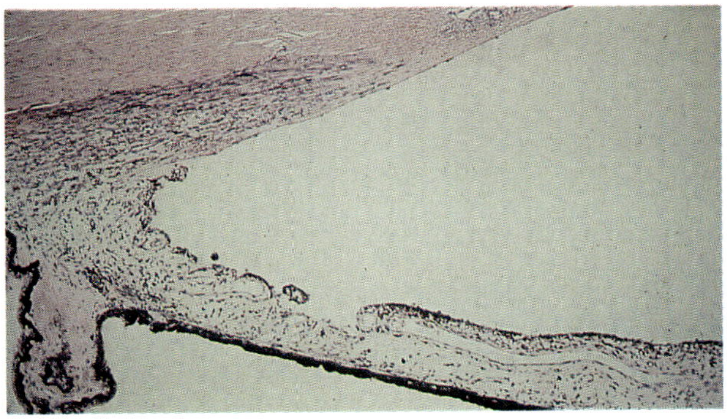

8.64 | Recessed anterior chamber angle after blunt trauma, showing widened angle, posterior attachment of iris, and collapsed scarred trabecular meshwork with overlying endothelial cells (arrows).

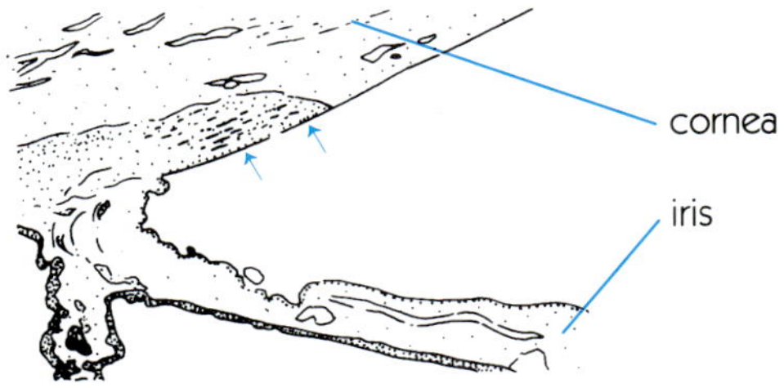

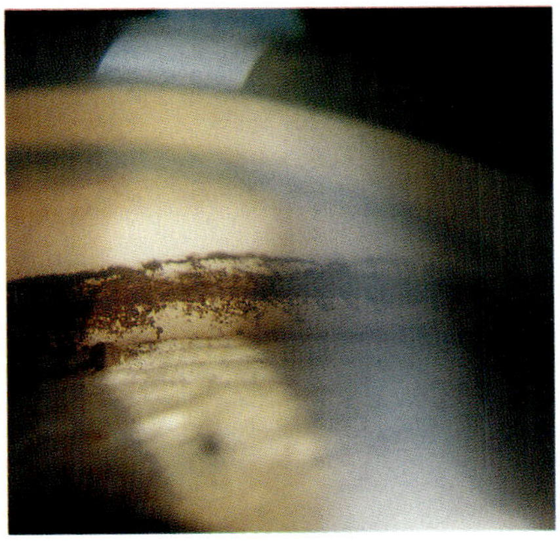

8.65 | Uveal pigment matted and clumped on trabecular meshwork surface after blunt trauma. Angle recession is present but partially obscured by pigment.

on the extent of angle recession. By the same token, direct injury to the trabecular meshwork further compromises aqueous humor outflow (Fig. 8.66). Although glaucoma commonly occurs early after injury, it may not be manifest for many years.[198] On the other hand, if the angle disruption is so extensive as to develop cyclodialysis (see Fig. 8.62), the traumatized eye may develop hypotony. In either case, the eye may also manifest disruption of the lenticular zonula with phakodonesis, lens subluxation, or dislocation. Long-forgotten blunt trauma should be considered in any eye with unilateral glaucoma.[198]

Ocular contusion or angle-recession glaucoma should be managed as an open-angle glaucoma with conventional hypotensive agents. However, cholinergic agents are less likely to be effective in angle recession because of the disruption of the ciliary muscle. If the conjunctiva is satisfactory, such cases should respond well to conventional filtration surgery, although the persistence of inflammation, lens injury, aphakia, or relative youth may indicate adjunctive antimetabolite therapy.

PENETRATING TRAUMA

Glaucoma diagnosis and management after penetrating ocular trauma is based on the extent of injury, but is in general similar to that appropriate for blunt trauma. Such injuries are often also associated with severe inflammation, chronic peripheral anterior synechiae from collapse of the anterior chamber, or inflammation and lens disruption. The aphakic eye in a young person with disruption of the anterior segment has a poor prognosis for filtration surgery but can be managed with adjunctive antimetabolite therapy. When no satis-

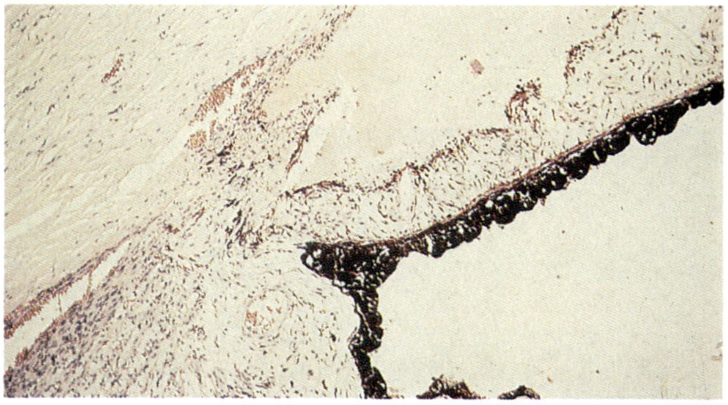

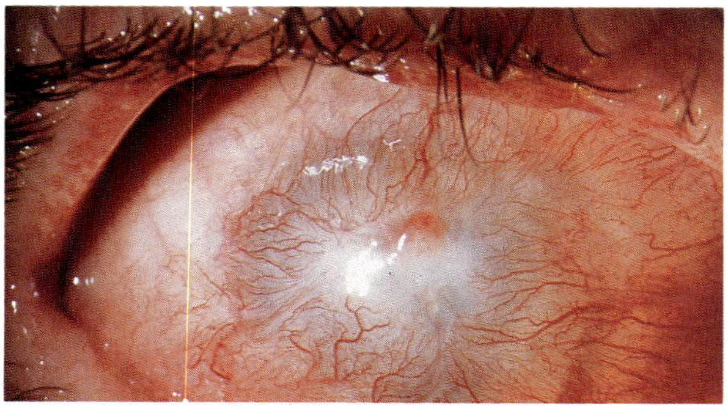

8.66 | Tear in trabecular meshwork associated with perforating injury. SC = Schlemm's canal with red blood cells in lumen. T = torn trabecular meshwork. P = extravasated protein in anterior chamber. SS = scleral spur. CM = ciliary muscle.

8.67 | Alkali burn of cornea and conjunctiva.

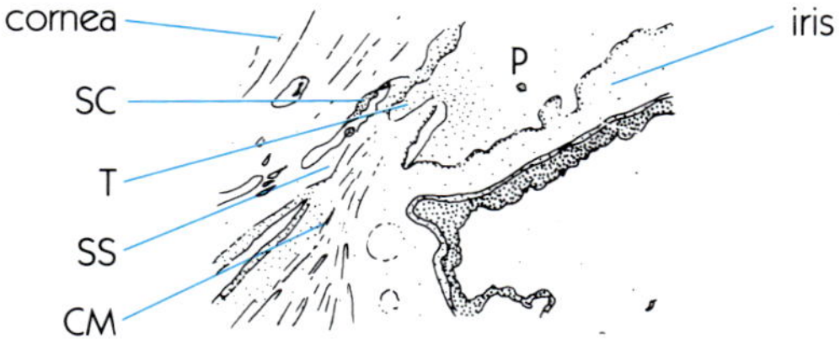

factory site for conventional filtration surgery can be identified, a tube, valve, or seton implant can be indicated. Eyes with poor visual potential are probably better managed with the less invasive cyclodestructive procedures.

CHEMICAL BURNS

Chemical burns to the eye may lead to collagenous contracture and disruption of the intrascleral outflow pathways and glaucoma. Such injuries, particularly alkaline burns, can be profoundly destructive and may lead to intractable glaucoma[199,200] (Fig. 8.67). Such eyes respond poorly to medical and/or laser therapy because the obstruction is downstream from the trabecular meshwork. In addition, severe conjunctival burns make conventional filtration surgery exceedingly difficult, necessitating filtration with adjunctive antimetabolite therapy or a tube implant, depending on the visual potential of the eye.

GLAUCOMA WITH UVEITIS

Although reduced IOP is commonly cited as a sign of acute anterior uveitis (iridocyclitis), uveitis often leads to severe glaucoma (Fig. 8.68). Iridocyclitis may lead to reduced aqueous humor production or increased uveoscleral outflow,[201] but at the same time the ciliary process blood–aqueous barrier is disrupted. The latter may lead to an outpouring of plasma protein into the posterior chamber, with consequent increased aqueous humor viscosity, influx of associated growth factors, and increased outflow resistance.[202] Inflammatory cells themselves may also obstruct the aqueous humor pathways.

Pigment may be spattered on the inner surface of the meshwork, giving it a dirty, muddy appearance[203] (Fig. 8.69). In other cases, the inflammatory

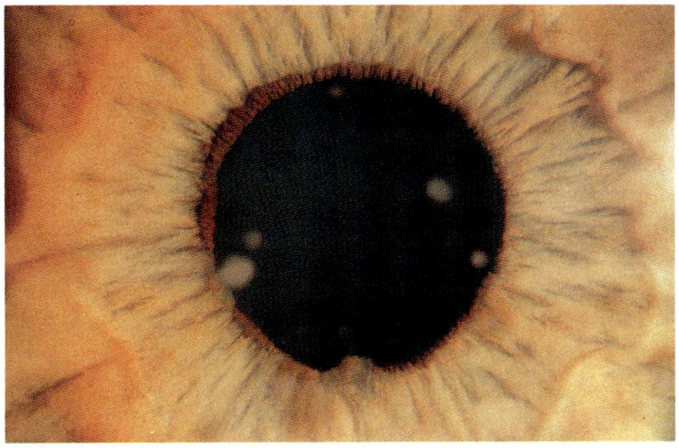

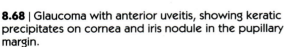

8.68 | Glaucoma with anterior uveitis, showing keratic precipitates on cornea and iris nodule in the pupillary margin.

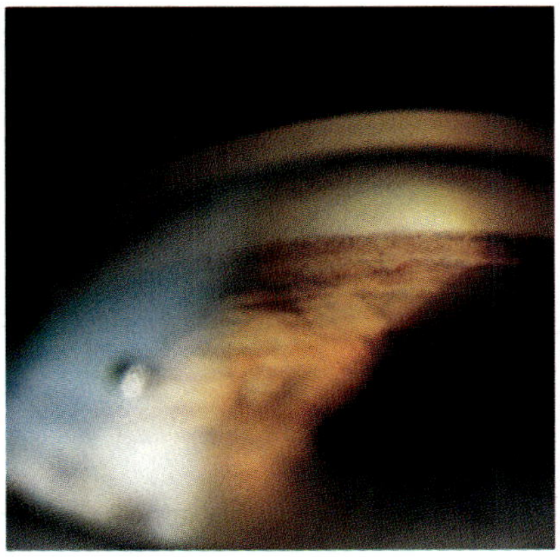

8.69 | Low-grade, smoldering uveitis with pigment spattered on trabecular meshwork surface.

precipitates that are commonly manifested on the cornea (keratic precipitates) may accumulate on the surface of the meshwork itself, leading to an open-angle glaucoma associated with precipitates on the trabecular meshwork.[204] Finally, in more severe, smoldering, particularly granulomatous uveitis, the trabecular meshwork may become occluded by the presence of peripheral anterior synechiae (Fig. 8.70). By the same token, posterior synechiae (adhesions between the iris and lens), manifesting as an irregular, sometimes cloverleaf-shaped pupil, may entirely block aqueous flow, leading to iris bombé and secondary angle-closure glaucoma (Fig. 8.71). Granulomatous uveitis, such as that associated with sarcoidosis or tuberculosis, typically exhibits severe anterior synechiae and glaucoma. Other cases may be much less severe, manifesting only a few cells in the anterior chamber with a mild perilimbal erythematous flush, without synechiae or other gonioscopic abnormalities. This is the more common appearance in nongranulomatous uveitis, particularly that associated with pars planitis in young adults.[205]

Herpes simplex or herpes zoster keratouveitis may be associated with hypopyon and severe glaucoma[206]; herpes zoster keratouveitis usually manifests fewer peripheral anterior synechiae than expected, but posterior synechiae and large geographic patches of stromal iris atrophy are typical and hypopyon may occur.[207]

The therapy of glaucoma with uveitis should be directed towards the uveitis itself. An evaluation for cause may be undertaken, as outlined in other volumes. Corticosteroids form the bulwark of therapy. Ocular hypotensive agents may supplement anti-inflammatory therapy. Aqueous secretory suppressants are usually most effective, but epinephrine may also work in some cases. Cholinergics typically exacerbate inflammation and should be used only as a last resort. Glaucoma associated with uveitis does not respond to argon laser trabeculoplasty. Filtration surgery can be employed, but the uveitis should be minimized as much as possible preoperatively and the postoperative course should usually be supplemented with increased anti-inflammatory drugs. Adjunctive antimetabolite therapy should be given serious consideration.

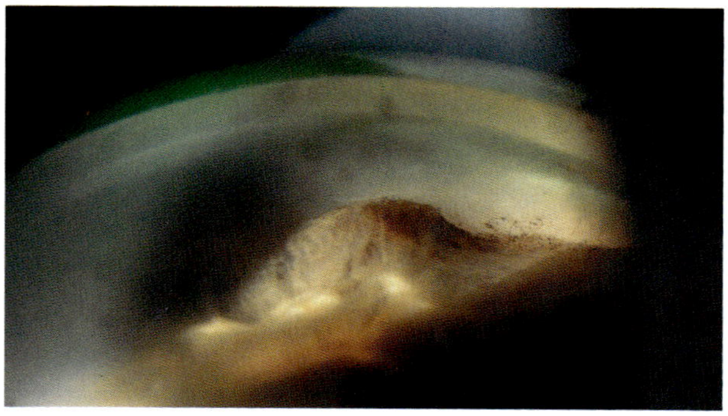

8.70 | Granulomatous uveitis with peripheral anterior synechiae covering trabecular meshwork.

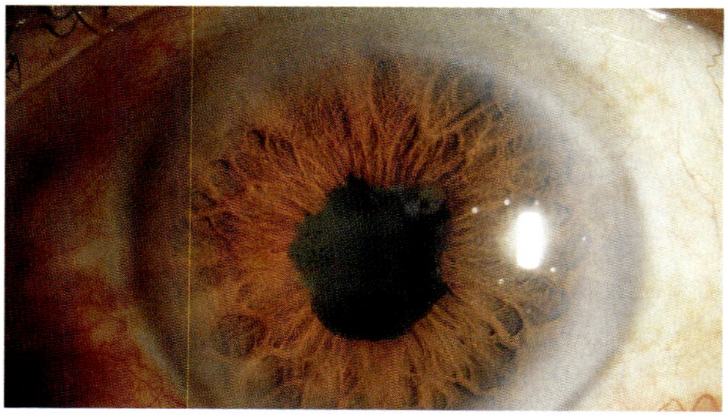

8.71 | Posterior synechiae with nearly occluded pupil in granulomatous uveitis.

SPECIAL VARIETIES OF GLAUCOMA ASSOCIATED WITH OCULAR INFLAMMATION

Glaucomatocyclitic crisis (Posner–Schlossman syndrome) is an uncommon variety, manifesting in young to middle-aged adults with sudden attacks of acute glaucoma, mild to moderate ocular pain, blurred vision, and corneal edema with rainbow-like halos around lights.[208] Glaucoma in these patients may be confused with acute angle-closure glaucoma, but the differentiation is easily based on the absence of a closed chamber angle.[209] Glaucomatocyclitic crisis is typically unilateral, but subsequent attacks may occur in either eye. The eyes show a mild anterior uveitis with a few cells and flare, and occasional very fine keratic precipitates. The chamber angle remains open despite a history of multiple attacks, and typically remains free of peripheral anterior synechiae. These acute attacks are typically self-limited, but can be reduced both in duration and severity, although not in frequency, with topical corticosteroids and aqueous secretory suppressants. Occasionally, a residual glaucoma develops between attacks, requiring filtration surgery.[210]

An unusual and poorly understood variety of glaucoma suggestive of an association with inflammation is Fuchs' *heterochromic iridocyclitis*.[211,212] It is usually unilateral but may be bilateral. The affected eyes exhibit signs of a mild anterior uveitis, with cells in the aqueous humor and anterior vitreous humor, which is relatively resistant to conventional anti-inflammatory therapy with corticosteroids. The affected eye is usually but not always hypochromic relative to the fellow eye (Fig. 8.72). The iris usually manifests a thin, mottled atrophic fibular appearance to the stroma, even in the absence of hypochromia, and a fine, wispy neovascularization at its root that does not progress nor lead to chronic peripheral anterior synechiae.[213,214] These vessels often bleed slightly into the chamber angle when the IOP is abruptly reduced during intraocular surgery.[215] Perhaps the most characteristic features of Fuchs' heterochromic iridocyclitis are the rather extensive stellate, keratic pre-

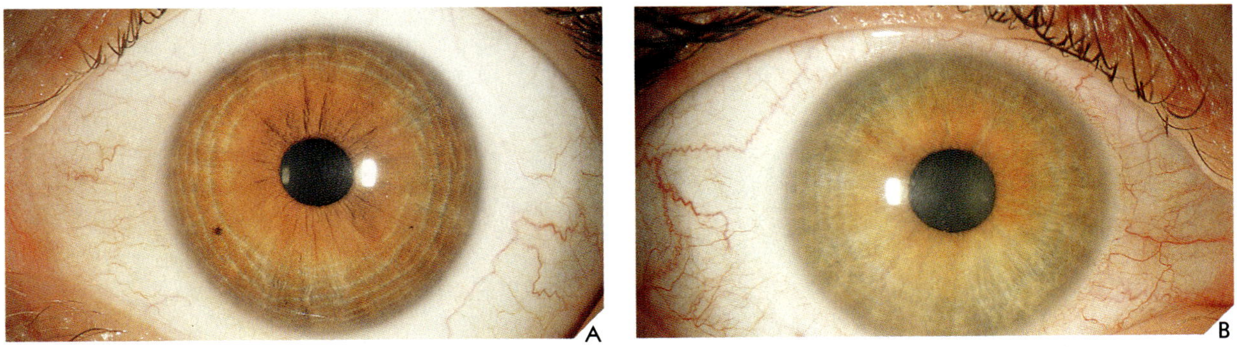

8.72 | Fuchs' heterochromic iridocyclitis, showing more darkly pigmented, normal eye *(A)* and more lightly pigmented, mottled iris in affected eye *(B)*.

cipitates on the cornea that send long tendrils to contiguous deposits (Fig. 8.73). Ipsilateral cataract commonly develops with or without corticosteroid therapy. Although cataract surgery is often technically uneventful, the postoperative chronic inflammation and glaucoma sometimes compromise the ultimate visual result.

Uveitis associated with luetic interstitial keratitis can also cause a variety of acute and chronic glaucomas. These may relate to exacerbation of the anterior uveitis associated with luetic keratouveitis (Fig. 8.74). In congenital lues the anterior segment is small, increasing the risk of angle-closure glaucoma.[216] Luetic interstitial keratitis has also been associated with a secondary open-angle glaucoma accompanied by an irregular trabecular pigmentation and a glassy pretrabecular membrane, as sometimes occurs in smoldering nongranulomatous uveitis.[217]

Episcleritis and scleritis are associated with an open-angle glaucoma in about 10% of cases, usually related to inflammation and edema in the trabecular meshwork and the intrascleral outflow pathways. Angle-closure glaucoma has been described resulting from pupillary dilatation in predisposed eyes or from edema of the ciliary body associated with posterior scleritis.[218]

LENS-INDUCED GLAUCOMAS

Although cataract commonly occurs in elderly glaucoma patients, only under unusual circumstances do abnormalities of the lens directly lead to glaucoma.[219] Some factors associated with angle-closure glaucomas can derive, in varying degrees, from the size or location of the crystalline lens. In classic angle-closure glaucoma, relative pupillary block occurs when the posterior chamber aqueous humor cannot escape between the lens and the pupillary margin to enter the anterior chamber.[220] This process can become acutely exacerbated with sudden enlargement of the lens or when the lens–iris diaphragm has shifted forward, as sometimes occurs after occlusion of the central retinal vein.[221,222] Dislocated or subluxed lenses may also migrate forward to become entrapped in the pupil, leading to angle-closure glaucoma.[223,224] They may also dislocate entirely into the anterior chamber,

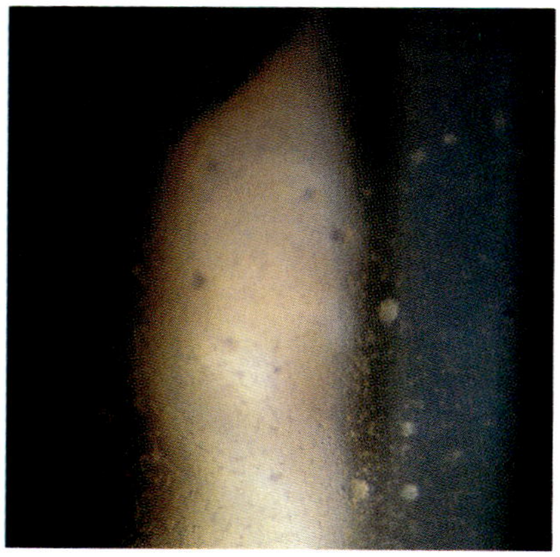

8.73 | Stellate keratic precipitates on corneal endothelium in Fuchs' heterochromic iridocyclitis.

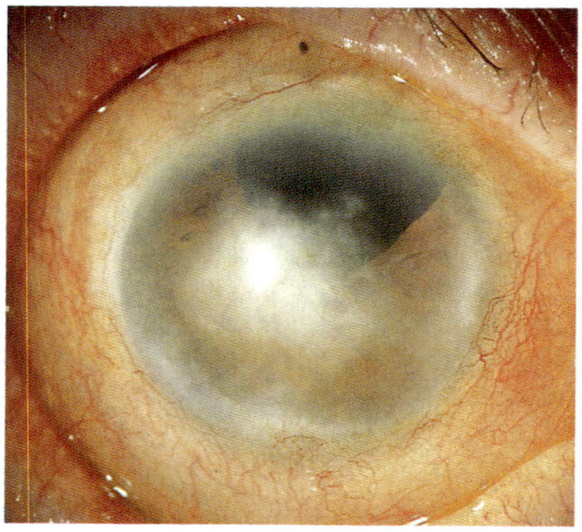

8.74 | Glaucoma associated with luetic interstitial keratitis and uveitis.

causing not only inflammation but also reverse pupillary block, with the pupil compressed against the back surface of the lens (Fig. 8.75). Spherophakia, as in Weill–Marchesani syndrome, may allow the small, spherical lens to become entrapped in the pupil, leading to pupillary block and angle closure glaucoma[225] (Fig. 8.76). These can be corrected by peripheral iridectomy or by lens extraction when indicated.

Lenses dislocated into the posterior segment may also become hypermature and develop a wrinkled, leaky capsule, leading to the phacolytic varieties of glaucoma discussed below (Fig. 8.77).

A spectrum of glaucomas under the circumstances of a leaking lens, usually mature or hypermature, has been described.[226] These include phacolytic glaucoma, lens-induced uveitis, and obstruction of the trabeculum by lens protein or particles—either lens fragments or fine iridescent calcium oxalate crystals.[226,227] *Phacolytic glaucoma* classically presents in an eye with poor visual acuity and a longstanding mature cataract. These eyes acutely develop high IOP, pain, erythema, and corneal edema but have an open anterior chamber angle (Fig. 8.78). The hypermature cataract, usually with a wrinkled lens capsule, exudes proteinaceous material that circulates in the anterior chamber along with macrophages engorged with ingested lens

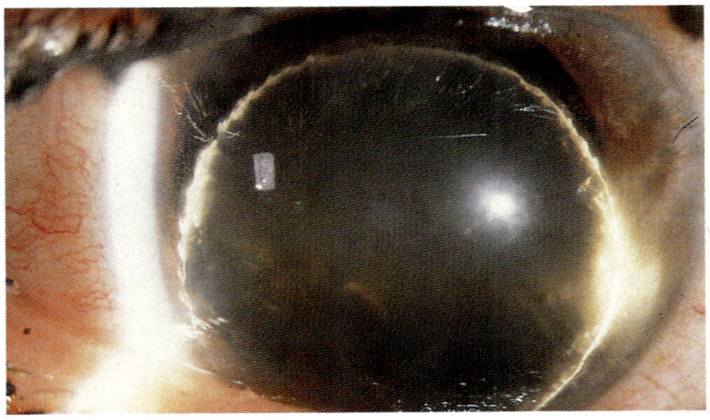

8.75 | Crystalline lens dislocated into anterior chamber.

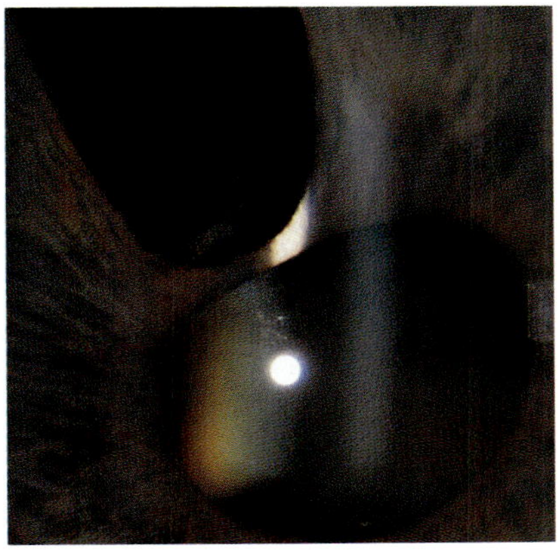

8.76 | Angle-closure glaucoma in Weill–Marchesani syndrome with spherophakia. A peripheral iridectomy has been performed.

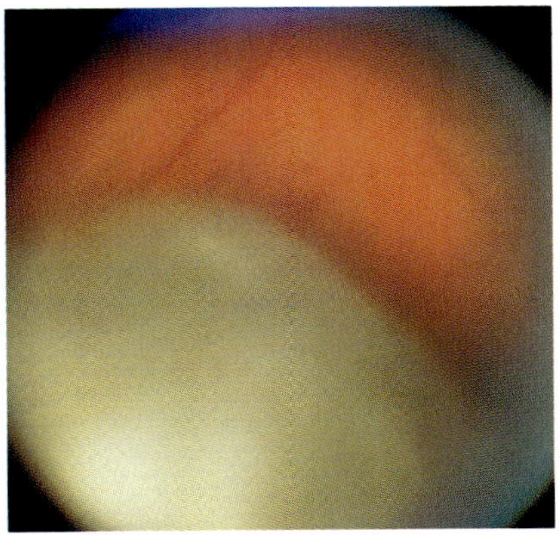

8.77 | Dislocated hypermature cataract. Note milky white color and irregular wrinkled capsule, with retina and choroid just posterior.

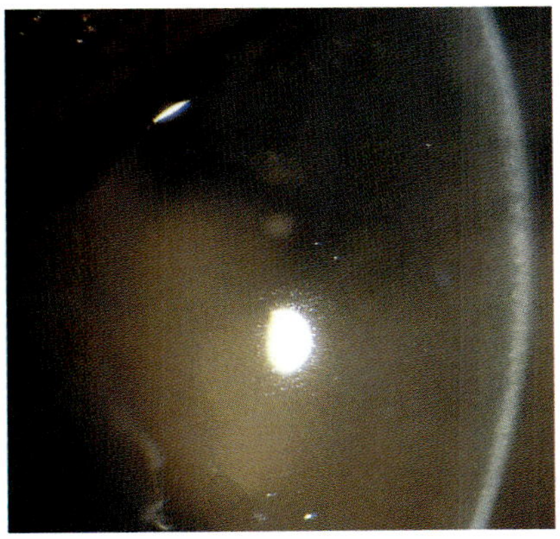

8.78 | Phacolytic glaucoma. The anterior chamber is virtually filled with white, proteinaceous lens material; corneal edema and acute glaucoma are present.

material (see Fig. 8.78). A pseudohypopyon may be present, formed by the protein and macrophages. Conventional hypotensive and anti-inflammatory therapy is often ineffective, but lens extraction usually relieves the IOP and the inflammation. Milder forms of inflammatory glaucoma associated with a leaking but immature lens may also occur. Occasionally, the lens may leak through an unrecognized rent in the posterior capsule while the anterior capsule remains unwrinkled in early stages, making early diagnosis difficult.

Excessive amounts of retained lens cortex after extracapsular cataract extraction may exacerbate postoperative glaucoma (Fig. 8.79). This may lead to chronic postoperative uveitis which by itself can result in glaucoma, or to direct outflow obstruction by lens material. Although this material usually absorbs spontaneously, unacceptably high IOPs after cataract surgery may require evacuation of the retained material. Longstanding uveitis associated with residual glaucoma may respond to topical corticosteroids and ocular hypotensive agents.

Phacoanaphylactic endophthalmitis is a largely histologic diagnosis that describes an immune response to released lens protein. Either a latent period after release of the protein or prior sensitization to lens protein, normally immunologically sequestered in the lens capsule, is required. Polymorphonuclear leukocytes pour into the aqueous and anterior chamber.

IRIDOCORNEAL ENDOTHELIALIZATION SYNDROMES

Clinical entities only recently ascribed to a single spectrum of disorders, the *iridocorneal endothelialization (ICE) syndrome,* were described separately in the early to mid-twentieth century.[228,231] These include Chandler syndrome, essential iris atrophy, and the iris–nevus syndrome of Cogan–Reese.[232,233] Although the individual clinical picture varies slightly at first presentation to the ophthalmologist, the syndromes share an abnormality of the corneal endothelium, the chamber angle, and the iris. Eventually, many of these eyes will develop glaucoma and corneal edema, with bullous keratopathy and corneal opacification. The patients usually first present in early to middle adulthood with corneal edema, ocular pain, various degrees of corectopia, iris atrophy, or visual blurring (Fig. 8.80). These disorders are nearly always unilateral and are more common in women. The underlying pathophysiologic anomaly with iridocorneal endothelialization syndrome appears to be corneal endothelial degeneration with fine guttata-like changes resembling beaten silver, similar to but finer than the changes of Fuchs' endothelial dystrophy[233] (see Fig. 8.80). This anomalous endothelium migrates over the anterior chamber angle, the trabecular meshwork, and onto the surface of the iris.

In Chandler syndrome the corneal changes predominate, with only mild iris stromal atrophy and corectopia (see Fig. 8.80). Corneal edema tends

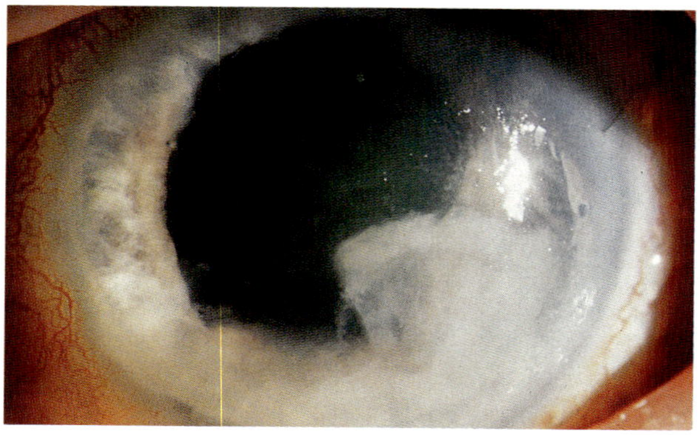

8.79 | Retained lens cortex after extracapsular cataract extraction associated with uveitis and glaucoma.

to be severe even at normal IOP, often requiring corneal transplantation. In essential iris atrophy the iris changes predominate, with marked progressive stromal iris atrophy and then through-and-through holes, marked corectopia, and polycoria (Figs. 8.81 and 8.82). As the endothelial membrane con-

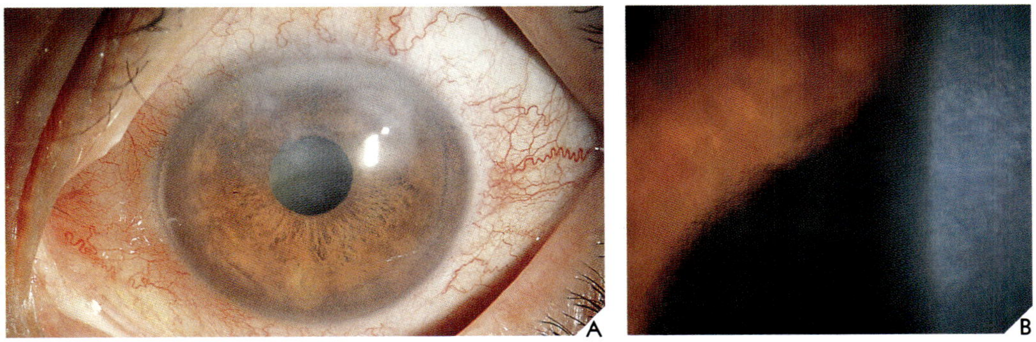

8.80 | Chandler syndrome with unilateral corneal epithelial edema *(A)* and fine, "beaten silver" changes of the corneal endothelium *(B)*.

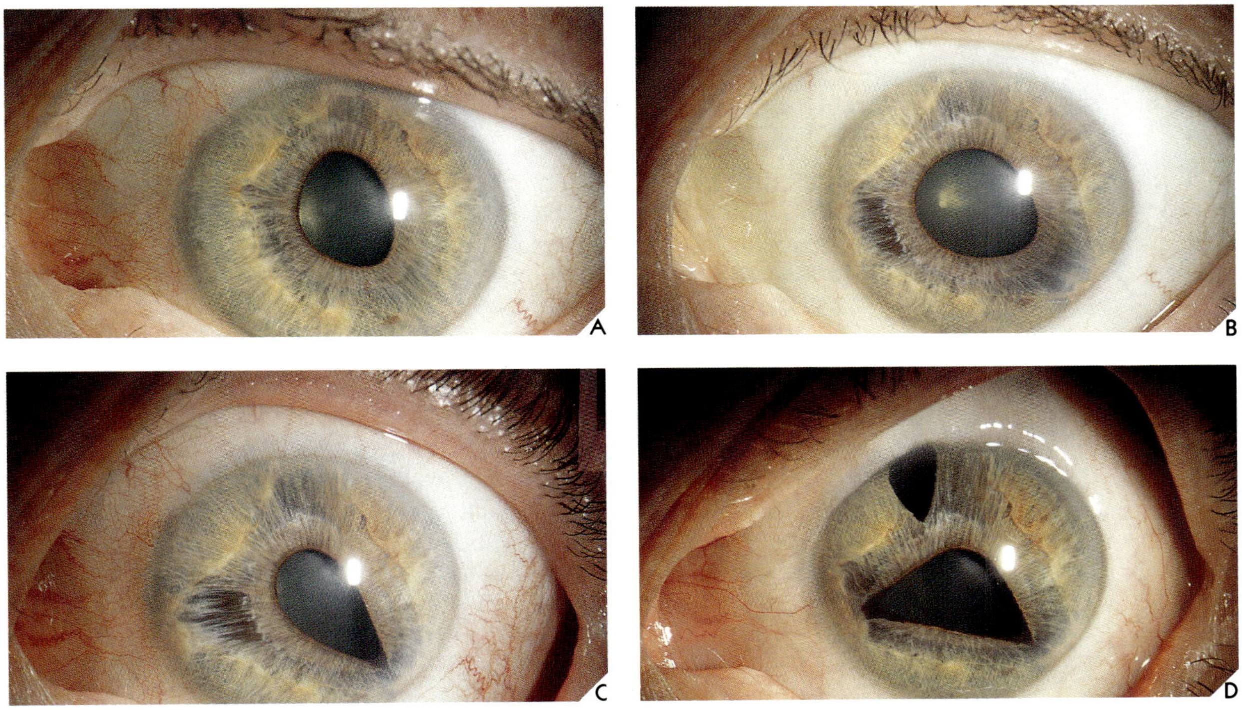

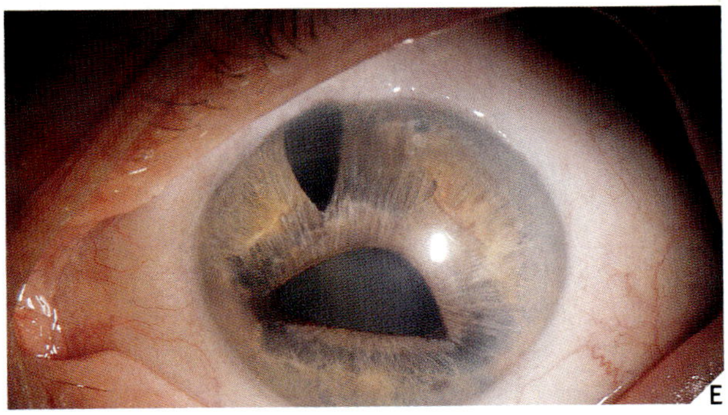

8.81 | Progressive corectopia and iris atrophy in ICE syndrome, initially manifesting as Chandler syndrome in 1982 *(A)*. By 1984, some stromal atrophy with mild distortion of the pupil is present *(B)*. Peripheral anterior synechiae are present inferotemporally by 1985 *(C)*, and inferotemporally and inferonasally with glaucoma requiring filtration surgery by 1988 *(D)* and corneal edema requiring penetrating keratoplasty by 1990 *(E)*.

tracts towards the chamber angle it pulls the pupil with it, markedly stretching the iris on the opposite side, leading to so-called stretch holes. Eventually, little may be left of the iris except for a few stromal strands in the iris sphincter (see Fig. 8.82). In addition, small, round melting holes may also develop in unstretched areas of iris.

In actual clinical practice, the majority of ICE patients present somewhere between the two classic extremes of these disorders, with some signs of both entities (see Fig. 8.81). With progressive peripheral synechiae, the IOP can be controlled initially with medical therapy but filtration often becomes necessary as aqueous humor outflow becomes further compromised. Endothelialization may also occur over a filtration fistula or within the bleb itself.

The Cogan–Reese iris–nevus syndrome manifests corneal edema, iris atrophy, and angle changes similar to those typical of the ICE syndrome (Fig. 8.83). In addition, these patients develop multiple, discrete, pigmented nodules or diffuse nevus-like areas on the iris surface, but histologically these nodules are believed to be areas of iris stroma extruding through holes in the ectopic endothelial membrane that covers the iris surface.

Posterior polymorphous dystrophy exhibits some of the signs of the iridocorneal endothelialization syndrome but possesses distinctive features that distinguish it from ICE.[234] It is almost always bilateral and is familial, being inherited as an autosomal dominant trait. Unlike the ICE syndrome it is manifest from childhood, but usually does not become clinically apparent until early adult life. It is primarily a disorder of the corneal endothelium, with multiple vessels and crater-like abnormalities visible with the slit lamp. The lesions are much larger and more discrete than those of the ICE syndrome. Most patients have normal irides. Some may develop iridocorneal adhesions and about 15% develop glaucoma.

GLAUCOMA FROM INTRAOCULAR HEMORRHAGE

Intraocular bleeding usually follows injury or surgery but may occur spontaneously as the result of intraocular neovascularization, tumors, or iris vascular tufts. Whatever the source, blood in the aqueous humor can eventually obstruct the aqueous outflow pathways, leading to glaucoma. Hyphema from blunt injury may manifest only as a small layer of red cells in the inferior portion of the chamber angle, or may entirely replace the aqueous humor. Most intracameral hemorrhages clear spontaneously with rest, but about

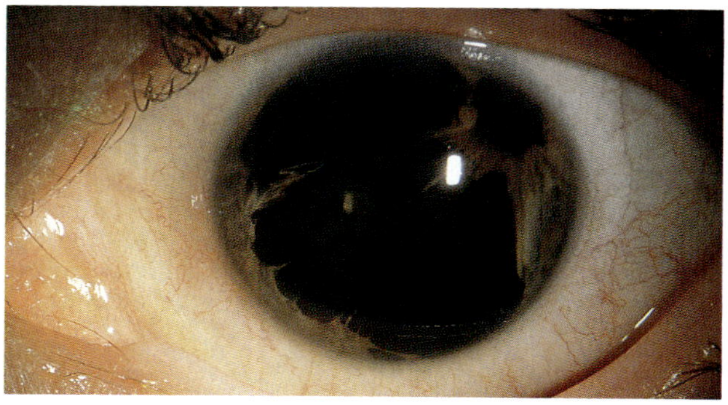

8.82 | Essential iris atrophy with almost complete absence of iris tissue.

8.83 | Cogan–Reese iris nevi syndrome, showing iris nodules.

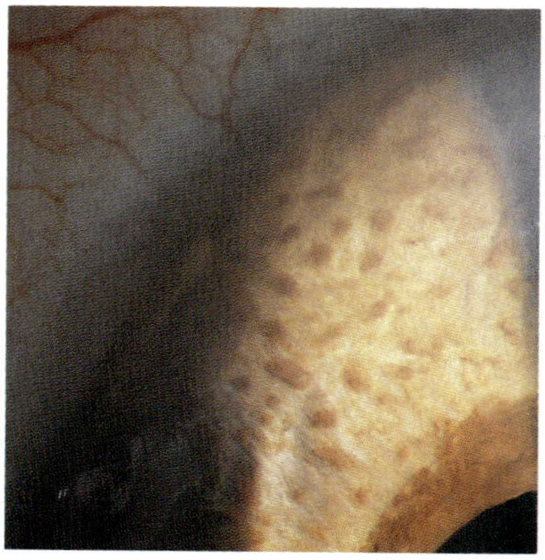

10–30% rebleed, usually within the first week.[235,236] Recurrent hemorrhage is more likely to fill the anterior chamber completely, leading to glaucoma and/or blood staining of the cornea[235,237–239] (Fig. 8.84).

Rebleeding most likely occurs when a hyphema undergoes clotting, or during clot retraction, 3 to 10 days later.[235] The blood may gradually be absorbed, or a large intracameral clot associated with degenerative blood components may appear as a large, blackened mass, the so called "eight-ball" hyphema, almost always associated with severe glaucoma (Fig. 8.85). Degenerative erythrocytic forms such as red cell ghosts or sickle cells are not nearly as malleable as fresh erythrocytes and are more likely to obstruct aqueous humor outflow and cause glaucoma.[240–243] Red cells with hemoglobin S tend to sickle in the relatively hypoxic environment of aqueous humor, leading to severe glaucoma even with very small hyphemas.[240]

Small, fine vascular tufts may occur at the pupillary margin in an otherwise normal eye. These may bleed spontaneously, leading to intermittent attacks of blurred vision and increased intraocular pressure.[244] They can sometimes be obliterated with a laser to prevent recurrent bleeding. Spontaneous hyphemas may also occur as the result of iris neovascularization or of intraocular tumors, particularly juvenile xanthogranuloma. Rarely, they also signal the presence of malignant melanoma.

Persistent intraocular hemorrhage gradually undergoes degeneration of red cells into a variety of breakdown products. Red cell ghosts are greenish, khaki-colored, spherical, nonpliable degenerative red cell bodies that develop in longstanding vitreous hemorrhage. The rigid red cell ghosts do not pass through the trabecular meshwork, and thus lead to ghost-cell glaucoma, especially when the vitreous face is disrupted and these cells are released in large quantities into the anterior chamber. They can be seen circulating as greenish, almost iridescent bodies or, when concentrated enough, they create

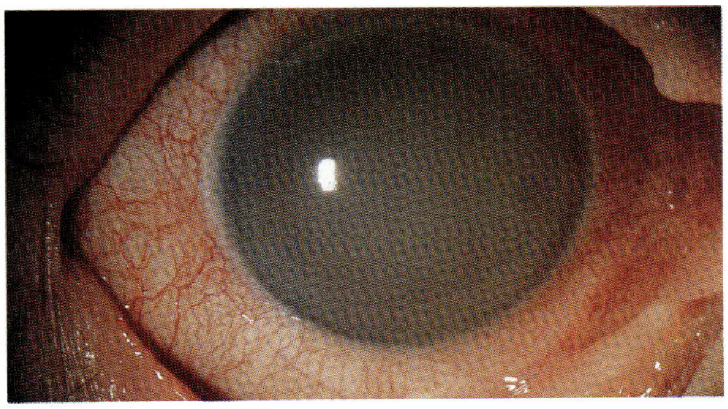

8.84 | Severe blood staining of the cornea after hyphema.

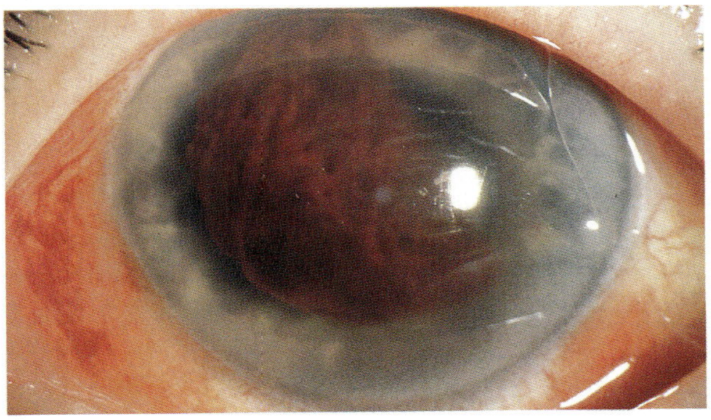

8.85 | Retracting blood clot almost filling anterior chamber, associated with repeated hyphema and glaucoma. In some instances, the clot may blacken into the so-called eight-ball hyphema.

a tan colored pseudohypopyon in the inferior anterior chamber angle[243] (Fig. 8.86). Other degenerative red cell fragments may be ingested by macrophages, which themselves can obstruct the trabecular meshwork, a syndrome known as hemolytic glaucoma.[245] Vitreous or aqueous aspirates in such cases usually demonstrate a variety of red cell products, macrophages, and red cell ghosts.

GLAUCOMA ASSOCIATED WITH INCREASED VENOUS PRESSURE

Aqueous humor exits the eye primarily by way of the trabecular meshwork, Schlemm's canal, and aqueous veins, which in turn drain to the episcleral veins. Under most conditions, episcleral venous pressure is in the range of 8–10 mm Hg, but may be increased under physiologic and pathologic conditions, leading to elevation of the IOP.[246] Simple breath holding, Valsalva maneuvers, or compression of neck veins increase episcleral venous pressure.

Increased episcleral venous pressure may occur pathologically from obstruction of orbital venous drainage, increased central venous pressure, arteriovenous fistulas, or idiopathically. Clinically, markedly dilated, tortuous, and prominent episcleral veins characterize these eyes and proptosis and chemosis may also be present, especially with high-flow arteriovenous fistulas.[247] Such findings may be mistaken for an infectious "red" eye (Fig. 8.87). These patients often complain of hearing pulsations, and an ocular bruit may be heard over the eye or orbit. The chamber angle is usually open, often with blood reflux into Schlemm's canal. On rare occasions neovascularization

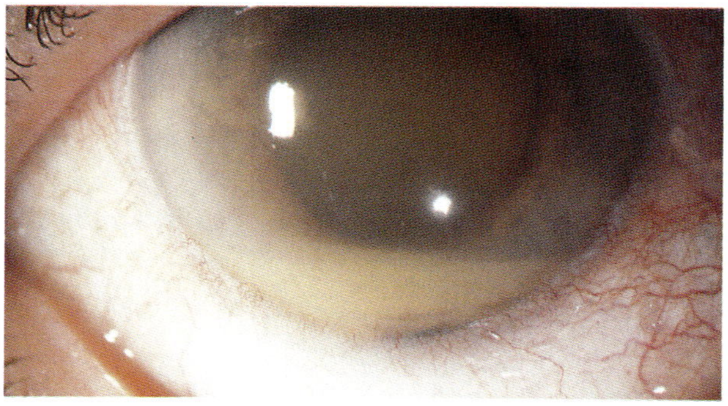

8.86 | Khaki-colored fluid level in inferior anterior chamber with ghost-cell glaucoma.

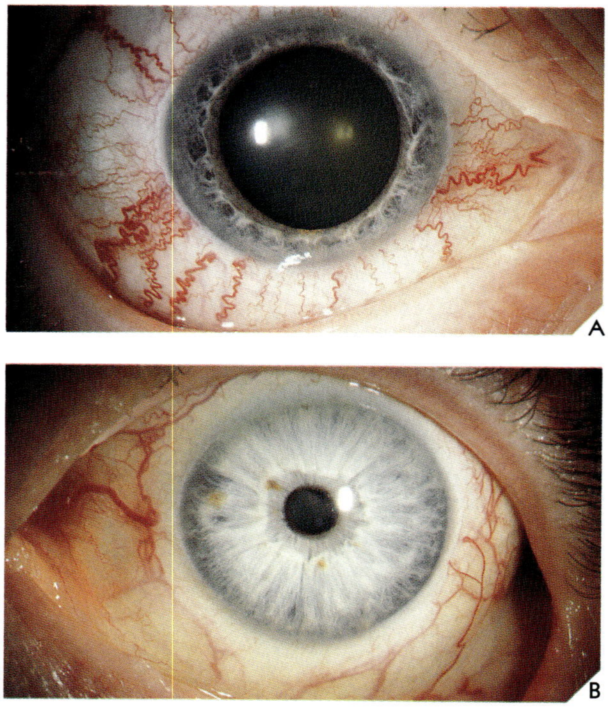

8.87 | *A:* Traumatic carotid-cavernous sinus fistula with increased episcleral venous pressure, proptosis, chemosis, and glaucoma. *B:* Low-flow external carotid artery arteriovenous shunt with glaucoma.

occurs, apparently on an ischemic basis.[248] Trabecular outflow facility is normal unless blood reflux or other anomalies block the trabecular meshwork.

Venous obstruction may occur with retrobulbar tumors or from distal obstruction associated with increased pressure in the superior vena cava. More common is dysthyroid ophthalmopathy with orbital congestion, proptosis, lid retraction, and chemosis. Arteriovenous fistulas classically occur between the carotid artery and the cavernous sinus, especially after blunt trauma[249] (see Fig. 8.87A). These typically are high-flow shunts, usually of acute onset, associated with high venous pressure, severe proptosis, chemosis, bruits over the head and orbit, and severe glaucoma. The majority of arteriovenous fistulas are traumatic in origin. However, those encountered in the ophthalmologist's office more typically are low-flow, low-volume shunts associated with other intracranial, often dural, vessels with less prominent clinical findings except for a "red eye"[247,249] (see Fig. 8.87B). An idiopathic, sometimes familial syndrome of prominent episcleral veins and glaucoma can also be observed with no demonstrable arteriovenous shunt or other cause for the increased episcleral venous pressure.[250,251]

Sturge–Weber oculofacial hemangioma syndrome may also manifest increased episcleral venous pressure associated with episcleral hemangiomas.[252] These are characteristic of the adult variety of Sturge–Weber glaucoma and usually have finer, less discrete episcleral veins than those associated with arteriovenous fistulas, exhibiting a fleshy, vascular appearance to the episclera (Fig. 8.88).

These eyes are often resistant to conventional medical therapy as well as to laser glaucoma therapy, and trabeculectomy or other filtration surgery is often necessary. These eyes are also prone to intraoperative or immediate postoperative uveal effusion and suprachoroidal hemorrhage because of the increased intraocular venous pressure.[253] Prophylactic posterior sclerotomy may prevent serious complications from suprachoroidal hemorrhage.

GLAUCOMA FROM INTRAOCULAR TUMORS

Intraocular tumors may lead to glaucoma of either the open angle or closed angle types.[254] Glaucoma is a poor prognostic sign for intraocular tumor.[255] Metastatic tumors and malignant melanomas present most often, but hemangiomas, neurofibromas, and leukemia, among others, also occasionally lead

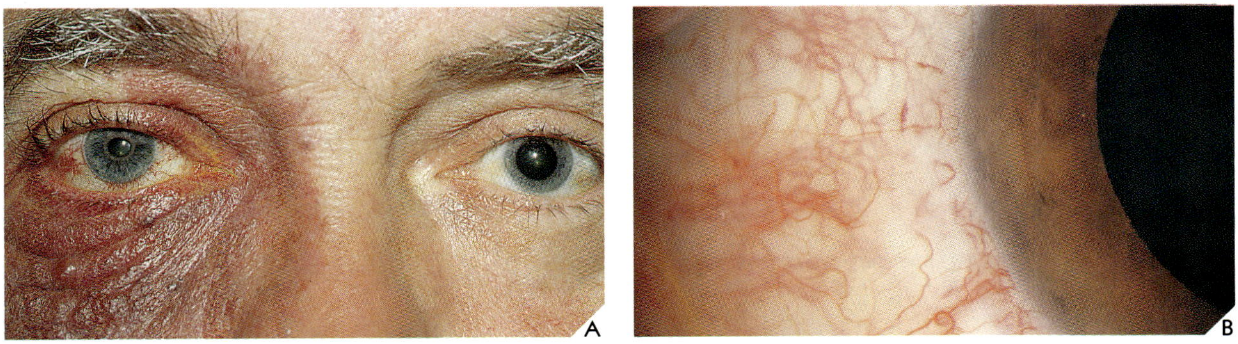

8.88 | *A:* Adult Sturge–Weber oculofacial hemangioma with prominent episcleral veins and adult-onset glaucoma. *B:* Dilated racemose, tortuous episcleral veins with adult onset Sturge–Weber glaucoma.

to glaucoma. Most iris nevi are benign, requiring only photography and careful follow-up for assessment of growth and angle invasion.[256] Anterior segment tumors tend to invade the open angle directly (Fig. 8.89), whereas posterior segment masses more commonly lead to angle-closure glaucoma by anterior displacement of the lens–iris diaphragm. Neovascular glaucoma also sometimes complicates intraocular tumors.

Ocular tumors may be misdiagnosed as uveitis, rubeosis, or even primary angle-closure glaucoma. Longstanding visual loss, unilateral shallowing of the anterior chamber, unilateral irregular chamber angle pigmentation, or a poor view of the fundus all suggest the possibility of tumor. When cataract obscures visualization of the fundus, transillumination and ultrasonography are diagnostically helpful.

The most common intraocular tumor in adults, uveal melanoma, accounts for the majority of tumor-induced glaucomas.[254] Expanding posterior segment melanomas can lead to angle-closure glaucoma by anteriorly displacing the vitreous, lens, ciliary body, or iris. Although intraocular tumors should be considered diagnostically in any unilateral angle-closure glaucoma, melanomas of the anterior segment, iris, or ciliary body are more likely to be associated with open-angle glaucoma. Direct extension of tumor from iris or ciliary body may infiltrate the chamber angle[255] (see Fig. 8.89). The trabecular meshwork can provide a fertile template for rapid expansion of some iris or ciliary body tumors, which can extend from a localized nidus to fill the entire trabecular meshwork leading to a ring-shaped melanoma (Fig. 8.90). Extension of an intraocular melanoma into the anterior chamber angle is a poor prognostic sign, often requiring enucleation.

Another rare melanoma-induced glaucoma is melanomalytic glaucoma. This develops when necrotic tumors, usually of the ciliary body, release pigmented debris that is ingested by macrophages.[257] Large, tumor-laden, densely pigmented macrophages are visible circulating in the aqueous humor and become enmeshed in the interstices of the trabecular meshwork, leading to glaucoma[258] (see Fig. 8.51A, Ritch and Liebmann, this chapter).

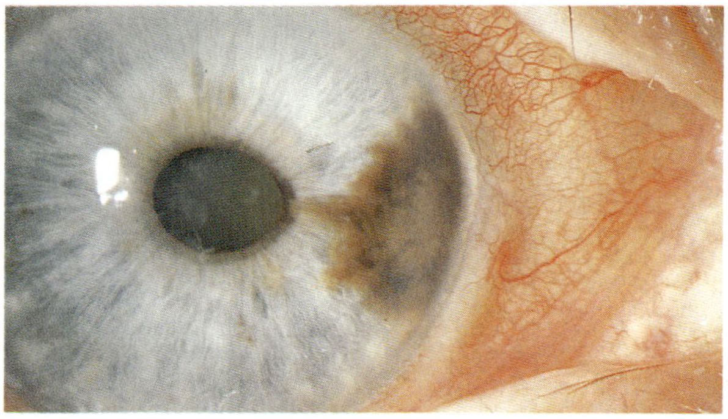

8.89 | Iris melanoma directly invading anterior chamber angle.

8.90 | Gonioscopic view of malignant ring melanoma involving entire circumference of trabecular meshwork, with pigmented seeding on meshwork surface.

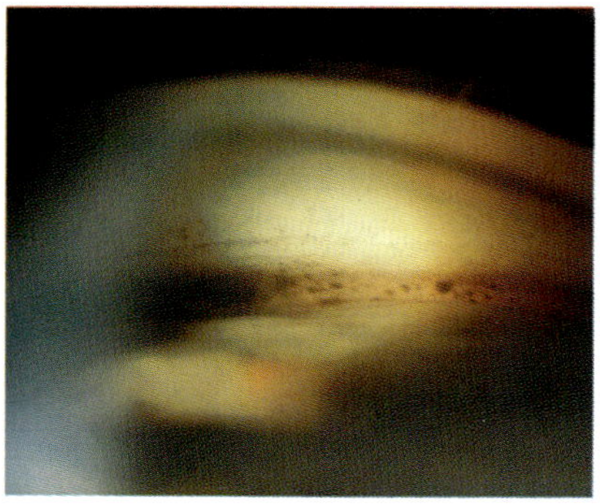

SECTION IX

PEDIATRIC GLAUCOMA

Michael J. Sakamoto
John R. Hetherington, Jr.

All forms of glaucoma in infants and children are very rare. It has been estimated that a general ophthalmologist would see only two new cases every five years. Despite this low incidence, the impact can be dramatic, as severe visual disability is often the consequence of these disorders. Early diagnosis and treatment can prevent blindness in a majority of these patients.

Optimal therapy is determined by the specific type of glaucoma present. Childhood glaucoma can be divided into two main categories, depending on whether the pathogenesis is primary or secondary. A primary glaucoma is due to the maldevelopment of the anterior segment of the eye and is often of genetic origin. This category can be further subdivided into primary congenital glaucoma, in which the developmental anomaly is restricted to the trabecular meshwork, and those glaucomas associated with other ocular or systemic congenital abnormalities (Fig. 8.95). The secondary glaucomas

Figure 8.95. Conditions Associated with Developmental Glaucomas

Aniridia	Peter's anomaly	Pierre Robin syndrome	Microspherophakia
Sturge–Weber syndrome	Rubella	Congenital iris hypoplasia	Broad thumb syndrome
Neurofibromatosis	Turner syndrome	Weill–Marchesani syndrome	Homocystinuria
Goniodysgenesis syndromes	Trisomy 21	Oculodentodigital dysplasia	Congenital ectropion uveae
Axenfeld's anomaly	Trisomy 13	Lowe syndrome	Zellwegger syndrome
Rieger's syndrome	Trisomy 18	Microcornea	Anomalous superficial iris vessels
	Trisomy 29		
	Marfan syndrome		

are acquired as the result of other ocular and systemic problems, such as inflammation, trauma, or neoplasia[269] (Fig. 8.96).

This chapter will focus on the major primary childhood glaucomas, which are developmental in nature.

CLINICAL PRESENTATION

The signs and symptoms of glaucoma in children are variable and are dependent on the age of the child and the rapidity and severity of intraocular pressure elevation.

The newborn eye is elastic, in comparison with older eyes, and it stretches under the influence of elevated IOP. Corneal stretch disturbs the epithelium and causes symptoms of epiphora, photophobia, and blepharospasm. The cornea may become hazy, and as the eye stretches further there is corneal enlargement (Fig. 8.97) and deepening of the anterior chamber. Tears in Descemet's membrane (Haab's striae) (Fig. 8.98) may occur suddenly and cause

Figure 8.96. Secondary Pediatric Glaucomas

- Retinopathy of prematurity
- Persistent hyperplastic primary vitreous
- Tumors
  - Retinoblastoma
  - Juvenile xanthogranuloma
- Inflammation
  - Rubella
  - Herpes simplex
  - Juvenile rheumatoid arthritis
- Trauma

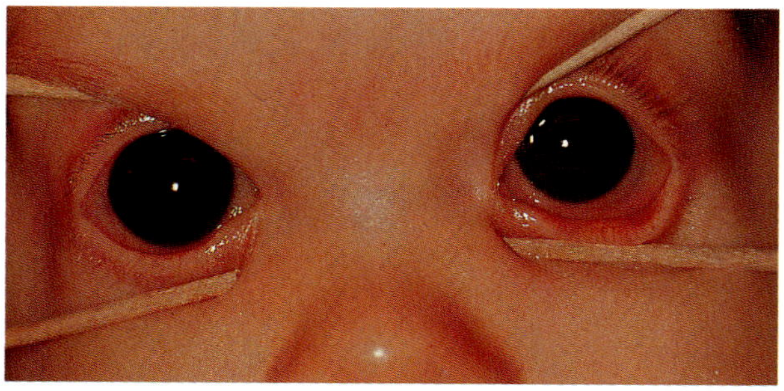

8.97 | Enlarged corneal diameters in bilateral primary infantile glaucoma.

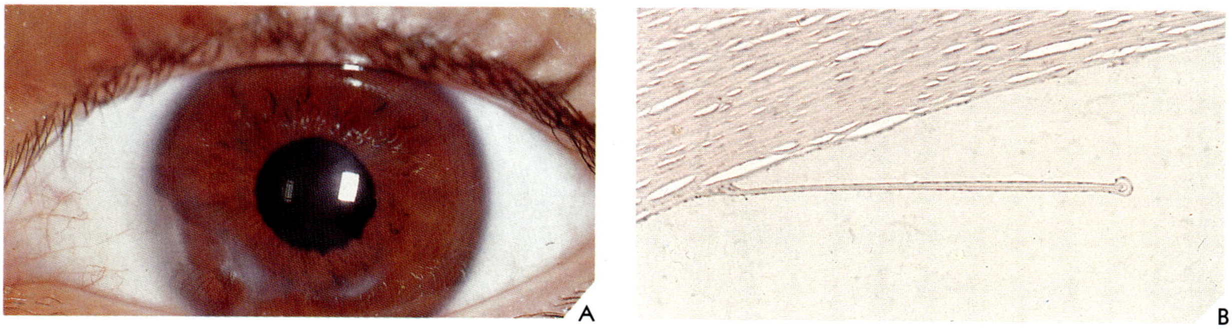

8.98 | Haab's striae. *A:* Clinical appearance showing localized corneal edema in area of ruptures in Descemet's membrane. *B:* The ruptured ends of Descemet's membrane have sealed over. The ends, which extend into the anterior chamber, are scroll-like and covered by endothelium. (*B*, from Yanoff M, Fine BS: *Ocular Pathology. A Color Atlas*, ed 2. New York: Gower Medical Publishing, 1992, 16.3.)

increased stromal edema and increased ocular irritation. If left untreated, continued stretching can lead to permanent corneal scarring, erosions, and ulcerations. Stretching of the zonules may cause lens subluxation.

Glaucoma developing in older children (older than 3–4 years) may reveal few symptoms or anterior segment changes. Slowly progressing myopia may occur.

EXAMINATION

A reasonably good office examination can be obtained in some children, depending on their age and their degree of cooperation. A mild sedative such as chloral hydrate (25–50 mg/kg) is useful in some cases. Most infants require general anesthesia for a reliable evaluation. Surgery, if necessary, can then immediately follow the examination.

The evaluation for glaucoma is similar to the usual complete pediatric examination, with special emphasis in certain areas.[270]

INTRAOCULAR PRESSURE

Most anesthetics lower the IOP. The exception to this is ketamine, which may slightly increase it. Measurement of IOP with as little medication as possible is preferable but is often difficult to accomplish. When anesthesia is used, the IOP should be measured as soon as the child is safely quiet, to obtain the most reliable measurement.[271,272]

Tonometry can be performed by Schiotz tonometer, Tonopen, or handheld applanation tonometer.

The normal IOP in an infant is reported to be slightly lower than that in an adult. A pressure reading higher than 21 mm Hg is suggestive of glaucoma, despite the potential inaccuracy of measurement.[273] Normal IOP, however, does not rule out glaucoma. Other signs and symptoms must be considered (Fig. 8.99).

GENERAL ANTERIOR SEGMENT EXAMINATION

Nasolacrimal duct obstruction should be evaluated as a possible cause of epiphora. Details of this examination will not be discussed here.

Corneal diameter is then measured in the horizontal plane with calipers. The normal corneal diameter in a neonate is 10–10.5 mm, which may increase by 1 mm at 1 year of age. Measurements greater than 12 mm

Figure 8.99. Initial IOP in Infants Under Anesthesia With and Without Glaucoma

IOP (mm Hg)	Normal Eyes n (%)	Glaucomatous Eyes n (%)
<15	26 (35)	0 (0)
15–21	39 (53)	14 (9)
21–24	4 (5)	0 (0)
>24	5 (7)	145 (91)
Total	74 (100)	159 (100)

(Adapted from Hoskins HD, et al: Developmental glaucomas: diagnosis and classification, in Cairns J, et al (eds): New Orleans Academy of Ophthalmology: Symposium on Glaucoma. St. Louis: CV Mosby, 1981, 172.)

are suggestive of glaucoma during this time. The cornea is then evaluated for haziness, developmental anomalies, and tears in Descemet's membrane.

The anterior chamber is often deeper than normal in childhood glaucoma, and the iris and lens must also be evaluated for developmental abnormalities.

GONIOSCOPY

Gonioscopy is performed with a smooth-domed Koeppe lens, a hand-held microscope, and a Barkan light, or with any direct gonioscopy lens and an operating microscope. When edematous corneal epithelium is present it can be removed by careful scraping with a knife or a cotton swab soaked in 70% alcohol.

In a normal newborn, the angle recess is absent and the iris inserts flatly into the ciliary body posterior to the scleral spur. Alterations in the angle are a clue to the type of glaucoma that may be present and also to its prognosis.[274,275]

OPHTHALMOSCOPY

Ophthalmoscopy is best carried out via a direct ophthalmoscope with a smooth-domed Koeppe lens. Increased cupping of the optic nerve is an early sign of increased intraocular pressure[276] (Fig. 8.100). This enlargement of the cup occurs more rapidly and at lower pressures in infants than in adults. A C/D ratio greater than 0.3 or an asymmetry of cupping greater than 0.2 is unusual in infants and should arouse suspicion of glaucoma (Fig. 8.101).

Reversal of early increased cupping is likely when the IOP is lowered early enough.[277] Careful documentation of optic nerve anatomy is important in monitoring progression.

REFRACTION

Visual acuity monitoring, when possible, and cycloplegic refraction should be determined and observed. A rapid increase in myopia may be a sign of glaucoma progression. Amblyopia may also occur and, when found, should be treated.

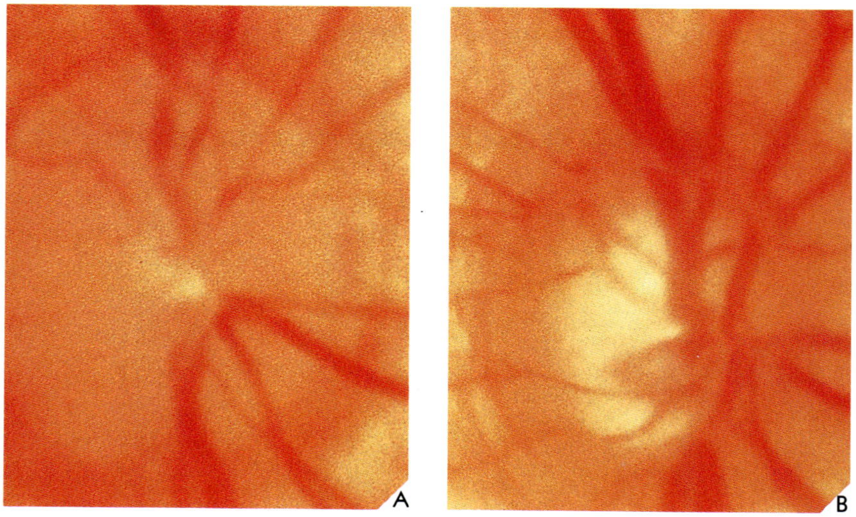

8.100 | Normal *(A)* and pathologically cupped *(B)* infant optic nerve heads.

Some of the clinical features that define the pediatric glaucomas can be seen in other ocular conditions. A differential diagnosis must therefore be considered to determine the diagnosis of glaucoma. A partial list of other ocular pathologies that can mimic glaucoma is shown in Figure 8.102.

Figure 8.101. Cup/Disc Ratios at Birth to 3 Years

Glaucomatous Eyes		Normal Eyes	
C/D Ratio	No. of Eyes (%)	C/D Ratio	No. of Eyes (%)
>0.6	67 (71)	>0.5	2 (4)
0.5	12 (13)	0.4	4 (9)
0.4	12 (13)	0.3	4 (9)
0.3	3 (3)	0.2	3 (7)
0.2	1 (1)	0–0.1	33 (72)
Total	95 (100)		46 (100)

(Adapted from Hoskins HD, et al: Developmental glaucomas: diagnosis and classification, in Cairns J, et al (eds): New Orleans Academy of Ophthalmology: Symposium on Glaucoma. St. Louis: CV Mosby, 1981, 172.)

Figure 8.102. Differential Diagnosis of Pediatric Glaucoma Symptoms and Signs

Epiphora
- Tear hypersecretion due to such causes as conjunctivitis, uveitis, exposure, corneal abrasion, or corneal dystrophy
- Inadequacy of the lacrimal drainage system due to such causes as congenital abnormalities, dacryocystitis, tumor, or trauma

Photosensitivity
- May be secondary to the same causes as epiphora by hypersecretion

Corneal Enlargement
- Myopia
- Megalocornea
- Marfan syndrome
- Metabolic disorders
- Anterior chamber cleavage syndrome

Haab's Striae
- Birth trauma (forceps)
- Keratoconus

Optic Nerve Cupping
- Tumor
- Congenital
  - Coloboma/pit
  - Oblique optic nerve insertion
  - Familial

Myopia

Corneal Opacification and Edema
- Congenital
  - Anterior chamber cleavage syndrome
  - Sclerocornea
  - Dermoid
- Trauma (particularly at birth)
- Corneal dystrophies
- Inflammation secondary to HSV, rubella, interstitial keratitis, or uveitis
- Inborn errors of metabolism, such as the mucopolysaccharidoses
- Chromosomal abnormalities, such as a trisomy

TYPES OF CHILDHOOD GLAUCOMA

PRIMARY GLAUCOMA

Primary congenital glaucoma is the most common form of childhood glaucoma and accounts for approximately 50% of these cases. It usually presents early in life, and is diagnosed by the age of 1 year 80% of the time. This disease is bilateral in 70% of patients and affects males and females with a 3:2 ratio. Inheritance is multifactorial in 90% and autosomal recessive in the remaining 10% of patients. The natural course of this glaucoma produces blindness.[278]

Pathogenesis is probably due to the isolated maldevelopment of the trabecular meshwork drainage system. Gonioscopy usually reveals anterior iris insertion into the ciliary body and an increased translucent appearance to the trabecular meshwork (Fig. 8.103). Clinical features include the classic signs and symptoms of congenital glaucoma described above.

Surgery is the definitive treatment, and goniotomy or trabeculotomy is the procedure of choice. Early management decreases IOP and produces a cure rate of greater than 80%, but more than one procedure is often necessary.

In the late-onset form of this disease, elevated IOP occurs after the age of 3 years, when distensibility of the eye decreases. The onset of this glaucoma is usually slow, and the patient is asymptomatic and the examination findings are similar to adult open-angle glaucoma. Management is difficult, and surgery is often unsuccessful owing to the greater propensity for rapid healing in the young.

OTHER DEVELOPMENTAL GLAUCOMAS

Aniridia is a bilateral congenital disorder characterized by the absence of the iris except for a remnant of its root.[279] There is a frequent association with other ocular abnormalities such as cataracts, ectopia lentis, corneal pannus, and foveal hypoplasia (Fig. 8.104). Underdevelopment of the macula may

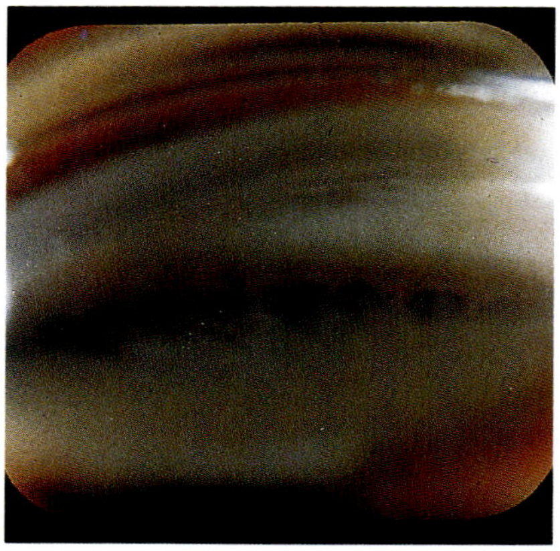

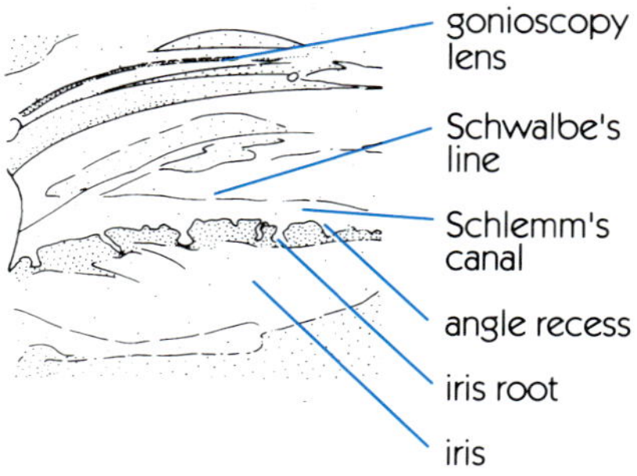

8.103 | Gonioscopic appearance of anterior chamber angle in primary infantile glaucoma. (From Hoskins HD Jr, Kass M: *Becker-Shaffer's Diagnosis and Therapy of the Glaucomas*, ed 6. St. Louis: CV Mosby, 1989.)

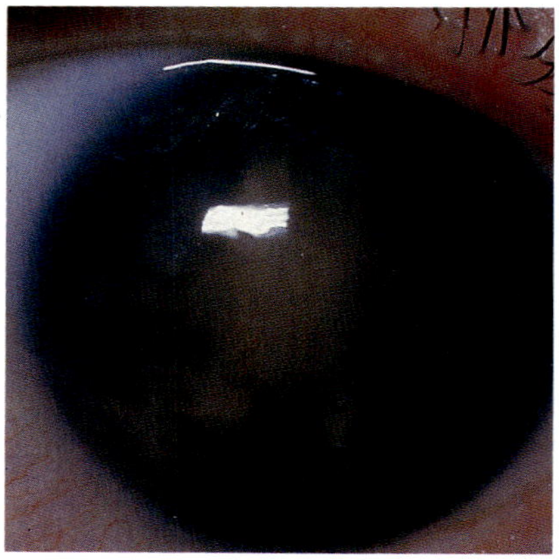

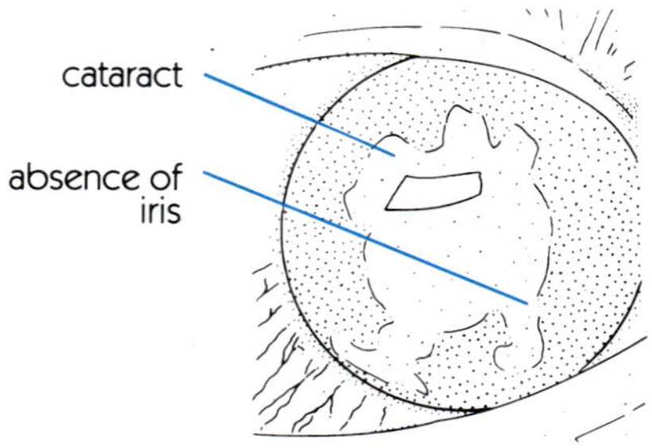

8.104 | Aniridia with cataract. Note corneal pannus.

lead to reduced vision and nystagmus. Systemic aspects of this syndrome include mental retardation and genitourinary anomalies. It is a hereditary disease, transmitted as an autosomal dominant trait in two out of three cases. The remaining third of cases are sporadic and are believed to be the result of point mutation. The sporadic cases are associated with a 20% incidence of Wilms' tumor. Glaucoma occurs in 50% of patients with aniridia, usually late in childhood, and is believed due to vestigial iris blockage of the trabecular meshwork. Therapy of this glaucoma is difficult. In younger children goniotomy can be considered. In older children, medical management or filtering surgery works best, but the prognosis is poor.

Sturge–Weber syndrome is characterized by a facial hemangioma associated with the distribution of the trigeminal nerve (Fig. 8.105). Hemangiomas may also be found in the meninges and can cause seizures. Ocular involvement may be seen in the conjunctiva, episcleral vessels, iris, angle, choroid, or retina. This disease is usually unilateral. The mode of genetic transmission is unclear. Glaucoma usually occurs when a hemangioma involves the lid or conjunctiva. Elevated IOP appears to be caused by trabeculodysgenesis or elevated episcleral venous pressure.[280,281] The treatment of choice is unclear, but medical treatment can be attempted. If this fails, goniotomy and guarded filtering surgery can be tried. Postoperative complications are common and the prognosis is poor.

Neurofibromatosis (von Recklinghausen's disease) is a systemic disorder characterized by multiple café-au-lait spots, absence of part of the sphenoid bone, and by neurofibromas of the viscera, skin, peripheral and central nervous systems, and iris. Transmission is usually autosomal dominant with variable expression, although some cases are the result of spontaneous mutation. Glaucoma occurs most frequently when the neurofibromas involve the eye or eyelid. The pathogenesis of the glaucoma appears to be due to trabeculodysgenesis.[282] The best form of treatment is unclear, but goniotomy is usually considered to be the first step in management.

Goniodysgenesis is the improper development of the mesodermal structures of the anterior segment of the eye. This results in abnormalities of the cornea, iris, and angle. Three forms of goniodysgenesis predispose the patient to glaucoma.[283]

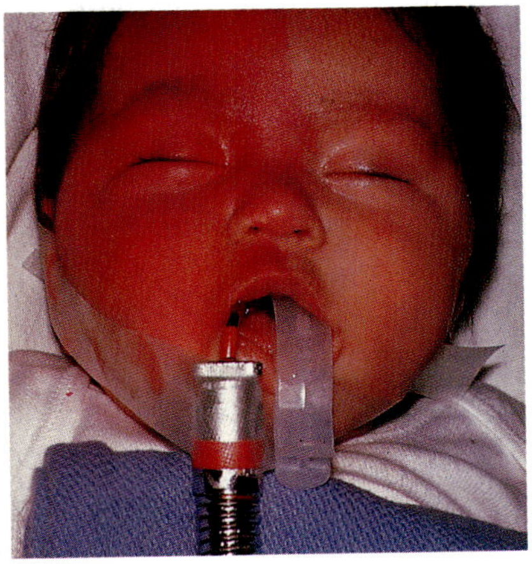

8.105 | Sturge–Weber syndrome. Note right-sided facial hemangioma involving eyelids in this infant with unilateral glaucoma.

Axenfeld's anomaly is characterized by a thickened and anteriorly displaced Schwalbe's line (termed posterior embryotoxon), with iris strands attached to the posterior embryotoxon (Fig. 8.106).

Rieger's syndrome involves a spectrum of ocular findings consisting of posterior embryotoxon, midperipheral iris adhesions (leukomas) to the cornea, iris hypoplasia, and defects of the pupil. Microcornea and macrocornea may accompany this condition. Coexistence with dental or facial abnormalities may occur.

Peter's anomaly is characterized by central corneal opacification and thinning. Frequently there are adhesions of lens and iris to the cornea.

All of these anomalies are inherited as autosomal dominant traits, are bilateral, and have a 50% incidence of glaucoma. Treatment options range from medical therapy to goniotomy and filtering procedures.

Rubella in the newborn can cause cataracts, keratitis, uveitis, microcornea, retinopathy, and glaucoma, as well as systemic manifestations (Fig. 8.107). Glaucoma may be primary, due to trabeculodysgenesis, or secondary, due to uveitis.[284] The treatments of choice are goniotomy or steroids, depending on the cause of the glaucoma. Medical treatment of the glaucoma may also be necessary.

Chromosomal abnormalities associated with pediatric glaucomas include Turner syndrome, trisomy 21, trisomy 13, trisomy 18, and trisomy 29. Therapy must be individualized to each patient.

Pediatric glaucomas are also associated with other rare congenital and inherited abnormalities such as Marfan syndrome, Pierre Robin syndrome, homocystinuria, Lowe syndrome, microcornea, spherophakia, persistent hyperplastic primary vitreous, and broad thumb (Rubinstein–Taybi) syndrome.

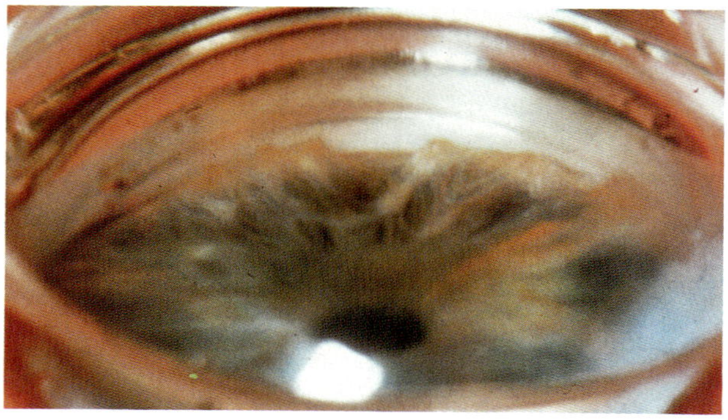

8.106 | Axenfeld's anomaly. Note broad iridial bands extending to anteriorly displaced Schwalbe's line. Chamber angle structures can be seen at the left and center of the photograph.

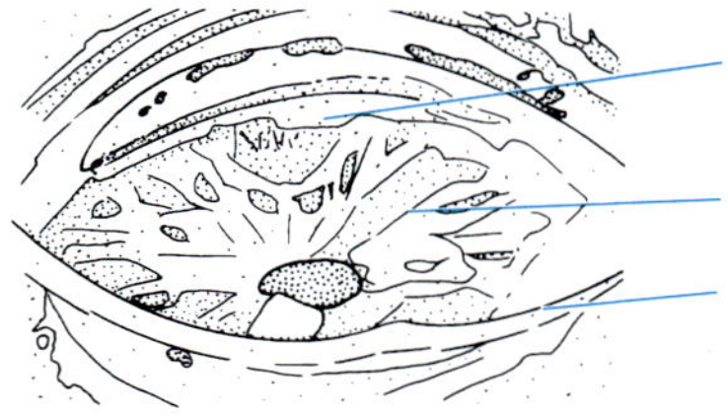

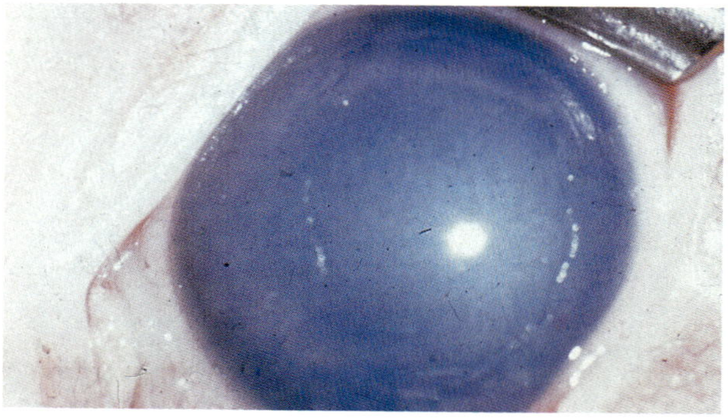

8.107 | Congenital rubella. Note keratitis.

MANAGEMENT

The goal of glaucoma therapy is to reduce IOP below the level that causes damage to the eye. Surgery is the preferred therapy in primary congenital glaucoma and for most other congenital glaucomas, for the following reasons: surgery is often curative; medications are difficult to administer to children; risks of long-term side effects of antiglaucoma medications in children are not established; and medications are often ineffective. Therefore, medical therapy with beta-adrenergic blocking agents, cholinergic agents, adrenergic agents, and carbonic anhydrase inhibitors is used primarily in an adjunctive role in pediatric glaucomas.[285,286] Preoperative medications are used to temporize and to clear the cornea for surgery. Postoperative medications are used in patients who have not responded to surgery.

The preferred type of glaucoma surgery depends on the form of congenital anomaly present and on the clarity of the cornea. In general, the most effective operations for pediatric glaucoma are goniotomy and trabeculotomy. Trabeculectomy is required when the above surgeries fail, as frequently occurs in glaucomas that present with multiple congenital defects.

Goniotomy (Fig. 8.108) consists of a shallow incision into the trabecular meshwork under direct visualization with an operating microscope and gonioscopy lens. A goniotomy knife is passed through the cornea and across the anterior chamber to the opposite angle. The blade is subsequently swept 90–120° along the anterior meshwork with the aid of an assistant who rotates the eye clockwise and counterclockwise, or with the eye stabilized by fixation sutures.[287,288]

The mechanism for the effect of goniotomy is unclear. Perfusion studies show increased aqueous flow into Schlemm's canal. The goniotomy incision recesses the point of iris insertion into the ciliary body and perhaps decompresses the trabecular meshwork. The increased facility of outflow tends to lower IOP. Goniotomy can be repeated three to four times in untreated areas of the eye when further IOP reduction is necessary, as often occurs.[289,290]

Trabeculotomy is a procedure that produces results similar to those of goniotomy.[291,292] It has an added advantage in that it can be performed when corneal clouding prevents adequate visualization of the anterior chamber angle. Trabeculotomy begins with the dissection of a small limbal-based conjunctival flap. A partial-thickness scleral flap, which is hinged at the limbus, is created. An incision into Schlemm's canal is then made by careful, gradual deepening of a radial cut at the gray-white limbus transitional zone. A tra-

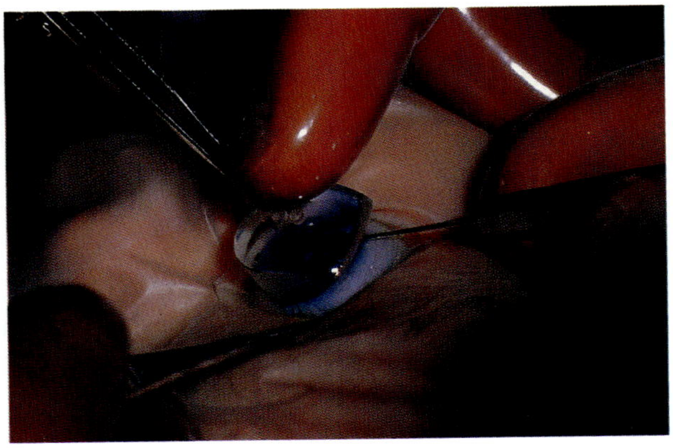

8.108 | Goniotomy with Barkan lens. Goniotomy knife enters cornea near limbus, and is seen through the gonioscopy lens approaching the opposite chamber angle.

beculotome is inserted into one end of Schlemm's canal and is rotated into the anterior chamber, rupturing the trabecular meshwork. The same maneuver is repeated in the opposite direction. The scleral flap is then sutured into place, and the conjunctiva is closed. Normally, some hyphema is seen postoperatively. This procedure, like goniotomy, can be repeated in virgin areas if a further decrease in IOP is necessary. Trabeculotomy can also be combined with trabeculectomy.

In general, goniotomy is the first procedure of choice for the developmental glaucomas. Trabeculotomy is an alternative and can also be performed if the goniotomies fail. Should the above procedures be unsuccessful, trabeculectomy or full-thickness filtering surgery would be the next step.[293–295] Use of a wound-modifying agent such as 5-fluorouracil after or mitomycin-C during filtering surgery is recommended to improve the chances for surgical success, although the former, requiring daily or alternate day subconjunctival injections is problematic in this age group. If despite these interventions the glaucoma remains uncontrolled, a seton procedure can be considered.[296] Cyclodestructive procedures remain the last viable option.[297]

SUMMARY

The pediatric glaucomas are an important cause of childhood visual disability. Increased IOP can cause optic nerve damage, corneal scarring, and amblyopia, producing loss of sight.[298] Individual prognosis depends on the type of glaucoma present. Early diagnosis and appropriate diligent therapy can make a substantial difference in the visual outcome for these difficult patients.

9 THERAPY OF GLAUCOMA

SECTION I

TREATMENT OF GLAUCOMA BY LOWERING INTRAOCULAR PRESSURE

Todd W. Perkins

EVIDENCE

Once a diagnosis of glaucoma has been made, it is necessary to formulate a treatment strategy. This strategy usually involves selecting a target intraocular pressure (IOP) that will slow or stop further progression of the disease.[1] But what is the evidence that lowering IOP arrests the progression of glaucoma?

Throughout different periods of history, ophthalmologists have placed varying degrees of importance on the role of IOP in glaucoma. Views have ranged from an exclusive emphasis on pressure to a total neglect of pressure. In the late nineteenth century, von Graefe explained the excavation of the disc as the consequence of high IOP. Later, however, Schnabel described caverns of the optic nerve as characteristics of glaucoma that he supposed to be independent from IOP and of a "primary" nature.[2] In the past two decades, academic discussion of glaucoma has tended to neglect the importance of IOP. Recently, however, there has been more emphasis on IOP in the literature.[3,4] The approach to therapy of elevated pressure in glaucoma tends to mirror the importance placed on IOP as a causative factor in the disease.

There is good evidence that IOP is a risk factor for glaucomatous damage. Elevated IOP is present in the majority of glaucoma cases.[5,6] The effect of IOP in unilateral secondary glaucoma is obvious to any practitioner. Even in normal-tension glaucoma (low-tension glaucoma), IOP has been implicated as a contributing factor.[7,8] In experimental animal models, it has been shown that elevated IOP causes a glaucomatous pattern of damage.[9]

On the basis of such observations and historical clinical evidence, most ophthalmologists assume that lowering IOP by medical means helps in the treatment of glaucoma. Recently, however, this assumption has been challenged. A position paper has suggested that "...there is virtually no usable evidence about the effectiveness of medical treatment for glaucoma."[10] In fact, the evidence for the efficacy of glaucoma treatment is relatively weak. Despite the history of glaucoma being variably related to IOP, few if any controlled clinical trials have demonstrated that treating glaucoma alters the course of disease. Our only evidence comes from collating a patchwork of clinical observations, studies of conditions related to glaucoma, and small retrospective studies of glaucoma therapy.

Many studies point indirectly to the beneficial effects of lowering IOP. It has been shown that a decrease in IOP may lead to reversal of optic nerve cupping, suggesting such reversal as a therapeutic endpoint.[11,12] Although ethical reasons preclude a randomized trial of treatment versus no treatment in primary open-angle glaucoma (POAG), no such limitation prevents studies in the related condition of ocular hypertension. Several investigators have found that lowering of IOP in ocular hypertensives was associated with less progression of optic nerve and visual field changes.[13–15] However, other investigators found no such effect.[16,17] Similarly, in a study of normal-tension (low-tension) glaucoma, a related condition, eyes that had undergone surgery had an 8% rate of visual field progression at a pressure of 12 mm Hg, while contralateral control eyes on medical therapy had a 44% rate of progression at a pressure of 18 mm Hg over a 3-year period.[18]

RETROSPECTIVE EVIDENCE FOR THE EFFICACY OF LOWERING IOP

The best evidence we have that lowering IOP arrests the progression of optic nerve and visual field damage comes from reviewing studies that have examined the effectiveness of three modes of glaucoma therapy: medical, combined medical and surgical, and surgical. By looking at the role of IOP in these studies, it is possible to draw some rough conclusions about management of pressure in glaucoma patients.

MEDICAL THERAPY

The results of long-term medical treatment of glaucoma are relatively poor. A number of studies have shown that over half of medically treated patients continue to suffer progressive visual field loss when followed long term (Fig. 9.1). However, these patients are probably far better off than untreated patients. Although no randomized prospective trial exists to give us a true

Figure 9.1. Visual Field Loss in Medically Treated Primary Open-Angle Glaucoma

Investigator	Field Progression (%)	Follow-Up (Yr)	IOP (mm Hg)	"Annual Rate" (%)
Hart, Becker[19]	73	10	20.4	7.3
Mikelberg et al[20]	76	7.6	—	10
Kolker[21]	59	4	19.5	15
Leydhecker, Gramer[22]	21	5	19	4
Mao et al[3]	50	4	19	12

untreated control group of glaucoma patients, an estimate can be made from a study of suboptimally treated patients. In 1974, a study of phenytoin for stabilization of visual fields in glaucoma was completed. Although phenytoin was shown to be ineffective in stabilizing fields, the study was helpful in providing a conservative estimate of the incidence of field loss in suboptimally treated POAG. Visual field loss occurred at an annual rate of 32% in these partially treated glaucoma patients.[1] The results of the studies of medical treatment for glaucoma suggest that the "annual rates" of field progression are much less than 32% (see Fig. 9.1).

More convincing evidence for the efficacy of lowering IOP comes from studies of the role of IOP in preventing disease progression. A strong correlation has been found between low IOP and retention of fixation in visual fields of advanced glaucoma patients.[2] Twenty-nine percent of patients with IOPs of 23 mm Hg or greater lost fixation, 19% did so at IOPs of 18–22 mm Hg, and only 4% lost fixation at IOPs of 17 mm Hg or less. In such advanced disease, it is well accepted that little benefit of pressure control is seen unless pressure is reduced to very low levels.

Recent studies using photographic and automated perimetric methods suggest that even in early disease visual field stability occurs only at pressures in the low-to-mid teens. One study[3] noted that *none* of their patients with IOPs ≤16 mm Hg progressed, whereas *all* of the patients with pressures ≥22 mm Hg worsened over a 4–11-year follow-up. At IOPs between 17 and 21 mm Hg, 50% of patients progressed (Fig. 9.2). Another study found that the rate of annual visual field decay was twice as great for mean IOPs >18 compared with IOPs <18, while for IOPs >22, the rate was four times greater.[23] Therefore, it may be that medical therapy could be more effective if used to reduce IOP to the lower teens. Apart from the absolute level of IOP, increased variation in IOP has also been shown to correlate with an increased rate of visual field loss.[4,24,25]

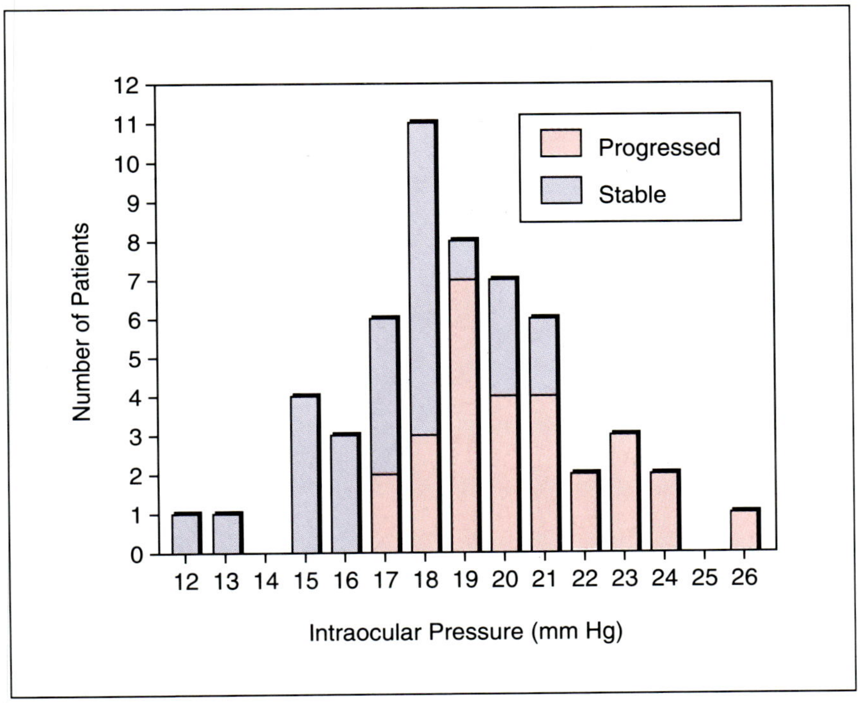

9.2 | Mean IOP of patients who remained stable or had progressive glaucomatous changes during the follow-up period. (From Mao LK, Stewart WC, Shields MB: Correlation between intraocular pressure control and progressive glaucomatous damage in primary open-angle glaucoma. *Am J Ophthalmol 1991;111:51–55.*) Published with permission from the *American Journal of Ophthalmology*. Copyright by the Ophthalmic Publishing Company.

Perhaps most important, several authors have noted a greater rate of automated visual field deterioration in *early* disease,[3,4,26] contrary to reports from earlier observers who noted that early disease tended to progress more slowly.[27] It may be that current methods of photographic optic nerve evaluation and automated perimetry allow detection of more subtle early defects. This finding may have important therapeutic ramifications.

STUDIES OF MEDICATION AND SURGERY

Additional evidence that reducing IOP to the low teens provides significant protection against progression comes from studies of combined medical and surgical management of glaucoma. One investigator has shown a dose–response relationship for IOP in causing visual field deterioration in a group of advanced glaucoma patients treated both medically and surgically.[28] Only patients with IOP consistently <15 mm Hg had a better than 50% chance of remaining stable (Fig. 9.3).

Another investigator showed that visual field progression occurred in only 10.5% of his surgically treated patients while their IOPs averaged 15.7 mm Hg.[21] Other investigators have reported long-term visual field progression in only 12.5% of eyes with IOPs of 14 mm Hg over an 8–42-year period.[29] These findings are consistent with observations that pressures in the high teens often led to blindness in advanced disease, whereas vision was usually retained when pressures remained in the lower teens.[27]

SURGICAL TREATMENT

Even more convincing evidence for the effectiveness of lowering IOP comes from studies of the efficacy of trabeculectomy in arresting visual field damage.[34] A randomized controlled trial of steroid use after trabeculectomy[30] suggested that visual field progression is dramatically reduced in patients with IOPs <15 mm Hg. It was found that patients treated with steroids had an average postoperative IOP of 14.4 mm Hg and had only a 6% incidence of visual field progression over a 5-year period. Patients not receiving steroids had an average pressure of 19.3 mm Hg and a 58% rate of progression.

Collectively, other studies of trabeculectomy results suggest the same rough dose–response effect of IOP[31] (Fig. 9.4). In addition, it appears that results of trabeculectomy are superior to those of medical treatment, perhaps conse-

Figure 9.3. Progression of Visual Field Loss Related to IOP in Advanced Medically or Surgically Treated Glaucoma

IOP (mm Hg)*	Eyes (N)	Progressed (%)
All ≤15	9	33
10–20, mostly ≤15	17	47
10–20, mostly >15	11	82
Some ≥20	37	84
All ≥21	5	100

*On multiple occasions.

(From Odberg T: Visual field prognosis in advanced glaucoma. *Acta Ophthalmol 1987; 65(suppl 182):27–29.)*

quent to the lower IOP usually achieved by trabeculectomy. Within several individual studies, the authors noted a similar dose–response effect of pressure. One study noted that 70% of patients with peak IOPs >21 mm Hg progressed, while only 21% of patients with peaks <22 mm Hg showed further visual field loss.[32] Another found that 56% of patients progressed with mean IOPs >21 mm Hg, but only 29% progressed with mean IOPs <21 mm Hg.[33] As with medications, less variation in IOP was also associated with less progression after surgery.[32]

IMPLICATIONS FOR THERAPY

On the basis of these observations, what therapeutic conclusions can be drawn? As shown above, in long-term follow-up the current therapeutic approach with medications only protects 25–50% of patients from further progression. But we have seen that IOPs controlled below 15 mm Hg preserve visual field in the large majority of patients in the presence of advanced disease. There is also some evidence that lowering IOP is effective in halting damage in normal-tension glaucoma.[18] Therefore, it is likely that lowering IOP in glaucoma is beneficial, and that if IOP is brought low enough most patients may be protected from deterioration. Pressure has been considered one risk factor for damage in glaucoma; the aim of therapy is to decrease this risk.[35] Because each patient presents with a different pressure, it may be reasonable to lower pressure by a significant percentage,[35] e.g., 30%. The data presented above suggest that IOP needs to be brought to 15 mm Hg or lower to offer substantial protection to the optic nerve. Even though we have traditionally reserved such low IOPs for advanced disease, it may be that visual field progression in early disease is actually more rapid than in advanced disease.[3,4] It may be helpful to keep in mind that "normalizing" IOP really means bringing it to the true normal mean of 15–16 mm Hg, not the upper limit of "normal."[2] Conversely, if a patient presents with maximum IOP of 16 mm Hg, it is probably necessary to reduce it to 10 or 12 mm Hg to reduce significantly the risk of progression from pressure.

Surgery reduces the risk of visual field progression to about 10–35% in most of the studies cited above. Some clinicians have concluded that primary surgery offers better protection to the optic nerve than medical therapy.[36] Medications have several disadvantages that may adversely affect success. Compliance is required. In addition, diurnal variation is not dampened as greatly as with surgery.[18,36] Wider fluctuations in IOP are associated with

Figure 9.4. Visual Field Deterioration After Trabeculectomy for Glaucoma

Investigator	Average IOP (mm Hg)	Field Loss Worse (%)	Follow-up (Yrs)	Number of Patients
Roth et al[30]	14.4	6	5	33
Kidd, O'Connor[31]	15.0	18	5	60
Kolker[21]	15.7	10	4+	22
Werner et al[32]	16.0	35	3.5	24
Greve, Dake[33]	17.3	35	4	42
Rollins, Drance[34]	18.1	29	5	48
Roth et al[30]	19.1	58	5	19

greater progression, and many of these fluctuations occur outside of office hours and are unknown to the physician.[37] The major advantage of medications is that operative complications are avoided.

APPROACH TO THERAPY

The general therapeutic approach to the glaucoma patient should be first to determine a target IOP.[1] Typically, this will require a significant reduction of pressure.[35] Depending on the other risk factors present and the response to therapy, an initial reduction of 30% seems to be a reasonable target. Some clinicians feel that the reduction should aim for a pressure closer to 15 mm Hg, based on the long-term data presented above. The target can be adjusted depending on the response to therapy and the anticipated iatrogenic risk of the next intervention.

Once the target pressure is reached, the patient is then evaluated over time to determine whether the target is low enough to halt progression of damage. Frequent examinations are made to ascertain the level of damage and to detect any further deterioration.[35]

Medications are still the first line of therapy but can be used more effectively than in the past. A monocular therapeutic trial is performed to determine efficacy and acceptance by the patient.[1] Generous amounts of encouragement and education will help to stimulate compliance and acceptance by the patient. Most important, practitioners must resist "target slippage"—the temptation to allow slight elevations of IOP above target to accumulate without further intervention so that a higher target has been chosen de facto.

Laser trabeculoplasty is usually the next line of treatment, although some proponents suggest primary laser treatment,[37] and many often omit it as poorly effective in advanced cases.

Trabeculectomy with suture lysis or removable sutures is presently the surgical procedure of choice. Advocates for primary surgery note lower and more stable IOP with surgery,[36] although most clinicians still feel that the risks outweigh those benefits.[1] Chemical wound healing retardants, such as 5-fluorouracil and mitomycin-C, have become routine adjuvants in high-risk cases. Current investigation of laser sclerostomy suggests a place for this simpler procedure, although its ultimate role will be determined by studies of complications and long-term effectiveness.

Once trabeculectomy with adjuvant chemotherapy has failed, a drainage device is then used. The Molteno implant[38] was the first such device, and serves as the archetype for many new implants now available.

Ciliodestructive procedures, such as transscleral cyclophotocoagulation, are usually the last line of intervention in recalcitrant glaucoma. This procedure has largely supplanted cyclocryotherapy and is used by some in lieu of drainage devices.

The details of each of these treatments in the glaucoma armamentarium will be discussed in the sections that follow. However, as with any weapon, the target must be kept in mind. The data discussed above suggest that this target will entail a significant pressure reduction of 20–30% and perhaps to a level close to 15 mm Hg in the majority of primary open-angle glaucoma patients. Beyond these rough guidelines, management of patients with these therapeutic agents must be tailored to each individual. Risks of both intervening and not intervening are weighed in the context of the patient's life situation and life expectancy. A large "gray area" exists in glaucoma decision making, frustrating the novice and challenging the expert. Such is the art of glaucoma practice.

SECTION II

MEDICAL THERAPY OF GLAUCOMA

Paul L. Kaufman
Thomas W. Mittag

GENERAL CONSIDERATIONS

Primary-open angle glaucoma (POAG) is a multifactorial disease for which a variety of risk factors have been identified (e.g., age, race, family history, diabetes, blood pressure, and intraocular pressure) (see Wilensky, Chapter 8). Other types of primary glaucoma (e.g., angle-closure, infantile) and a large array of secondary glaucomas have different pathophysiologies and risk factors, but all glaucomas produce visual loss in the same manner: a characteristic type of optic neuropathy (see Radius, Higginbotham, and Caprioli and Weinreb, Chapter 6) resulting in progressive and characteristic loss of the visual field (see Heijl, Chapter 7). Our understanding of the pathophysiology of this optic neuropathy is so limited at present that therapy in all cases is restricted to manipulation of only one parameter, the intraocular pressure (IOP). All glaucoma therapeutic modalities—pharmacologic, laser or incisional surgical—are designed to lower IOP.

The hydraulics of aqueous humor dynamics are described by the modified Goldmann equation, as follows:[39]

$$F = C_{trab}\,(IOP - Pe) + U$$

where F = aqueous humor flow, C_{trab} = facility of outflow from the anterior chamber via the trabecular meshwork and Schlemm's canal, IOP = intraocular pressure, Pe = episcleral venous pressure (the pressure against which fluid leaving the anterior chamber via the trabecular–canalicular route must drain), U = uveoscleral outflow.

The physiology of these various parameters has been considered in detail in other sections of this chapter, and will not be repeated here. Nevertheless, if we rearrange the equation such that

$$IOP = \frac{F-U}{C_{trab}} + Pe$$

it is apparent that for a modality (e.g., a drug) to lower IOP it must either decrease F or Pe, or increase C_{trab} or U.[39]

DRUG DELIVERY

The eye's external location affords it a unique opportunity to receive pharmacologic agents directly via topical rather than via systemic administration. This reduces but, unfortunately, does not eliminate the risk of systemic side effects from the very potent drugs used to treat glaucoma. Given the 10 μl capacity of the human conjunctival sac and the limited rate at which most drugs cross the cornea to enter the anterior chamber, it is not surprising that drug solutions of very high concentration must be administered topically to achieve therapeutically effective intraocular concentrations. Most topical drops are 25–50 μl and therefore 60–80% of the dose overflows immediately into the lacrimal drainage. (Despite the fact that a 10–15-μl drop size would be more desirable, a practical and simple device to deliver such small volumes without touching the eye has yet to be devised.) The drug dose initially retained by the conjunctival sac (10 μl) leaves the eye at approximately 15% per minute due to normal tear formation, blinking, and lacrimal drainage. Therefore, to maximize absorption a second dose should be given no sooner than 5–7 minutes after the first.

Even with maneuvers designed to enhance corneal penetration and increase corneal contact time (e.g., adjusting pH, prodrugs, increasing viscosity, wetting agents, lacrimal punctal occlusion, eyelid closure), the majority of any drug applied topically leaves the conjunctival sac via the lacrimal drainage system and reaches the nasopharyngeal mucosa, whence it is rapidly absorbed into the general circulation. Therefore, it is important to understand the potential systemic as well as the adverse ocular effects of antiglaucoma drugs, and the interaction of the drugs with other agents the patients may be taking for other medical conditions. Because the majority of POAG patients are elderly (see Wilensky, Chapter 8) and may well be under treatment for cardiovascular and pulmonary diseases, this is of more than theoretical importance.

DRUG RESPONSE MECHANISMS

Drugs presently used as glaucoma therapy alter cellular functions in the eye by direct interaction either with receptors or with certain specific enzymes. Although no presently used therapeutic glaucoma agent is known to interact directly with ion channels of cells, as outlined below, channels are probably important effectors of responses initiated by glaucoma drugs acting via receptors.

Signal transduction mediated by drug receptors is a rapidly expanding field. New knowledge and increased understanding of this field are advancing in two areas. The first area, resulting mostly from application of molecular biology techniques, concerns the discovery of new subtypes of receptors. These advances include several families of receptors relevant to current glaucoma therapy. At the time of writing, this group includes three forms of β-adrenergic receptor (β_1, β_2, and β_3), six types of α-adrenergic receptors (α_{1A}, α_{1B}, α_{1C}, α_{2A}, α_{2B}, and α_{2C}), five types of dopamine receptors (D1–D5), and at least five types of muscarinic acetylcholine receptors (AChR-M_1–M_5). The new subtypes of receptors have been identified from their mRNA sequences. Unfortunately, our knowledge of the physiologic or pharmacologic significance of these subtypes lags far behind the knowledge of their structural identity. However, these new findings hold promise for future development of more selective drugs targeted to specific subtypes of receptors expressed on specific cell types.

The second area of rapidly expanding knowledge concerns the biochemical events of signal transduction initiated by receptor activation. The general pattern for signal transduction is given by the headings at the left in Figure 9.5, and can be described as follows. Interaction of the primary signal

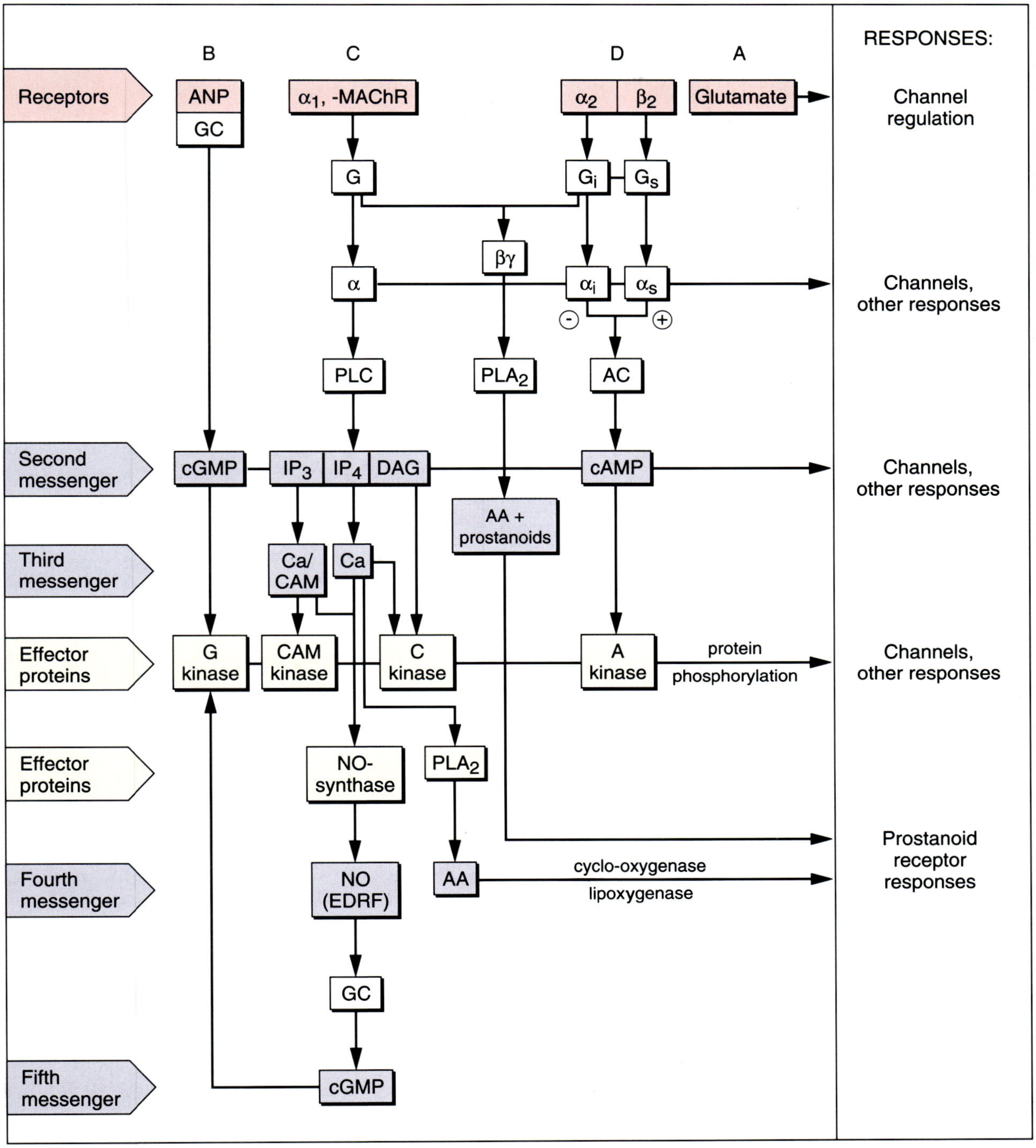

9.5 | Representative receptor/signal pathway cascades A–D (see text). General sequence denoted by headings at left and responses at right of figure. ANP = atrial natriuretic peptide. MACh-R = muscarinic acetylcholine receptor. α_1, α_2, β_2 = subtypes of adrenergic receptors. G = guanylyl nucleotide binding protein. α_i, α_s = subunit of G-protein. $\beta\gamma$ = subunit complex of G-protein. GC = guanylyl cyclase. AC = adenylyl cyclase. PLC = phospholipase C. PLA_2 = phospholipase A_2. IP_3, IP_4 = inositol phosphates. AA = arachidonic acid. DAG = diacylglycerol. CAM = calmodulin. NO (EDRF) = nitric oxide.

molecule (the first messenger) with its specific receptor triggers a cascade of one or more amplification steps involving small intermediate signal molecules (second and third messengers), which culminates in the regulation of a specific effector protein at the end of the first stage of the signal pathway. The active effector protein(s) (usually an enzyme such as a kinase) may directly mediate the cell response (e.g., regulate closing of ion channels by protein phosphorylation), may activate additional regulatory proteins which act by further protein–protein interactions, or may generate the second, third, and even a fourth messenger. Several components of a signal transduction cascade, including small molecule messengers, effector proteins, or regulatory proteins, can contribute to the overall final cell response(s). Most of our present knowledge involves the biochemical steps from receptor to effector protein (enzyme). Much less is known of the specific events from the effector protein to the final cell response, but specific protein phosphorylation and dephosphorylation seems to be one major mechanism.

These general concepts are further illustrated by individual schemes diagrammed in Figure 9.5, which shows four major types of signal transduction cascade. These signal pathways have been fairly well established from studies in a variety of mammalian tissues and, as can be seen from the types of receptors involved, most of them are relevant to drugs used in glaucoma (discussed in more detail under specific drug sections of this chapter). Because similar signal pathways occur in many different cell types it is important to recognize that the same signal transduction pathway can give quite different responses in different cells. A well-known example of this is the effect of the β-adrenergic agonist isoproterenol acting via the β-receptor/cAMP signal pathway, which in cardiac muscle cells increases contraction, whereas in most smooth muscle cells this pathway decreases contraction, i.e., causes relaxation. Such differences in response usually result from different pathways beyond the effector protein (enzyme) step of the signal cascade, i.e., that part of the signal cascade of which current understanding is limited.

CASCADE A

The number of steps in a signal transduction pathway can vary greatly. The shortest pathways fall into the category of ligand operated channels (see Fig. 9.5, scheme A), where the channel and the receptor are integral. No second messenger is involved and the response is directly controlled by the primary signal molecule. Examples of this type are mostly found in electrically excitable cells such as those in the CNS, where excitatory amino acid receptors (glycine, GABA-A, glutamate)[40] can operate anion or cation channels. Receptors of this type have not been investigated in target tissues involved in glaucoma therapy.

CASCADE B

The next level of complexity is illustrated by the signal pathway for the atrial natriuretic peptide (ANP; see Fig. 9.5, scheme B), where the receptor is integral with the enzyme for second messenger generation.[41] Thus, ANP acting as the primary signal directly controls a guanylyl cyclase activity, which generates cGMP. Although not yet demonstrated in the primate eye, this pathway probably has relevance in ocular hemodynamics and/or aqueous humor dynamics,[42] since ANP[43] and its receptor are present in anterior segment structures[44,45] (e.g., ciliary processes) and may also be expressed in other fluid-transporting tissues (e.g., kidney[46]). The second messenger of this cascade, cGMP, plays several roles, including regulation of cation channels directly in some sensory cells (e.g., photoreceptors).[47] Cyclic GMP also activates the enzyme G-kinase. G-kinase is an important mediator of relaxation in vascular smooth muscle cells and pericytes. Because of these actions cGMP and G-kinase could play a role in the regulation of tone and responsiveness of intraocular muscles (iris and ciliary muscle) and intraocular vascular beds (ciliary, choroidal circulation) or the venous drainage vessels of the eye.

CASCADE C
Autacoid and Other Responses

This is an important general pathway which has branch points at the second and third messenger level and mediates a variety of responses.

G-kinase-mediated relaxation of vascular smooth muscle, an endpoint of cascade B, can also be achieved via the signal transduction cascade illustrated in Figure 9.5, scheme C. This is one of the longest pathways thus far delineated, involving five messenger molecules. Receptors on vascular endothelial cells (for example, AChR-M or α_1-adrenergic receptors) can be the initiating signal that leads to a rise in intracellular calcium. Beginning at the endothelial cell (first cell), the agonist-stimulated receptor activates a G-protein which dissociates into its β–γ component and α-subunit. The specific α-subunit of the G-protein coupled to the specific receptor activates phospholipase-C (PLC) to produce inositol phosphates (IP_3 or IP_4), the second messenger. IP_3 releases internal stores of calcium ions and/or mediates influx of calcium ions from outside the cell.

This rise in intracellular calcium (third messenger), together with calmodulin, activates an enzyme, NO-synthase,[48] which acts on arginine to produce nitric oxide (NO) or an NO-derivative (fourth messenger). This labile mediator (known as endothelium derived relaxing factor, EDRF[49]) can diffuse to adjacent smooth muscle cells (second cell) and activate guanylyl cyclase (a different isoenzyme from the ANP receptor/enzyme in cascade B). The cGMP thus formed (fifth messenger) activates G-kinase, which mediates smooth muscle relaxation.

An important feature of this type of signal pathway is that mediators generated by one cell affect adjacent or neighboring cells. This represents a general signal scheme for responses to locally produced (autacoid) substances. Prostanoids, which are another important class of autacoid substances with relevance to glaucoma therapy (see below), can be produced by a similar pathway. This is diagrammed by the right-hand branch from the Ca^{2+} third messenger step at the bottom of cascade C. In this case, the rise of intracellular calcium in the first cell activates a phospholipase A_2 enzyme (PLA_2) which causes the formation of arachidonic acid (AA). The AA or its active prostanoid metabolites (fourth messenger) can diffuse to adjacent cells (second cell) to initiate responses via the cyclooxygenase or lipoxygenase products of arachidonic acid. Because drugs that can activate AChR-M (e.g., pilocarpine) and α_1-adrenergic (e.g., epinephrine) receptors are important antiglaucoma agents (see below), both of these autacoid-generating pathways may play a role in the ocular response to such agents (see section on prostaglandins).

Calcium/Contractile Responses

Activation of cascade C by AChR-M and α_1-adrenergic receptors has a further important role because it mediates contractile responses of many cells. Contractile responses involve the second messengers IP_3, IP_4, and diacylglycerol (DAG), third messengers $[Ca^{2+}]_i$ or its complex with calmodulin (CAM), and the effector enzymes protein kinase C and Ca^{2+}/CAM-activated kinase enzymes. In smooth muscle (and other cells) calcium ion can be released from internal stores. There are at least two types of internal stores, one in which a large calcium release is triggered by a small increase in internal [Ca^{2+}] (this store is characterized by release of its calcium by caffeine), and a second type of internal calcium store in which IP_3 induces the release of calcium. The proportion of these two types of internal store varies widely from one type of smooth muscle to another and has not been characterized in iris or ciliary muscle cells. This signal pathway can also trigger the entry of calcium from outside the cell via Ca^{2+} channels. In some cells, IP_3 or IP_4 seems to be the direct regulator of such channels, but they are more usually regulated via the second messenger DAG, which activates protein kinase C. These mechanisms to control intracellular Ca^{2+} ions are clearly important in the contractile responses of vascular, ciliary, and iris muscle cells (e.g., responses to pilocarpine or epinephrine) and perhaps also for contractile elements in the trabecular outflow apparatus.

CASCADE D

The signal cascade illustrated in Figure 9.5, scheme D, is an important pathway for antiglaucoma drugs. Receptors acting via these routes (α_2, β_2-adrenergic) are coupled to G-proteins that either positively or negatively[50] regulate adenylyl cyclase, but these G-proteins can also have direct functions. For example, in cardiac myocytes the active form of the Gs protein (αs) by itself activates a calcium channel[51] as well as activating the enzyme adenylyl cyclase, which in turn regulates several channels via cAMP (a K^+ channel,[52] a second and possibly different type of Ca^{2+} channel,[53] and a Cl^- channel[54]). In addition, this pathway illustrates the important concept that different intermediates of a particular signal cascade can have independent regulatory functions. The second messenger cAMP itself can directly activate cation channels (as in heart[52] or olfactory sensory neurons[55]), and it also activates cellular cAMP-dependent protein kinase. This class of kinase (A-kinase) apparently regulates many cell responses, including some important and widely distributed cellular ion channels, such as activation of "big-K" calcium-dependent potassium channels[53] and activation of chloride channels in epithelial cells.[56] Multiple channel regulation that can be effected by mediators of the cAMP pathway (cascades C and D) are indicated in Figure 9.5 at right and have direct relevance to possible mechanisms of ocular hypotensive drugs (e.g., β-blockers, epinephrine, apraclonidine) that interact with β- and/or α_2-adrenergic receptors. These possible mechanisms will be discussed under specific drug types in the following sections of this chapter.

Very recent studies implicate both of the functional subunits of G-proteins in signal transduction. The families of G-proteins represented in pathways C and D differ in their α-subunits but have common β and γ components. Activation of a G-protein by receptor stimulation leads to dissociation into the GTP-bound α-subunit (the active form) and the β–γ component. β–γ has been found to activate a PLA_2 enzyme, generating free AA from which prostanoid second messengers are formed.[57] (This interconnecting pathway is indicated in Fig. 9.5 between the C and D cascades.) The PLA_2 involved is likely to be different from the Ca^{2+}-regulated PLA_2 enzyme indicated further down in pathway C. This newly discovered pathway for the formation of prostanoids has potential relevance to the generation of prostaglandins in anterior segment tissues.

SPECIFIC AGENTS
CHOLINOMIMETICS

Cholinomimetics (Fig. 9.6) lower IOP by increasing trabecular outflow facility. Classically, this effect is thought to be mediated by muscarinic receptors in the ciliary muscle. When the receptors are stimulated, the muscle contracts. Contraction is mediated by free intracellular Ca^{2+} ions. Although not studied specifically in ciliary muscle fibers, this probably occurs via cascade C (see Fig. 9.5) with IP_3, IP_4, or DAG as second messengers leading to Ca

Figure 9.6. Cholinomimetics*

Drug	Delivery/Duration/ Frequency	Side Effects: Ocular	Side Effects: Systemic
Direct acting—imitate acetylcholine (ACh)			
Pilocarpine Isopto Carpine Ocusert Pilo, Pilogel SNO Pilo Minims Pilocarpine	Eye drops 0.5–10% sol'n; 4% usually maximal q.6hr Gel (Pilopine HS®) 4% pilocarpine in gel applied q.h.s. 24-hr effect? Ocusert 20 µg/hr, 40 µg/hr constant release rate 7-day duration equivalent to 1–2%, 3–4% drops	Ciliary and conjunctival congestion Ocular and periocular pain Accommodative myopia Pupillary constriction (decreased acuity with lens changes) Iris cysts (with ChE inhibitors; prevented by phenylephrine) Increased pupillary block: angle closure (stronger miotics) Iritis (especially anticholinesterases)	Nausea Vomiting Diarrhea Bradycardia Salivation Sweating CNS (depression, delusions) Apnea (anticholinesterases, if succinylcholine used during general anesthesia)
Carbachol Isopto Carbachol	0.75–3% sol'n q. 6 or 8 hr	Posterior synechiae (even without overt iritis)	
Indirect acting—anticholinesterases—bind acetylcholinesterase		Retinal detachment (especially with strong miotics in aphakes) Lacrimal canalicular stenosis (especially anticholinesterase)	
Echothiophate (Phospholine Iodide®) (Phospholine Iodide)	0.03–0.25% sol'n q.12 or 24 hr	Allergic conjunctivitis and dermatitis (unusual)	
Demecarium (no more sol)	0.125-0.25% sol'n q.12 or 24 hr	Irritative conjunctivitis and follicular hypertrophy (eserine) Cataracts (anticholinesterases) Decreased ocular rigidity (anticholinesterases)	

*Additive to all other currently available antiglaucoma drugs.

release/entry. The fact that ciliary muscles are capable of graded sustained contractions (as in accommodation) indicates that Ca^{2+} entry via channels is probably an important mechanism in these specialized muscle fibers. Because of the intimate anatomic association between the anterior tendons of the muscle and the trabecular meshwork and inner wall of Schlemm's canal (see Rohen and Lütjen-Drecoll, Chapter 1), this contraction mechanically deforms the meshwork and widens the canal in such a way that the resistance to aqueous outflow is decreased (see Nilsson and Bill, Chapter 1). However, when the ciliary muscle contracts, the spaces between the muscle bundles are obliterated, obstructing the drainage of aqueous humor via the uveoscleral route (see Nilsson and Bill, Chapter 1). In general, the enhancement of trabecular drainage outweighs the obstruction of uveoscleral drainage, so that the net effect is decreased IOP.

The other major consequence of ciliary muscle contraction is accommodation, so that near rather than distant objects are in focus. The accommodative myopia induced by cholinomimetic antiglaucoma drugs is a major drawback to their use, especially in younger patients. However, recent anatomic and physiologic evidence suggests that there may be some regionalization of the accommodative and outflow functions within the ciliary muscle.[58] Muscle fiber bundles appear to be grouped in three major orientations, and the directional force exerted by each group is therefore likely to be different. Studies are now in progress to characterize better such regionalization and to determine whether the accommodative and outflow functions might be mediated by different subtypes of AChR-M. If the latter is the case, it may be possible to employ subtype-specific agonists to maximize contraction mediating the outflow effect while minimizing contraction mediating the accommodative effect. The same strategy could prove useful in minimizing the pupillary constriction produced by the action of cholinomimetic drugs on the iris sphincter muscle. The latter is presently a serious drawback to the use of such agents in elderly patients with incipient cataracts, in whom the induced miosis can significantly compromise visual acuity. However, the miotic action of cholinergic agonists is of use in the treatment of various angle closure glaucoma situations (e.g., pupillary block, plateau iris) to pull the iris root away from the trabecular meshwork (see Skuta, Chapter 8).

The possibility of targeting cholinomimetic drugs to reduce iris responses seems quite promising. It is already well known that some muscarinic antagonist drugs are partially selective for mydriasis as compared with cycloplegia (e.g., tropicamide), suggesting a difference in receptors on the two muscles. Although the dominant contractile control of the pupil is via AChR-M, a second cholinergic component causing iris dilator relaxation has been reported.[59] This suggests that when a cholinergic miosis occurs, sphincter muscle contraction and dilator fiber relaxation work together. Cholinergic relaxation occurs in some other primate sphincter muscles by opening of a K^+ channel, possibly via a different subtype of AChR-M than that mediating muscle contractions. Although cholinergic relaxation has not been specifically shown for primate iris dilator muscles, one could postulate a decreased miotic effect for a cholinergic agonist that does not cause iris dilator fibers to relax.

Very recently, the presence of muscarinic receptors, primarily of subtype M3, has been identified in human and bovine trabecular endothelial cells.[58] In addition, cells containing smooth muscle actin and myosin have been identified in the human meshwork, and preliminary studies in bovine tissue have suggested that the meshwork itself may have contractile properties, perhaps independent of the ciliary muscle.[58] Neither the physiologic nor the therapeutic implications of these findings are clear at present, but it may prove possible to devise a therapeutically useful cholinomimetic that acts on the meshwork itself. At present, however, we must view all cholinomimetic effects on aqueous humor dynamics as consequent to the mechanical effects of ciliary muscle contraction. Muscarinic receptors are also present in ciliary processes and other anterior segment structures,[60] but there is no evidence for a meaningful cholinergic effect on the rate of aqueous humor production or on episcleral venous pressure in the human eye.[58]

The topically active cholinergic agonists in common clinical use—carbachol and pilocarpine—have somewhat different characteristics. Carbamylcholine (carbachol) is the methylcarbamyl ester of choline. It is therefore permanently positively charged (quaternary ammonium group) and must be used at high concentrations (0.75–3%) to achieve effective penetration across the cornea. It is just as effective as ACh directly at the receptors, but because of its carbamyl group it is also a weak suicide substrate for acetylcholinesterase (AChE) (see below). Thus, carbamylcholine has a dual action: mostly direct, but partly indirect.

Pilocarpine acts only on AChR-M. The drug effectively penetrates the cornea in its uncharged form, but because it is only a partial agonist (i.e., the maximal response is less than can be obtained with a full agonist such as carbamylcholine) it must be administered in about the same concentration as carbachol to be therapeutically effective.

INDIRECT-ACTING CHOLINERGIC AGENTS

This group of drugs (physostigmine, demecarium, echothiophate, isoflurophate) all block cholinesterase (AChE) and prevent metabolic inactivation of ACh released from parasympathetic nerve endings. None of these drugs has any affinity for MACh receptors. The first two agents block AChE by carbamylating and the second two by phosphorylating the enzyme. Thus, they act somewhat like ACh itself, which acetylates the enzyme, with the significant difference that the acetyl-enzyme has a half-life on the order of microseconds, whereas the $t_{1/2}$ for the carbamyl-E is hours, and days for the phosphoryl-E. These drugs are thus suicide substrates of AChE and some of their effects can last for days or weeks.

When AChE is blocked by such a suicide substrate the concentration of endogenously released ACh and its time of action is increased. Thus, endogenous cholinergic response (tone) is increased and prolonged. The use of AChE inhibitors to treat glaucoma is declining because of their substantial adverse ocular effects (see Fig. 9.6).

ADRENERGIC AGONISTS

From a glaucoma therapeutic perspective, two types of adrenergic agonists are of interest—α_2 and β_2 (Fig. 9.7).

The α_2-adrenergic agonists are powerful inhibitors of aqueous humor formation, reducing fluorophotometrically determined aqueous flow by 35–40% in the conscious human.[61] In some ocular normotensive subjects, the final IOP becomes so low (10 mm Hg) as to suggest that a parameter of aqueous humor outflow is also affected.[62] Since tonographic studies have shown no α_2-agonist effect on outflow facility,[62] and in view of the very low pressures achieved, such an additional effect presumably would be on episcleral venous pressure or uveoscleral outflow. This issue is presently unresolved and further studies are needed. Even considering only ciliary epithelial cells as the site of drug action, it remains unclear whether the α_2-receptors mediating the decrease in aqueous formation are presynaptic (i.e., on sympathetic nerve endings that normally innervate the ciliary processes—indeed, it is unclear whether in the primate the ciliary epithelium actually

Figure 9.7. Adrenergic Agonists*

Drug	Delivery/Duration/Frequency	Side Effects: Ocular	Side Effects: Systemic
α_2			
Apraclonidine (Iopidine®)	1% sol'n-drops Single application or q.12 hr	Allergic blepharo-conjunctivitis Mydriasis Eyelid retraction Conjunctival blanching	Dry nose and mouth Minimal adverse cardio-vascular effects
Brimonidine (in clinical trials)	0.5% sol'n-drops Single application or q.12 hr	To be determined	To be determined
β_2			
Epinephrine	0.25–2% sol'n-drops q.12 hr	Reactive hyperemia Brow ache Headache Allergic blepharo-conjunctivitis Adrenochrome deposits on conjunctiva, cornea Corneal haze and edema Blurred vision and halos Maculopathy in aphakes (20% incidence) Madarosis	Blood pressure elevation Extrasystoles Tachycardia Cerebrovascular accident
Dipivefrin (Propine®)	0.1% sol'n-drops q.12 hr	Mydriasis Angle closure	

*α_2-agonists additive to all other antiglaucoma drugs; β_2-agonists only marginally additive to β_2-antagonists.

receives a sympathetic innervation), postjunctional (i.e., located on the ciliary epithelial cell side of a sympathetic synapse), or are isolated receptors on noninnervated ciliary epithelial cells, or some combination thereof. However, the high density of these receptors found in ciliary processes in animal species suggests that the majority of them are likely to be isolated noninnervated receptors.[63] It is also unresolved whether these agents act solely via α_2-adrenergic receptors. Many drugs in the α_2-adrenergic agonist class have appreciable affinity for dopamine D2-receptors in many tissues. Because dopamine receptors are present in ciliary processes[64] and other anterior segment tissues in some species, drugs classed as "α_2-adrenergic agonists" may also act via D2-receptors in the eye. The signal transduction pathway for α_2-receptor drugs in epithelial cells is also not well understood. Both D2 and α_2-receptors are often found negatively coupled to adenylyl cyclase (see Fig. 9.5, cascade D, left side) but probably activate other signal pathways.

It is hypothesized that activation of these receptors decreases cAMP levels and turns off cAMP-dependent systems responsible for maintaining aqueous humor secretion.[65] This hypothesis is intellectually satisfying because it fits with the mechanism postulated for β-blockers turning off aqueous humor formation.[66] However, other mechanisms are also possible. It has been recently shown that α_2-receptors can control K^+-channel activity independently of cAMP,[67] and channel regulation is likely to be a major control point for aqueous humor formation. Another postulated mechanism for α_2-adrenergic response is activation of presynaptic receptors on sympathetic or peptidergic nerve endings.[68,69] This depresses release of neurohormones or neuropeptides, presumably decreasing the physiologic tone responsible for maintaining the rate of aqueous secretion.[70] However, it is not known whether these mechanisms apply to the human eye.

At present, only one α_2-agonist, apraclonidine, is employed clinically in the United States, and only to prevent or blunt the acute IOP rise caused by anterior segment laser surgical procedures.[62] Studies of the applicability of this drug class for more chronic glaucoma therapy are in progress. In Europe, the parent compound clonidine is used for long-term therapy, but its CNS activity is a major drawback. It causes significant systemic arterial hypotension even when given topically, by interfering with central sympathetic outflow.[62] Indeed, clonidine is used worldwide to treat systemic hypertension.

β_2-adrenergic receptors are present in the cells of the ciliary epithelium,[71] the ciliary muscle,[72] and the trabecular meshwork,[73] so that β_2-agonists have complex effects on aqueous humor dynamics. Although epinephrine is by no means a specific β_2-agonist, its effects on aqueous dynamics are presently all thought to be consequent to its β_2-agonist properties (but see also Nilsson and Bill, Chapter 1). Indeed, it and its prodrug congener dipivifrin are the only such agonists used to treat glaucoma.

Epinephrine increases trabecular outflow facility in rabbit, monkey, and human eyes, probably via a β_2-receptor–cyclic AMP-mediated mechanism (see Fig. 9.5, cascade D, right).[74] Neither the trabecular endothelial cell function nor the consequent physical change in the meshwork responsible for the increased hydraulic conductivity is known. Alteration in composition or turnover of resistance-producing extracellular matrix in the meshwork has been a longstanding hypothesis. Recently, a change in endothelial cell shape, perhaps mediated by cytoskeletal alterations, has emerged as another possibility.[75] Changes in composition of the extracellular matrix could be a specialized response in trabecular cells mediated via cAMP-dependent protein kinase, acting at the level of gene transcription (see Acott, Chapter 1). The hormonal induction of transcription of many eukaryotic genes is an important function of cAMP not normally considered in signal pathways for acute responses such as those shown in Figure 9.5. However, when epinephrine is used chronically, it is possible that "remodeling" of the trabecular meshwork extracellular matrix occurs via gene transcriptional activity, resulting in a decreased outflow resistance.

Epinephrine also increases uveoscleral outflow in monkey[76] and human[77] eyes. Classically, this has been thought consequent to β_2-receptor mediated relaxation of the ciliary muscle[76] (i.e., as with bronchiolar smooth muscle), with widening of the intermuscle spaces. More recent evidence suggests that epinephrine may promote prostaglandin release within ciliary muscle or nonmuscle interstitial cells and that prostanoid-mediated effects on the connective tissue within the intermuscular spaces may enhance uveoscleral outflow (see below).[78–82] Two possible mechanisms for epinephrine-induced formation of arachidonic acid/prostanoids are shown in Figure 9.5. The α-receptor pathway (cascade C) acts via a Ca^{2+}-stimulated PLA_2 enzyme and may occur in nonmuscle cells in the ciliary body, while the β-adrenergic receptor pathway (cascade D) in ciliary muscle cells may act via a different β–γ-stimulated PLA_2 enzyme, as previously discussed.

Finally, epinephrine acutely stimulates aqueous secretion by the ciliary epithelium,[83] leading to an ≈15–20% increase in the rate of aqueous humor production in the conscious human. Aqueous flow in the sleeping human is ≈30–40% less than in the conscious state, the reduction of aqueous flow by complete β-blockade in the human is also ≈30–40%, and β-blockers produce no further suppression of aqueous flow in the asleep state[84] (see below). Therefore, it appears that maximum β-adrenergic stimulation of the ciliary epithelium approximately doubles the rate of aqueous formation over its basal nonstimulated level. It is not clear whether the ciliary epithelial β_2-receptors mediating this stimulatable component of aqueous production are innervated or not; i.e., whether under normal conditions they are responding to neuronally released norepinephrine or to locally released (paracrine) or circulating epinephrine. In any event, this initial epinephrine-induced increase in aqueous production tends to blunt the IOP-lowering effect produced by enhancement of trabecular and uveoscleral outflow, but seems to decline with additional doses. It is possible that the effect on aqueous production rapidly desensitizes,[85] leaving the trabecular and uveoscleral mechanisms as the major responses to chronic therapy. The specific effect of chronic epinephrine administration on aqueous production in the human remains unclear. Classically thought to reduce aqueous formation, such treatment has shown little or no effect in more recent, methodologically superior studies.[83] More work is required in this area to explain the apparent lack of response of ciliary processes, which have a high density of β-receptors.

ADRENERGIC ANTAGONISTS

The α_1-adrenergic receptor antagonists (Fig. 9.8) induce miosis by preventing the α_1-receptor-mediated contraction of the iris dilator muscle produced by norepinephrine released from sympathetic nerve endings. The α_1-antagonists can also reverse the iatrogenic mydriasis produced by α_1-agonists such as phenylephrine, which are used to facilitate funduscopy. Such "therapeutic" miosis is employed primarily to lessen the intensity and duration of the photophobia associated with mydriasis, but may also be useful in preventing or reversing iatrogenic angle closure in susceptible patients.

Figure 9.8. Adrenergic Antagonists

Drug	Delivery/Duration/Frequency	Side Effects: Ocular	Side Effects: Systemic
α_1			
Dapiprazole	0.5% sol'n-drops, single application For reversing mydriasis	Conjunctival injection, burning, ptosis, lid erythema, lid edema, chemosis, itching, punctate keratitis, corneal edema, brow ache, photophobia and headaches	—
Nonselective β (block β_1 or β_2)			
Timolol (Timoptic®)	0.25–0.5% sol'n-drops q.12 or 24 hr 12–24 hr duration Some effect 2–4 weeks after chronic treatment is stopped	Drugs generally well tolerated, side effects rare SPK, corneal anesthesia Increased mydriasis with epinephrine Stinging and burning, primarily with betaxolol solution Allergic blepharoconjunctivitis Decreased tear production	**Cardiovascular** Bradycardia Hypotension Syncope CHF **Respiratory** Bronchiolar constriction Exacerbation of asthma COPD **CNS** Fatigue Lethargy Somnolence Disorientation Confusion Weakness Dissociation Memory loss Apnea? **Other (rare)** GI distress Impotence Exacerbation of myasthenia Allergic dermatitis Alopecia Prolonged hypoglycemia with insulin
Levobunolol (Betagan®)			
Metipranolol (Optipranolol®) Minims Metipranolol	0.3%q.12 hr		
Carteolol (Ocupress®) TEOPTIC	1.0%q.12 hr		
Relatively β_1 selective			
Betaxolol (Betoptic®)	0.5% solution or 0.25% microsuspension drops q.12 hr duration Magnitude of effect less than nonselective agents in some patients		

Nonselective β-blockers are additive to all other antiglaucoma medications, but only marginally to β_2-agonists; betaxolol shows better additivity to β_2-agonists.

Special considerations:

1) lower incidence of systemic side effects with betaxolol.
   - a: low affinity for β_2-receptor spares bronchioles, perhaps CNS.
   - b: relatively low β_2-blocking activity in plasma—less systemic absorption; more plasma protein binding.
2) patients receiving systemic β-blockers (hypertension, myocardial infarction) or at higher risk (asthma, heart or lung disease) for β-blocker-related side effects.

Putatively by blocking β_2-adrenergic receptors on the ciliary nonpigmented epithelial (NPE) cells,[71,82] β_2-antagonists (see Fig. 9.8) reduce the rate of aqueous formation by ≈30% in the conscious human.[84] The β-blockers are ineffective during sleep,[84] presumably because there is insufficient neural or humoral adrenergic tone on the ciliary epithelium to stimulate aqueous production (i.e., blockade of the receptors produces no further reduction in such tone). Some authorities question whether the action of β-blockers in reducing aqueous secretion is related to their pharmacologic activity at β-adrenergic receptors.[87,88] The best evidence to support this view is the fact that subjects with Horner syndrome (i.e., cervical sympathectomy), who have no neuronally-mediated sympathetic tone, nevertheless have normal IOP and aqueous secretion rates.[89] However, these findings are not definitive support, because the source of the endogenous catecholamine(s) which maintains secretory tone could be other than from the cervical autonomic neural trunk.

The β-antagonist drugs have no effect on outflow facility in humans or monkeys, indicating that even in the conscious primate there is no facility-effective tone present on the trabecular endothelium.[90] Although β-antagonists may reduce uveoscleral outflow slightly by inhibiting β-receptors in the ciliary muscle and thus causing weak muscular contraction (as in the bronchioles),[91] the effect on secretion predominates, producing a net reduction in IOP in most patients.

Studies of the effects of β-blockers, β-agonists (epinephrine), and α_2-agonists on aqueous humor secretion clearly show that important components of the transport system can be regulated by receptors. The main driving mechanisms for aqueous secretion are the two enzymes Na^+/K^+-ATPase and carbonic anhydrase (see Nilsson and Bill, Maren, Chapter 1), neither of which is thought to be directly regulated by receptor-mediated signals. Figure 9.9 depicts one of the simplest hypothetical models for aqueous humor secretion mechanisms formulated as the transport of NaCl into the posterior chamber. An equivalent amount of H^+, HCO_3^- is transported to the stromal side and the CO_2 is recycled. Because the bulk of aqueous volume is determined by epithelial secretion of NaCl, the activity of the two driving enzymes must in some way be coupled to the separate entry of Na^+ (e.g., by H^+/Na^+ exchange) and Cl^- (e.g., by HCO_3^-/Cl^- exchange) as illustrated in Figure 9.9, or their cotransport (e.g., by Na^+, K^+, $2Cl^-$ symport) on the stromal side. Similarly, on the basolateral membrane of epithelial cells facing the posterior chamber there need to be mechanisms for egress of anions (HCO_3^- or Cl^-) as well as for the K^+ ions needed to "prime" the sodium pump (see Fig. 9.9). The information obtained from other types of cells indicates the importance of channel regulation via receptors (see Introduction and Fig. 9.5). Such channels and exchangers or their equivalents depicted in the model shown in Figure 9.9 are, therefore, likely targets for receptor-mediated control in epithelial cells because they can be rate-limiting for aqueous humor secretion. For example, inactivation of a K^+ channel on the basolateral membrane opposing or blocking the egress of K^+ ions could slow down the sodium pump. This is a possible mechanism for α_2-adrenergic agonists, which have been recently shown to regulate K^+ channels in other cells. Similarly, Cl^- (or other anion) channels on the basolateral membrane could be activated by increased cAMP levels (e.g., the acute response to epinephrine) causing increased secretion, or deactivated by decreased cAMP levels (response to α_2-agonists or β-blockers). These conjectures indicate the lack of specific knowledge relating the receptors and ion channels in human ciliary epithelial cells, but considerable progress has been made in studies on both subprimate[92] and monkey[93] ciliary epithelium.

The β-antagonists are the most widely used antiglaucoma drugs worldwide by virtue of their efficacy and low incidence of ocular side effects. Five agents are in use in the United States (see Fig. 9.8), and several additional β-blockers are used in foreign countries (e.g., pindolol). The β-blockers approved for clinical use are not partial agonists except for carteolol (i.e., have no intrinsic sympathomimetic activity), have little local anesthetic action, have very weak activity at α-adrenergic receptors and, perhaps most important, have an appropriate lipophilic/hydrophilic balance to penetrate the cornea well. However, they can produce significant systemic side effects, especially in elderly patients with cardiovascular or obstructive pulmonary disease, in asthmatics, and in patients already receiving β-blockers systemically for nonocular conditions.

The risk of systemic side effects can be minimized by the use of relatively β_1-selective antagonists.[94] These compounds have enough β_2-blocking activity to inhibit aqueous formation at their high intraocular concentrations after topical application, but not enough to produce major systemic problems at the concentration reached in the general circulation. Interestingly, because of differences in ocular versus systemic absorption and binding to plasma proteins, betaxolol, a relatively selective β_1-antagonist, also seems to have less propensity to produce cardiovascular effects than do the nonselective agents such as timolol or levobunolol. However, β_1-antagonists are in general less effective than β_2-blockers in lowering IOP, so the added safety comes at a price. Therefore, the choice of agent must be individualized to the situation of the specific patient.

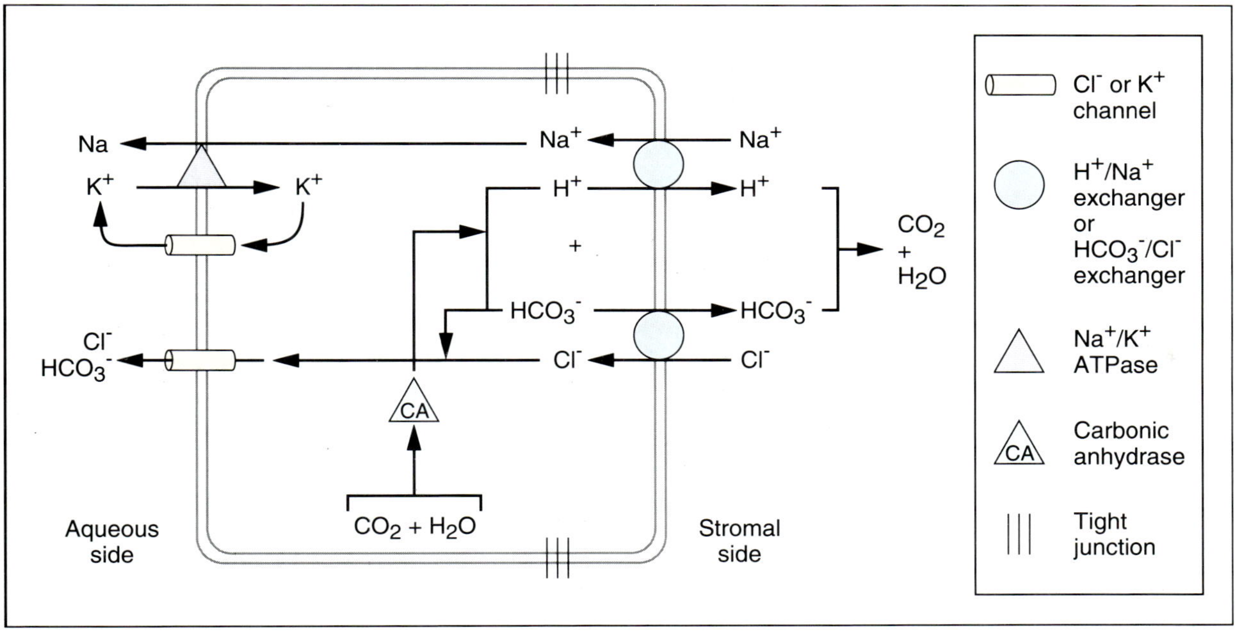

9.9 | Simple model for ciliary epithelial aqueous humor secretion formulated as Na^+Cl^- transport to the aqueous side and $H^+HCO_3^-$ to the stromal side.

The question of therapeutic additivity between epinephrine and the β-blockers has been widely discussed. In most patients, β-blockers are more effective ocular hypotensives than are epinephrine or dipivefrin. When epinephrine is added to the drug regimen of a patient already receiving a nonspecific β-antagonist, the additional IOP lowering is either minimal or nil,[95] since the β_2-adrenergic receptors are blocked. In patients receiving betaxolol the effect may be greater, because epinephrine can still exert its effect on outflow facility.[90] Apparently, the β_2-receptors in the ciliary epithelium are more effectively blocked by this agent than are those in the trabecular endothelium, or perhaps there are pharmacokinetic differences in drug distribution. However, because betaxolol is somewhat less effective as a secretory inhibitor than the nonspecific antagonists,[96] one can view the combination of betaxolol + epinephrine or betaxolol + dipivefrin as having about the same efficacy as timolol or levobunolol alone. The risk of particular side effects in a specific clinical situation may govern the choice.

Although maneuvers to reduce systemic absorption of topically applied drugs (e.g., digital punctal occlusion, eyelid closure, prodrugs) can be validly directed towards all topical antiglaucoma medications, they would be most helpful if applied to the β-blockers. A prodrug in this category would be especially welcome.

CARBONIC ANHYDRASE INHIBITORS

The enzyme carbonic anhydrase is present in high concentration in the ciliary nonpigmented epithelium,[39] where it plays a vital role in the formation of aqueous humor (see Fig. 9.9 and Maren, Chapter 1). For a table describing carbonic anhydrase inhibitors (CAIs) see Figure 9.10. Complete inhibition of ciliary epithelial carbonic anhydrase can reduce the rate of aqueous formation by 40–50%.[39] This is to some extent a different "component" of aqueous secretion than that blocked by β-adrenergic antagonists, because the effect of these two drug classes is at least partly additive.[97] However, to produce *any* inhibition of aqueous formation at least 99% of the ciliary enzyme must be blocked,[39] and therein lies the cause of the major therapeutic problem facing the CAIs. Until very recently, pharmacokinetic, pharmacodynamic, and solubility factors militated against their topical use; the drugs simply could not reach the ciliary epithelium in high enough concentrations to be effective. CAIs are therefore given systemically. Although they are very effective at lowering IOP when given by this route, their inhibition of red cell, renal, and other CA produces side effects of sufficient frequency and severity that perhaps 50% of the patients started on CAIs must eventually discontinue them. Some of the metabolic effects which are not necessarily severe in themselves (e.g., metabolic acidosis, potassium depletion) may be much more serious in the presence of concurrent illness or other drugs (e.g., hypokalemia if the patient is also taking another salt-depleting diuretic, and cardiac arrhythmia if the hypokalemia occurs in the presence of a cardiac glycoside).

More recently, major breakthroughs have occurred in CAI drug design such that their pharmacokinetic, pharmacodynamic, and solubility profiles now permit their effective topical use. Several such compounds have proven effective in human clinical trials, with apparently few or no side effects, and it seems likely that a topical agent will be generally available within the next two years.[98] Depending on the results of longer trials in elderly patients, such an agent may not only become a first-line drug but may also affect medical versus surgical decision-making.

Figure 9.10. Carbonic Anhydrase Inhibitors

Drug	Delivery/Duration/Frequency	Side Effects: Ocular	Side Effects: Systemic
Acetazolamide (Diamox®)	125 or 250 mg tablets q.6-12 hr 500 mg sustained-released capsules q.12 or 24 hr	Transient myopia	Paresthesias Metabolic acidosis Ureteral calculi Hypokalemia (with potassium-depleting diuretic) Allergic dermatitis Metallic taste from carbonated beverages Bone marrow depression Possible teratogenicity Precipitation of acute hepatic failure (preexisting liver disease) Salicylism (concurrent ASA therapy) Anorexia Weight loss Lethargy Fatigue Somnolence Generalized malaise Loss of libido Depression Confusion Disorientation
Methazolamide (Neptazane®)	50 mg tablets; 25 mg q.12 hr–100 mg q.8 hr		
Dichlorphenamide (Daranide®)	50 mg tablets; 50 mg q.12 hr–100 mg q.6-8 hr		
MK 927, MK 417, MK 507/ Dorzolamide* (TRUSOPT)	2% drops q.8–12 hr		

*Undergoing clinical trials.

Additive to all other antiglaucoma drugs.

Special considerations:

1) renal disease—CAI builds up in plasma.
2) hepatic disease—increased plasma ammonia.

A low dose of methazolamide (25 mg q.12 hr) will produce no effect on renal or erythrocyte CA, and therefore no acidosis, but will still lower IOP. Such dissociation of ocular and renal effects is not possible with acetazolamide at any dose.

HYPEROSMOTIC AGENTS

Unlike the other pharmacologic classes discussed, hyperosmotic agents (Fig. 9.11) do not affect the usual parameters of aqueous humor formation and drainage. Administered systemically, hyperosmotic agents create an osmotic gradient of about 30 mOsm between the blood and the vitreous, so that water leaves the vitreous cavity and enters the ocular vasculature. This produces the most rapid and marked IOP-lowering of all the antiglaucoma drugs. Indeed, it is quite common to see an IOP decrease of 40–50 mm Hg within 30 minutes after intravenous administration of a hyperosmotic agent in cases of acute angle-closure glaucoma. Because the efficacy of these drugs depends on the osmotic gradient between the blood and the vitreous, it stands to reason that such drugs will be least effective in conditions of severely altered ocular vascular permeability, in which the systemically administered drug will enter the vitreous humor more easily (e.g., neovascular glaucoma).[99]

In addition to drawing fluid out of the eye, the hypertonicity of the blood also draws extra- and intracellular water from many organs and tissues into the general circulation. This circulatory overload can have serious consequences, especially in patients who are elderly and may already have cardiovascular diseases. For this reason, these potentially lethal drugs must be used with great caution and selectivity. They can be immensely helpful and even sight-saving in desperate situations when the IOP is so high as to threaten the retinal circulation or to make intraocular surgery hazardous because of

Figure 9.11. Hyperosmotic Agents

Drug	Molecular Weight	Usual Dose*	Distribution	Advantages	Disadvantages	Side Effects
Glycerol	92	1–1.5 g/kg orally as 50% sol'n	Extracellular	Less diuresis Penetrates eye poorly Stable	Nausea and vomiting Metabolism, calories, ↑ blood glucose Slower pressure fall than intravenous	Headaches and back pain Dehydration Nausea, vomiting Vertigo, chills Agitation Disorientation
Isosorbide	146	1–2 g/kg orally as 45% sol'n	Total water	Well tolerated No caloric value Rapid absorption Stable Nonmetabolized	Penetrates eye (slowly) Slower pressure fall than intravenous	Chest pain Congestive failure Pulmonary edema
Mannitol	182	1–1.5 g/kg I.V. as 20% sol'n	Extracellular	Rapid action Stable Nonmetabolized Less irritating Penetrates eye poorly	Large volume Cellular dehydration Diuresis	Diuresis Urinary retention Subdural hematoma

*Additive to all other antiglaucoma medications.

sudden decompression. However, their appropriate use in most cases is as a single-dose weapon to buy a few hours of time while a more definitive, longer-term attack on the elevated IOP is mounted.

PROSTAGLANDINS

Prostaglandins (PGs), and most especially congeners of $PGF_{2\alpha}$ (Fig. 9.12), are the most potent and efficacious topical ocular hypotensive agents currently known. At a maximally effective topical dose of only 5 µg or less of the isopropylester prodrug, IOP in a normal monkey is typically reduced to <5 mm Hg, well below any rational value for episcleral venous pressure.[100] There is little or no effect on aqueous humor formation[101] or trabecular outflow facility[102] and, based on studies in the cat, on episcleral venous pressure.[103,104] Rather, there is a severalfold enhancement of uveoscleral outflow, sufficient to account for the profound IOP fall.[80,81] In addition, there is a major redirection of outflow from the trabecular to the uveoscleral route,[80,81] which probably explains why the IOP can fall to levels much lower than those achieved with drugs that enhance trabecular outflow or suppress aqueous formation. In the latter two instances, aqueous still drains against an episcleral venous pressure of ≈10 mm Hg, which therefore represents the floor to which IOP can fall. However, the uveoscleral route drains towards an intraorbital pressure of ≈0 mm Hg, which becomes the floor for the IOP when the resistance through the intraocular portion of the uveoscleral pathway is largely eliminated.[81]

The mechanism by which PGs enhance uveoscleral outflow is not well understood. There appears to be a narrowing of the ciliary muscle fiber bundles,[82] a widening of the intermuscle spaces,[82] and an enzymatically mediated lysis of the intermuscular connective tissue,[105] all of which could enhance the movement of fluid from the anterior chamber through the muscle and into the suprachoroid. Such a system must serve some purpose in nature. Because prostaglandins are released by various ocular tissues during many types of ocular inflammation, the system may represent a back-up for a trabecular meshwork compromised by inflammation or obstructed by inflammatory debris, with prostaglandins being the "messenger." This would be consistent with the view of prostaglandins as autacoids—hormones that are synthesized, released, and active locally. This could also explain the very low IOP that often accompanies uveitis; indeed, during experimental iridocyclitis in monkeys, uveoscleral outflow is increased approximately fourfold.[106] Finally, this overall conceptualization would be consistent with the view that the uveoscleral outflow route serves as the equivalent of a lymphatic

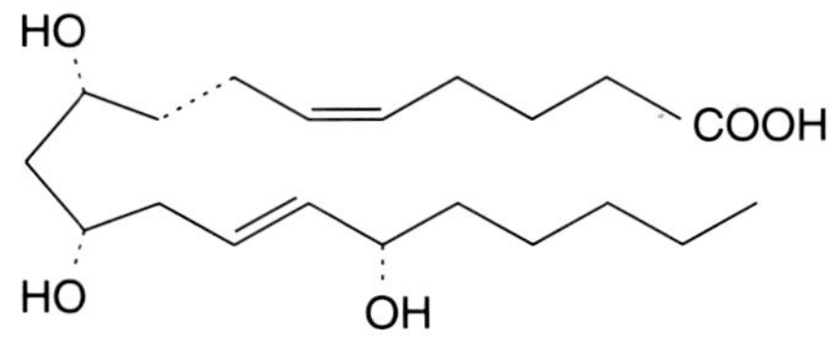

9.12 | Structure of prostaglandin $F_{2\alpha}$.

drainage pathway for the eye.[106] Although the issue is not entirely settled, neither the eye nor the orbital contents within the extraocular muscle cone appear to have true lymphatics.[107] Uveoscleral outflow provides for exit of larger proteins and other tissue constituents from the uvea,[108] which is situated too far posteriorly to be drained via anterior chamber aqueous exiting through the canal of Schlemm, and can also be "turned up" by prostaglandins to handle virtually all of the aqueous drainage when the meshwork is compromised and the aqueous is especially laden with proteins and other inflammatory debris.

$PGF_{2\alpha}$ effectively reduces IOP in both normal and glaucomatous human eyes[109] (Fig. 9.13). Because the complete dose–response relationship has not yet been determined in humans, it is not clear whether the maximum possible IOP reduction will be as great as in subhuman primates. Furthermore, a number of other issues must be resolved before PGs can be considered for routine clinical use. IOP-effective doses of $PGF_{2\alpha}$, even given in as small an amount of 0.25 μg of the isopropylester prodrug, cause clinically unacceptable conjunctival hyperemia and irritation.[109] Alternative formulations, congeners, or delivery systems may be needed, or perhaps a separation by receptor subtype of the IOP-lowering from the extraocular vasodilatory responses. Finally, the interaction of PGs with other antiglaucoma drugs must be explored. For example, pretreatment with pilocarpine completely inhibits the IOP-lowering effect of $PGF_{2\alpha}$ in monkeys, presumably by obliterating the intermuscle spaces in the ciliary muscle and preventing uveoscleral drainage.[110] Despite these caveats, PGs have exciting potential for antiglaucoma therapy in the future.

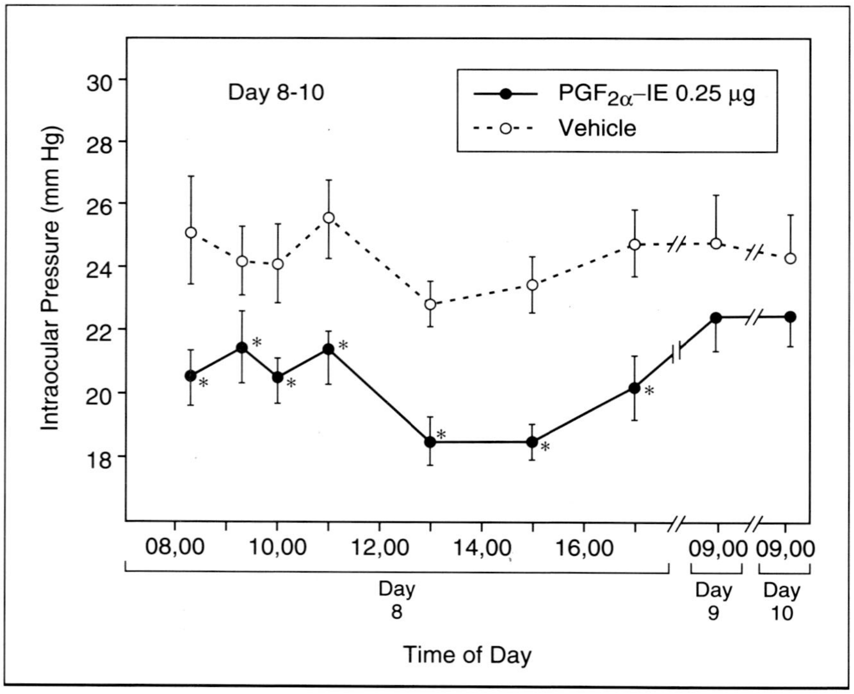

9.13 | Effects on IOP before and after the last (fifteenth consecutive) 0.25-μg dose of $PGF_{2\alpha}$ IE (•) or its vehicle (o) given twice daily for 8 days in 11 ocular hypertensive or glaucoma patients. The 8:30 AM values on day 8 were taken 11.5 hours after the previous dose. Day 9 and 10 measurements were obtained 24 and 48 hours, respectively, after the last dose. Points represent means, and the limits ± standard error of the mean. *Indicates measurements significantly ($p < 0.05$) different from contralateral controls using two-tailed, paired *t*-test. (From Camras CB, Siebold EC, Lustgarten JS, et al: Maintained reduction of intraocular pressure by prostglandin $F_{2\alpha}$1-isopropylester applied in multiple doses in ocular hypertensive and glaucoma patients. *Ophthalmology 1989;96:1329–1335.*)

NA+/K+-ATPase INHIBITORS

Na^+/K^+-ATPase catalyzes the degradation of ATP to AMP + inorganic phosphate.[39] This reaction is accompanied by the release of the energy required for many cellular metabolic functions. The enzyme is present in high concentration in the basolateral infoldings of ciliary NPE, where it is thought to generate the energy needed to actively transport Na^+ into the posterior chamber. This transport of Na^+, passively followed by H_2O, constitutes the basis for the secretion of aqueous humor (see Fig. 9.9). Inhibition of the ciliary process enzyme reduces aqueous formation by up to 50% in several species, including human. However, topical administration of most inhibiting drugs affects a similar transport system in the corneal endothelium, producing corneal edema. Systemic administration of such drugs produces significant cardiac effects, analogous to the cardiac glycosides. Consequently, this class of compound cannot presently be used to lower IOP in the clinical setting. However, more specific drugs, along with pharmacokinetic and pharmacodynamic improvements, may allow the future use of this approach.

CYTOSKELETAL-ACTIVE AGENTS

Trabecular and Schlemm's canal inner wall endothelial cells contain cytoplasmic actin microfilaments and possess contractile properties.[74] The inner wall endothelial cells are joined by tight junctions, providing a barrier to paracellular movement of fluid in either direction between the meshwork and canal lumen (see Rohen and Lütjen-Drecoll, Chapter 1). The juxtacanalicular region of the meshwork, which harbors most of the resistance to aqueous outflow, consists of five or six layers of endothelial cells, whose cytoplasmic processes contact one another, which secrete and are imbedded in an extracellular matrix consisting of glycosaminoglycans, proteoglycans, and various other macromolecules (see Rohen and Lütjen-Drecoll, Chapter 1). Given this anatomic substrate, it is not surprising that compounds that alter cell junctions and contractile proteins could produce alterations in the shape of cells in the juxtacanalicular meshwork and inner canal wall, in turn promoting washout of resistance-producing extracellular material.

Cytochalasins B and D inhibit the polymerization of globular cytoplasmic actin into actin microfilaments, the calcium chelators EDTA and EGTA disrupt cell-to-cell junctional complexes, and ethacrynic acid and related compounds bind sulfhydryl groups on the cell membrane. Intracameral infusion of these agents produces separation of meshwork and inner wall cells, washout of extracellular material, and increased outflow facility. Much work remains before such agents can be considered for clinical use (e.g., corneal endothelial effects, duration of action, topical versus intracameral administration), but the concept of such a "pharmacologic trabeculocanalotomy" is exciting.

GENERAL TREATMENT STRATEGY

The question of when to initiate IOP-lowering therapy in open-angle glaucoma generates much discussion. IOP is only one of probably many risk factors that predispose to glaucomatous optic neuropathy, and only a few of those risk factors are known (race, age, IOP, family history, diabetes mellitus, glaucoma in the contralateral eye, hypertension) (see Wilensky, Chapter 8). No IOP, regardless how low, carries a 0% risk, and no IOP, no matter how high, carries a 100% risk, of causing optic nerve damage. Therefore, IOP-lowering therapy is usually not initiated without some evidence that: (1) the eye is not tolerating the present IOP (i.e., functional or anatomic nerve damage is already apparent); (2) the IOP is so high that, based on experience, the risk of damage is judged to be great (i.e., IOP >30 mm Hg); or (3) the presence of other risk factors suggests that the present IOP, even if not inordinately high, will probably produce damage in the not too distant future (i.e., a history of glaucoma developing in first-order blood relatives at a similar age, and IOP). The best indication for lowering the ambient IOP in an eye, of course, is evidence that the eye has already suffered damage at that IOP.[111]

It is important to keep these general principles in mind and to individualize the indications for therapy rather than making a decision based on some statistical population-based concept of "normal" IOP. On a single given occasion, one third of all POAG patients will have an IOP ≤21 mm Hg, i.e., within two standard deviations of the population mean (see Wilensky, Chapter 8). Although many of these POAG patients will reveal higher IOP on multiple measurements (certainly a much higher percentage of initially "normotensive" POAG patients than non-POAG patients will do so),[112] there are some POAG patients whose IOP is virtually always in the so-called "normal" range. Even for these patients, however, IOP may have a pathophysiologic role in their glaucomatous optic neuropathy, and because at present it is the only risk factor we can manipulate, it should be decreased.

As in all therapeutic decision making throughout the practice of medicine, risk must be weighed against benefit. All medical (and surgical) therapeutic modalities have the potential to produce adverse ocular and/or systemic effects. The best predictor of what will happen to a given eye at a given IOP in the near future is what has happened to that eye at that IOP in the recent past,[111] and if damage has occurred at a given IOP, reducing IOP by only 2 or 3 mm Hg will probably be insufficient to prevent further damage. If the patient is very elderly and, based on general medical status, has limited life expectancy and only minimal glaucomatous damage with evidence of very slow progression, it may not be wise to be so aggressive with treatment as to create significant ocular or systemic side effects; the glaucomatous damage probably will not be clinically relevant within the patient's lifetime. Conversely, substantial damage and rapid progression in a younger, otherwise healthy individual demands more aggressive treatment.[111]

In commencing IOP-reducing therapy, one currently can choose among three classes of topical ocular medications: cholinomimetics, β-adrenergic agonists, and β-adrenergic antagonists. Systemic CAIs, because of their propensity to produce adverse systemic effects, are reserved for use when topical agents are insufficient or produce unacceptable side effects. However, when topical CAIs become generally available they may assume a primary role. The choice among the different drug classes should, again, be individualized to the patient. An elderly patient with posterior subcapsular or nuclear cataract may not do well on pilocarpine drops, because the pupillary constriction may decrease the light reaching the retina and degrade the visual acuity. A young person may have difficulty because of the fluctuating accommodative myopia. However, a 50-year-old presbyope with clear lenses may do beautifully with pilocarpine, assuming the ability to comply with the regimen of four daily doses. Such a patient, and younger patients, may also do well with the pilocarpine Ocusert®; this eliminates the need for repetitive drop administration, and the zero-order kinetics produce only a mild, stable myopia, which can be compensated by spectacles. With aphakes and pseudophakes, the miosis and accommodative myopia are not of concern.

Dipivefrin has virtually eliminated the risk of systemic cardiovascular side effects that can occur with topical epinephrine. If the patient is not at risk for angle closure, this can be a good initial choice. However, external ocular allergy or irritation can still occur, as can macular edema in aphakes. Although many patients do not achieve as large an IOP fall with dipivefrin as with pilocarpine or β-antagonists, for responsive patients this can be a good choice.

Most patients who require treatment are begun with a topical β-adrenergic antagonist, because these compounds are so effective, produce so little in the way of ocular side effects, and need be used only once or twice daily. The biggest concern is systemic side effects, and again careful history and knowledge of the patient's particular situation are important in rational decision making. The unstable asthmatic or the patient in third-degree heart block may not be an ideal candidate for these compounds. Using only the smallest dose necessary, taking steps to minimize systemic drug absorption (punctal occlusion, eyelid closure), and choice of the agent with the better systemic safety profile (i.e., betaxolol) may help. When there is a question regarding systemic safety in a particular patient, consultation with the patient's general physician is often wise, and certainly is never wrong. Even when the ophthalmologist feels comfortable making the decision to use potentially systemic-acting drugs without such consultation, informing the general physician after the fact is still advisable; problems may arise late and may be reported by the patient to the general physician rather than to the ophthalmologist, but the patient may not remember to tell the physician about the eye medications.

Finally, one must consider as primary therapy agents that have no propensity to produce systemic effects: laser trabeculoplasty (ALT) or incisional surgery. Although ALT by itself does not seem to be a long-term solution for most patients, it appears to be as effective as timolol for initial therapy (see Wilensky, Chapter 9). There are also data suggesting not only that incisional surgery as primary therapy may be more effective at lowering IOP and preserving vision,[113] but also that it may improve "quality of life" by reducing or eliminating the need for bothersome polypharmacy therapy. Some ophthalmologists also feel that many patients will eventually come to surgery anyway when they escape from medical or laser control, and that the surgery is more likely to succeed if they have not been pharmacologically assaulted previously. The resolution of such issues awaits the outcome of prospective, randomized multicenter clinical trials now being designed.

This entire discussion is, of course, predicated on the assumption that reducing IOP will prevent further optic nerve damage or, in high-risk ocular hypertensives, will prevent or delay its initial occurrence. This "conventional clinical wisdom" was called into question several years ago, because the data supporting it did not meet modern biostatistical and epidemiological/clinical trial design criteria. Some,[114] albeit not all,[115] more recent and careful prospective trials have confirmed the concept, and although more work is needed (and is being undertaken) to sharpen the indications and the efficacy data, it seems clear not only that IOP is a major risk factor in development and progression of glaucoma but also that reducing IOP can prevent or retard its development and progression in at least some individuals at risk (see also Perkins, this chapter). The possibility that such a beneficial effect of IOP-lowering medications could be due to some action other than IOP-lowering, such as an IOP-independent effect on optic nerve circulation, must be considered[116]; trials of laser or incisional surgery as primary therapy may provide information on this point. Of course, a drug might lower IOP yet accelerate disease progression via some other mechanism affecting the circulation, metabolism, or connective tissue of the optic nerve; this may occur with the α_2-adrenergic agonist clonidine, putatively because of its effect on the systemic and local ocular circulation.[62]

The decision as to when and how to escalate therapy involves many of the same issues as that to undertake treatment initially. IOP level is used only to indicate that a given therapeutic change has affected its target parameter, IOP, to a degree *likely* to be of benefit. Careful monitoring of the appearance of the optic nerve head, nerve fiber layer and, if they prove clinically valid and accessible, other measures of nerve and nerve fiber layer topography, as well as functional status as determined by various perimetric, contrast sensitivity, color vision, electrophysiologic, and other techniques (perimetry currently being the benchmark method), will indicate whether the nerve deterioration has been arrested. If escalation is required, one must choose between a higher concentration or more frequent dosing of an agent already being used (e.g., 0.5% versus 0.25% timolol) versus addition of another class of compound, again based on assessment of individual responses, known dose–response relationships, and the patient's overall health status. It may also be useful to withdraw a therapeutic agent after a long period of use if the patient's IOP is on the rise; it may be that the patient is no longer responsive to it. Indeed, it can be difficult to tell whether a patient is no longer responsive to a given drug because of induced subsensitivity, tachyphylaxis, desensitization or the like, or whether the outflow obstruction is increasing in the natural course of the disease.

Patient compliance is an important consideration and a major problem in medical therapy of glaucoma.[117] Patients may have difficulty remembering dosing schedules for multiple medications, especially when the two eyes receive different regimens, when the patient is also on medications for other systemic conditions, or when the patient is elderly, forgetful, or in an occupational setting where multiple dosing is disruptive. Such poor compliance may consist of too few or too many medications or doses, incorrect timing of medications or doses, or use of the wrong medication. In addition, POAG patients are asymptomatic from their disease, but are often symptomatic from their often expensive glaucoma medications, giving them many disincentives to treatment. Therefore, patient understanding of the disease and of the rationale and importance of correct therapy is crucial. Noncompliance is common regardless of education, ethnic background, or socioeconomic status, and can render even a physiologically and pharmacologically "perfect" medication useless. Efforts to develop improved therapeutic modalities, and choices among currently existing ones, should be made with this issue in mind.

SECTION III

LASER TRABECULOPLASTY

Jacob T. Wilensky

The first utilization of laser energy in the treatment of glaucoma involved attempts to create holes from the anterior chamber through the trabecular meshwork into Schlemm's canal, in a manner somewhat analogous to trabeculotomy. Krasnov in Russia,[118] using a Q-switched ruby laser, and Worthen and Wickham[119] of the United States, using an argon laser, reported beneficial intraocular pressure (IOP) responses to treatment. Within a year of Worthen's report, however, Gaasterland and Kupfer[120] reported that an experimental glaucoma could be created in monkey eyes by applying laser energy to the trabecular meshwork. This report somewhat dampened the enthusiasm for laser treatment of glaucoma and delayed further clinical work.

In 1979, Wise and Witter reported the results of a somewhat different laser treatment for glaucoma.[121] In their treatment, a series of approximately 100 argon laser burns were scattered over the whole 360° of the trabecular meshwork. These burns were not of sufficient intensity to create penetrating holes through the trabecular meshwork, but rather caused a local area of coagulation and a decrease in IOP. Their work was quickly confirmed by other investigators,[122,123] and argon laser trabeculoplasty (ALT), as the technique came to be called, rapidly gained widespread acceptance within the ophthalmic community as a treatment for open-angle glaucoma.

MECHANISMS OF ACTION

The mechanism by which laser trabeculoplasty lowers IOP is still the subject of debate.[124] Wise[121] proposed that the coagulation caused by the laser burns results in a contracture of the adjacent tissues, thereby tightening the trabecular ring and perhaps widening the adjacent trabecular pores. A second theory is that the laser induces physiologic changes in the activity of the trabecular cells. Differences in cellular glycosaminoglycan biosynthesis measured by [^{35}S]-sulfate incorporation were detected in treated autopsy eyes. Others have reported increased phagocytic activity of meshwork cells in laser-treated eyes.[125] A third theory is that ALT induces division of trabecular meshwork cells, as has been demonstrated in human organ culture systems.[126] Whatever the mechanism by which it is accomplished, multiple observers have documented that ALT increases tonographic facility of aqueous outflow from the anterior chamber,[122,123] and this is how IOP is lowered.

TREATMENT TECHNIQUE

The initial Wise and Witter treatment protocol consisted of placing 100 burns in the middle of the pigmented meshwork. The burns were 50 µm in size and 0.1 second in duration at an initial power level of 1,000 mw, increasing to 1,500 mw, depending on the tissue response. Since then, there have been multiple articles reporting the results of various alterations in this technique. Even today, there is still not complete consensus about all the treatment parameters.[127]

PROPORTION OF ANGLE TREATED

One early study reported that a significant IOP response could be achieved with treatment of as little as 90° of the meshwork with 25 laser burns. Increasing the amount of meshwork treated to 180° seemed to achieve greater lowering of IOP. Studies have compared treatment of 180° versus 360° of the trabecular meshwork. Most have failed to show any significant difference in the response, at least over the short term. Wise feels that after 2 or more years, eyes receiving full treatment maintain the pressure-lowering effect better than those that had only half the angle treated.

LOCATION OF THE LASER BURNS

Different investigators have placed their burns over almost all aspects of the trabecular meshwork, ranging from anteriorly in the nonpigmented trabecular meshwork just below Schwalbe's line all the way to the ciliary body band posteriorly. In general, there does not seem to be any major difference in pressure-lowering effect, but with more posteriorly placed burns there was more patient discomfort, inflammatory response, and late synechia formation. For these reasons, we recommend placing the burns anteriorly at the junction between the pigmented and the nonpigmented meshwork (Fig. 9.14).

ENERGY DENSITY

Energy density is determined by a combination of the duration, power, and diameter of the burns placed. There have been reports of 0.2-second burns, but they seem to offer no advantage over the 0.1-second standard. Although Wise initially treated with 1,000 mw or more, other investigators determined that a pressure-lowering response could be achieved with energy levels as low as 500 mw. Rouhianen and co-workers found no difference in pressure lowering when the laser power was varied from 500 to 800 mw.[128] Although the majority of investigators have treated to a tissue reaction of either blanching or small bubble formation and have varied the energy level to achieve such a reaction, others have found that good pressure lowering can be achieved even in the absence of a visible tissue response, and advocate a standard 800 mw power setting for all eyes.

When the diameter of the laser beam is doubled at a constant power setting, the energy density is reduced by a factor of four. Therefore, it is important to make sure the aiming beam is sharply focused on the trabecular meshwork during the treatment. If the gonioscopy lens is tilted or if the slit lamp itself is not parfocal with the aiming beam, the density of the energy delivered at the level of the trabecular meshwork will be reduced significantly.

PATIENT FACTORS INFLUENCING TREATMENT RESULTS

TYPE OF GLAUCOMA

Most observers have found that the greatest absolute percentage of IOP reduction has occurred in eyes with exfoliation syndrome glaucoma.[129] It is not unusual to achieve IOP decreases of 20 mm Hg. However, there seems to be a much greater "rebound" of IOP in eyes with exfoliation syndrome.[130] In 2 or 3 years, a significant percentage of patients may be back near their pretreatment IOP level or even higher.

In primary open-angle glaucoma (POAG) most studies have indicated that one can expect a reduction of 20–30%.[122,123] Although the absolute magnitude of the pressure drop will be greater the higher the initial IOP, the percentage drop seems to be fairly constant over a wide pressure range. A number of studies have suggested that ALT is much less effective in aphakic open-angle glaucoma.[122,129] There have been relatively few reports on the results of ALT in pseudophakic eyes, but there is a suggestion that the results are better in pseudophakia than in aphakia. The beneficial effects of ALT are not diminished by subsequent cataract extraction.[131]

Good results have also been reported in patients with pigmentary glaucoma, but laser treatment may be less effective in the older, somewhat atypical pigmentary glaucoma patient.[132]

ALT is somewhat less beneficial and more risky in a number of the secondary glaucomas. In uveitic glaucoma, even where there is sufficient open angle to allow treatment, there is a risk that the trabeculoplasty may cause a

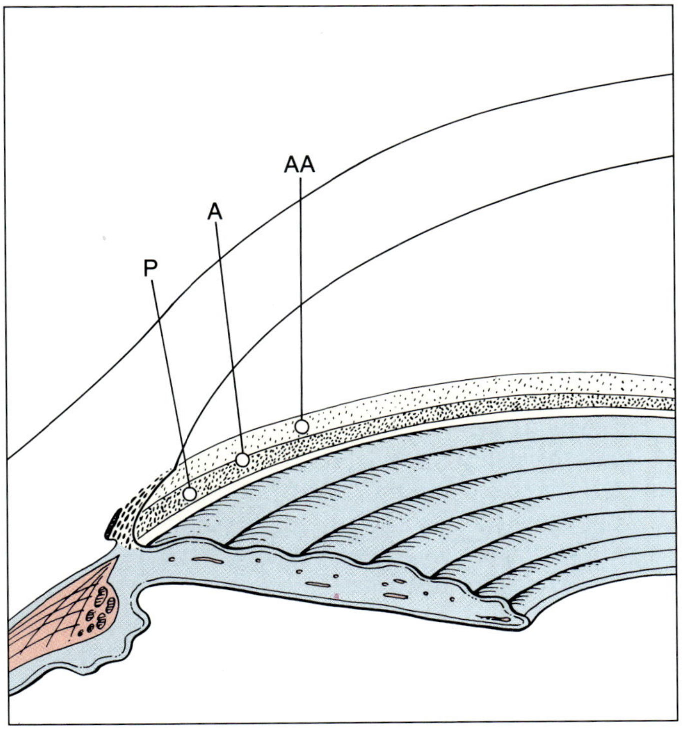

9.14 | Placement of laser burns in the angle. The preferred site A is at the junction of the pigmented and nonpigment trabecular meshwork. Burn AA is more anterior, completely in the nonpigmented meshwork, while burn P is more posterior, completely in the pigmented meshwork. (Reproduced from *Ophthalmology Times,* Feb. 1, 1983, with permission of Ophthalmology Times, Inc.)

flare-up of the uveitis, and some experience suggests that there is a greater risk of peripheral anterior synechia formation. Similarly, very mixed results have been reported in angle recession glaucoma. Severe acute pressure rises have been seen after such treatment, although a beneficial response occurs in a small number of eyes. There is also a lower response rate and significant complications in juvenile-glaucoma patients.[133]

PATIENT AGE

ALT is more effective in older individuals than in younger ones.[134] In addition, a higher complication rate has been reported in younger patients. Whether this is truly related to age or to the type of glaucoma is not completely clear.

PIGMENTATION OF THE TRABECULAR MESHWORK

Many studies have tried to correlate the degree of trabecular pigmentation with the effectiveness of ALT.[135] Several, but not all, reports have indicated a higher success rate in eyes with greater pigmentation. It has been suggested that the pigmentation of the trabecular meshwork allows a sharper or more precise focusing of the laser beam, and that the pigmentation better absorbs the laser energy so that less energy is required to obtain a tissue response. However, two entities showing a particularly good response to ALT, exfoliation-syndrome glaucoma and pigmentary glaucoma, both have densely pigmented trabecular meshworks, and one could argue that the disease entity rather than the presence of the pigment promotes the good result.

PRETREATMENT INTRAOCULAR PRESSURE

As with all therapeutic modalities, the greatest reduction in IOP occurs in eyes with the highest initial pressures. However, if one defines success as the absence of progression of visual field loss or cupping, then eyes with lower initial pressures will probably achieve this criterion more often.

RESULTS IN THE FELLOW EYE

POAG and many of the secondary glaucomas are usually bilateral diseases, although they may be somewhat asymmetric in their presentation. Accordingly, a reasonable number of patients will require ALT bilaterally. Most investigators feel that there is a fairly strong correlation between the responses in the two eyes,[136] so that a favorable response in the first eye portends a good result in the second. Similarly, a lack of response in the first eye tends to predict a poor response in the second eye.

COMPLICATIONS OF TREATMENT

PRESSURE ELEVATION

The single most common complication of ALT is an acute rise in IOP immediately after the treatment. Depending on the treatment technique and other variables, from 10–30% of patients may experience a rise in IOP ≥10 mm Hg 1–7 hours after the treatment.[137] In most studies the rise has occurred within the first 3 hours, but there have been a few reports of a delayed IOP elevation. A number of studies have suggested that both the incidence and magnitude of the pressure rise can be reduced by treating only 180° of the trabecular meshwork with approximately 50 burns instead of treating the entire circumference of the eye with 100 burns at one session.[138]

The pathophysiology of this acute pressure rise is unclear. No strong experimental evidence exists to support any of the theories. Steroidal and nonsteroidal antiinflammatory drugs have not prevented the pressure rise. One study suggests that the use of additional pilocarpine at the time of the laser treatment blunts the pressure elevation,[139] as does the α_2-adrenergic agonist apraclonidine.[140]

There also have been several reports of more long-term pressure elevations after ALT. They have occurred days to weeks after the treatment and have persisted for weeks to months. In an early series, 3% of patients were found to have IOP greater than their pretreatment value at one month.[129] In at least some of these eyes, the elevated pressure has been associated with the development of post-treatment uveitis.

LOSS OF CENTRAL VISION

There have been several reports of central vision loss immediately after ALT.[129,138] Most of these reports appeared early in the history of ALT and appeared to be associated with acute pressure elevations that were not aggressively treated. There have not been similar reports during the last few years, indicating that close monitoring of the IOP, and aggressive intervention with apraclonidine, carbonic anhydrase inhibitors, and osmotics when needed, protect even vulnerable small central islands of vision.

PERIPHERAL ANTERIOR SYNECHIAE

Peripheral anterior synechiae (PAS) have been reported in 12–47% of eyes that have undergone ALT. In the Glaucoma Laser Trial, PAS to the level of the pigmented trabecular meshwork were seen in 33% of eyes.[137] In that study, the only factor that correlated with a higher incidence of PAS formation was denser pigmentation of the trabecular meshwork. There was no correlation with laser power. Other studies have suggested a higher incidence of PAS formation when the laser burns were placed more posteriorly in the angle.[132] To date there have been no data to support any detrimental effects from these small PAS, and the effectiveness of the treatment is comparable in patients both with and without PAS formation.

UVEITIS

Mild iritis is an almost universal sequela of ALT. Rarely, severe iritis after laser treatment may persist for months.[122] Eyes in which "significant" iritis develops are more prone to PAS formation.[141] Most clinicians use topical corticosteroids during the immediate post-treatment period in an attempt to minimize this problem.

SYNCOPE

An unusual and unexpected complication of ALT has been syncope, with the patient "passing out" at the laser or within minutes of the treatment.[142] Most of the patients who experienced syncopal episodes have been younger men with no apparent cardiac disease or other predisposing illnesses.

ROLE OF RETREATMENT

The effects of ALT appear to diminish with time. In one study, 77% of the eyes were considered to be successfully controlled 2 years after treatment, but this had decreased to only 46% at the end of 5 years. The results were worse in black patients (32% success rate) than in white patients.[136] In another, larger series the mean decrease in IOP after 5 years was about the same as after one year (9.3 versus 10.3 mm Hg), but only 44% of the eyes treated initially were considered to have successful IOP control. These investigators state that, although failure was most common in the first year after treatment (23%), additional eyes failed at a rate of 7–10% per year.[143] Whether these late failures represent a true reduction in the effectiveness of the treatment or a continual progression of the underlying disease is not clear.

A natural question was whether repeat trabeculoplasty might be beneficial in these patients. In less selective early series, only approximately a third of individuals showed a significant beneficial response to retreatment, and several patients appeared to have been made worse.[144,145] When retreatment was restricted to individuals who had shown a very good initial response to ALT that had persisted for at least a year or two, the success rate for retreatment was, at least initially, higher.[146] Even in these patients, however, there seemed to be a fairly rapid loss of adequate IOP control. Therefore, retreatment does not appear to be a major long-term option for most patients.

CLINICAL USE OF LASER TRABECULOPLASTY

INDICATIONS FOR TREATMENT

Laser trabeculoplasty should be considered in most patients with primary open-angle glaucoma, exfoliation-syndrome glaucoma, pigmentary glaucoma, and angle-closure glaucoma successfully treated with laser iridotomy but having residual elevated IOP. It also may be indicated in many cases of normotensive (low-tension) glaucoma and aphakic/pseudophakic glaucoma. It is much less commonly indicated in uveitic glaucoma, angle-recession glaucoma, and juvenile glaucoma, and then only with the patient being aware that there is a substantial risk that the treatment will worsen the glaucoma.

Other factors in addition to the glaucoma diagnosis must be taken into consideration in deciding whether to use ALT. In general, the older the patient, the lower the IOP, and the less advanced the glaucoma damage, the greater the likelihood that ALT will be successful in controlling the glaucoma. Conversely, the younger the patient, the higher the IOP, and the more advanced the damage, the less likely that ALT will be adequate treatment.

Initially, ALT was used only in eyes uncontrolled on maximal medical therapy. With experience there is a trend towards using it earlier in the therapeutic regimen. It is now often used before carbonic anhydrase inhibitors, as a substitute for miotics in symptomatic patients, or before cataract extraction in otherwise controlled eyes. With the growing number of reports of the successful use of ALT as an initial treatment for glaucoma,[147,148] and especially the results of the Glaucoma Laser Trial,[149] it may become a first-line treatment in many glaucoma patients, although there are still many glaucoma specialists who believe that medical therapy should be tried first.

CURRENT TREATMENT TECHNIQUE

Because many patients achieve a significant (and sometimes maximal) IOP reduction with treatment of only half of the angle with a reduced risk of post-treatment IOP elevation, ALT is now usually performed in two sessions. The second treatment is usually performed about 1 month after the initial one, but occasionally the IOP reduction exceeds the treatment objective and the second treatment session can be deferred.

The laser burns should be placed anteriorly, straddling the border of the pigmented and nonpigmented trabecular meshwork. This seems to result in less pain during treatment, fewer PAS, and less postoperative inflammation than do more posteriorly placed burns. A 50-μm laser spot and a duration of 0.1 second should be used. Some physicians use a standard power setting (e.g., 800 mw) for all treatments, but if even one chooses to treat to a tissue reaction (blanch or small bubble formation), the laser power should not exceed 1,000 mw.

After the laser treatment patients continue their usual glaucoma medications. In eyes with very advanced visual field loss and/or cupping of the optic nerve head, a drop of apraclonidine is instilled in the eye before and/or after the laser treatment. In all patients the IOP is measured hourly for 2–4 hours. If a significant elevation of IOP is detected (generally defined as a rise of ≥10 mm Hg), apraclonidine, a carbonic anhydrase inhibitor, and/or a hyperosmotic agent are administered. In all cases, topical corticosteroids are administered several times daily for several days, and the patient is seen again 1–2 weeks later.

SECTION IV

LASER IRIDOTOMY AND IRIDOPLASTY

Gregory L. Skuta

LASER IRIDOTOMY

In most angle-closure glaucomas with associated pupillary block, argon or Nd:YAG laser iridotomy is the definitive procedure of choice (Fig. 9.15). Before laser iridotomy with either modality, pilocarpine drops (2–4% for two to three doses) are given to make the pupil miotic and place the iris on stretch. A topical anesthetic is then applied. For laser iridotomy, an Abraham iridotomy lens (or similar lens) is placed on the eye. This lens (Fig. 9.16) consists of a +66 diopter planoconvex button bonded to a glass plate. The lens increases magnification, provides limited control of ocular movement, serves as a lid speculum, decreases the likelihood of corneal epithelial burns, and decreases the effective beam spot size by 50% while increasing the power density by a factor of four.[150,151]

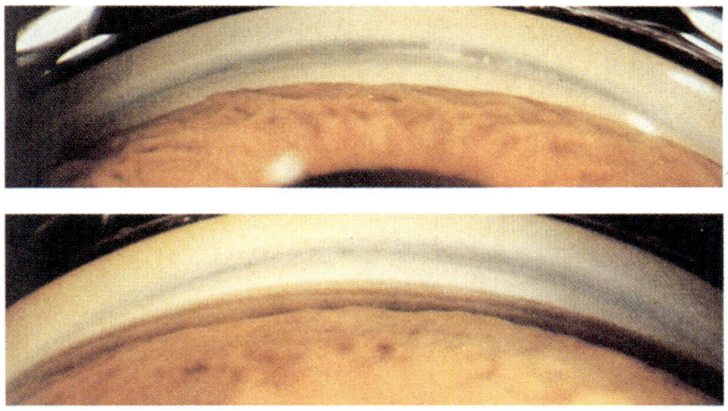

9.15 | Closed anterior chamber angle (above) has deepened markedly (below) after laser iridotomy. (From Van Buskirk EM: *Clinical Atlas of Glaucoma.* Philadelphia: WB Saunders, 1986, 49.)

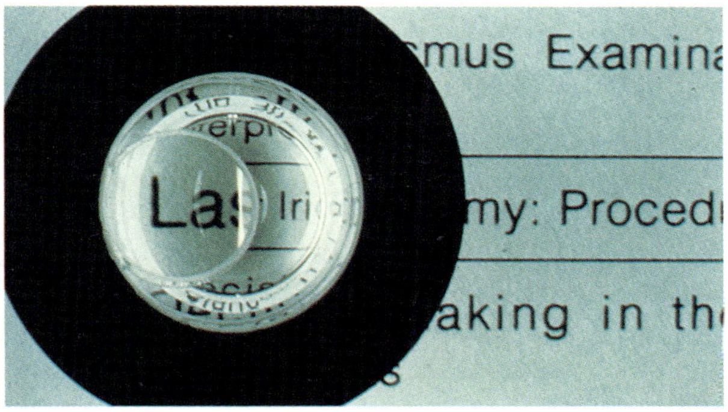

9.16 | Abraham lens used in performing laser iridotomy. (Courtesy of Dr. Eve J. Higginbotham.)

In performing laser iridotomy, one usually chooses to treat the outer third of the iris in the region of an iris crypt, most commonly superonasally or superotemporally.[150–152] Traditionally, the superonasal quadrant has been chosen to reduce the likelihood of macular injury with the argon laser. Treatment directly at the 12 o'clock position should be avoided, as air bubbles (Fig. 9.17) may collect and prevent completion of the iridotomy at that site. As penetration of the iris is achieved, one usually sees a burst of pigment from the iridotomy site. The anterior lens capsule can also usually be seen.

With the argon laser, thermal and disruptive effects result in creation of an iridotomy. Because of the coagulative properties of argon laser energy, bleeding is not associated with argon laser iridotomy. Common parameters for treatment with the argon laser include 50–100 μm spot size, 500–2,000 mw power, and 0.05–0.2 second duration. Settings may depend on iris pigmentation and thickness of the iris stroma. Blue irides typically require the greatest amount of energy to achieve penetration. A chipping technique using short-duration applications may be particularly effective in the treatment of thick brown irides. Variations in technique are described in more detail in Figure 9.18 and in other texts.[150–152]

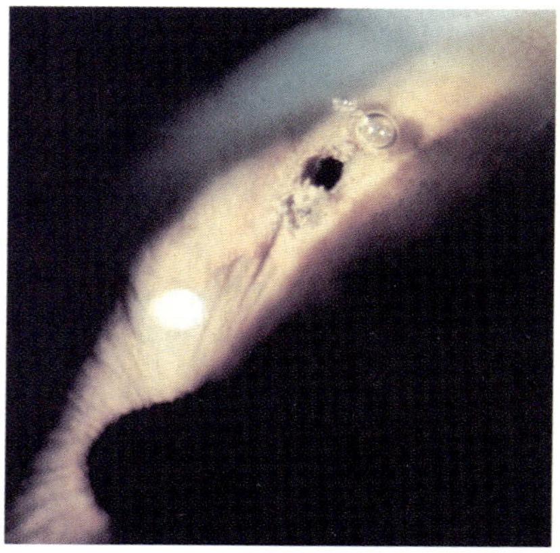

9.17 | Air bubbles adjacent to superonasal iridotomy site. If iridotomy is attempted at 12 o'clock position, bubbles may collect and prevent completion of treatment at that site. (Courtesy of Dr. Eve J. Higginbotham.)

Figure 9.18. Parameters for Argon Laser Iridotomy

Burn Type	Power (mw)	Spot Size (μm)	Duration (sec)
Stretch	200–500	200–500	0.2–0.5
Penetration	600–1,500	50	0.1–0.2
Chip	600–1,500	50	0.01–0.10

(Modified from Higginbotham EJ, Shahbazi MF: Laser therapy in glaucoma: An overview and update. *Int Ophthalmol Clin 1990;30:189.*)

With the Nd:YAG laser, the iridotomy is created by photodisruption of the target tissue (Fig. 9.19). Because the Q-switched Nd:YAG laser possesses no coagulative properties, bleeding may occur.[150–152] Therefore, one should avoid treatment on or near an iris vessel. Usual parameters include 3–10 mj power and one to three pulses per burst (Fig. 9.20). The total energy delivered during YAG laser iridotomy is less than with argon therapy.[152]

Complications of argon laser iridotomy include corneal epithelial and/or endothelial burns (Fig. 9.21).[150,151] With the Nd:YAG laser, endothelial injury is characterized by a shattered-glass appearance. Rare cases of corneal decompensation after argon laser iridotomy have been described.[153]

Nonprogressive focal lenticular opacities are not uncommonly seen after argon laser iridotomy due to thermal effects on the anterior lens capsule

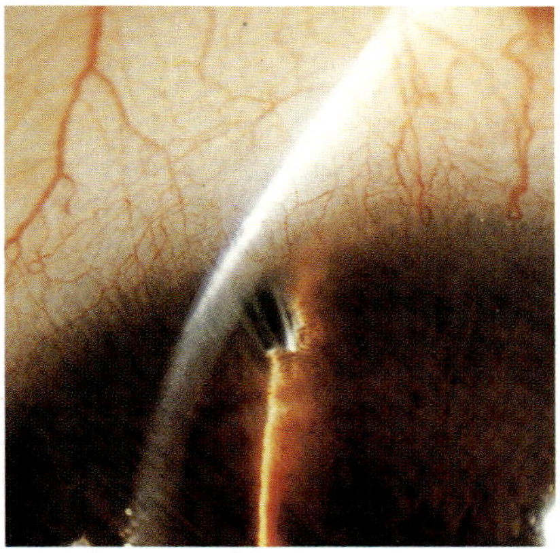

9.19 | Patent Nd:YAG laser iridotomy. Note more slit-like opening in comparison with argon laser iridotomy (see Fig. 9.17).

Figure 9.20. Parameters for Nd:YAG Laser Iridotomy

Energy of pulse	3–10 mj
Spot size	70 µm*
Pulses per burst	1–3
Number of pulses	1–10

*Size at focal spot dependent on contact lens used.
(Modified from Higginbotham EJ, Shahbazi MF: Laser therapy in glaucoma: An overview and update. *Int Ophthalmol Clin 1990;30:189.*)

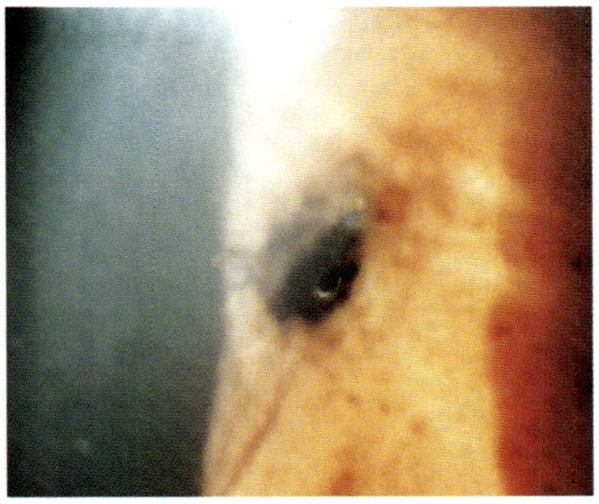

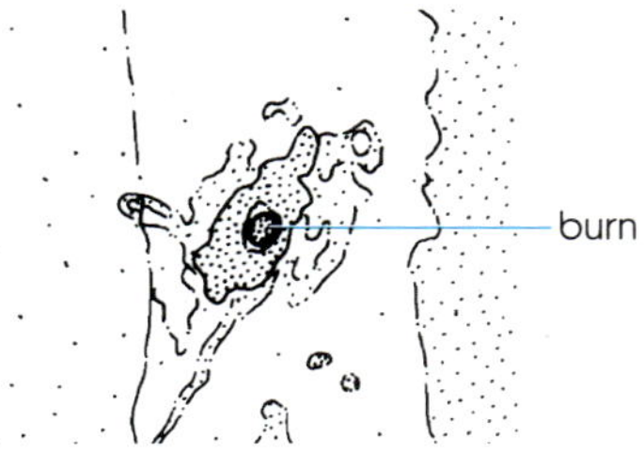

9.21 | Focal corneal endothelial burn after argon laser iridotomy.

(Fig. 9.22).[150–152] With the Nd:YAG laser, an additional potential risk includes photodisruption of the anterior lens capsule although, again, no progressive cataracts have been reported.[152]

Transient elevations of intraocular pressure (IOP) are common after argon and Nd:YAG laser iridotomy, presumably due to decreased outflow related to inflammation and debris created by the treatment. One study described an IOP rise of 8 mm Hg or more in 31.6% of Nd:YAG-treated eyes and 34.2% of argon-treated eyes.[154] IOP should therefore be monitored for at least 1–2 hours after treatment. Topical apraclonidine hydrochloride has been shown to be particularly effective in blunting the postoperative IOP rise,[155] although other medications have also been used.

Postoperative inflammation may increase the likelihood of developing posterior synechiae (Fig. 9.23), especially when the argon laser is used.[156] The use of postoperative topical corticosteroids for 4–7 days after treatment may therefore be helpful.

As already noted above, Nd:YAG iridotomy may be associated with bleeding (Fig. 9.24), with an incidence reported as 59% in an overview of several series.[157] This complication is more likely to be observed in inflamed eyes. The bleeding can usually be controlled by gentle pressure on the eye with the Abraham lens. However, a clinically significant hyphema may occasionally develop. To decrease the risk of bleeding during Nd:YAG iridotomy, some investigators have recommended pretreatment with the argon laser.[157]

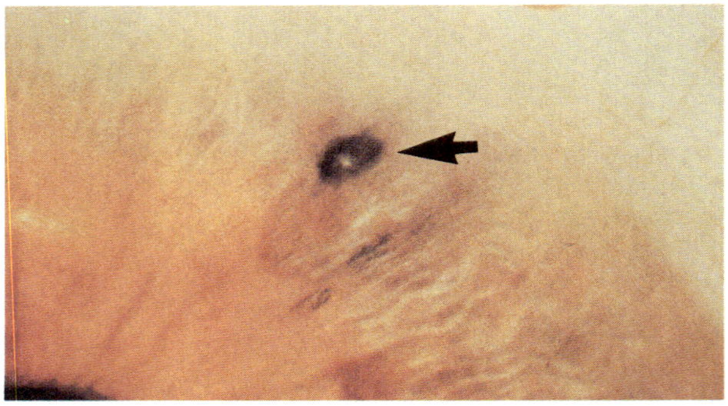

9.22 | Focal nonprogressive lenticular opacity (arrow) after argon laser iridotomy. (From Van Buskirk EM: *Clinical Atlas of Glaucoma.* Philadelphia: WB Saunders, 1986, 107.)

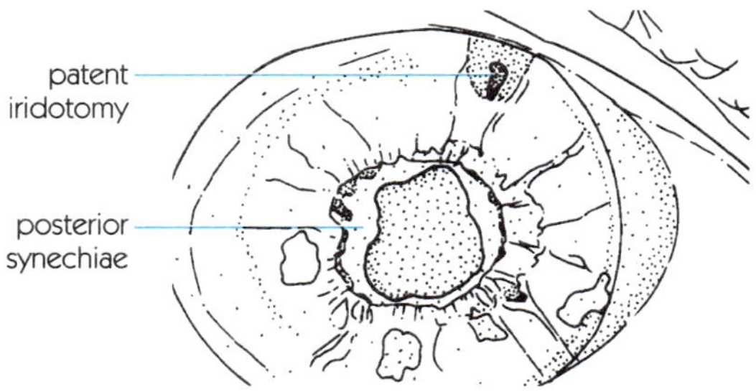

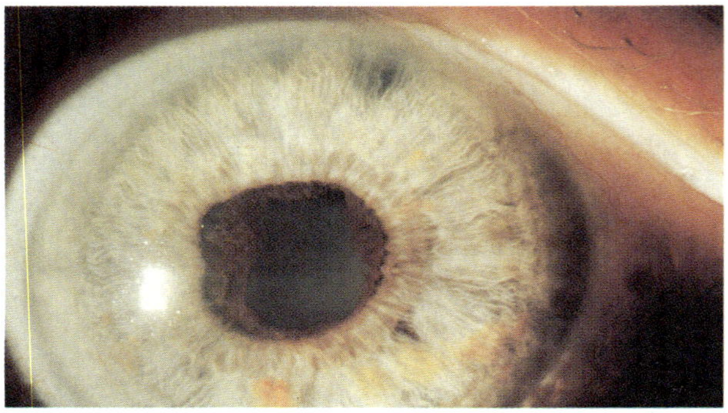

9.23 | Dense posterior synechiae which developed after argon laser iridotomy. Note patent iridotomy site superiorly. (Courtesy of Dr. Terry J. Bergstrom.)

Postoperative closure of the iridotomy site has been reported in up to 30% of eyes undergoing argon laser iridotomy.[154,156] This is secondary to proliferation of the iris pigment epithelium (Fig. 9.25), which can usually be easily eliminated with light retreatment at the iridotomy site. Because of the possibility of closure, some investigators have recommended the placement of two iridotomies at the time of initial treatment. After Nd:YAG laser iridotomy, the incidence of closure is less than 1%.

PERIPHERAL IRIDOPLASTY (GONIOPLASTY)

In the treatment of some angle-closure glaucomas, including plateau iris syndrome, lens-related angle-closure glaucoma, nanophthalmos, and angle closure following scleral buckling surgery, peripheral laser iridoplasty or gonioplasty may help to eliminate appositional closure and to open or widen the angle.[150–152,158,159] It may also occasionally be needed in conjunction with argon laser trabeculoplasty in areas where the angle is narrow or when prominent iris rolls are present.

The peripheral iris is treated with the aid of a contact lens to create moderate stromal burns and subsequent contracture of the surrounding iris

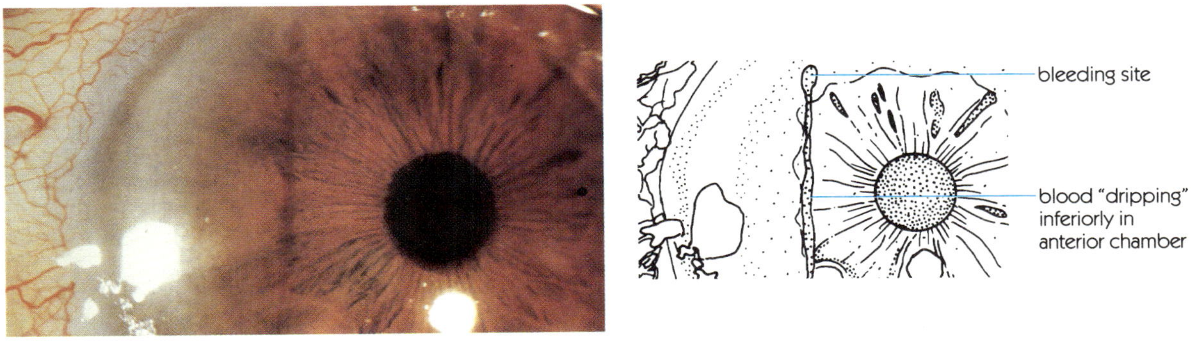

9.24 | Bleeding from Nd:YAG laser iridotomy site. (Courtesy of Dr. Paul R. Lichter.)

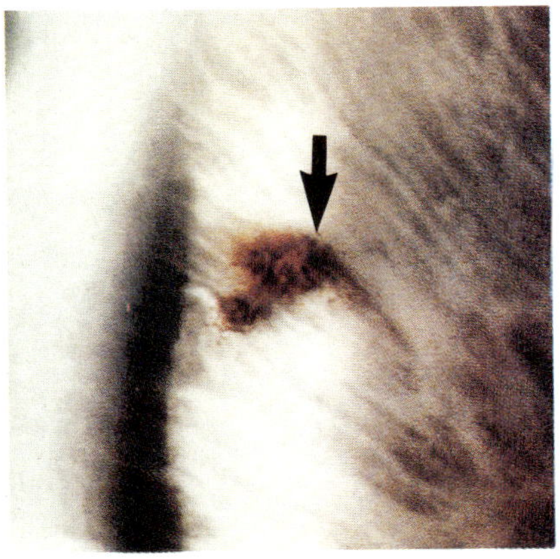

9.25 | Closure of argon laser iridotomy site secondary to proliferation of iris pigment epithelium (arrow). (From Van Buskirk EM: *Clinical Atlas of Glaucoma*. Philadelphia: WB Saunders, 1986, 107.)

(Fig. 9.26). Typically, 10–15 burns are placed in each quadrant with relatively long burns of low energy intensity (e.g., 200–500 µm spot size, 200–400 mw power, and 0.2–0.5 second duration). Confluence of the burns should be avoided to prevent significant iris ischemia and secondary atrophy. Other possible complications include mild iritis, transient ocular irritation, corneal endothelial burns, and transient postoperative IOP elevation.[150–152]

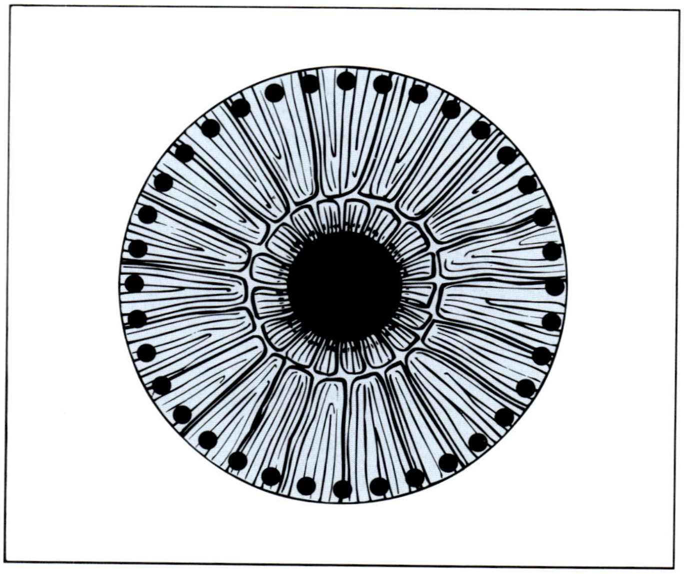

9.26 | Diagram shows appropriate placement of contraction burns in peripheral iridoplasty. (Adapted from Ritch R, Liebmann J, Solomon IS: Laser iridectomy and iridoplasty, in Ritch R, Shields MB, Krupin T (eds): *The Glaucomas.* St. Louis: CV Mosby, 1989, 599.)

SECTION V

FILTRATION SURGERY

Barbara A. Smythe
Jonathan Herschler

Since the late nineteenth century, when it was determined that glaucoma damage was caused by elevated intraocular pressure (IOP), filtration surgery in one form or another has formed the basis for surgical intervention in the treatment of glaucomas of all kinds. In present-day practice, when standard medical and laser therapy have proven inadequate to control IOP satisfactorily, filtration surgery is the treatment of choice.

The basic concept behind filtration surgery is the creation of a fistula between the inside of the eye (usually the anterior chamber) and the subconjunctival space. The potential space available for fluid beneath the conjunctiva and/or Tenon's capsule allows a filtering bleb to form from which the intraocular fluids can either be absorbed by aqueous vein-like structures[160] or, in some cases where the conjunctiva is quite thin, pass directly into the tear film.[161] The earliest fistulizing procedures are represented by the full-thickness sclerectomy[162] or trephination procedure.[163] A subconjunctival dissection is carried out using a limbus-based approach, and a full-thickness segment of corneal/limbal tissues is excised, with an iridectomy being performed. The conjunctival flap is resutured in place. Although the success rates for these procedures are as high as for any other modification of filtration surgery, the complications associated with the early hypotony and shallowing of the chamber, including cataract and corneal decompensation, led to the development of many modifications.

The first major development in terms of decreasing the rate of flow through the filtering ostium during the early postoperative period was the use of the iris as a wick to act as a partial plug.[164] This procedure, known as iridencleisis, was popular for a number of years and did indeed decrease the complications of early postoperative hypotony. However, the updrawn pupil created by the incarceration of the iris in the filtering wound, and the small but real risk of sympathetic ophthalmia due to uveal tissue being placed extrasclerally, led ultimately to the decrease in its popularity.

The concept of a seton to maintain the patency of the internal filtering ostium by keeping the edges permanently separated has been attempted in many forms. Materials ranging from horsehair to metals (titanium) to plastics such as polyethylene have been utilized.[165] All these attempts are based on the belief that failures of filtration surgery occur because of closure of the internal filtering window. In fact, closure of the internal window is not a frequent cause of failure. When decreased filtration occurs after filtering surgery the villain is usually scar tissue forming in the subconjunctival space, which tends to delimit the area available for aqueous absorption and ultimately lessens the flow of fluid through the filtering ostia. The latter ultimately allows closure of the internal window.

The most popular modification of filtering surgery in the present day is the use of a partial-thickness, loosely sutured scleral flap overlying the internal ostium to provide some resistance to outflow of fluid (Fig. 9.27). This procedure, known as trabeculectomy, was first described in the late 1960s.[166] Its name derives from the incorrect concept that removal of a portion of the trabecular meshwork would allow flow into the cut ends of Schlemm's canal. In the adult human there is very little evidence that circumferential flow of fluid occurs within Schlemm's canal.[167] The actual pressure-lowering effect of partial-thickness filtering procedures is based on aqueous flow through the loosely closed edges of the scleral flap into the subconjunctival space, with perhaps some flow directly through the scleral flap if it is very thin.[168] The partial-thickness trabeculectomy filtering procedure is slightly less effective in reducing IOP than a full-thickness procedure.[169] Typical final postoperative IOP readings are in the mid to high teens after partial-thickness surgery, in contrast to pressures in the mid to low teens on average with the full-

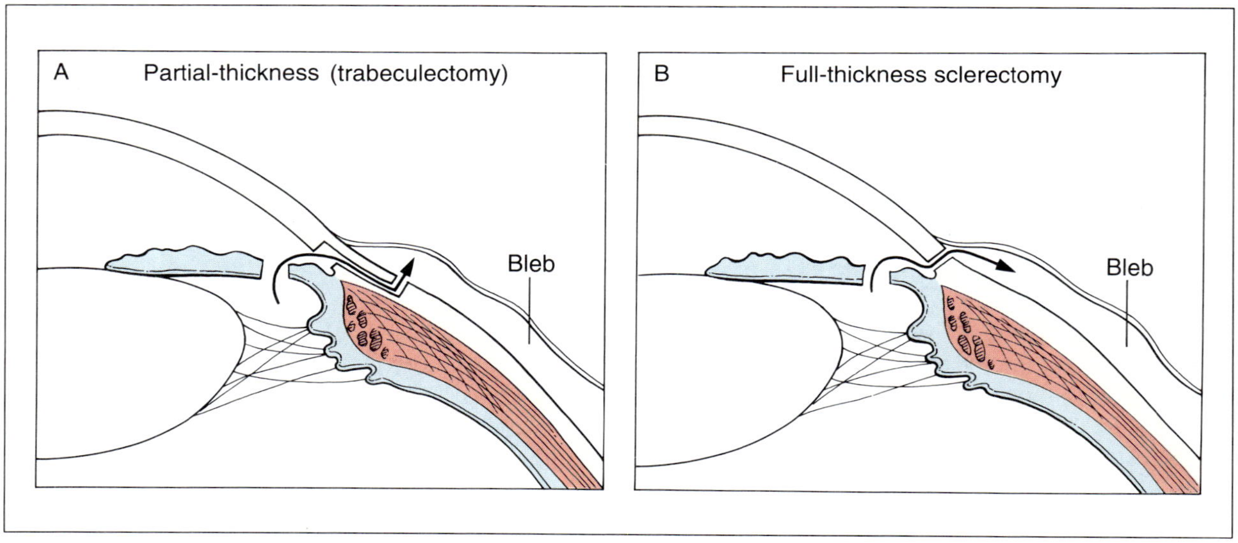

9.27 | *A:* Trabeculectomy with partial thickness scleral flap in place. Aqueous drains through the edges of the flap into the subconjunctival space. *B:* Full-thickness sclerectomy. Aqueous drains directly into the subconjunctival space.

thickness filtration procedures. This difference in final IOP has led to enthusiasm for a modified trabeculectomy, which mimics the full-thickness filtration procedure, in patients with severely damaged optic nerves or those suffering glaucoma damage at relatively low IOPs. Such modifications include fashioning a smaller scleral flap only slightly larger than the internal ostium and/or releasing or lysing (with the argon laser) the sutures holding the scleral flap in place shortly after surgery.

The bulk of research in filtration surgery has focused on ways to obtain successful filtering procedures in patients shown to have a high risk of failure. Glaucoma associated with inflammation or growth of new blood vessels in the anterior segment, glaucoma in youthful patients, patients who are aphakic, and patients who have had previous failures in filtration surgery attempts all have greatly increased chances of failure when filtration surgery is performed. For the most part, the research with regard to these failing filtration procedures has overlooked the mechanism by which filtration surgery *succeeds* in the vast majority of patients. There is some evidence that normal aqueous humor contains a mixture of bioactive factors, some that stimulate and others that inhibit the growth of fibroblasts.[170] The net result is that tissues bathed in this normal aqueous humor tend not to proliferate or to form scar tissue. However, after surgical intervention or trauma, aqueous humor tends to change its biochemical constituents (or their ratios) so that the predominant effect of the fluid is to stimulate fibroblast proliferation[171] and migration.[172] This may derive from the addition of nutrient material to support fibroblast growth, or from inactivation of inhibitors normally present in aqueous humor.[171] Thus far it has proven difficult to isolate and characterize the aqueous constituents that tend to have the inhibitory effect. Therefore, the current approach to increasing success rates with filtration surgery has been to use antimetabolite-type drugs that tend to prevent the growth of the fibroblasts during the time in which the aqueous humor contains the stimulatory properties. The antimetabolite drug 5-fluorouracil has been proven clinically effective in suppressing formation of subconjunctival scar tissue and increasing the rate of success of filtration surgery in high-risk patients.[173] As one might expect, because this antimetabolite is nonspecific in its effect (i.e., not targeted solely at proliferating fibroblasts) there is a significant morbidity to the normally replicating tissues involved in ocular metabolism.[173] The most common complication from subconjunctivally injected 5-fluorouracil is a corneal epithelial disturbance. Fortunately, these defects tend to resolve after the antimetabolite medication is discontinued (see Wright and Parrish, this chapter).

Another approach to managing high-risk patients has been the use of a seton tube connected to a large plastic plate, with the plate being sewn externally to the sclera postequatorially. Such devices work by virtue of the very large surface area of the plastic episcleral plate. Even though scar tissue forms around the plate and the layers of scar tissue are relatively impermeable, so that the rate of flow per square millimeter across the scar tissue is small, the surface area exposed to the aqueous is so large that the total flow is often sufficient to lower IOP. As with standard filtration surgery, adjunctive medications may be required during the postoperative period to maintain acceptable levels of IOP. However, the ultimate pressures obtained, even with adjunctive medications, are usually not as low as with standard filtration surgery (see Krupin, this chapter).

SURGICAL TECHNIQUES

It is worthwhile to highlight some general technical concepts in filtration surgery. The conjunctival flap should be prepared in the least traumatic fashion possible. Conjunctival flaps can be either limbal- or fornix-based (Fig. 9.28). If a limbus-based flap is employed, the flap is started posteriorly in the fornix, usually approximately 10 mm from the limbus, with the dissection confined to one intermuscle quadrant. Care should be taken not to slant the periphery of the incision towards the limbus, as the conjunctival incision will tend to form a barrier scar that will ultimately delimit the bleb that has formed. Usually the conjunctiva and Tenon's capsule tissue are dissected as one.[163] Some authorities favor excision of the Tenon's tissue, based on the notion that it is Tenon's tissue that is the source of the scar. However, it is more likely that the episclera is the source of the fibroblasts that cause scar tissue formation.[172] If a fornix-based approach is utilized, it is important to incise the conjunctiva directly at its insertion into the cornea so as not to leave a tag of adherent conjunctiva attached to the cornea; this could act as an impediment to conjunctival reattachment. The fornix-based approach requires less dissection, is faster, and makes the sclera more accessible, but there is a greater tendency for leaks to develop underneath the edges of the conjunctival flap during the early postoperative period.[174]

Closure of the fornix-based approach is simpler; usually a single wing-type suture at each extremity of the incision is placed to stretch the conjuncti-

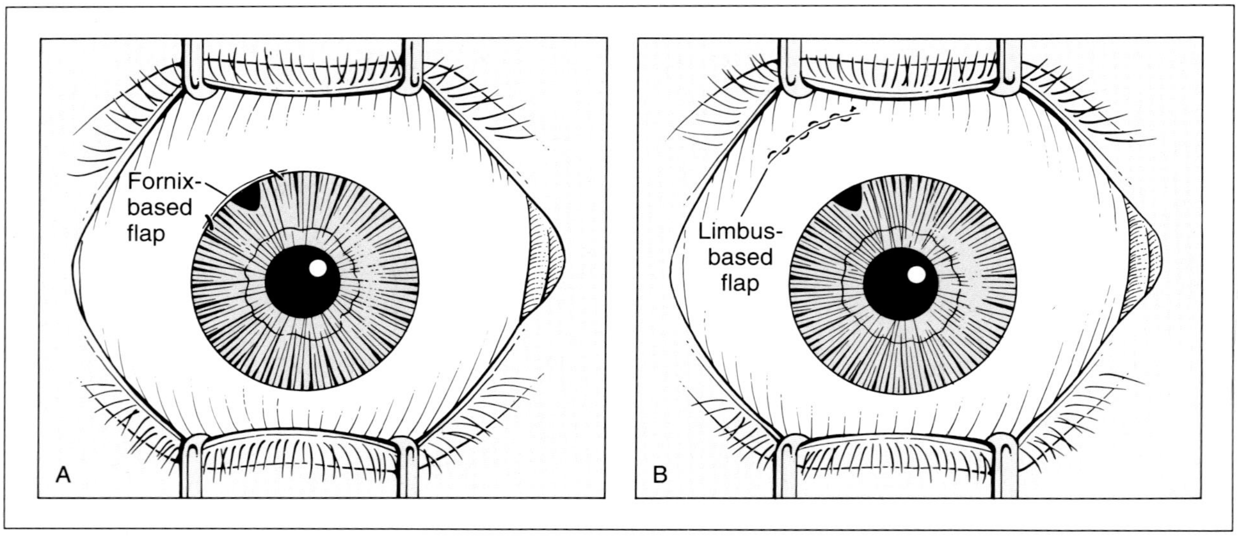

9.28 | Closure of the conjunctival flap after trabeculectomy. *A:* Fornix-based flap with wing suture at either end of the incision. The conjunctiva is stretched tightly across the peripheral cornea. *B:* Limbus-based flap with continuous running suture to close conjunctiva and Tenon's layer, either separately or together.

va in a tight cord across the peripheral cornea so that there is resistance to flow in the early phase before the conjunctiva has actually physically adhered to the cornea (see Fig. 9.28A). Some authorities recommend applying light cautery to the surface of the exposed peripheral cornea to encourage conjunctival adherence. At a minimum, the cornea needs to be locally de-epithelized to provide a good surface for adherence of the flap. Suturing of the limbus-based flap requires careful closure of both the conjunctiva and Tenon's tissue, either together or separately in two layers. With either limbal- or fornix-based flaps, the watertightness of the conjunctival closure should be checked by injecting fluid into the anterior chamber through a previously placed paracentesis tract to be sure that there is good flow into the bleb and that there is not significant leakage along the conjunctival incision line (Fig. 9.29).

The surgical technique (Fig. 9.30) for making the opening into the anterior chamber, whether full thickness or underneath the scleral flap, varies according to the surgeon's preference. Commonly, a rectangular block of tissue is excised with a sharp blade and angled Vannas scissors.[174] An alternative is the use of a small punch, such as a Kelly Descemet punch, which removes a semicircular segment of the posterior lip of the incision once the anterior chamber has been entered with a sharp blade. However, making a linear incision and then retracting the edge of the incision with a cautery is also acceptable. Once the deep sclerectomy has been performed, a peripheral iridectomy must be made. It is important to obtain a full-thickness hole in the iris, and it is desirable that the hole in the peripheral iris be slightly larger than the hole in the overlying limbal tissue. This can be accomplished by gently elevating the peripheral iris with forceps and cutting through the exposed iris tissue with a scissors, making two individual cuts at 45° to one another. This tends to make a broad hole in the iris, which is larger at its base

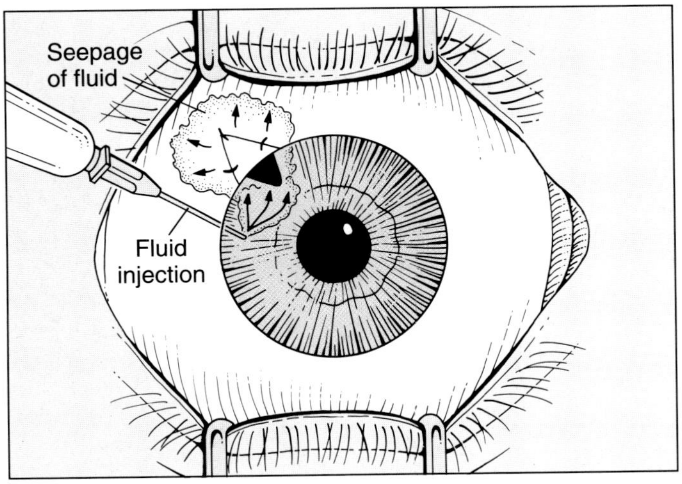

9.29 | Testing the conjunctival closure. At the conclusion of the procedure fluid is injected into the anterior chamber to assess flow across the scleral flap and tightness of the conjunctival wound.

than the sclerectomy (Fig. 9.30). Some authors have proposed placing a viscoelastic substance, such as hyaluronate, in the anterior chamber at the start of the procedure to prevent shallowing during the intraoperative and postoperative period.[175]

COMPLICATIONS

There are potential complications after filtering surgery. Hypotony may result from overfiltration, particularly in the case of full-thickness procedures, but also may occur in the presence of a loosely sutured scleral flap. A conjunctival wound leak further contributes to overfiltration. Significant or prolonged hypotony, in turn, promotes the development of choroidal effusion, a complication that is most frequently found in aphakia. Choroidal detachment with ensuing ciliary body shutdown acts to reinforce the hypotony and thus maintains the detachment. This cycle can be interrupted with steroids and cycloplegic agents aimed to reduce inflammation of the ciliary body, hence promoting its recovery. Occasionally, surgical intervention is required and involves the drainage of suprachoroidal fluid and reformation of the anterior chamber.

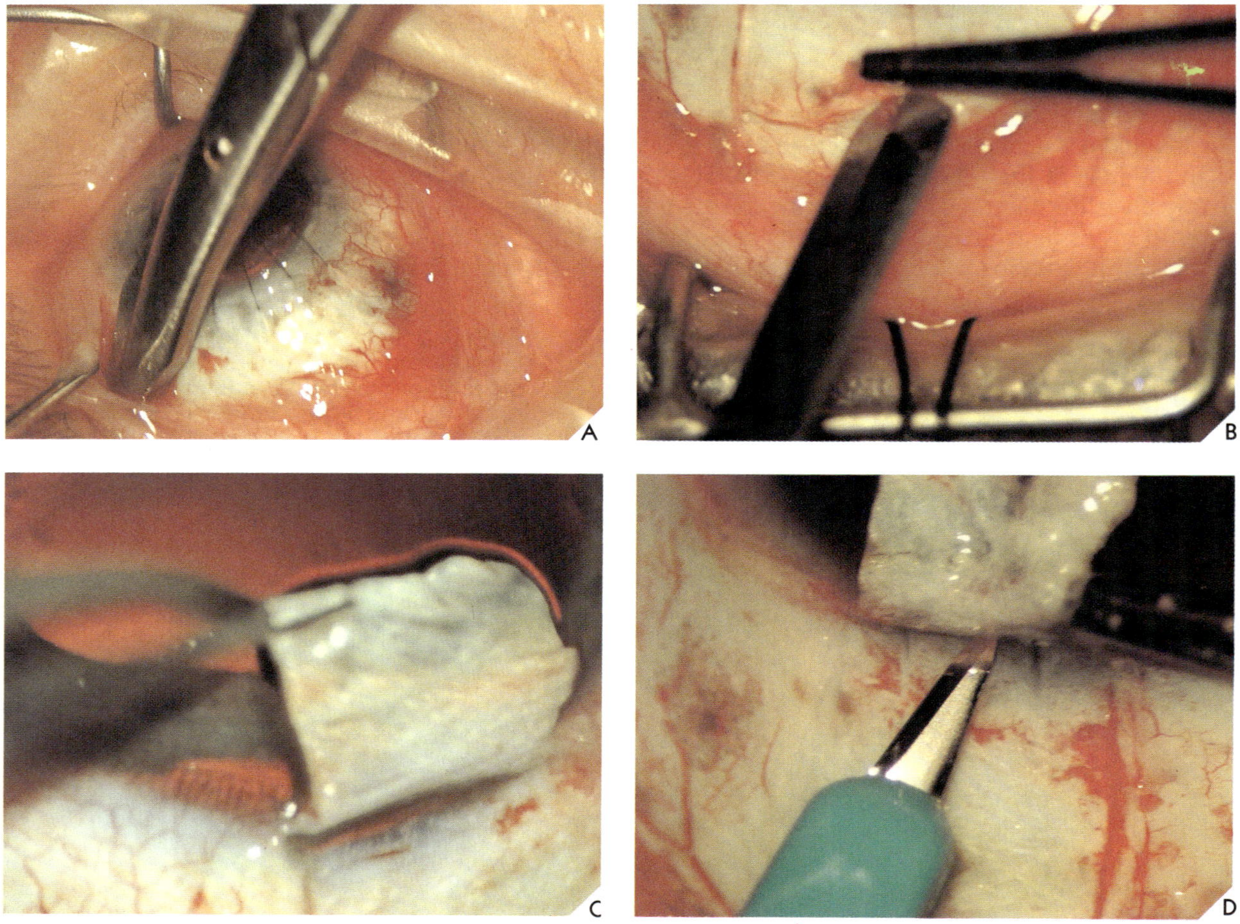

9.30 | Partial thickness (guarded) trabeculectomy. *A:* The conjunctiva is opened to expose the limbus. A fornix-based approach is shown here. Care is taken to avoid buttonholing (perforating) the tissue. *B:* The flap is outlined on the sclera extending to 1/2 to 2/3 scleral depth. *C:* Flap is dissected forward into clear corneal tissue. *D:* A rectangular block of tissue is excised from underneath the scleral flap. This block may consist of cornea only or may include trabecular meshwork.

On the other hand, IOP may be elevated postoperatively. This is commonly due to a tight scleral flap, but may occur from occlusion of the ostium by blood, pigment, or uveal tissue. Appropriate diagnosis requires gonioscopic examination of the filtering cleft, followed by efforts to force fluid through the cleft by massaging the globe. Suture lysis may be required. In the case of obstructing debris, Nd:YAG laser energy can disrupt the material and reestablish aqueous outflow.

Postoperative pressure elevation may unusually arise from ciliary block. In this case appropriate medical therapy should be instituted promptly, and includes topical cycloplegic–mydriatic agents and steroids, as well as oral hyperosmotic agents and carbonic anhydrase inhibitors. This complex regimen is followed for up to 4 days before surgical measures are undertaken. In the aphakic or pseudophakic patient, attempts to disrupt the hyaloid face by means of the Nd:YAG laser often successfully relieve the block. In some cases, however, a full vitrectomy is required.

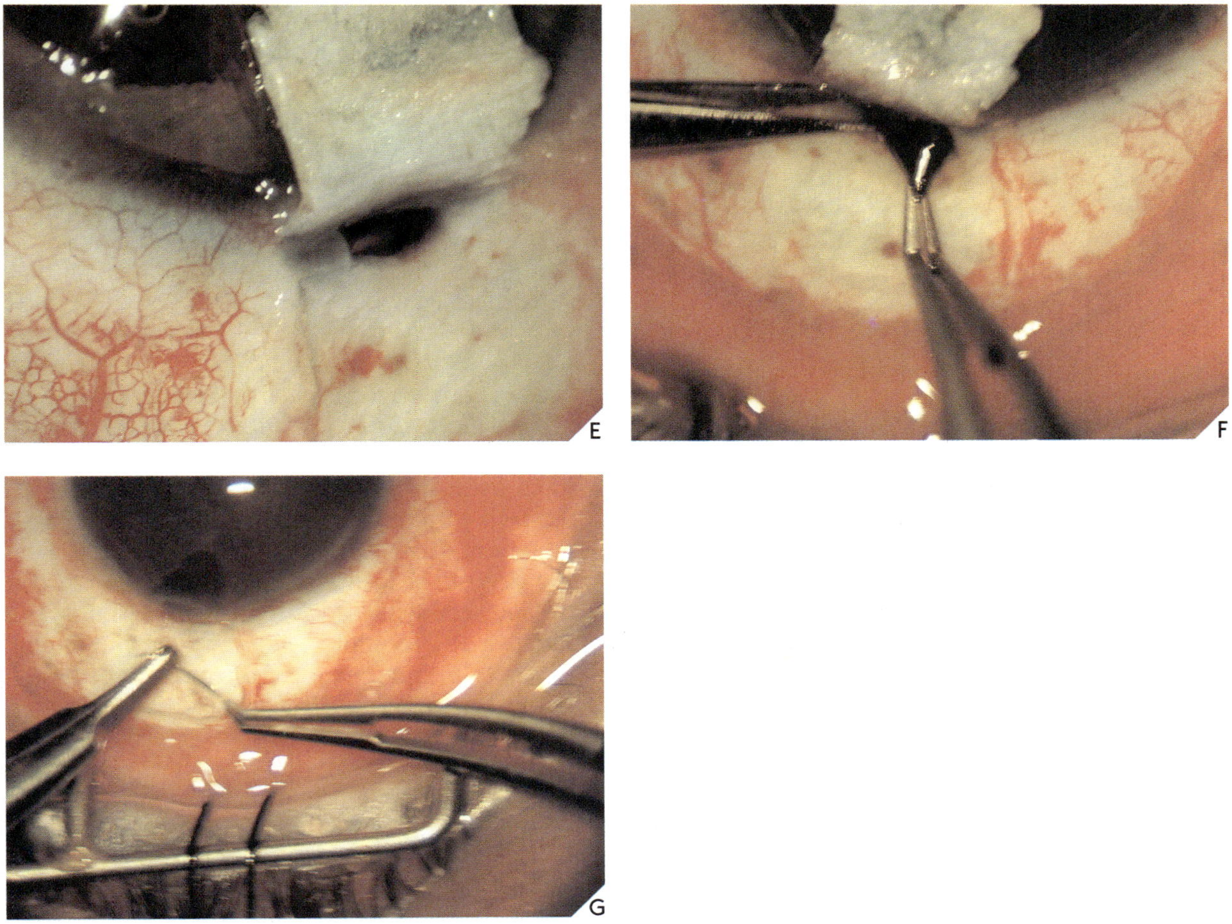

9.30 | (Cont'd) *E:* Completed fistula. *F:* Peripheral iris is drawn through the fistula and an iridectomy is created. *G:* Scleral flap is sutured, followed by suturing of conjunctival flap. (From Nardin G, Zimmerman TJ: Surgery for glaucoma and related conditions, in Jaffe NS: *Atlas of Ophthalmic Surgery*. New York: Gower Medical Publishing, 1990.)

A rare but potentially devastating complication of filtering surgery is the loss of a small remaining island of central vision. This may occur in the face of apparently uneventful surgery and satisfactory postoperative IOP control. The phenomenon occurs characteristically in patients whose useful preoperative vision is a central island splitting fixation along the horizontal meridian.

Postoperative endophthalmitis may develop after filtering procedures. This complication, although rare, is seen more frequently after full-thickness sclerostomy procedures with their associated thin-walled conjunctival bleb. The organisms involved are typically streptococcal and staphylococcal strains. Unusually severe anterior chamber inflammatory reaction and/or conjunctival hyperemia unresponsive to steroid treatment warrants investigation for an infectious process.

Finally, the appearance of lens opacities at variable intervals after filtering surgery is commonly described. This phenomenon of cataract formation may occur after an apparently uneventful procedure, and the underlying pathophysiology for this process is unclear. The concomitant loss of visual acuity poses a challenge in terms of saving a successful filter while addressing the cataract. Surgical approaches for cataract extraction entail either entering the eye through a clear corneal incision (anterior to the filtering cleft) or approaching the limbus along its temporal aspect.

A period of elevated IOP to the mid 20s range is commonly encountered 4–6 weeks after filtering surgery and may be difficult to distinguish from early bleb failure. Efforts are directed towards promoting fluid flow through the ostium and across the episclera by massage. This maneuver, more accurately termed compression, is done by applying direct, firm, steady digital pressure on the globe at a site away from the conjunctival bleb. Massage can be done several times daily but such pressure should be interrupted approximately every 10 seconds to avoid prolonged retinal arterial occlusion.

IOP elevation that persists for several weeks or that progresses into the high-twenties range mandates a more rigorous approach to salvage the filter. The site of outflow resistance may be within the episcleral tissue of the bleb or across the filtering ostium itself. In the former situation, a thick-walled, relatively well-vascularized bleb with few conjunctival microcysts is seen; this is the more frequent problem. In the less common latter case, a membrane spanning the filtering cleft can be identified during gonioscopic examination. Incising thickened episcleral tissue is easily done by passing a thin needle through the conjunctiva at a location well away from the filtering bleb. The needle is then advanced within the subconjunctival space, through the episclera, and into the filtering reservoir. Fluid withdrawn at this point confirms adequate placement of the needle.

Puncturing a membrane that covers the trabeculectomy cleft can be done with either a needle or goniotomy knife. This procedure, known as goniopuncture, involves gonioscopically-assisted manipulation under microscopic visualization. It is most adequately done in the operating room with use of, e.g., the Swan–Jacob lens. The eye and lens are positioned appropriately, and then a needle or goniotomy knife is introduced into the anterior chamber at a position 180° away from the cleft. It is advanced transcamerally until the cleft is reached, and then is pushed through the membrane and up into the bleb. The knife tip can be directly viewed within the subconjunctival space at this time and care is required to avoid conjunctival perforation. The subconjunctival injection of viscoelastic or balanced salt solution before manipulation will elevate the bleb and protect against buttonholing the tissue in the final step of the procedure. The knife is then withdrawn along the same tract and a corneal suture is placed at the paracentesis site if necessary.

In occasional situations a full surgical revision is needed to maintain a functional filter. For instance, a bleb that has migrated onto the corneal surface is exposed to continuous disturbance by the blinking eyelids. The tissue may become thinned and may potentially perforate; or it may become irritated and secondarily thickened. In either case the process is interrupted only after the bleb is excised and fresh conjunctiva is advanced across the filtering site.

At present, research involving the use of lasers and internal trephination devices to cut sclerectomies without having to incise the overlying conjunctiva is under way (see March, this chapter). This may further increase the rate of success with filtration surgery. However, basic research must be done into understanding how patent fistulas are maintained by the biologic interaction of the aqueous humor and the scleral tissues, and how pressure is regulated after fistulizing surgery. It is a wonder that one can drill a hole in the limbal tissues of the eye and cover it with conjunctival tissue so that the end result is a normalization of IOP. A better understanding of how that process occurs will greatly facilitate intelligent improvements in our surgical techniques and results.

Section VI

Antimetabolites in Filtering Surgery

Martha M. Wright
Richard K. Parrish

Glaucoma filtering surgery in primary open-angle glaucoma has an estimated success rate of 80–90%,[176,177] but filtering procedures in other types of glaucoma are not as successful. In particular, aphakia,[178–180] previous unsuccessful filtering surgery,[176,180] anterior segment neovascularization,[181–183] youth,[184,185] and possibly black race[178,186] are believed to have a poor prognosis with filtering surgery. Filter failure can occur at three locations. First, the surgery may fail because the internal ostium of the filter is blocked, usually by prolapse of iris, lens, ciliary body, or vitreous. Second, failure may occur at the level of the sclera when the sclerostomy created at surgery is too small. Third, extraocular failures occur when subconjunctival scarring eliminates the filtering bleb.[187] The majority of filter failures are of the extraocular type. Antimetabolites, which limit fibroblast proliferation and the formation of subconjunctival fibrosis, have been used after filtering surgery in an attempt to prevent filter failure.[188]

5-Fluorouracil

5-Fluorouracil (5-FU), a pyrimidine analogue, has been the most widely used antimetabolite in conjunction with filtering surgery. 5-FU acts by competitive inhibition of the enzyme thymidylate synthetase and is cell-cycle specific, interfering with the S-phase of cell replication[189,190] (Fig. 9.31). This specificity makes 5-FU more toxic to replicating cells than to nonproliferating cells; therefore, 5-FU interferes with fibroblast proliferation and subsequent scar tissue formation. The replication of normal epithelial cells of the cornea and conjunctiva is also inhibited by 5-FU, making epithelial toxicity the most commonly reported side effect of subconjunctival 5-FU administration after filtering surgery.

Subconjunctivally injected 5-FU after trabeculectomy was shown in a randomized, prospective multicenter trial to improve significantly the chance of intraocular pressure (IOP) control for at least 1 year in eyes that have undergone previous cataract or filtering surgery.[191] Possible uses for postoperative subconjunctival 5-FU not tested in the multicenter trial include uveitic glaucoma, neovascular glaucoma, primary phakic filters, combined cataract and glaucoma surgery, cataract surgery in an eye with a functioning filter, and childhood glaucomas; however, the long-term safety and efficacy of 5-FU in these conditions remains to be proven.

The optimal dose and frequency of 5-FU administration has yet to be determined. The dose given in the multicenter trial (5 mg twice daily during postoperative days 1–7, and once daily on postoperative days 8–14) may have been more than the maximal effective dose, and a recent report suggests that a lower dose may be equally effective with less corneal toxicity.[192] At present, a daily subconjunctival injection of 5 mg of 5-FU is given for the first postoperative week, then every other day during the second week, for a total of 10 doses (50 mg). Although topical 5-FU would be more convenient to administer than subconjunctival injections, the topical application of 5-FU drops is more toxic to the cornea than is subconjunctival administration. Alternate delivery systems for 5-FU that would obviate the need for daily injections are under investigation. Sustained release systems currently under study include liposomes, membranes, and bioerodible polymers containing 5-FU.[188]

PATIENT SELECTION

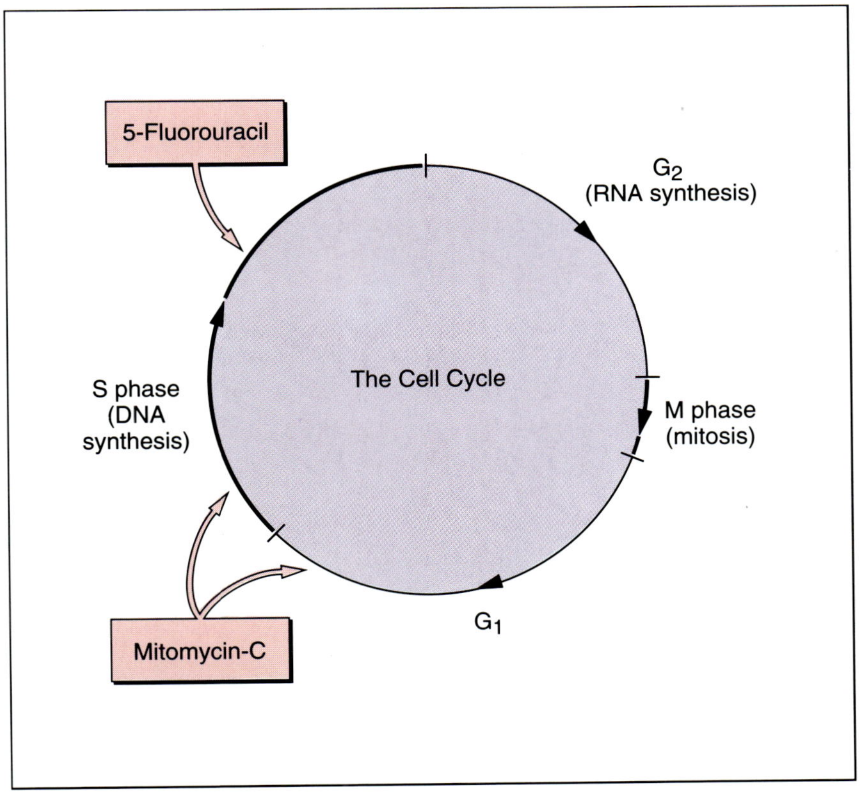

9.31 | The cell cycle. 5-Fluorouracil interferes with the S-phase (DNA synthesis) of cell replication.

SURGICAL PROCEDURE

A detailed description of trabeculectomy is given by Smythe and Herschler in this chapter, but special attention to selection and exposure of the surgical site and to wound closure is required when the postoperative use of 5-FU is planned.

The surgical site should be placed in an area of unscarred, freely movable conjunctiva. If the surgeon prefers to operate in a position that includes a previous surgical site, lack of scarring at the limbus can be determined by injecting balanced salt solution through a 25- or 30-gauge needle, 8–10 mm posterior to the limbus in the proposed incision line. If the conjunctiva elevates easily to the limbus, proceed with trabeculectomy; however, if there is scarring of the episcleral tissue, as may occur with previous cataract surgery, an inferotemporal or inferonasal site should be chosen (Fig. 9.32). Exposure of the inferior conjunctiva is achieved by a 7-0 polyglactin (Vicryl 910®) corneal traction suture, placed in peripheral clear cornea directly in front of the planned filtering site (Fig. 9.33).

Meticulous wound closure is crucial for postoperative use of 5-FU. The trabeculectomy is performed with a limbus-based conjunctival flap to ensure a watertight closure. Avoidance of conjunctival tears or buttonholes is critical. The conjunctival incision is closed with 8-0 braided or 9-0 monofilament polyglactin on a taper-point needle (BV 130-4 or BV 100-3),

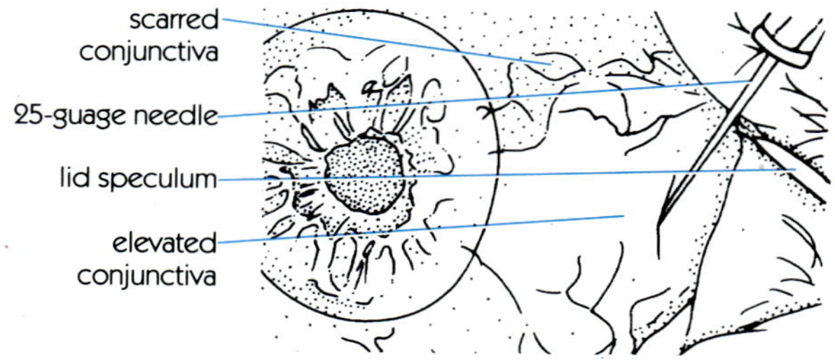

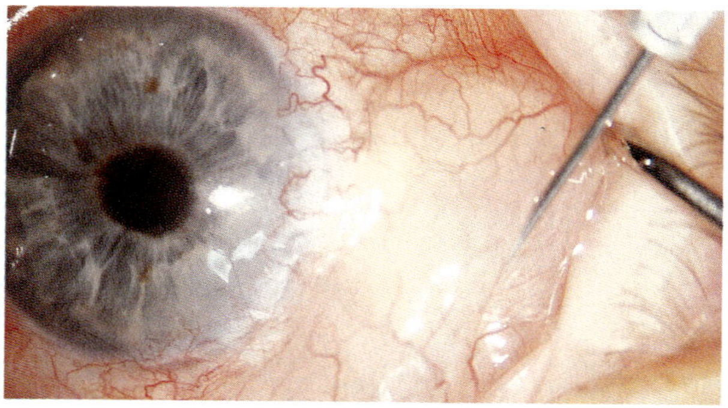

9.32 | Balanced salt solution is injected through a 25-gauge needle, 8–10 mm posterior to the limbus in the proposed incision line. Areas of scarred and areas of freely elevated conjunctiva are easily delineated. The unscarred area is chosen as the trabeculectomy site.

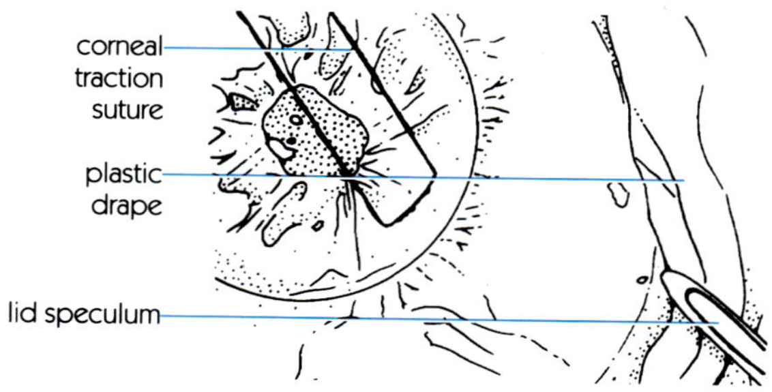

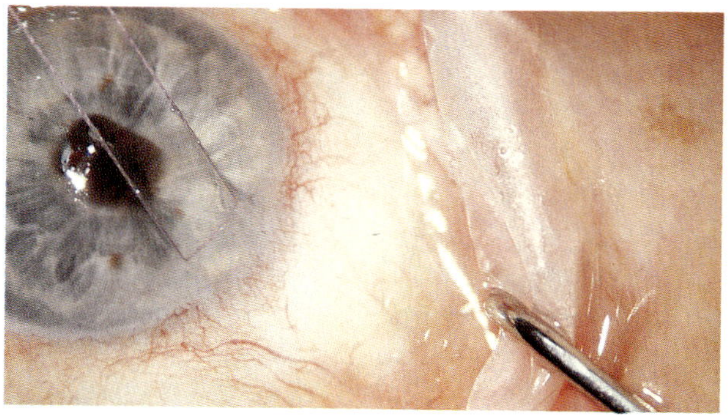

9.33 | A 7-0 polyglactin corneal traction suture is used to expose the inferotemporal conjunctiva.

or with 10-0 Prolene® or 10-0 nylon on a vascular needle. When possible, Tenon's tissue can be closed as a separate layer. Leaks along the incision line are minimized by using a suture on a taper-point (vascular) needle rather than a cutting needle, because the former makes a hole approximately the same size as the suture, whereas the latter makes a much larger hole (Fig. 9.34). Adequacy of conjunctival wound closure and integrity of the conjunctiva can be evaluated by injecting balanced salt solution through a paracentesis tract to elevate the bleb (Fig. 9.35). Cycloplegics and frequent

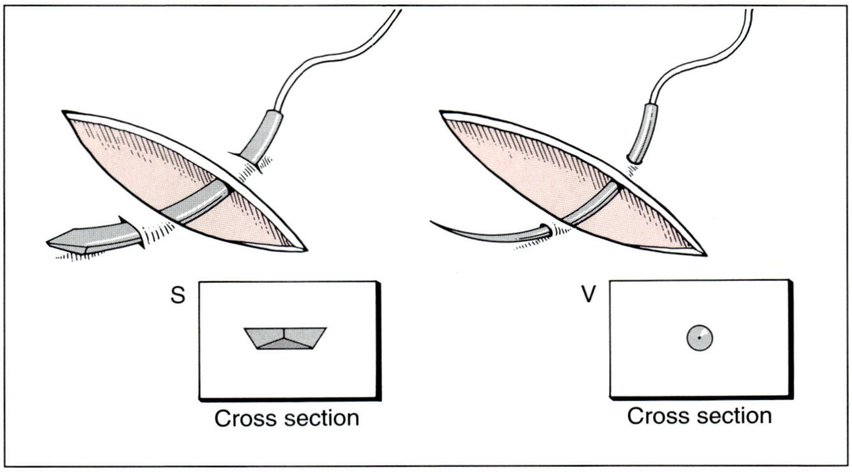

9.34 | Comparison of spatula/cutting needle (S) with a vascular/taper needle (V). A cross-sectional view is shown adjacent to each needle. The vascular needle creates a hole in the conjunctiva approximately the same size as the suture, whereas the spatula needle creates a larger slit that can cause postoperative wound leaks.

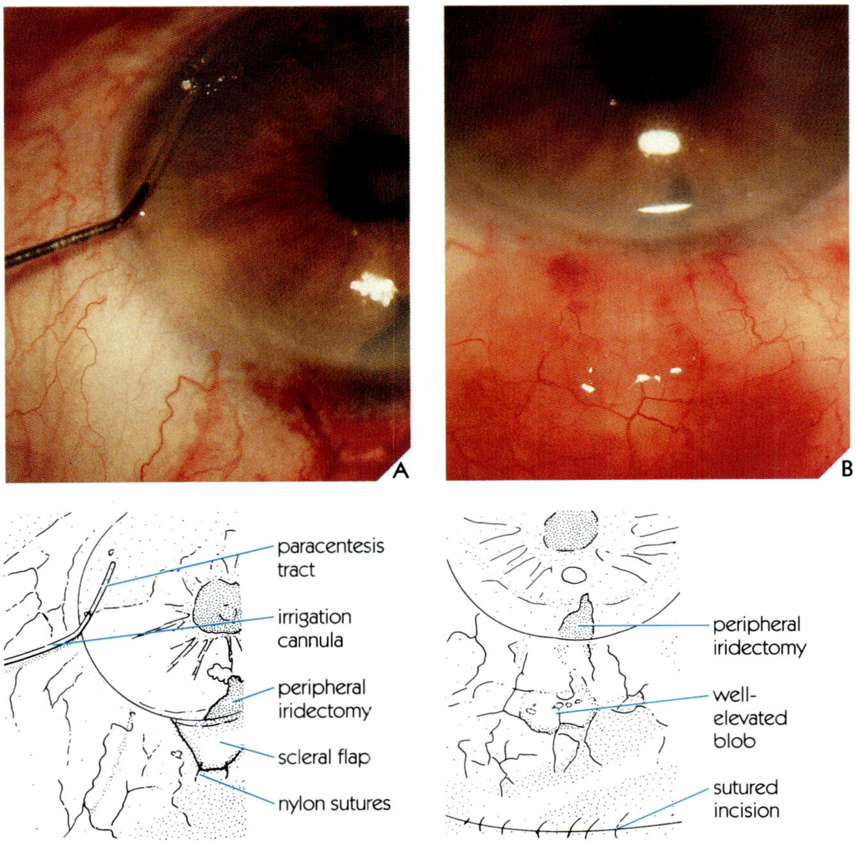

9.35 | *A:* Injection of balanced salt solution through the paracentesis tract causes elevation of the filtration bleb. *B:* No wound or bleb leak is seen.

(every 1–2 hours) topical steroids are used postoperatively. Lysis of the scleral flap sutures by the argon laser can be used to lower IOP during the first few weeks postoperatively (Fig. 9.36).

INJECTION OF 5-FLUOROURACIL

A careful eye examination is necessary before each 5-FU dose. Visual acuity is assessed. Slit-lamp examination of the cornea for punctate staining or epithelial defects is performed. Painting the bleb and incision line with fluorescein helps in the detection of aqueous leaks (Seidel testing) (Fig. 9.37). Intraocular pressure is measured and the fundus is examined.

The patient's head is stabilized against the exam chair headrest; this is facilitated by placing the chair in a reclining position (Fig. 9.38). After a drop of topical anesthetic (proparacaine) is placed in the eye, a cotton-tipped

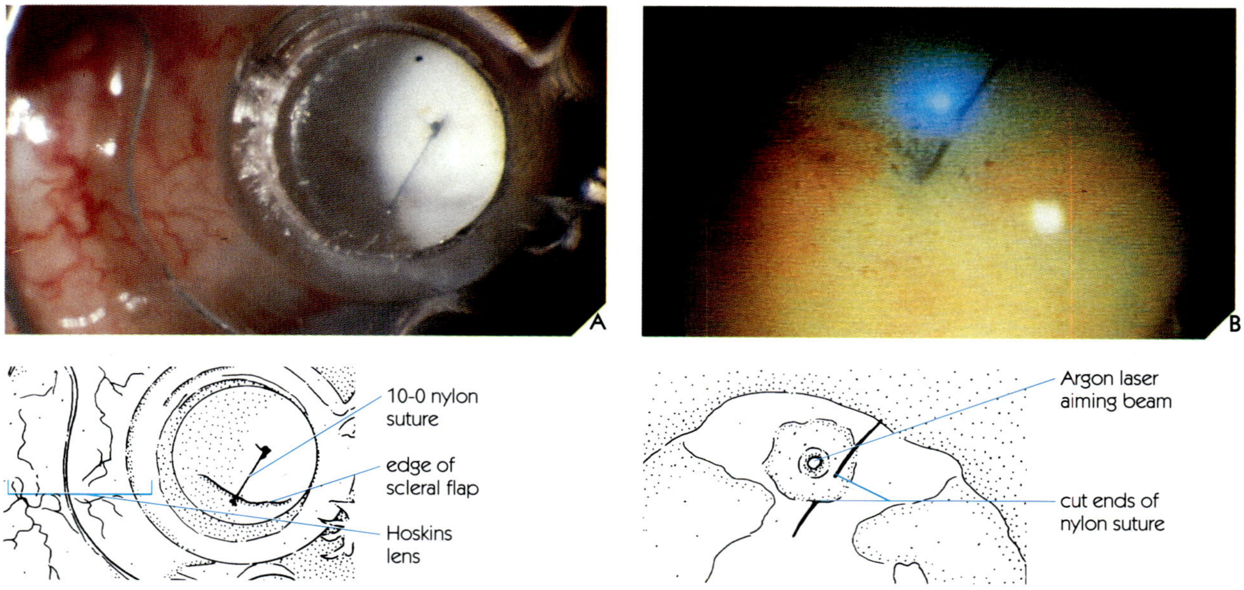

9.36 | *A:* Hoskins nylon suture laser lens used to compress the conjunctiva overlying the 10-0 nylon scleral flap suture. (Courtesy of Dr. A. Grajewski.) *B:* Once the scleral flap suture is well visualized it is cut with the Argon laser. (Courtesy of Dr. P. Palmberg.)

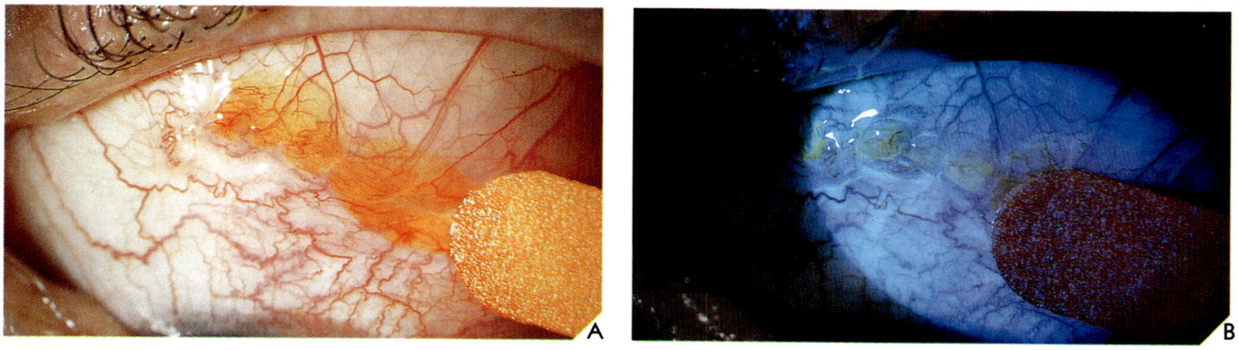

9.37 | *A:* A moistened fluorescein strip is used to paint the bleb and incision line. *B:* The cobalt blue light filter is used to check for leaking aqueous (Seidel testing).

applicator soaked in 4% lidocaine without epinephrine may be placed on the conjunctiva 90–180° from the trabeculectomy site for 1 minute or longer (Fig. 9.39). Five milligrams of 5-FU (0.5 ml of 10 mg/ml 5-FU diluted in unpreserved sterile saline or 0.1 ml of undiluted 50 mg/ml 5-FU) is drawn into a tuberculin syringe and a 30-gauge needle is placed on the syringe. Taking care to avoid the conjunctival blood vessels, the 5-FU is slowly injected subconjunctivally in the anesthetized area (Fig. 9.40).

At the discretion of the surgeon, 5-FU is withheld for incision or bleb leaks, large or expanding corneal epithelial defects, flat anterior chamber, or appositional ("kissing") choroidal effusions.

COMPLICATIONS

Many complications have been reported with subconjunctival 5-FU.[191–196] The most common side effect is epithelial toxicity. This can range from superficial punctate keratopathy to large epithelial defects of the cornea (Fig. 9.41) and

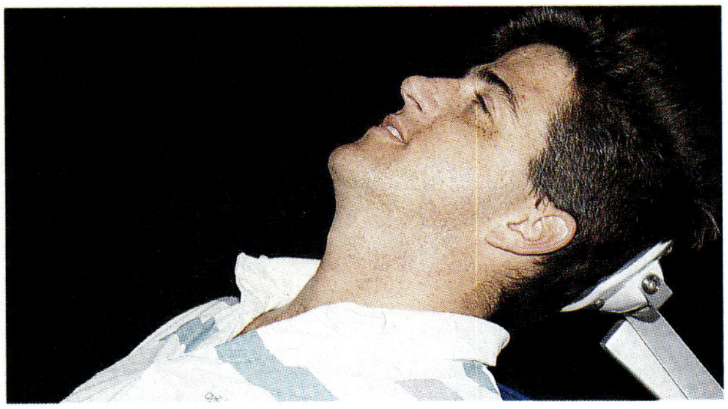

9.38 | Before injection of 5-FU, the patient's head is stabilized against the headrest and the chair is placed in a reclining position.

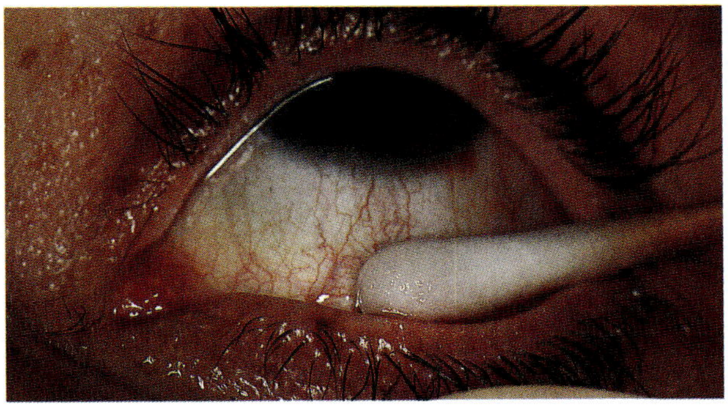

9.39 | A cotton-tipped applicator soaked in 4% lidocaine is placed on the conjunctiva 90–180° from the trabeculectomy site and held in place for 1 minute.

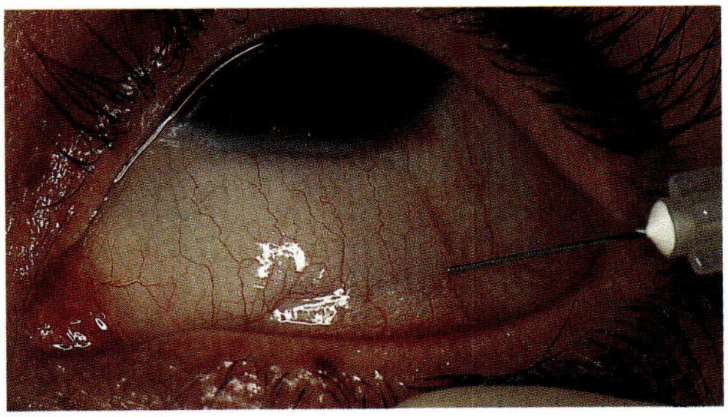

9.40 | 5-FU is injected slowly into the anesthetized area. Conjunctival blood vessels are avoided.

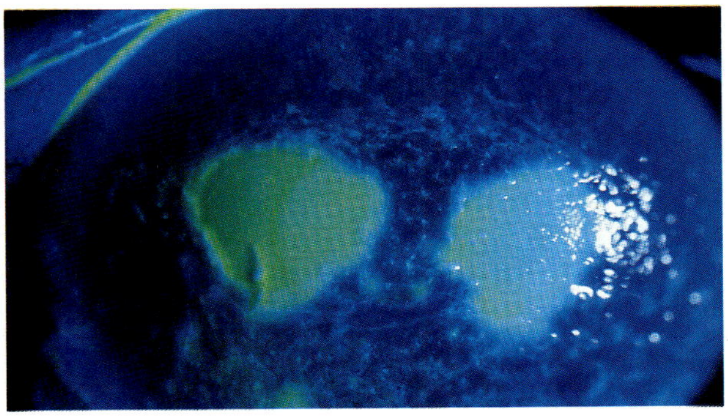

9.41 | Corneal epithelial defects with fluorescein.

conjunctiva (Fig. 9.42). Corneal filaments may develop (Fig. 9.43). Epithelial defects created by 5-FU, especially in the face of concomitant topical steroid use, may be slow to heal and (albeit rarely) can develop secondary infection (Fig. 9.44), scarring (Fig. 9.45), or perforation.[191,195] It should be used with

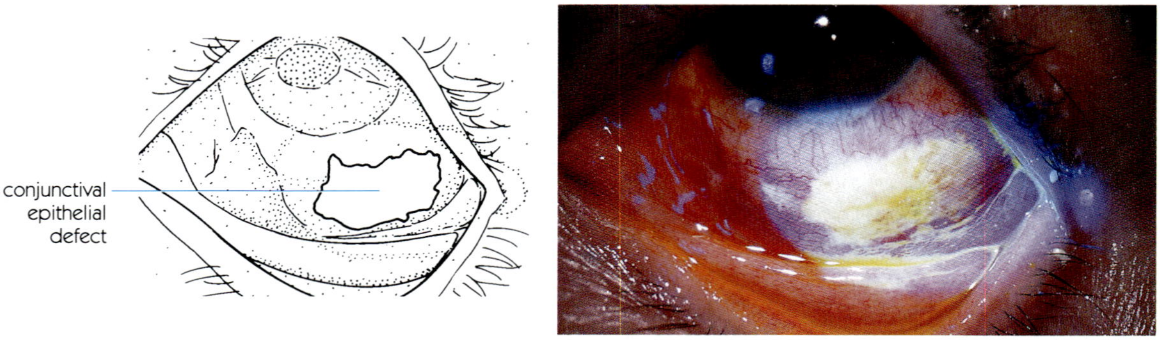

9.42 | Conjunctival epithelial defect at the site of 5-FU injection.

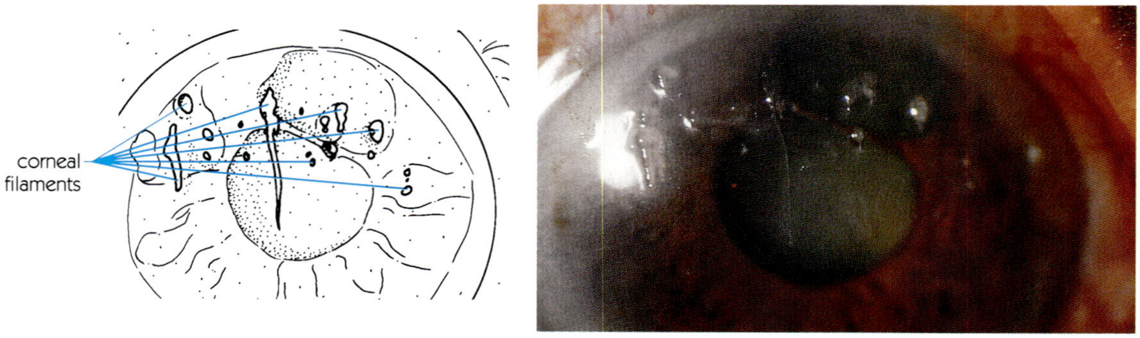

9.43 | Corneal filaments after 5-FU trabeculectomy.

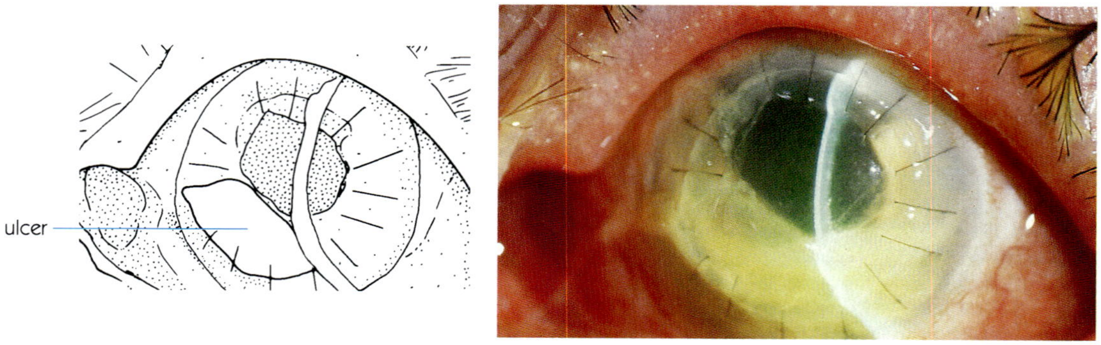

9.44 | Eye with a penetrating keratoplasty and a 5-FU trabeculectomy that developed a corneal ulcer. (Courtesy of Dr. A. Grajewski.)

extreme caution in eyes with preexisting corneal disease and in eyes with pemphigoid or pseudopemphigoid. Because it interferes with the normal healing process, 5-FU may cause conjunctival wound leaks both at the site of the surgical incision (Fig. 9.46) and along the needle tract at the injection site. The frequent subconjunctival injections required carry with them a risk of subconjunctival hemorrhage (Fig. 9.47). Excessive filtration can result in a

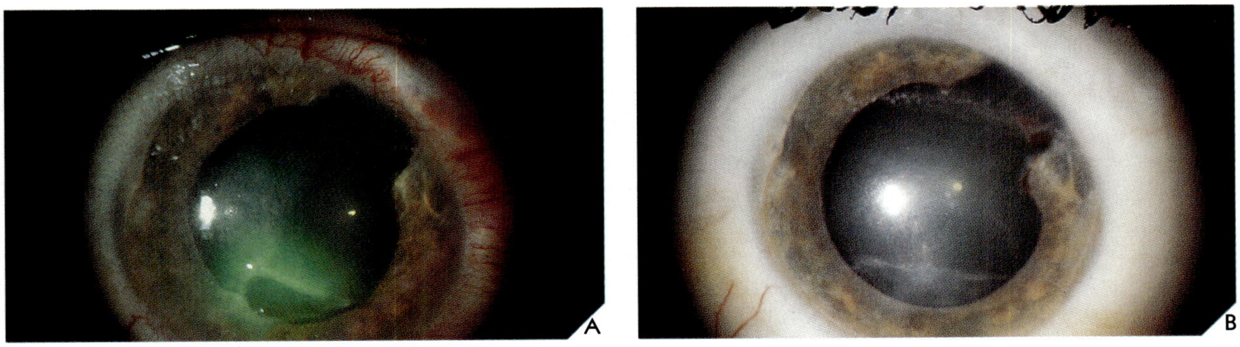

9.45 | Eye with a persistent epithelial defect after 5-FU *(A)* that resulted in corneal stromal scarring *(B)*.

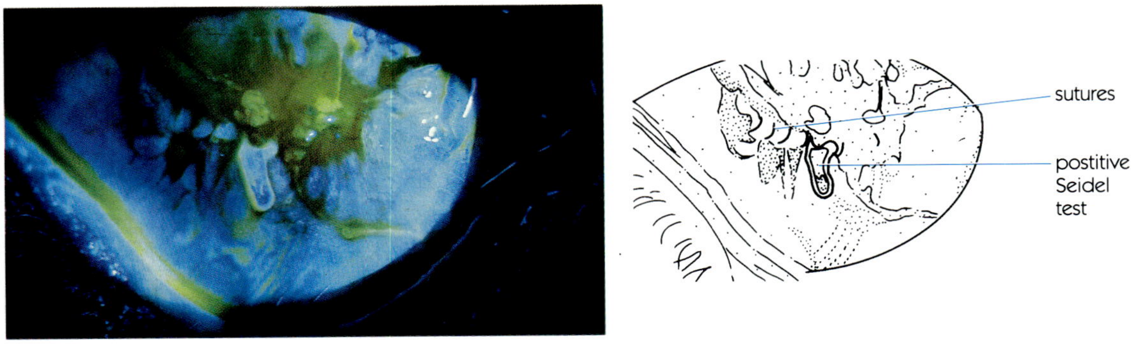

9.46 | Positive Seidel test at conjunctival incision site.

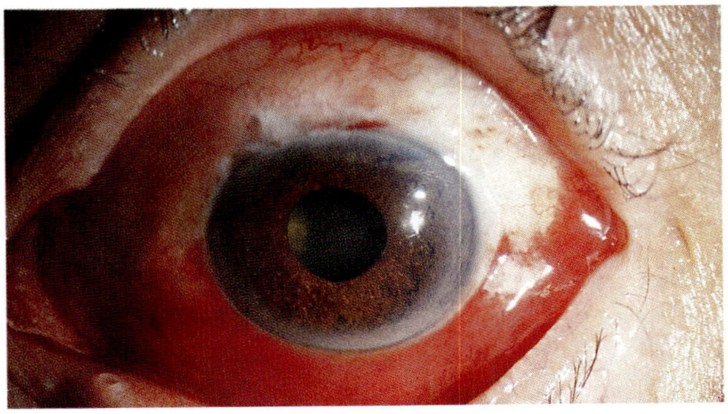

9.47 | Subconjunctival hemorrhage resulting from 5-FU injection.

shallow or flat anterior chamber and in choroidal effusion (Fig. 9.48). Longstanding hypotony with decreased vision has been reported after the use of 5-FU. The visual decline may persist after resolution of the hypotony.[197] The other complications shown in Figure 9.49 may occur in filtration surgery without the use of 5-FU,[177,178] and therefore may be due to the filtering procedure, rather than the 5-FU.

MITOMYCIN-C

Mitomycin-C is an antibiotic isolated from *Streptomyces caespitosus* which has been introduced as adjunctive therapy for trabeculectomy. Mitomycin acts in the late G_1 and early S-phase of the cell cycle to cross-link DNA and inhibit DNA synthesis (see Fig. 9.31). Like 5-FU, mitomycin is toxic to replicating cells and interferes with fibroblast proliferation.

Mitomycin has not been studied as extensively as 5-FU; however, one randomized prospective trial indicates that the two agents produce similar results in the first 6 months after surgery.[199] In addition, because mitomycin has less apparent corneal toxicity and does not require daily injections, it may be possible to use mitomycin when preexisting corneal disease or lack of patient cooperation precludes the use of 5-FU. Because mitomycin is applied only intraoperatively, it is more convenient for the patient and the physician.

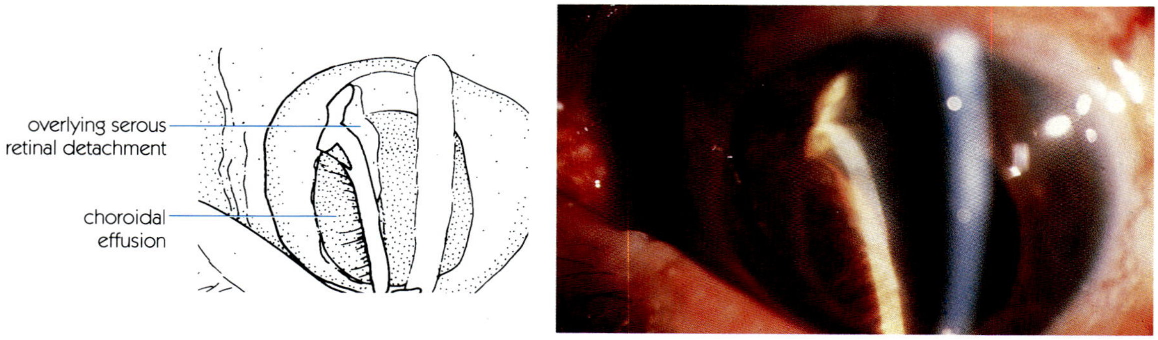

9.48 | Large choroidal effusion visible through the pupil. Shallow serous detachment of the retina overlies the choroidal effusion.

Figure 9.49. Complications of 5-FU in Filtering Surgery

Epithelial toxicity	Needle track leaks	Progression of cataract
Superficial punctate keratopathy	Subconjunctival hemorrhage	Choroidal detachment
Epithelial defects of the cornea and conjunctiva	Dellen formation	Suprachoroidal hemorrhage
Corneal ulcer	Aphakic bullous keratopathy	Late bleb leak or rupture
Corneal scarring	Hyphema	Vitreous hemorrhage
Corneal perforation	Shallow anterior chamber	Retinal detachment
Wound leaks at surgical incision	Flat anterior chamber	Endophthalmitis
	Ciliary block glaucoma	Phthisis

APPLICATION OF MITOMYCIN-C

After dissecting a limbus-based conjunctival flap and outlining the scleral flap, a 0.2–0.5 mg/ml solution of mitomycin-C on a cellulose sponge or gelfoam is placed over the scleral flap. The conjunctiva is pulled over the sponge (Fig. 9.50). After 2–5 minutes the sponge is removed and the eye is copiously irrigated with saline. Some authors describe dissecting the scleral flap before applying the mitomycin.[200,201] If the eye is entered inadvertently during the dissection, the mitomycin cannot be applied, for even a small amount in the anterior chamber is severely toxic to the endothelium. After irrigation of the eye, the trabeculectomy is completed as usual, with careful attention paid to wound closure as described for 5-FU. Complications with the ocular application of mitomycin are shown in Figure 9.51. Some of the complications listed were reported only with the topical application of mitomycin for the postoperative treatment of pterygium and have not been reported in the use of intraoperative mitomycin with trabeculectomy.[202] Hypotony and wound leaks are the most frequently reported complications of filtration surgery with intraoperative mitomycin.

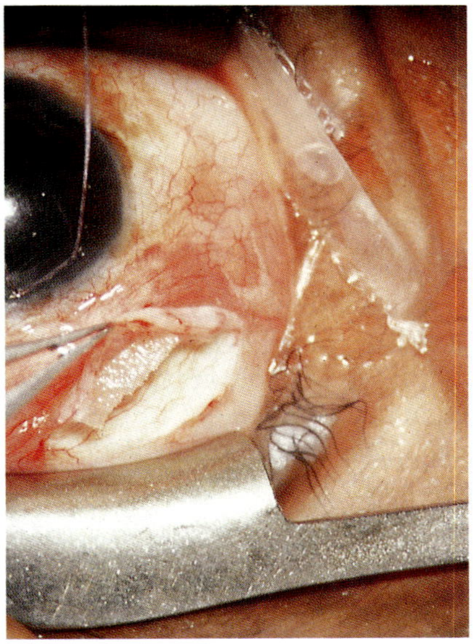

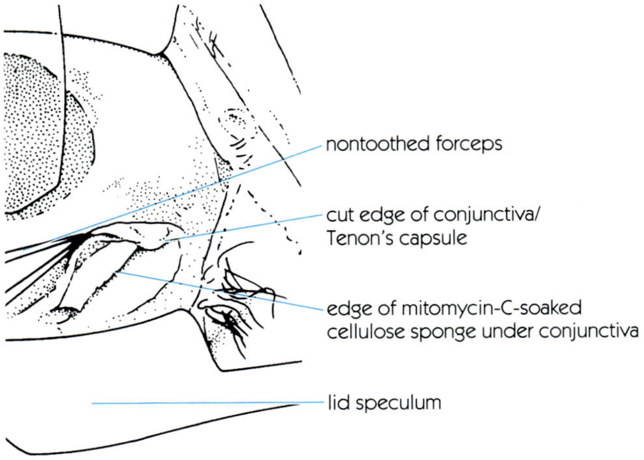

9.50 | Mitomycin-C-soaked cellulose sponge is placed between the sclera and the limbus-based conjunctival flap. Immediately following the application of mitomycin the eye is copiously irrigated with saline. (Courtesy of Dr. G. Skuta.)

Figure 9.51. Complications of Mitomycin-C in Ocular Use

- Wound leak
- Hypotony
- Corneal ulceration
- Scleral ulceration
- Scleromalacia
- Scleral calcification
- Symblepharon

SECTION VII

DRAINAGE IMPLANTS

Theodore Krupin
Lisa F. Rosenberg
Jon M. Ruderman

HISTORICAL REVIEW

The early 1900s introduced the classic glaucoma filtration procedures of sclerectomy,[203] iridencleisis,[204] and corneoscleral trephination.[205] Shortly thereafter it became apparent that these procedures did not always result in prolonged intraocular pressure (IOP) control. Surgical failures led to trials with the implantation of various types of foreign materials to facilitate drainage of aqueous humor. These early devices, which may be categorized as paracentesis drains, cyclodialysis implants, or sclerostomy implants, were usually reported only once and were characterized by limited experience and follow-up. In general, the long-term results were poor and the complications great, as a result of either excessive postoperative inflammation or foreign body reaction leading to bleb scarring.

PARACENTESIS DEVICES

Rollett and Moreau in 1906 described placing a horse hair across the anterior chamber through paracentesis incisions to treat two patients with painful absolute glaucoma.[206] Zorab described a procedure he called "aqueoplasty," in which he placed a double silk loop covered with a conjunctival flap through a superior keratome incision 2 mm behind the limbus.[207] Mayou[208] and Wood[209] modified this procedure and reported good results in patients with absolute glaucoma. A channelled silicone strip passed from the anterior chamber to the conjunctival sac was described in 1965 for therapy of neovascular glaucoma.[210] Vail reported in 1915 placing a silk thread in a tract from the vitreous cavity into the subconjunctival space.[211] The suture was removed at 3 months and the glaucoma did not return for the 2 years prior to the patient's death. However, long-term results with this group of devices was overall very poor due to infection, foreign body reaction, and inflammation.

CYCLODIALYSIS IMPLANTS

A multiplicity of materials have been placed within a cyclodialysis to maintain patency of the cleft. In 1934 Row reported placing a platinum wire and a horse hair within the cleft.[212] Troncosco originally used a magnesium strip[213] and later tantalum foil[214] as a cyclodialysis implant. A number of ophthalmologists subsequently used inert plastics (supramid, gelatin film, teflon) as implants.[210,212,215–217] While these later materials were well tolerated by the eye, long-term intraocular pressure lowering was poor, probably due to the overall poor results with cyclodialysis as a glaucoma surgical procedure.

SCLEROSTOMY SETONS

A silk thread was the first device to be placed translimbally from the anterior chamber to the subconjunctival space.[207] This was followed by the use of a variety of materials placed translimbally in attempts to prevent closure of the sclerostomy and to act as a "wick" promoting aqueous humor flow through the anterior chamber opening. These materials have included various plastic plates and rods, gold, tantalum, glass, and platinum.[217–221] Most of these devices were associated with postoperative inflammation and uniformly poor results.

ANTERIOR CHAMBER SHUNTS TO A DISTANT SITE

Tube shunts have been used to direct aqueous humor from the anterior chamber to a distant site. Mascati connected a plastic anterior chamber tube to the lacrimal sac,[222] and Rajah-Sivayoham connected a silicone anterior chamber tube to a superficial temporal vein.[223] An anterior chamber-venous shunt using a collagen tube inserted into the intrascleral portion of a vortex vein was described by Lee and Wong in 1974.[224] Initial results with these shunts were good; however, there have been no long-term follow-up studies, and to our knowledge they are no longer in use. Obvious difficulties with these devices include erosion of the extraocular portion of the tube and reflux of contents into the anterior chamber.

TRANSLIMBAL TUBE SHUNTS

Open plastic tubes have been inserted at the limbus into the anterior chamber. Before the introduction of subscleral filtration procedures, the external end of the tube is fixated to the sclera and covered with conjunctiva.[210,217,221] The open end of the anterior chamber tube, and not the entry incision, becomes the effective "sclerostomy." When the external end of the tube is covered with conjunctiva, scarring usually occurs. However, placement of the external portion under a partial-thickness scleral flap reduces external scarring. Two such translimbal tube shunts include the open tube reported by Honrubia et al[225] and the pressure-sensitive glaucoma valve implant described by Krupin et al.[226–228]

The device described by Honrubia et al requires the insertion of a silicone tube into the anterior chamber. The external end of the tube is placed under a scleral flap to allow aqueous egress into the subconjunctival space. Complications associated with an open anterior chamber tube (e.g., excessive aqueous humor flow, flat chamber, choroidal detachment) occur with this procedure. An implant containing a pressure-sensitive and unidirectional valve was described by Krupin et al in 1976. This device consists of an open Supramid tube which is placed into the anterior chamber. The valve-end of the implant remains outside the eye under a scleral lamellar flap. Translimbal implants result in an anterior limbal bleb. Both procedures do not address the major cause for filtration failure, external scarring of the bleb. Postoperative bleb scarring and reduced filtration success, as well as surgical limitations in eyes with excessive perilimbal scarring, have limited the use of these implants. The currently used posterior tube shunt implants address the problem of external bleb scarring by incorporating this process into the procedure with the creation of a large encapsulated area for filtration of aqueous humor posterior to the limbus.

POSTERIOR TUBE SHUNTS

Early studies by Molteno were directed towards designing an implant that would promote formation of a functioning bleb.[229] This was in contrast to prior work in the field which had focused on using devices to maintain a patent communication between the anterior chamber and the subconjunctival space. Molteno's implant consisted of a circular (8 mm diameter) episcleral plate sutured to the sclera a few millimeters posterior to the limbus. In addition, Molteno used pharmacological drugs to modulate bleb inflammation and fibrosis. Postoperatively he administered topical and systemic corticosteroids, a systemic prostaglandin synthetase inhibitor (fluphenamic acid), and a systemic antimitotic agent (colchicine).[230] The large area of limbal encapsulation caused a number of problems, including discomfort and formation of corneal dellen. Therefore, the location of the external explant was moved posteriorly to the equator, allowing a larger episcleral disc and resulting in a large posterior bleb. This pioneering work led to the currently used posterior tube shunt implant procedures.

Molteno's concept has been incorporated into three other devices as described by Schocket et al,[231] Krupin et al,[232] and Joseph et al.[233] All of these implants consist of an open tube which is placed into the anterior chamber to shunt aqueous humor posteriorly into an area of encapsulation around an

Figure 9.52. Posterior Tube Seton Implants

IMPLANT	ANTERIOR CHAMBER TUBE	SCLERAL EXPLANT
Molteno	Silicone (OD 0.63, ID 0.3 mm), unrestricted tube	Polypropylene rigid plate, 13-mm diameter, single or double plates
Joseph	Silicone (OD 0.64, ID 0.3 mm), slit valve on side of tube with opening pressure between 4–20 mm Hg	Silicone strap, 9-mm wide, 1-mm thick, 180–360° in length
Schocket	Silastic (OD 0.64, ID 0.3 mm), unrestricted tube	Silicone No. 20 band, 360° in length
Krupin	Silastic (OD 0.58, ID 0.38 mm), slit valve on posterior end of the tube: opening pressure 11 mm Hg, closing pressure 9 mm Hg	Silicone No. 220 band, 180–360° in length Silicone oval disc, 13 x 18 mm, 1.75-mm high

episcleral explant. Differences exist regarding the presence or absence of a flow-limiting valve and the type of episcleral explant (Fig. 9.52). General concepts common to all four devices will be presented, with the specifics of each device discussed separately.

PRINCIPLES OF POSTERIOR TUBE SHUNT IMPLANTS

ANTERIOR CHAMBER TUBE AND POSTERIOR EXPLANT ENCAPSULATION

The open anterior chamber tube functions as the effective sclerostomy, can be inserted beyond areas of peripheral anterior synechiae, and prevents sclerostomy closure. The tube functions as a conduit for aqueous humor flow from the anterior chamber to the attached episcleral explant.

The posterior episcleral explant stimulates a fibrous encapsulation[234,235] which functions as a filtration bleb, avoiding the limbal bleb formation associated with conventional filtration surgery. This has an advantage in eyes with prior limbal surgery and conjunctival scarring.

The internal surface of the encapsulation is an open, collagenous meshwork which is not lined by continuous layers of cells. The capsular wall becomes progressively more dense externally and is covered by an external fibrovascular layer. The capsule appears to develop as a separate layer from Tenon's capsule.[235]

POSTERIOR FILTRATION BLEB

Minckler et al, using the nonrestrictive Molteno implant in animal eyes, have shown that pressure within the bleb is similar to that within the anterior chamber.[235] Perfusion studies have demonstrated linear pressure–flow relationships in the range of 10–50 mm Hg, indicating that the main resistance to flow is the capsular wall. Latex microspheres as large as 0.2 μm in diameter pass freely through the capsular wall,[235] and horseradish peroxidase (molecular weight 50,000) moves between the collagenous bundles and reaches the capillaries in the vascular layer. Horseradish peroxidase moves similarly across the encapsulated space surrounding the encircling silicone explant used in the Schocket procedure.[236]

Reduction of intraocular pressure involves passive pressure-dependent flow of fluid across the resistance of the capsular wall. The thinner the capsule and the larger the total surface area of encapsulation, the lower the pressure.

INDICATIONS

Posterior tube shunt implants are indicated in patients with an elevated IOP despite maximal tolerated medical therapy and prior failure with filtration surgery. These implants are used in primary open-angle, closed-angle, and congenital glaucomas, and a variety of secondary glaucomas including aphakic, pseudophakic, and neovascular glaucoma. Primary implantation of a shunt device is advised in eyes with neovascular glaucoma or closed-angle glaucoma with anteriorly located synechiae that prevent a limbal sclerostomy from communicating with the anterior chamber. In most other eyes, filtration surgery with postoperative use of 5-fluorouracil or intraoperative mitomycin-C (see Wright and Parrish, this chapter) should be attempted before a posterior tube shunt implant.[237]

POSTERIOR TUBE SHUNT PROCEDURES

MOLTENO IMPLANT

The Molteno implant is presently the most frequently used. It consists of a circular, 13-mm diameter, convex, rigid polypropylene episcleral plate with a smooth, elevated rim and a scleral surface area of 133 mm^2 (Fig. 9.53). Holes within the plate aid in suturing the device to the sclera. A valveless silicone tube (outside diameter 0.63 mm, inside diameter 0.3 mm) passes through the rim and opens onto the convex outer surface of the plate. The open end of the tube is placed in the anterior chamber through a paracentesis wound.

Several variations of the Molteno implant are available. A double-plate system with twice the surface area has two polypropylene plates connected to each other by a 10-mm long silicone tube (see Fig. 9.53). Both right- and left-eyed versions of the double-plate Molteno system are available. An 8-mm diameter plate is available for small eyes.

Surgical Implantation

Molteno originally inserted the implant as a one-stage procedure: the episcleral plate was fixated to the globe and the tube was inserted into the anterior chamber. Because of a high incidence of choroidal detachment and flat anterior chamber, he converted to a two-staged implantation: fixation of the plate, followed by tube insertion into the anterior chamber at a second, later, operation. Encapsulation of the episcleral plate occurs between the two surgical stages. Current application of the Molteno implant utilizes either of these approaches (see below).

Single-Plate Implantation

As with all of the posterior tube implant procedures, a surgical assistant is highly recommended. The type of conjunctival incision depends on the surgeon's preference and on the degree of conjunctival scarring present. A scarred limbal conjunctiva presents a more difficult dissection and less conjunctival elasticity. For these cases, a fornix-based conjunctival flap with the peritomy extending slightly greater than one quadrant in length is preferable. A relaxing incision on either side of the flap improves scleral exposure. When there is minimal conjunctival scarring, a limbus-based flap can be performed with the incision approximately 6–8 mm posterior to the limbus. A limbus-based conjunctival flap permits a smaller conjunctival incision with improved posterior scleral exposure between adjacent rectus muscles.

Adequate scleral exposure must be obtained so that the anterior edge of the episcleral plate is at least 8 mm (and preferably 10 mm) posterior to the limbus. Traction sutures under the rectus muscles improve exposure. The

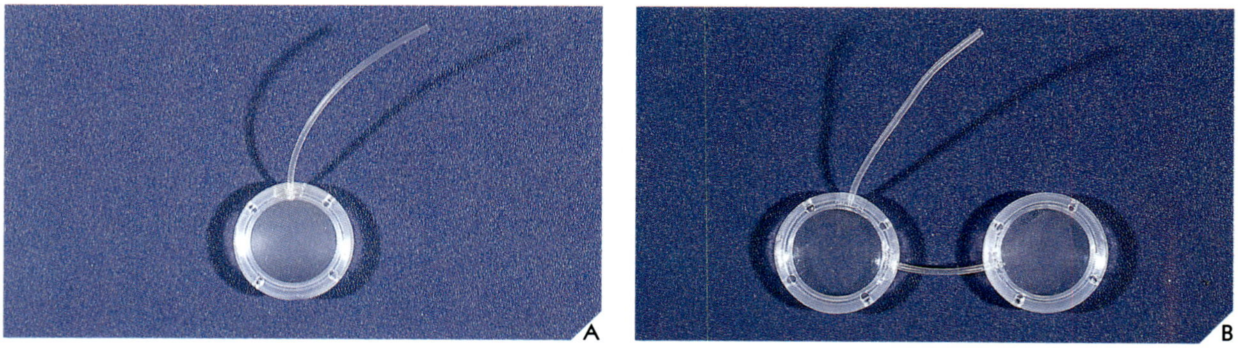

9.53 | The single-plate *(A)* and the double-plate *(B)* Molteno implants. The silicone rubber anterior chamber tube is attached to, and opens onto, the upper surface of a 13-mm diameter rigid episcleral plate.

plate is positioned between any two rectus muscles with the tube extending in a radial direction towards the limbus. Nonabsorbable sutures are passed through the fixation holes on the episcleral plate and sutured to the episclera (Fig. 9.54). These sutures prevent plate (and therefore tube) migration. In order to facilitate suture placement, the position of the plate and fixation holes are marked with a surgical pen. The plate is then removed, the sutures are placed through the fixation holes, and passed through the episclera at the appropriately marked places. The plate is inserted onto the surface of the eye and the sutures are tied. The silicone tube is trimmed, bevel up, to extend 2–3 mm into the anterior chamber, the length estimated by laying the tube across the cornea.

A separate corneal paracentesis tract is made before the limbal entry incision, and a viscoelastic agent is injected into the anterior chamber. Two types of limbal entry incision are possible: full thickness or, preferably, within the bed of a 4 x 4-mm half-thickness lamellar scleral flap. The flap is dissected into clear cornea, improving visualization of the limbal anatomy and allowing more accurate tube placement into the anterior chamber. A full-thickness entry tract is indicated if the sclera is extremely thin, making dissection of a flap difficult. The entry tract for the anterior chamber tube is made with a 22- or 23-gauge hypodermic needle, creating a tight entry wound, preventing leakage around the tube, and immobilizing it. The tract is made either under the scleral flap in clear cornea or at the limbus through the full thickness of the tissue. Care must be taken to ensure that the latter incision is limbal and not corneal. A through-and-through corneal incision may predispose to epithelial ingrowth (see below). With either approach, a 2–3-mm long entry tract is made at an oblique angle, parallel to the plane of the iris. Proper position of the tube after insertion is in the middle of the anterior chamber without contacting the iris, lens, or cornea.

Episcleral sutures (10-0 nylon) are placed near the limbus and tied around the tube to reduce side-to-side tube movement. If a scleral lamellar

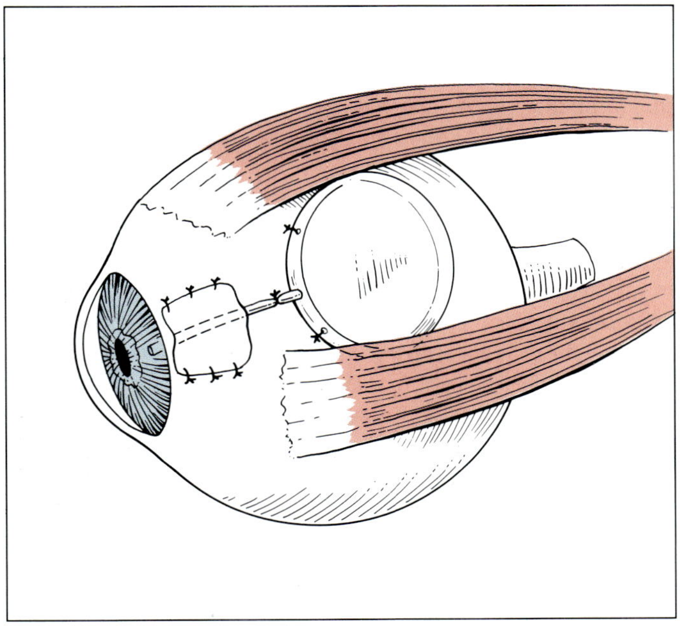

9.54 | Illustration of an installed single plate Molteno implant. Two interrupted sutures anchor the scleral explant to the episclera. A scleral graft is sutured over the anterior portion of the tube. A temporary ligature is tied around the tube at the posterior edge of the graft. (Adapted from Krupin T: Setons in glaucoma surgery, in Waltman SR, Keates RH, Hoyt CS, et al (eds): *Surgery of the Eye.* New York: Churchill Livingstone, 1988, 382.)

flap was used, it is reapproximated over the tube with the corners recessed slightly inward to prevent tension. A donor scleral patch graft (at least 4 x 4 mm) is used to cover the flap and the limbal portion of the tube. These maneuvers reduce the possibility of postoperative erosion of the tube.

The presence of vitreous in the anterior chamber may result in internal blockage of the tube. Therefore, an automated vitrectomy is performed using a separate entry site. An alternative approach in an eye with a shallow anterior chamber and a cataract is to perform both an anterior and posterior vitrectomy with a lensectomy. This allows tube placement posterior to the iris through the pars plana.

The conjunctiva is closed either by reapproximation to the limbus (fornix-based flap) or by a continuous suture (limbus-based flap) with an absorbable suture (e.g., 8-0 Vicryl®). Balanced salt solution is irrigated through the corneal paracentesis site until the chamber has re-formed to normal depth. Sodium fluorescein is used to detect wound leaks. Topical atropine drops and subconjunctival injection of antibiotics and corticosteroids are administered at the end of the procedure, and topical atropine and corticosteroids are administered several times a day. Postoperatively, therapy is slowly reduced as anterior chamber inflammation subsides.

Double-Plate Implantation

Insertion of the Molteno double plate requires additional surgery and modifications. A 180° conjunctival flap is required to expose two scleral quadrants between three rectus muscles. The tube connecting the two episcleral plates can be placed under or over a rectus muscle.

Two-Stage Insertion

During the first stage, the explant(s) is attached to the episclera while the open end of the anterior chamber tube is placed under the episcleral plate or beneath an adjacent rectus muscle and sutured to the episclera. Because this operation does not reduce IOP, a trabeculectomy is frequently performed for interim IOP control at a different site from where the tube will later be inserted into the anterior chamber. Tenon's capsule and conjunctiva are sutured closed. Medical antiglaucoma therapy is administered as required to lower IOP. The second operative stage, insertion of the tube into the anterior chamber, is performed 2 to 6 weeks later. The two-stage procedure is recommended in patients at high risk for suprachoroidal hemorrhage or flat anterior chamber, such as aphakic or pseudophakic glaucoma (especially if there has been prior vitreous loss), high myopia, congenital glaucoma, shallow anterior chambers, and closed-angle glaucoma.

Flow of aqueous humor through the tube creates a posterior filtration bleb by dissecting the fibrous encapsulation off the surface of the episcleral plate. During this interval, IOP is frequently elevated to preoperative (or even higher) levels and marked inflammation is observed in the region of the posterior bleb. Antiglaucoma medications and topical corticosteroids are administered during this transient hypertensive phase, which may last several weeks.[234,239] Gradually IOP declines and the bleb inflammation resolves, permitting withdrawal of antiglaucoma medications. The magnitude of the hypertensive phase is reduced with the double-plate Molteno system.[240]

One-Stage Insertion

The one-stage operation consists of attaching the episcleral plate(s) and inserting the anterior chamber tube during the same procedure. Advantages of this method compared with the two-stage insertion include avoidance of a second operation, more rapid IOP control by eliminating the period of uncontrolled glaucoma during the interval of the two-stage technique, and reduction of the hypertensive phase observed after completion of the two-stage insertion. However, the one-stage technique is associated with hypotony-related complications.

Techniques to Prevent Postoperative Hypotony

Various methods have been used during a one-stage insertion to prevent or decrease the incidence of postoperative hypotony. These techniques temporarily occlude the flow of aqueous humor through the anterior chamber tube until the episcleral plate becomes encapsulated.

1. **Buried tube ligature.** The tube is occluded with a suture ligature placed around the tube posterior to the scleral flap or donor graft. A 7-0 or 8-0 Vicryl suture will usually dissolve in 2–4 weeks. Argon laser or direct incisional lysis is performed if earlier release is needed or if the suture incompletely dissolves.
2. **Exposed tube ligature.** A releasable nylon suture is tied around the tube and exposed externally.[241] Care must be taken when this suture is removed not to dislodge the tube. Potential complications include infection.
3. **Anterior chamber tube ligature.** Before inserting the distal end of the tube into the anterior chamber, a polypropylene suture is tied to the wall of the tube and then around it as a ligature.[242] If IOP is elevated, the argon laser is used to cut the suture, opening the tube but still leaving the suture attached to its wall.
4. **Exposed tube occlusion.** The internal lumen of the tube is occluded with a 4-0 chromic suture which exits the conjunctiva, and is, therefore, exposed, over the episcleral plate. The tube occlusion is removed at a later date by pulling the externalized suture.[243] This "rip-cord" technique may promote inflammation or serve as a conduit to infection.[244]

If a double-plate Molteno device is used for a one-stage procedure, the tube between the two plates can be tied with a black silk suture at the time of insertion, in addition to one of the above techniques, to restrict flow through the anterior chamber tube. Flow is initially established by removing the anterior chamber tube occlusion. The silk suture between the plates is removed later if IOP is not sufficiently lowered by the first plate.

Surgical Considerations in the Pediatric Patient

Ultrasonography is performed in pediatric patients to determine the size of the eye. The pediatric-size Molteno implant is used if the globe is small. Alternatively, the adult implant can be reduced in size by removing the posterior one-third of the plate with cautery. The anterior chamber tube is cut longer than usual to compensate for future growth of the eye. If bilateral surgery is required, both eyes may be operated on during the same anesthesia, changing instruments, gowns, and gloves between eyes. We recommend performing a two-stage procedure on one eye and a one-stage implantation with a suture ligature around the anterior chamber tube on the fellow eye. Three to four weeks later, the tube is inserted into the anterior chamber to complete the two-stage operation and the suture ligature is cut in the eye undergoing the one-stage implant.

Surgical Considerations in Eyes with Prior Corneal Transplant

Molteno implantation in eyes with a prior penetrating corneal keratoplasty shows IOP control in about 71% of patients, although there is a high incidence of graft failure (30%) after tube implantation.[245] Placement of the anterior chamber tube may be more difficult in keratoplasty patients, because peripheral corneal opacification makes it difficult to judge the position of the tube within the anterior chamber. In addition, the iridocorneal angle in these eyes is frequently closed by peripheral synechiae or fibrous ingrowth.

Results

A review from various reports using either the single- or double-plate Molteno implant indicates a success rate between 60–80% if an IOP less than 21 mm Hg is taken as the measure of success.[234,239,240,296] Less than 33% of successful cases have controlled IOP without the additional use of antiglaucoma medications. IOPs after a successful Molteno implant tend to be higher than after a successful trabeculectomy or full-thickness procedure, either with or without the postoperative use of subconjunctival 5-FU injections.

The success rate for IOP control is dependent on the type of glaucoma. The highest success rates occur in eyes with open- or closed-angle glaucoma, either phakic or aphakic/pseudophakic, and in eyes with prior failure after limbal filtration surgery. Success rates are lower (40–50%) in eyes with neovascular and other types of secondary glaucoma (e.g., uveitic glaucoma) and in the pediatric patient.

A recent prospective study comparing the single- and double-plate Molteno implant demonstrated higher success and lower IOP with the double-plate implant.[240] In addition, the double-plate implant tends to reduce the hypertensive phase observed after the two-stage single-plate implantation technique. These results confirm the belief that the postoperative level of IOP with all of the posterior shunt filtration procedures relates partially to the surface area of the encapsulated bleb.

Late postoperative visual acuity is similar to preoperative vision in approximately two thirds of patients undergoing implantation of the Molteno device. Reduced vision is most likely from corneal opacification, cataract formation, or macular edema.

KRUPIN–DENVER LONG VALVE IMPLANT

The original external end of the short glaucoma valve implant was placed under a lamellar scleral flap at the limbus.[226] This portion contained the unidirectional and pressure-sensitive slit valve with an opening pressure between 10–12 mm Hg and a closing pressure between 8–10 mm Hg. The major cause for failure was external scarring at the limbus.

The long glaucoma valve implant (Fig. 9.55) consists of a Silastic anterior chamber tube with an outside diameter of 0.58 mm and an inside diameter of 0.38 mm. The tube is approximately 20 mm long. The distal end of the tube is sealed and contains the slit valve. Two different types of external scleral explants have been used with the long glaucoma valve implant.

1. **No. 220 Silastic band.** The external valve end of the tube is placed through the side wall of the band with the valve end fixated within the groove.
2. **Silastic disc.** A large oval disc, 13 mm x 18 mm, with a 1.75-mm high side wall has been fabricated to received the external valve end of the tube.

Surgical Implantation

A conjunctival peritomy is performed, the size dependent on the type of scleral explant to be used: either 180° or 360° for a similar-sized No. 220 band, or 90° to 110° for the disc. The band explant can be placed either superiorly or inferiorly, and the disc explant in any quadrant between two rectus muscles. The conjunctival flap is dissected posteriorly. Three rectus muscles are isolated for the 180° explant, four rectus muscles for the 360° explant, and two muscles for the disc. A limbus-based conjunctival flap can be used for the single-quadrant disc implant.

The No. 220 band explant is placed with the grooved side against the sclera: the 180° band beneath one rectus muscle with the band cut so that each end extends just up to the adjacent muscles, and the 360° band beneath all four muscles (see Fig. 9.55). The band is sutured to the sclera in each quadrant so that the anterior edge of the band is 8–10 mm from the limbus and the tube extends forward from the explant to one side of a rectus muscle.

The disc is placed horizontally between two rectus muscles with the flat surface against the sclera, and trimmed if it is too large. The anterior edge of the disc is placed 8–10 mm posterior to the limbus and sutured to the sclera, with the tube extending forward. Scleral flap and limbal dissection, tube insertion and fixation, scleral patch graft, conjunctival closure, and postoperative cycloplegic/antiinflammatory therapy are as described for the Molteno implant.

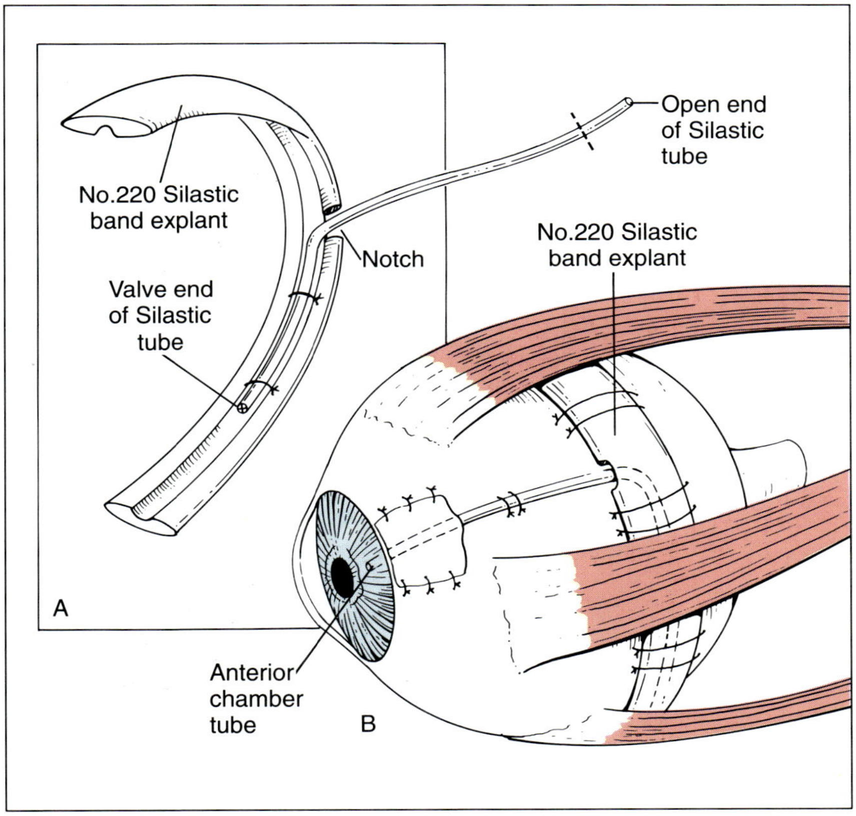

9.55 I Schematic of the 360° Krupin-Denver long glaucoma valve implant. *A:* The open end of the Silastic tube is trimmed (diagonal dashed line) for insertion into the anterior chamber. A notch is removed from the side wall of a No. 220 Silastic band explant and the valve end is sutured within the groove of the explant. *B:* The anterior chamber tube is placed into the anterior chamber under a scleral flap. Episcleral fixation sutures are tied around the tube. The No. 220 Silastic explant is placed beneath the rectus muscles. (Adapted from Krupin T: Setons in glaucoma surgery, in Waltman SR, Keates RH, Hoyt CS, et al (eds): *Surgery of the Eye.* New York: Churchill Livingstone, 1988, 384.)

The long glaucoma valve implant to an everted Silastic band results in a posterior bleb over the area of the scleral explant (Fig. 9.56). IOP less than 21 mm Hg occurs in 77% of eyes with neovascular glaucoma and in 82% of eyes with failure after prior filtration surgery. Antiglaucoma medications are required to achieve this level of IOP control in approximately 50% of eyes.[228] Experience with the long glaucoma valve disc implant is limited, but preliminary results are very encouraging. A large posterior bleb is present, and IOP is lower than with the band, with most eyes not requiring antiglaucoma medications.

SCHOCKET BAND IMPLANT

The Schocket anterior chamber tube to encircling band (ACTSEB) implant consists of a Silastic tube (30-mm long tube, 0.3-mm inner diameter, 0.64-mm outer diameter) sutured into the grooved portion of a 360° No. 20 or No. 220 silicone band[231,247] (Fig. 9.57). Smaller diameter Silastic tubing may help reduce the occurrence of hypotony and conjunctival erosion.[248] These materials are available in most ophthalmic operating rooms. The surgical technique is essentially the same as for the long Krupin valve, and manipulations to avoid postoperative hypotony are the same as for the Molteno implant.

Schocket et al report IOP control with or without antiglaucoma medications in 96% of eyes with neovascular glaucoma 2 years after surgery.[231,247] Other investigators have had similar success with this procedure.[248]

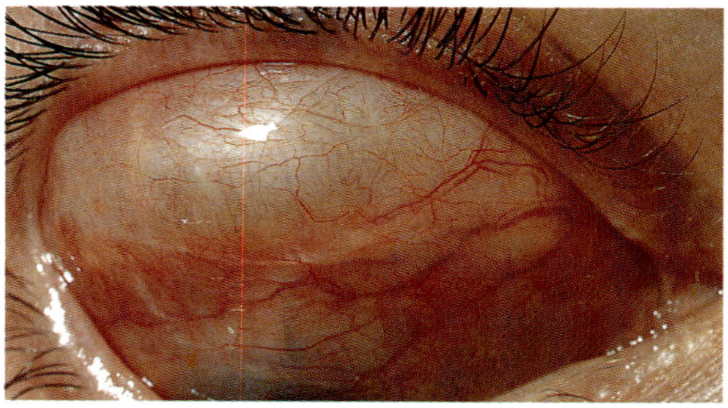

9.56 | Posterior filtration bleb over the area of the episcleral explant.

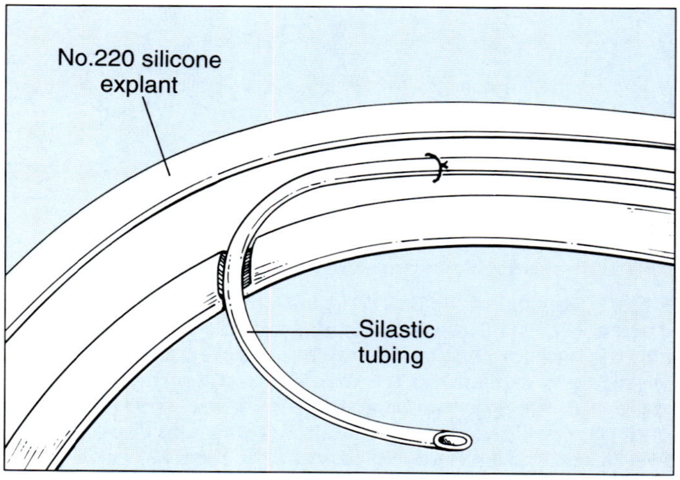

9.57 | Schocket implant. The Silastic tubing is sutured (10-0 nylon) within the groove of a No. 20 silicone explant. The tube exits through a punch excision in the side wall.

JOSEPH IMPLANT

Joseph et al designed a one-piece drainage device (Fig. 9.58) in an effort to overcome early postoperative complications associated with the Schocket device.[233,249] This implant consists of a curved length of silicone tubing (inner diameter 0.3 mm, outer diameter 0.64 mm) glued to the surface of a silicone plate curved to fit around the equator of the globe. The plate is 9-mm wide, 1-mm thick, and 85-mm long. A slit in the upper surface of the silicone tube functions as a valve with a reported opening pressure between 4–20 mm Hg. The technique for placement of this device is identical to that for the Schocket shunt.

Hitchings et al reported a 94% success rate 6 months after surgery in patients undergoing insertion of the strap implant.[250] The incidence of postoperative hypotony was reduced, but not eliminated, using the strap implant with a flow restrictive valve as compared with the Schocket shunt. Results were similar using either a 360° or a 180° band. The authors state that the surface area of the 180° strap is similar to the area of a 360° No. 20 band used in the Schocket procedure. The 180° strap size is recommended as sufficient to control intraocular pressure.

COMPLICATIONS OF POSTERIOR TUBE IMPLANT PROCEDURES

Filtration surgery with the posterior tube implant procedures is associated with operative and postoperative complications similar to those that occur after any intraocular procedure, e.g., anterior chamber or suprachoroidal hemorrhage, hypotony, and endophthalmitis. However, glaucoma-implant surgery is frequently associated with a higher rate of such complications owing to the severity of glaucoma and to the many prior surgical procedures.[251] Suprachoroidal hemorrhage occurs in 5–8% of such eyes, and the incidence of graft rejection in eyes with a previous penetrating keratoplasty may be increased. In addition, there are unique surgical and postoperative complications, which can occur with any of the four types.

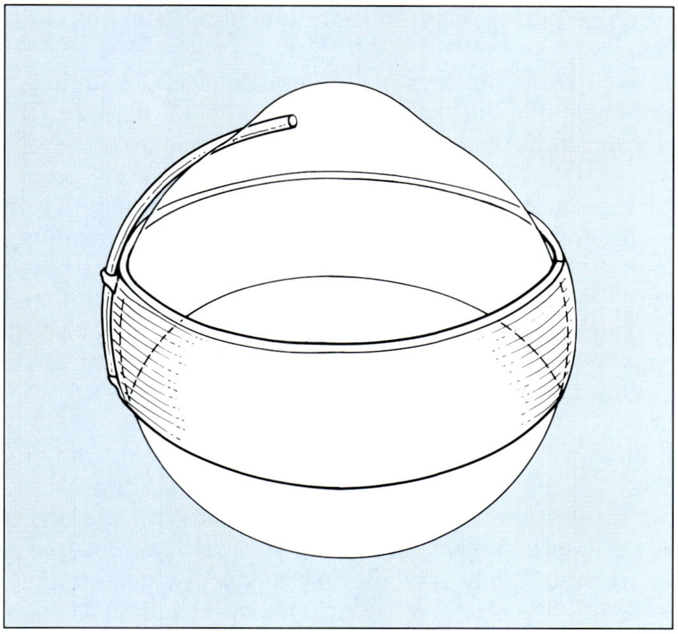

9.58 | Joseph one-piece tube and episcleral plate. (Adapted from Hitchings RA, Joseph NH, Sherwood MB, et al: Use of one-piece valved tube and variable surface area explant for glaucoma drainage surgery. Published courtesy of *Ophthalmology* 1987;94:1079–1084.)

OPERATIVE COMPLICATIONS

Special operative complications relate to insertion of the anterior chamber tube. Too large an entry incision predisposes to leakage around the tube, reducing aqueous humor flow through the tube to the posterior bleb. Sutures (10-0 nylon) should be used to close an incision that is too large. A 22- or 23-gauge needle or a microvitreal-retinal blade produces an adequate entry incision without aqueous humor leakage around the tube.

The correct direction for the anterior chamber tube entry incision is parallel to the plane of the iris, positioning the tube in the middle of the anterior chamber. Improper direction of the entry incision can allow the tube to damage the iris, lens, or cornea. In addition, these structures can occlude the open end of the tube. In this situation, we recommend making a new incision at a different site.

A full-thickness entry incision should be limbal in location. Entry through the cornea should be avoided. Insertion of the anterior chamber tube through a corneal incision may predispose to epithelial ingrowth.

EARLY POSTOPERATIVE COMPLICATIONS

Excessive flow of aqueous humor through an open tube before encapsulation around the posterior episcleral explant can result in a flat anterior chamber, hypotony, and choroidal detachment. These complications are more frequent after the use of devices that do not restrict flow of aqueous humor (e.g., single-stage Molteno or Schocket procedure). Reduction of aqueous humor flow by sutures placed within or around the tube (see preceding descriptions) until encapsulation has occurred, or implanting the device in two stages, decreases but does not eliminate these complications. The Joseph and Krupin devices contain a pressure-sensitive valve to restrict flow. Drainage of choroidal fluid and re-formation of the anterior chamber is recommended when the anterior chamber is flat and the tube is damaging the iris, cornea, or lens, or when there is corneal or lenticular decompensation.

Intraocular inflammation is usually more intense in eyes undergoing posterior tube implant surgery. Patients are placed on intensive topical corticosteroids and atropine postoperatively. Occasionally, systemic corticosteroids are required.

The open end of the anterior chamber tube can be blocked with fibrin, blood, or vitreous. In addition, iris tissue can enter and block the tube. The argon or Nd:YAG laser can be used to remove debris or tissue from the tube opening.

Elevated IOP can occur after insertion of the anterior chamber tube in the Molteno two-stage procedure or following opening of the tube in the Molteno one-stage or Schocket procedure by release or removal of the occluding suture. This elevation is transient, occurring while aqueous humor dissects the encapsulation surrounding the episcleral plate and creates a bleb. Aqueous humor suppressants (β-adrenergic blockers or carbonic anhydrase inhibitors) are continued during this period.

LATE POSTOPERATIVE COMPLICATIONS

Increased Intraocular Pressure

Late failure with increased IOP can be caused by blockage of the anterior chamber tube opening or tube migration out of the anterior chamber, blockage within the tube between the anterior chamber and the episcleral plate, or a nonfunctioning encapsulated bleb. Blockage of aqueous humor egress to the episcleral plate results in failure to produce a bleb, the overlying conjunctiva remaining flat against the plate. Visible occlusion of the tube at its opening can be eliminated with laser energy. If this is not successful or possible, surgical revision is necessary. Through a paracentesis incision, a 27-gauge blunt-tipped cannula is placed into the tube for injection of balanced salt solution. If the tube is patent, this maneuver may elevate the fibrous encapsulation off of the episcleral explant, with formation of a bleb. Resistance to irrigation through the tube may indicate a more distal tube obstruction. A wire (e.g., the stylet from a 25-gauge spinal needle) inserted through the paracentesis tract into the tube and advanced towards the plate may open an obstructed tube. Success is verified by repeat injection of balanced salt into the tube and formation of a bleb over the episcleral explant.

Inadequate anchoring of the tube to the episclera can result in fibrous tissue "pulling" the tube out of the anterior chamber. The tube will be kinked rather than having a straight course from the episcleral plate. In this situation, the tube is isolated by external dissection and repositioned into the chamber. Episcleral sutures are used to anchor the tube in place.

Migration of the tube either out of or into the anterior chamber can be due to movement of the episcleral plate. In this situation, the tube and anterior encapsulation around the plate are dissected, the plate repositioned so that the tube is in proper position within the anterior chamber, and the plate resutured to the sclera.

Elevated IOP with a thick, nonfunctioning encapsulation over the episcleral explant can be managed by bleb revision or by additional surgery with insertion of additional episcleral explants. Revision by needle puncture of the bleb (and withdrawal of aqueous humor) and 5-FU injections has a low success rate. Dissection of the area of encapsulation over the plate, excision of the fibrous wall, and postoperative 5-FU injections is preferred.

Implant Erosion

Late erosion of either the tube or episcleral plate can occur. Contact of the tube against the inner surface of the cornea can result in migration of the tube out through the entire thickness of the cornea. Melting of the scleral flap or the scleral patch graft results in the tube being covered only with conjunctiva, which can erode and expose the tube (Fig. 9.59). We do not repair this type of defect unless there is leakage of aqueous humor at the site (a positive Seidel test) or ocular irritation caused by the exposed tube. Exposed sutures that may be the cause of the erosion are removed. Repair of an exposed tube requires placement of a donor scleral graft over the site. Closure of conjunctiva alone over the tube is not adequate.

External erosion and exposure of the episcleral plate requires removal of the device. Erosion of the episcleral implant through the sclera into the globe is theoretically possible, but has not been reported.

This section was supported in part by an unrestricted grant from Research to Prevent Blindness Inc., New York, NY.

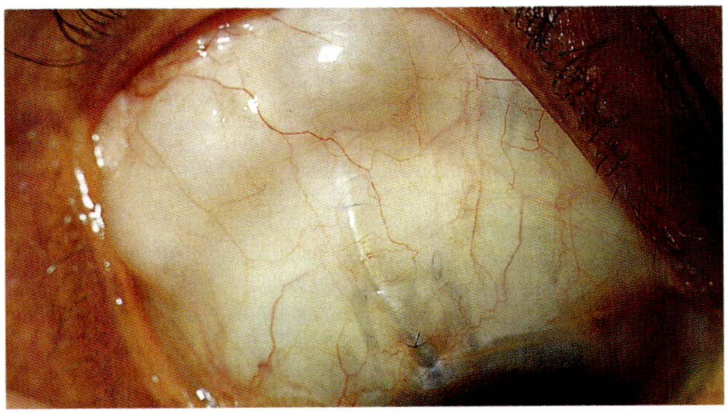

9.59 | Tube erosion through the scleral flap and conjunctiva at the limbus. An exposed 10-0 nylon suture is present. A Seidel test was negative. A large posterior bleb is present and the intraocular pressure is 15 mm Hg.

Section VIII

New Approaches to Glaucoma Filtration Surgery

Wayne F. March

To put this section in perspective, we should briefly review some old approaches to glaucoma filtration surgery. DeWecker first described the creation of the filtering fistula and the subsequent conjunctival "bleb" as a hallmark of success in 1895.[252] He used an internal approach with a puncture–counterpuncture technique using a Graefe knife. LaGrange showed that for filtering fistulas to function reproducibly, some sclera needed to be removed.[253] Because the removal of sclera was technically quite difficult with a scalpel from the internal approach, he inaugurated the external approach and the use of a suture.

The proper placement of the Elliot trephine was described in 1914 (Fig. 9.60) as being anterior to the plane of the iris. Elliot preserved the term "sclerostomy" out of deference to LaGrange but realized that he was, in fact, creating a corneosclerostomy.[254]

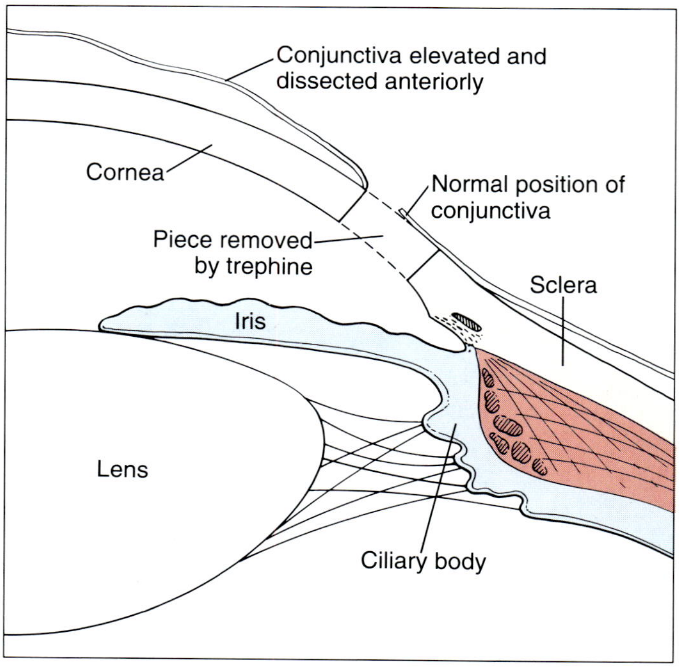

9.60 | Sclerocorneal trephining. (From Elliot RH: *Sclero-corneal Trephining in the Operative Treatment of Glaucoma,* ed 2. London: George Pulman & Sons, 1914, 78.)

TRABECUPHINE

An improvement on Elliot's trephine was made in 1982 by Brown et al,[255] who created an automated trephine known as the "trabecuphine." To avoid dissecting a conjunctival flap, Brown passed this trabecuphine across the anterior chamber in a similar manner to DeWecker's initial 1895 technique. The diameter of the tapered trephine cutting blade was 0.9 mm and the intraocular portion of the trabecuphine was equivalent to a 19-gauge needle. He confined his initial clinical studies to difficult end-stage cases of glaucoma that had previously failed glaucoma filtration procedures.[256] Considering his selection of cases, his results were quite good, but it is difficult to determine accurately if the results were in fact better than might be achieved by other forms of filtration surgery. The trabecuphine is presently in clinical use.

LASER SCLEROSTOMY

Laser sclerostomy refers to the use of a laser to create a filtering fistula between the anterior chamber and the subconjunctival space[257] (Fig. 9.61). The most successful approach to laser sclerostomy uses minimal laser power, because laser power and any other ocular trauma tends to stimulate inflammation, the first stage in the healing process. Several techniques have been used for laser sclerostomy and each in chronological turn appears to make the procedure easier, more practical, and to require less power.[258-261] Several invasive ab-interno approaches for laser sclerostomies have been recently investigated. Gaasterland et al[262] produced sclerostomies in bovine eyes using an argon laser. Jaffe et al[263] used a 15-watt argon laser passed internally across the anterior chamber to produce laser sclerostomies in rabbits. Wilson and co-workers[264,265] produced sclerostomies in animals and humans using a 60-watt continuous wave Nd:YAG laser coupled via a fiber optic to a 200-μm

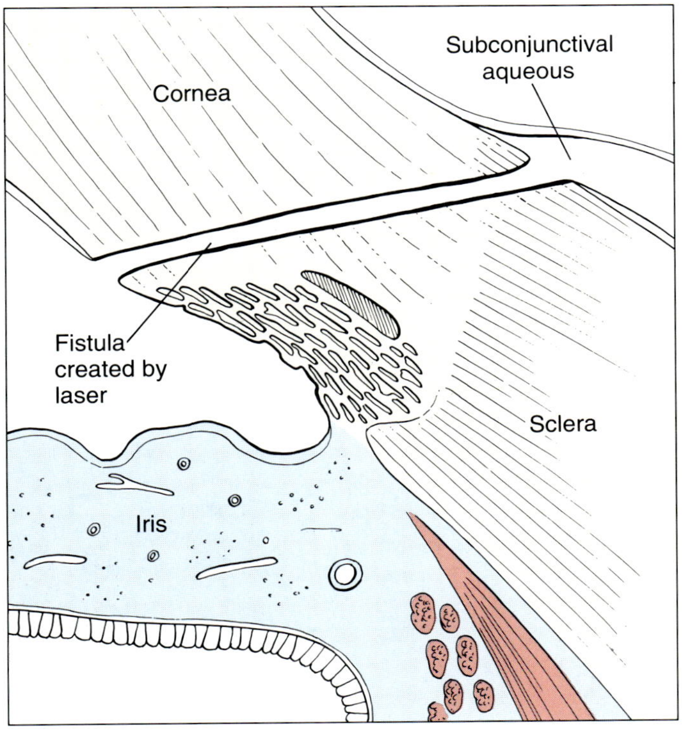

9.61 | Diagram of the filtering fistula in laser sclerostomy.

diameter sapphire tip, passed transcamerally to the sclerostomy site. This approach has received United States Food and Drug Administration approval.

However, it is inefficient to cut a transparent membrane such as the corneosclera with a light beam, so two approaches have been devised to facilitate the tasks and minimize the power required: (1) dyeing the sclera with nontoxic dye that absorbs the light beam; and (2) applying a light beam in the far infrared spectral region which is absorbed by the sclera. In the second case, the light beam must be delivered externally, rather than transcamerally via a goniolens, because the long-wavelength light will not pass through the cornea. We shall confine our discussion to one technique using a goniolens (the dye–laser technique) and another requiring an external approach (the holmium technique). These two approaches have had the most extensive clinical trials, and the holmium laser has recently been approved by the FDA for general clinical use. However, it is uncertain which will be the predominant technique in the long term.

DYE–LASER TECHNIQUE

The dye–laser technique[260] (Fig. 9.62) begins with the application of 1% methylene blue dye to the limbus for 4 minutes by iontophoresis[261] (Fig. 9.63). The conjunctiva is anesthetized by applying a swab with proparacaine at the blue spot for 4 minutes. The conjunctiva is then elevated at the intended exit site of the sclerocorneal fistula by subconjunctival injection of balanced salt solution or a viscoelastic agent with a 30-gauge needle. This ensures that the conjunctiva will not be inadvertently perforated.

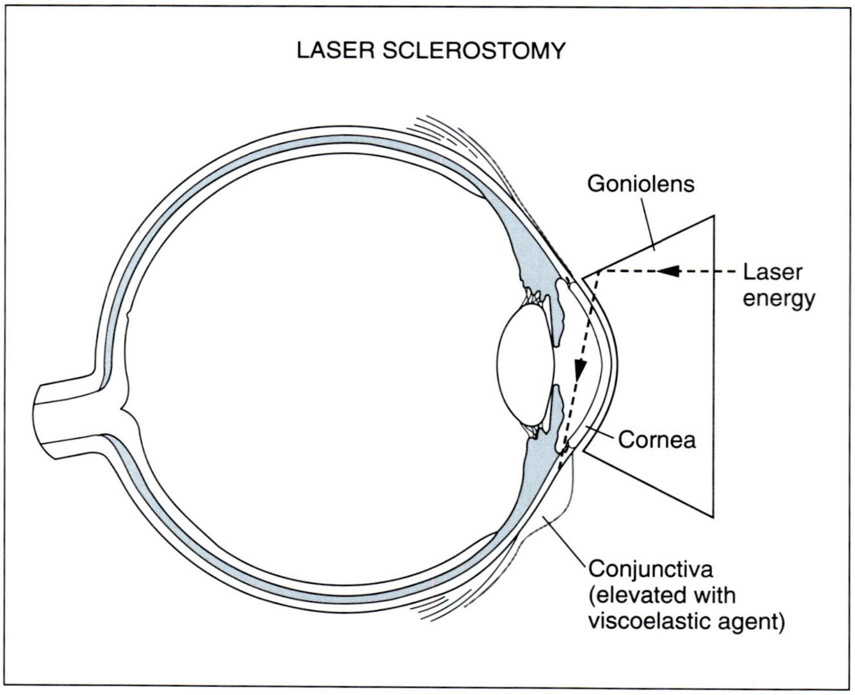

9.62 | Diagram of dye–laser sclerostomy performed at a wavelength of 668 nm through a goniolens.

The appropriate goniolens is then applied and the blue spot should be easily localized gonioscopically, showing that the blue dye has in fact completely penetrated the limbus (Fig. 9.64). The aiming beam of the dye laser is centered on the spot and a foot switch is pressed, releasing a single laser pulse at 668 nm. The process is continued until perforation occurs, as determined by shallowing of the chamber. The patient is given a mild steroid-antibiotic drop q.i.d. for 2 days following treatment. The inflammation is minor and is comparable to that produced by laser trabeculoplasty.

HOLMIUM LASER TECHNIQUE

The 26-gauge holmium laser probe currently in use for human patients, and first described by Dunbar Hoskins, is shown in Figure 9.65. The first step is to apply a 4% lidocaine-moistened swab for 4 minutes at the limbus. Retrobulbar anesthesia is not necessary. Any clock hour position may be used, and it is advantageous to go to an area of unused conjunctiva. A 30-gauge needle tip is touched to a Rose Bengal sterile strip to mark the site of conjunctival puncture. At least 8 mm from the intended site of entrance, the conjunctiva is grasped with smooth forceps and a 30-gauge needle is thrust

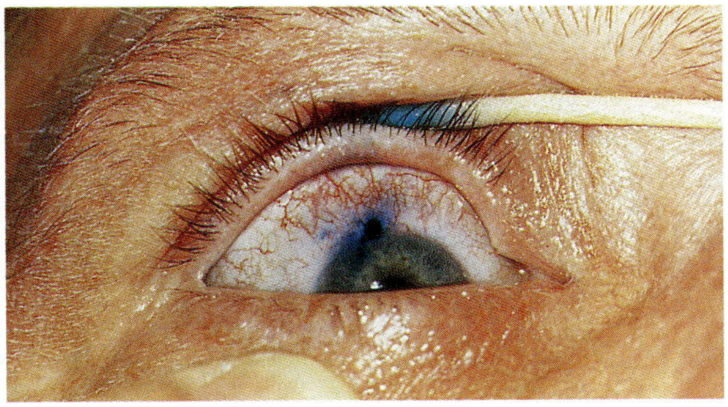

9.63 | Iontophoresis performed at the limbus with 1% methylene blue.

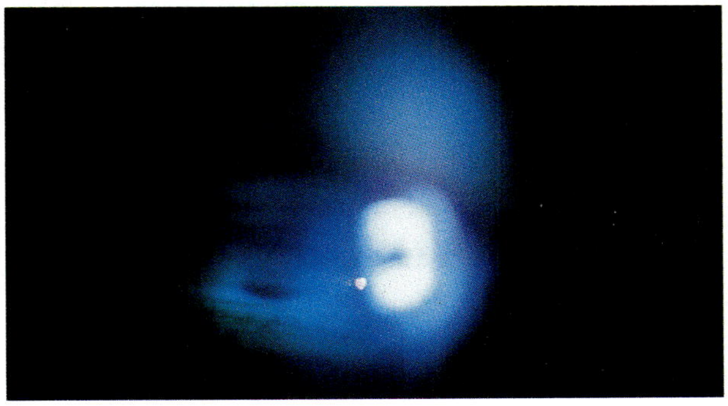

9.64 | Gonioscopic appearance of the methylene blue spot.

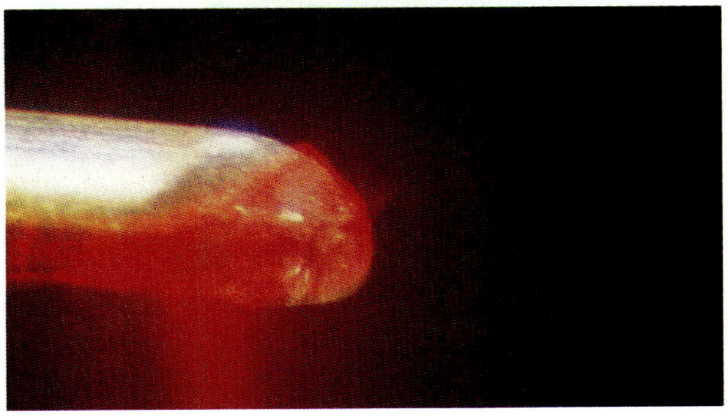

9.65 | Holmium laser probe used in sclerostomy.

through. A special "laser sclerostomy needle" for this procedure is shown in Figure 9.66. A regular 30-gauge needle can be used, but the advantage of the "laser sclerostomy needle" is its blunt tip and short bevel. The problem of inadvertent double perforation of the conjunctiva is thus avoided, and it is possible to dissect very far anteriorly and to inject a viscoelastic agent under the adherent corneal conjunctiva (a standard 30-gauge needle has too long a bevel to do this). The subconjunctival viscoelastic agent keeps the anterior chamber formed. The sterile probe (see Fig. 9.65) is then inserted to this hole

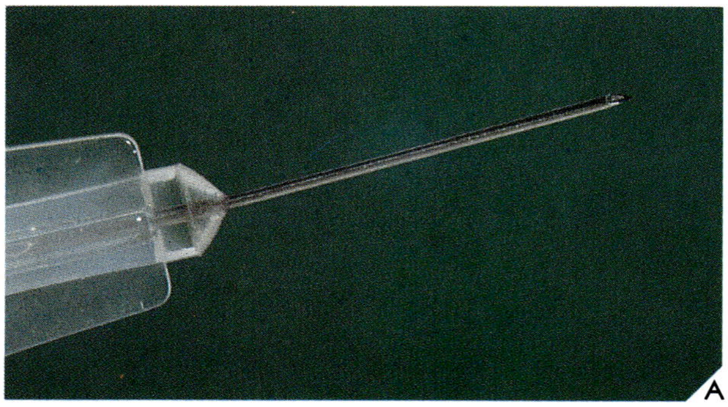

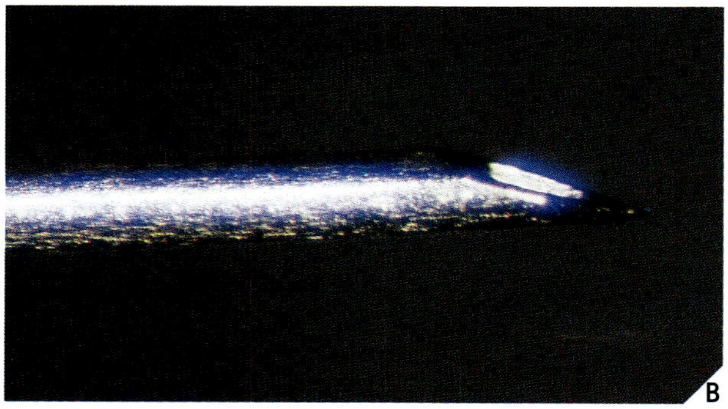

9.66 | *A:* Laser sclerostomy needle which may be used to gain anterior position for the probe by raising the adherent corneal conjunctiva. *B:* Detail of tip showing short bevel.

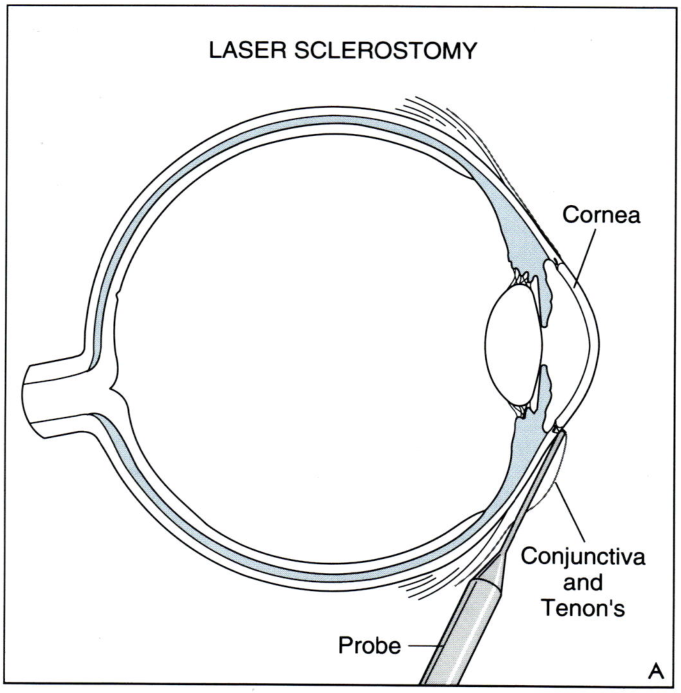

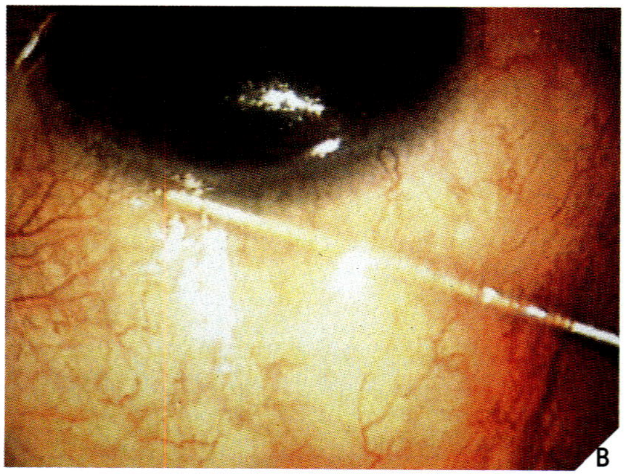

9.67 | *A,B:* Probe in proper position for holmium laser sclerostomy, perpendicular to the limbus. At this point the foot pedal is pressed to trigger the laser.

and worked to the limbus (Fig. 9.67). This is accomplished by noting the appearance of the aiming beam on either side of the correct position. The shape of the laser beam is shown in Figure 9.68. Energy of 140 mj per pulse or less can be used. The laser is then activated with a foot petal and, at the normal pulse repetition rate of 5 pulses/sec, the 300-msec pulse is applied for 40–60 pulses. Because the wavelength of the laser is 2.1 μm, the limbal tissue absorbs the laser energy well but the energy does not go beyond the aqueous humor, as water also absorbs this wavelength. The probe is then removed and the patient is treated in a similar manner as for dye-laser sclerostomy. A conjunctival suture is not required.

Among the potential complications with all current approaches to laser and transcameral sclerotomies are those relating to full-thickness as opposed to subscleral fistulization (see Smythe and Herschler, this chapter). Iris incarceration can usually be avoided, since an iridotomy can be produced many times or the iris freed postoperatively by argon/Nd:Yag laser photodisruption. However, caveats notwithstanding, laser fistulization techniques may signal a major advance in glaucoma therapy, and the holmium laser is the first truly practical method to become widely available. Since the days of LaGrange,[253] opthalmic surgeons have relied on scalpel, cautery, or scissors to perform glaucoma filtration surgery. Now, a more elegantly simple technique is available which adapts itself well to the outpatient surgical setting. Further refinements and alternatives for laser sclerostomy may lie ahead.

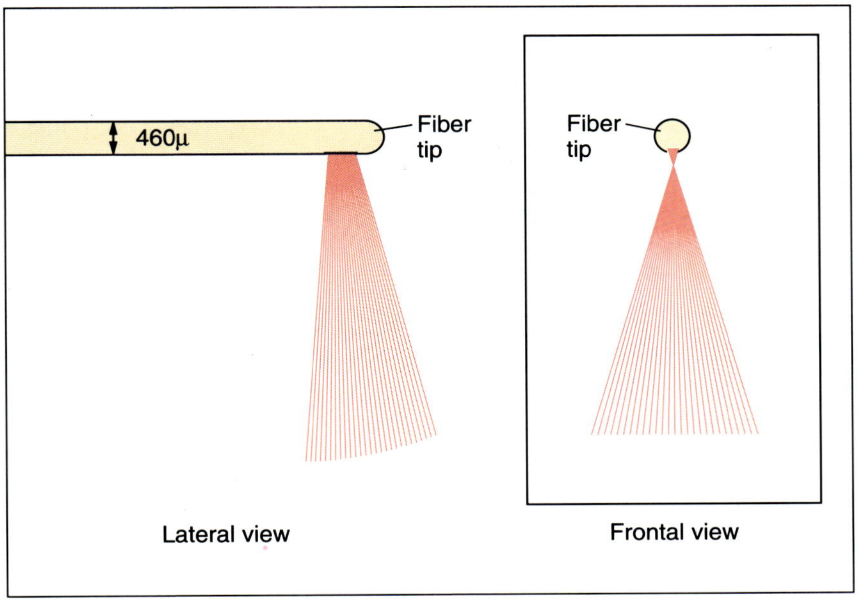

9.68 | Diagram of the laser beam as it exits from the probe in two views.

SECTION IX

CYCLODESTRUCTIVE PROCEDURES

M. Bruce Shields

All operations for the treatment of glaucoma are designed to lower the intraocular pressure (IOP) either by improving aqueous outflow or by reducing aqueous production. Techniques for the former, which include laser trabeculoplasty, iridotomy, and filtering surgery, constitute the first-line surgical defense in most cases. There are certain high risk situations, however, in which these procedures have a low probability of success. Included among the high-risk category are glaucoma in aphakia and pseudophakia, neovascular glaucoma, glaucoma associated with active inflammation, and glaucoma after multiple failed filtering procedures. It is within this group of patients that the alternative surgical technique of reducing aqueous production may be beneficial. These operations are referred to as cyclodestructive procedures because they reduce aqueous production through destruction of portions of the ciliary processes.

OVERVIEW OF CYCLODESTRUCTIVE PROCEDURES

In the 1930s and 1940s, several energy sources for cyclodestructive surgery were evaluated, including diathermy, β-irradiation, and electrolysis, although only cyclodiathermy achieved clinical acceptance. Cryotherapy was introduced in the 1950s and was the procedure of choice. Newer cyclodestructive elements that are currently being evaluated include laser, ultrasound, and microwaves, and recent experience suggests that laser cyclophotocoagulation is now the preferred cyclodestructive operation.

All of the cyclodestructive procedures described above utilize the transscleral route of energy delivery, in which the destructive element passes through conjunctiva, sclera, and ciliary muscle before reaching the ciliary processes. Transscleral cyclodestructive operations have the advantages of being noninvasive and relatively quick and easy, although significant disadvantages include the inability to visualize the processes being treated and damage to adjacent tissue, leading to unpredictable results and frequent complications. With the advent of laser energy as the cyclodestructive element, alternative delivery routes include transpupillary and intraocular approaches.

CYCLOCRYOTHERAPY

The use of a freezing source as the cyclodestructive element was suggested by Bietti in 1950.[266] The mechanism by which cryotherapy destroys ciliary processes appears to be a combination of intracellular ice crystal formation and ischemic necrosis.[267] The standard technique involves applying the cryoprobe over the conjunctiva with the anterior edge of the probe 1–1.5 mm from the limbus. The temperature is then reduced to -60° to -80°C, and this is maintained for approximately 60 seconds[268] (Fig. 9.69). Most surgeons treat two or three quadrants with three or four applications per quadrant. Postoperatively, the patient should be treated aggressively with topical and sub-Tenon's steroids and a mydriatic–cycloplegic, as well as with the preoperative glaucoma medications (with the exception of miotics). If the desired IOP level is not achieved after several weeks or months, additional cryotherapy can be performed.

Cyclocryotherapy is generally felt to be somewhat more predictable and less destructive than penetrating cyclodiathermy, and it has gradually replaced the latter technique as the most commonly used cyclodestructive operation. However, complications are significant with cryotherapy. A marked rise in IOP may occur during the freezing phase and also in the early postoperative period.[269] Patients may also have marked inflammation and severe pain during the early postoperative course. Additional complications include hyphema, hypotony, and phthisis. These serious complications have been responsible for the lack of popularity of cyclocryotherapy (as well as all cyclodestructive procedures) and have prompted the search for better cyclodestructive operations.

TRANSSCLERAL CYCLOPHOTOCOAGULATION

Weekers and associates, in 1961, first reported the use of light as the cyclodestructive element with the transscleral application of xenon arc photocoagulation over the ciliary body.[270] It was the introduction of the laser, however, that eventually led to the clinical application of cyclophotocoagulation. In 1969, Vucicevic and associates reported the use of transscleral cyclophotocoagulation in rabbits, using a ruby laser and a cytochemical to enhance laser absorption of the ciliary body.[271] In 1984, Beckman and Waeltermann reported a 10-year experience with 241 eyes treated by transscleral ruby laser cyclophotocoagulation.[272] However, it was not until the availability of specially designed Nd:YAG lasers that widespread interest in transscleral cyclophotocoagulation developed.

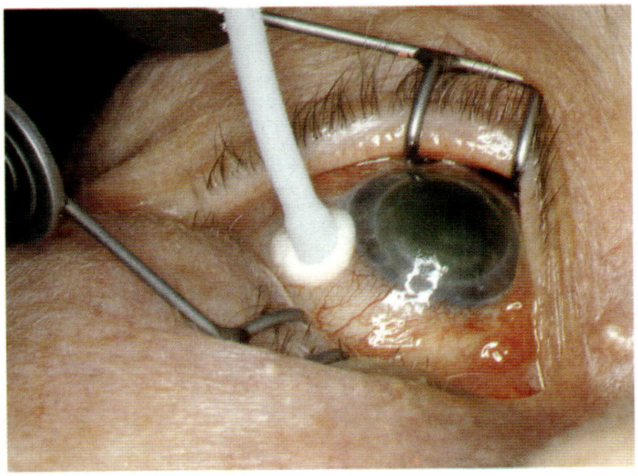

9.69 | Cyclocryotherapy, showing development of ice ball. (From Nardin G, Zimmerman TJ: Surgery for glaucoma and related conditions, in Jaffe NS: *Atlas of Ophthalmic Surgery*. New York: Gower Medical Publishing, 1990, 3.9.)

At the moment, two Nd:YAG lasers have been studied for transscleral cyclophotocoagulation. The first of these is the Lasag Microruptor 2, which uses noncontact, slit-lamp delivery with the laser in a free-running mode of 20-msec pulses. This laser also provides an adjustable offset between the focal points of the helium–neon aiming beam and the therapeutic beam so that the latter can be at a predetermined distance inside the eye when aiming on the conjunctiva. In addition, the laser is capable of operating at high energy levels of up to 8–9 joules. The other laser unit that has been extensively evaluated is the Surgical Laser Technologies (SLT) CL60, which provides contact probe delivery in a continuous-wave mode of 0.1–10 seconds. A 2.2-mm sapphire-tipped, hand-held probe (Fig. 9.70), which is focused at 1.5–2 mm in air, is coupled to a fiber optic delivery system. The unit can provide powers in excess of 10 watts. (Energy in joules equals power in watts times duration in seconds.)

With both of the lasers described above, the mechanism of reduced aqueous production is felt to be damage to the epithelial layers of the ciliary processes. With the noncontact system, histologic studies of human autopsy and living eyes reveal disrupted epithelium which is elevated blister-like from the stroma of the ciliary processes, with minimal damage to the overlying ciliary muscle and sclera [273,274] (Fig. 9.71). In contrast, the histologic appearance of lesions created by the contact, continuous-wave Nd:YAG laser is a smaller, more coagulative effect on the epithelium, with less blister-like elevation.[275] Alternative possibilities for the mechanism of reduced aqueous production by cyclophotocoagulation include ciliary vascular disruption with reduced inflow or chronic inflammation, which could influence either inflow or uveoscleral outflow.[276]

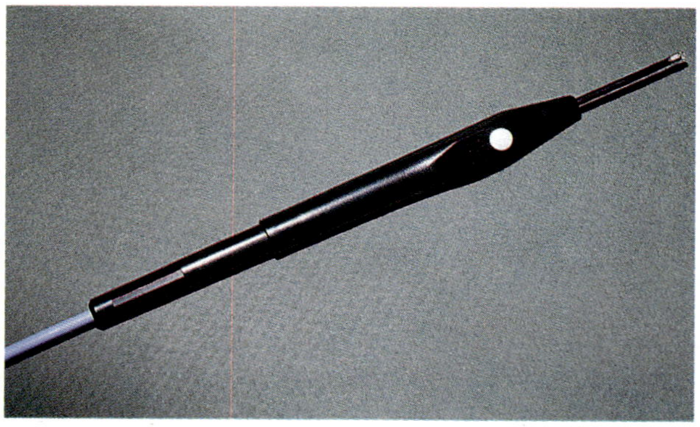

9.70 | Hand-held probe for contact transscleral Nd:YAG cyclophotocoagulation. (Courtesy of Dr. Paul L. Kaufman.)

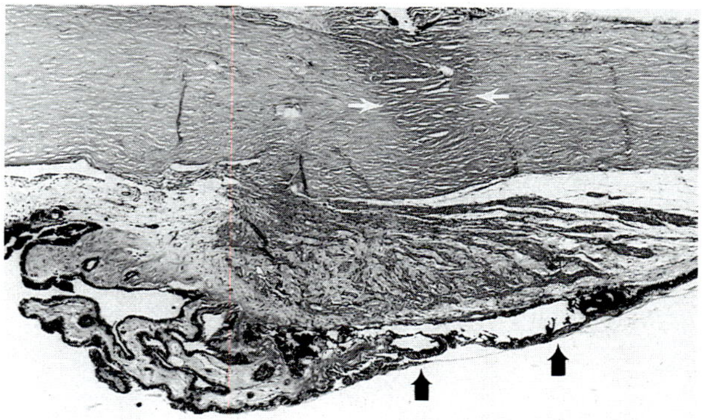

9.71 | Light microscopic view of human autopsy eye treated with noncontact, free-running transscleral Nd:YAG cyclophotocoagulation, showing blister-like elevation of disrupted ciliary epithelium (black arrows) with minimal ciliary muscle and scleral damage (white arrows). Defect on scleral surface was created by needle with India ink to mark center of laser track after laser application. (From Hampton C, Shields MB: Transscleral neodymium:YAG cyclophotocoagulation: A histologic study of human autopsy eyes. *Arch Ophthalmol 1988;106:1121.*)

Retrobulbar anesthesia is required with both transscleral cyclophotocoagulation procedures. With the noncontact, thermal mode technique, the patient is seated at the slit lamp. Standard settings include a pulse duration of 20 msec and a maximal offset between the aiming and therapeutic beams, which is 3.6 mm in air. Preferred energy levels vary considerably from 2–8 joules. The laser beam can be applied directly to the conjunctiva, or a contact lens can be used that separates the lids, compresses and blanches the conjunctiva, and provides measurements from the limbus.[277] Opinions differ regarding placement of the laser lesions, but most agree that focusing on the conjunctiva 1.0–1.5 mm behind the limbus is optimal for damaging the pars plicata. The total number of laser applications also varies among surgeons, with most using 30–40 evenly-spaced lesions over 360° (Fig. 9.72).

The contact, continuous-wave technique generally utilizes exposure times of 0.5–0.7 second. The laser focus is fixed by the design of the probe tip, which is held perpendicular to the surface of the conjunctiva with the anterior edge of the probe 0.5–1.5 mm behind the limbus. Power settings vary considerably among surgeons, with a range of approximately 4–9 watts (4 watts at 0.5 second provides an energy of 2 joules, while 9 watts at 0.7 second delivers 6.3 joules). The number of applications usually varies from 30 to 40 for 360°.

With both transscleral cyclophotocoagulation procedures, satisfactory IOP reduction is achieved in approximately two thirds or more of the cases after the initial session, with most of the remaining cases coming under control with one or more retreatments.[278,279] The contact technique requires less total energy and appears to have a slightly better IOP success rate. It also has the advantage of allowing treatment in a supine position, so that it can be performed under general anesthesia if necessary. Both cyclophotocoagulation procedures have significant advantages over cyclocryotherapy, including less rise in IOP, less inflammation, and less pain after treatment. However, reduced visual acuity remains a significant problem, although perhaps less so with the contact technique.

TRANSPUPILLARY CYCLOPHOTOCOAGULATION

Lee and Pomerantzeff, in 1971, introduced the concept of direct argon laser application to the ciliary processes via a transpupillary approach with the use of a goniolens.[280] This procedure is obviously limited to those eyes in which the ciliary processes can be visualized gonioscopically, as with a large iridectomy or retraction of the iris in advanced neovascular glaucoma

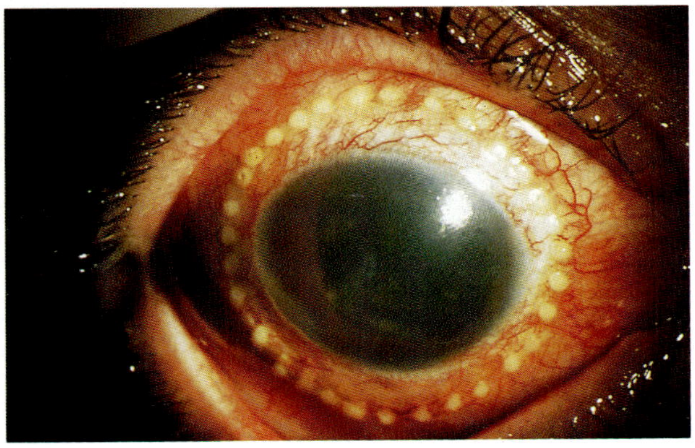

9.72 | Noncontact, free-running transscleral Nd:YAG cyclophotocoagulation showing conjunctival burns immediately after the procedure. (From Hampton C, Shields MB, Miller KM, Blasini M: Evaluation of a protocol for transscleral Nd:YAG photocoagulation in 100 patients. *Ophthalmology 1990;97:910.*)

(Fig. 9.73). Typical argon laser settings are 0.1–0.2 second, 100–200 μm, and an energy level that is sufficient to produce a white discoloration, as well as a brown concave burn of the ciliary process (usually 700–1,000 mw). All visible processes in up to two quadrants are usually treated at one session, with additional treatment at subsequent sessions if necessary. The success rate with transpupillary cyclophotocoagulation has been much lower than that with the transscleral approach.[281] Those cases in which the procedure fails may be due, in part, to the limited number of ciliary processes that can be visualized and treated. Another factor that may contribute to failure is the angle at which the processes are visualized gonioscopically. Even with scleral indentation, only the anterior tips of the ciliary ridges are usually exposed, preventing destruction of the entire ciliary process.

INTRAOCULAR CYCLOPHOTO-COAGULATION

It is also possible to apply laser energy directly to the ciliary processes, using an argon endophotocoagulator, through a pars plana incision. During the course of vitrectomy in an aphakic eye, it is possible to lower the IOP and to use scleral indentation to bring the ciliary processes into transpupillary view for the purpose of cyclophotocoagulation with the intraocular laser probe.[282] With an exposure time of 0.1–0.2 second, laser therapy is applied to individual ciliary processes, using an energy level that is sufficient to produce a white reaction and a shallow tissue disruption (usually 1,000 mw). Three to five laser exposures can be applied to each process in the two quadrants opposite the entry site. The primary value of this procedure is as an adjunct to pars plana vitrectomy in eyes with refractory glaucoma, although it has also been used alone in the treatment of difficult glaucoma cases.[283] An ocular endoscope with an attached laser fiber optic has also been used for direct visualization of the ciliary processes via the pars plana incision with simultaneous application of the laser energy.[284] However, the invasive nature and the relative risks of the procedure make it less promising than transscleral cyclophotocoagulation.

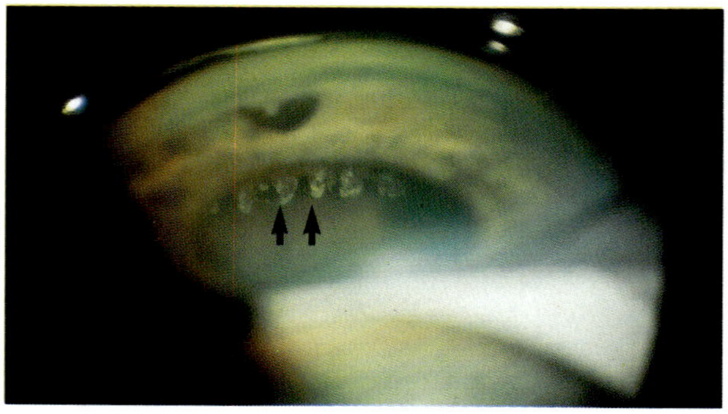

9.73 | Transpupillary cyclophotocoagulation, showing gonioscopic view of whitened ciliary processes (arrows). Exposure of processes in this eye is due to retraction of iris by fibrovascular membrane of neovascular glaucoma. (From Shields MB: *Textbook of Glaucoma.* Baltimore: Williams & Wilkins, 1987.)

THERAPEUTIC ULTRASOUND

In 1964, Purnell et al introduced the concept of using focused transscleral ultrasonic radiation to produce localized destruction of the ciliary body in rabbit eyes.[285] Coleman and associates have subsequently reported success in clinical trials with high-intensity focused ultrasound.[286] The basic technique involves delivering an average of six to seven exposures of ultrasound at an intensity level of 10 kw/cm^2 for 5 seconds each to scleral sites near the limbus (Fig. 9.74). Tissue destruction is more extensive than with cyclophotocoagulation, although the reported success rates and complications have been encouraging.

In summary, reduced aqueous production can be achieved by destroying a portion of the ciliary body with a variety of energy sources. Unpredictable results and high complication rates have limited the popularity of these operations in the past. As further experience is gained with transscleral cyclophotocoagulation, however, it may be that this surgical approach will assume an increasingly important role in the management of glaucoma.

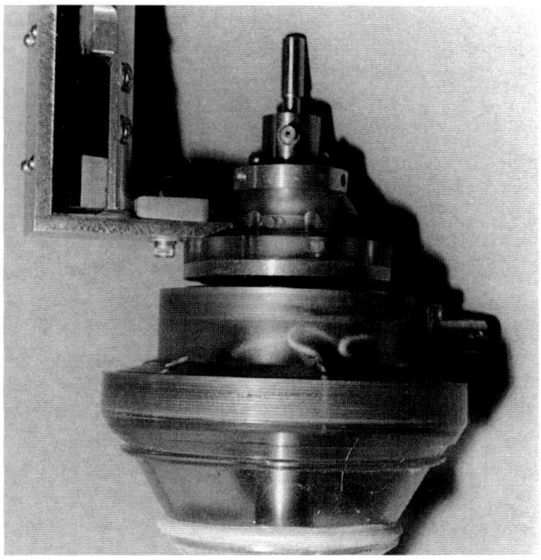

9.74 | Therapeutic ultrasound transducer assembly. (Courtesy of Dr. Wayne F. March.)

REFERENCES

CHAPTER 1
ANTERIOR SEGMENT

1. Brubaker RF: Measurements of aqueous flow by fluorophotometry, in Ritch R, Shields MB, Krupin T (eds): *The Glaucomas,* Vol I. St. Louis: CV Mosby, 1989, 337–344.
2. Morrison JC, van Buskirk EM: Ciliary process microvasculature of the primate eye. *Am J Ophthalmol 1984;97:372–384.*
3. Funk R, Rohen JW: *Functional Morphology of the Vasculature in the Anterior Eye Segment.* (Monograph series in Lütjen-Drecoll E, Rohen JW [eds]: *Basic Aspects of Glaucoma Research II.*) Stuttgart, New York: Schattauer Verlag, 1990, 1–179.
4. Funk R, Rohen JW: Scanning electron microscopic study on the vasculature of the human anterior eye segment. *Exp Eye Res 1990; 51:651–661.*
5. Hara K, Lütjen–Drecoll E, Prestele H, Rohen JW: Structural differences between regions of the ciliary body in primates. *Invest Ophthalmol Vis Sci 1977;16:912–924.*
6. Ober M, Rohen JW: Regional differences in the fine structure of the ciliary epithelium related to accommodation. *Invest Ophthalmol Vis Sci 1979;18:655–664.*
7. Lütjen–Drecoll E: Functional morphology of the ciliary epithelium, in Lütjen–Drecoll E (ed): *Basic Aspects of Glaucoma Research,* Vol I. Stuttgart, New York: Schattauer Verlag, 1982, 69–87.
8. Lütjen–Drecoll E, Lönnerholm G, Eichhorn M: Carbonic anhydrase distribution in the human and monkey eye by light and electron microscopy. *Graefes Arch Clin Exp Ophthalmol 1983;220:285–291.*
9. Lütjen–Drecoll E, Eichhorn M, Bárány EH: Carbonic anhydrase in epithelia and fenestrated juxtaepithelial capillaries of *Macaca fascicularis. Acta Physiol Scand 1985;124:295–307.*
10. Shiose, Y: Electron microscopic studies on blood retinal and blood-aqueous barriers. *Jpn J Ophthalmol 1970;14:73–87.*
11. Vegge T: An epithelial blood-aqueous barrier to horseradish peroxidase in the processes of the newt monkey (*Cercopithecus aethiops*). *Z Zellforsch Mikrosk Anat 1971;114:309–320.*
12. Raviola G: Effects of paracentesis on the blood-aqueous barrier: An electron microscope study on *Macaca mulatta* using horeseradish peroxidase as a tracer. *Invest Ophthalmol Vis Sci 1974;13:828–848.*
13. Raviola G: The structural basis of the blood-ocular barriers. *Exp Eye Res 1977;25(suppl):27–63.*
14. Raviola G, Raviola E : Intercellular junctions in the ciliary epithelium. *Invest Ophthalmol Vis Sci 1978;17:958–981.*
15. Rohen JW: Scanning electron microscopic studies of the zonular apparatus in human and monkey eyes. *Invest Ophthalmol Vis Sci 1979; 18:133–144.*
16. Tamm E, Lütjen–Drecoll E, Jungkunz W, Rohen JW: Posterior attachment of ciliary muscle in young, accommodating old, presbyopic monkeys. *Invest Ophthalmol Vis Sci 1991;32:1678–1692.*
17. Lütjen–Drecoll E, Kaufman PL: Echiothiophate-induced structural alterations in the anterior chamber angle of the cynomolgus monkey. *Invest Ophthalmol Vis Sci 1979;18:918–929.*
18. Lütjen–Drecoll E: Morphology of the pars plana region. *Dev Ophthalmol 1992;23:50-59.*
19. Flügel C, Lütjen–Drecoll E: Presence and distribution of Na^+K^+-ATPase in the ciliary epithelium of the rabbit. *Histochemistry 1988;88: 613–621.*
20. Bill A: The aqueous humor drainage mechanism in the cynomolgus monkey (*Macaca irus*) with evidence for unconventional routes. *Invest Ophthalmol 1965;4:911–919.*
21. Bill A: Conventional and uveo-scleral drainage of aqueous humour in the cynomolgus monkey (*Macaca irus*) at normal and high intraocular pressures. *Exp Eye Res 1966;5:45–54.*
22. Bill A, Phillips CI: Uveoscleral drainage of aqueous humor in human eyes. *Exp Eye Res 1971;12:275–281.*
23. Townsend DJ, Brubaker RF: Immediate effect of epinephrine on aqueous formation in the normal human eye as measured by fluorophotometry. *Invest Ophthalmol Vis Sci 1980;19:256–266.*

24. Lütjen–Drecoll E, Futa R, Rohen JW: Ultrahistochemical studies on tangential sections of the trabecular meshwork in normal and glaucomatous eyes. *Invest Ophthalmol Vis Sci 1981;21:563–573.*
25. Rohen JW, Futa R, Lütjen-Drecoll E: The fine structure of the cribriform meshwork in normal and glaucomatous eyes as seen in tangential sections. *Invest Ophthalmol Vis Sci 1981;21:574–585.*
26. Rohen JW: The evolution of the primate eye in relation to the problem of glaucoma, in Lütjen–Drecoll E (ed): *Basic Aspects of Glaucoma Research,* Vol I. Stuttgart, New York: Schattauer Verlag, 1982, 3–33.
27. Mäepea O, Bill A: The pressure in the episcleral veins, Schlemm's canal and the trabecular meshwork in monkeys: Effects of changes in intraocular pressure. *Exp Eye Res 1989;49:645–663.*
28. Bill A, Svedbergh B: Scanning electron microscopic studies of the trabecular meshwork and the canal of Schlemm. An attempt to localize the main resistance to outflow of aqueous humor in man. *Acta Ophthalmol 1972;50:295–320.*
29. Inomata H, Bill A, Smelser GK: Aqueous humor pathways through the trabecular meshwork and into Schlemm's canal in the cynomolgus monkey (*Macaca irus*). An electron microscopic study. *Am J Ophthalmol 1972;73:760–769.*
30. Johnstone MA, Grant WM: Pressure dependent changes in structures of the outflow system of human and monkey eyes. *Am J Ophthalmol 1973;75:365–383.*
31. Grierson I, Lee WR:Pressure effects on flow channels in the lining endothelium of Schlemm's canal. *Acta Ophthalmol 1978;56:935–952.*
32. Fink AI, Felix MD, Fletcher RC: Schlemm's canal and adjacent structures in glaucomatous patients. *Am J Ophthalmol 1972;74:893–906.*
33. Tripathi RC: The functional morphology of the outflow systems of ocular and cerebrospinal fluids. *Exp Eye Res 1977;25(Suppl):65–116.*
34. Epstein DL, Rohen JW: Morphology of the trabecular meshwork and inner wall endothelium after cationized ferritin perfusion in the monkey eye. *Invest Ophthalmol Vis Sci 1991;32:160–171.*
35. Lütjen–Drecoll E: Structural factors influencing outflow facility and its changeability under drugs, a study in *Macaca arctoides. Invest Ophthalmol Vis Sci 1973;12:280–294.*
36. Rohen JW, Lütjen E, Bárány E: The relation between the ciliary muscle and the trabecular meshwork and its importance for the effect of miotics on aqueous outflow resistance: A study in two contrasting monkey species, *Macaca irus* and *Cercopithecus aethiops. Graefes Arch Clin Exp Ophthalmol 1967;172:23–47.*
37. Rohen JW, Unger HH: *Zur Morphologie und Pathologie der Kammerbucht des Auges.* Wiesbaden: Steiner Verlag. (Abhandlungen Mainzer Akademie der Wissenschaft und Literaturzeitung: Mathematik-Naturwissenschaft Klasse vol 3, 1–206.)
38. Grierson I, Lee WR, Abraham S: Effects of pilocarpine on the morphology of the human outflow apparatus. *Br J Ophthalmol 1978;62: 302–313.*
39. Grierson I, Lee WR, Moseley H, Abraham S: The trabecular wall of Schlemm's canal: A study of the effects of pilocarpine by scanning electron microscopy. *Br J Ophthalmol 63:9–16.*
40. Lütjen-Drecoll E, Bárány EH: Functional and electron microscopic changes in the trabecular meshwork remaining after trabeculectomy in cynomolgus monkeys. *Invest Ophthalmol 1974;13:511–524.*
41. Rohen JW, van der Zypen E: The phagocytic activity of the trabecular meshwork endothelium. An electron microscopy study of the vervet (*Cercopithecus aethiops*). *Graefes Arch Clin Exp Ophthalmol 1968; 175:143–160.*
42. Grierson I, Lee WR: Erythrocyte phagocytosis in the human trabecular meshwork. *Br J Ophthalmol 1973;57:400–415.*
43. Svedbergh B, Lütjen-Drecoll E, Ober M, Kaufman PL: Cytochalasin B-induced structural changes in the anterior ocular segment of the cynomolgus monkey. *Invest Ophthalmol Vis Sci 1978;17:718–734.*

44. Rohen JW, Lütjen-Drecoll E: Biology of the trabecular meshwork, in Lütjen–Drecoll E (ed): *Basic Aspects of Glaucoma Research,* Vol I. Stuttgart, New York: Schattauer Verlag, 1982, 141–166.
45. Rohen JW, Lütjen-Drecoll E: Age changes of the trabecular meshwork in human and monkey eyes, in Bredt H, Rohen JW (eds): *Ageing and Development,* Vol I. Stuttgart, New York: Schattauer Verlag, 1971, 1–36.
46. Lütjen-Drecoll E, Shimizu T, Rohrbach M, Rohen JW: Quantitative analysis of "plaque material" in the inner and outer wall of Schlemm's canal in normal and glaucomatous eyes. *Exp Eye Res 1986; 42:443–455.*
47. Bill A: Physiology of the outflow mechanism, in Drance SM (ed): *Applied Pharmacology in the Medical Treatment of Glaucomas.* Orlando, FL: Grune & Stratton, 1984, 111.
48. Maepea O, Bill A: The pressures in the episcleral veins, Schlemm's canal and trabecular meshwork in monkeys: Effects of changes in intraocular pressure. *Exp Eye Res 1989;49:645–663.*
49. Bill A: Uveoscleral drainage of aqueous humor: Physiology and pharmacology, in Bito LZ, Stjernschantz J (eds): *The Ocular Effects of Prostaglandins and Other Eicosanoids.* New York: Alan R Liss, 1989, 417.
50. Bill A: Circulation in the eye, in Renkin EM, Michel CC (eds): *Handbook of Physiology—The Cardiovascular System IV.* Washington, DC: American Physiological Society, 1984, 1001.
51. Nilsson SFE: Studies on ocular blood flow and aqueous humor dynamics. Effects of VIP and PHI related to the effects of facial nerve stimulation. *Acta Univ Uppsala 1986;43:1–38.*
52. Nilsson SFE, Samuelsson M, Bill A, et al: Increased uveoscleral outflow as a possible mechanism of ocular hypotension caused by prostaglandin F_2a-1-isopropylester in the cynomolgus monkey. *Exp Eye Res 1989;48:707–716.*
53. Raviola G: The structural basis of the blood-ocular barriers. *Exp Eye Res 1977;25(suppl):27–63.*
54. Bill A: Basic physiology of the drainage of aqueous humor. *Exp Eye Res 1977;25(suppl):291–304.*
55. Bartels SP: Aqueous humor formation. Fluid production by a sodium pump, in Ritch E, Shields MB, Krupin T (eds): *The Glaucomas* St. Louis:CV Mosby, 1989, 199.
56. Bill A: Blood circulation and fluid dynamics in the eye. *Physiol Rev 1975;55:383–417.*
57. Green K, Bountra C, Georgiou P, et al: An electrophysiologic study of rabbit ciliary epithelium. *Invest Ophthalmol Vis Sci 1985;26:371–381.*
58. Wiederholt M, Zadunaisky JA: Membrane potentials and intracellular chloride activity in the ciliary body of the shark. *Pflügers Arch 1986;407 (suppl 2):S112–S115.*
59. Lütjen-Drecoll E: Functional morphology of the ciliary epithelium, in Lütjen–Drecoll E (ed): *Basic Aspects of Glaucoma Research.* Stuttgart, New York: Schattauer-Verlag, 1982, 69.
60. Wiederholt M, Helbig H, Korbmacher C: Ion transport across the ciliary epithelium: Lessons from cultured cells and proposed role of the carbonic anhydrase, in Botré F, Gross G, Storey BT (eds): *Carbonic Anhydrase.* New York, Basel, Cambridge:Weinheim, 1991, 232.
61. Ghosh S, Freitag AC, Martin-Vasallo P, et al: Cellular distribution and differential gene expression of the three a subunit isoforms of the Na,K-ATPase in the ocular ciliary epithelium. *J Biol Chem 1990;265: 2935–2940.*
62. Martin–Vasallo P, Ghosh S, Coca–Prados M: Expression of Na,K-ATPase alpha subunit isoforms in the human ciliary body and cultured ciliary epithelial cells. *J Cell Physiol 1989;141:243–252.*
63. Reddy VN: Biochemistry of aqueous humor, in Lütjen–Drecoll E (ed): *Basic Aspects of Glaucoma Research.* Stuttgart, New York: Schattauer-Verlag, 1982, 89.

64. Bito LZ, Wallenstein MC: Transport of prostaglandins across the blood-brain and blood-aqueous barriers and the physiological significance of these absorptive transport processes. *Exp Eye Res 1977; 25(suppl):229–243.*
65. Topper JE, Brubaker RF: Effects of timolol, epinephrine, and acetazolamide on aqueous flow during sleep. *Invest Ophthalmol Vis Sci 1985; 26:1315–1319.*
66. Gharagozloo NZ, Larson RS, Kullerstrand W, et al: Terbutaline stimulates aqueous humor flow in humans during sleep. *Arch Ophthalmol 1988;106:1218–1220.*
67. Stone RA, Kuwayama Y: The nervous system and intraocular pressure, in Ritch E, Shields MB, Krupin T (eds): *The Glaucomas.* St. Louis: CV Mosby, 1989, 257.
68. Bill A: Effects of norepinephrine, isoproterenol and sympathetic stimulation on aqueous humour dynamics in vervet monkeys. *Exp Eye Res 1970;10:31–46.*
69. Larson RS, Brubaker RF: Isoproterenol stimulates aqueous flow in humans with Homer's syndrome. *Invest Ophthalmol Vis Sci 1988; 29:621–625.*
70. Nilsson SFE, Mäepea O, Samuelsson M, et al: Effects of timolol on terbutaline- and VIP-stimulated aqueous humor flow in the cynomolgus monkey. *Curr Eye Res 1990;9:863–872.*
71. Lee DA, Topper JE, Brubaker RF: Effect of clonidine on aqueous humor flow in normal human eyes. *Exp Eye Res 1984;38:239–246.*
72. Gharagozloo NZ, Relf SJ, Brubaker RF: Aqueous flow is reduced by the alpha-adrenergic agonist, apraclonidine hydrochloride (ALO 2145). *Ophthalmologia 1988;95:1217–1220.*
73. Kaufman PL, Wiedman T, Robinson JR: Cholinergics, in Sears ML (ed): *Pharmacology of the Eye.* Berlin, Heidelberg: Springer-Verlag, 1984, 149.
74. Honkanen RE, Howard EF, Abdel-Latif AA: M3-muscarinic receptor subtype predominates in the bovine iris sphincter smooth muscle and ciliary processes. *Invest Ophthalmol Vis Sci 1990;31:590–593.*
75. Sears ML: Regulation of aqueous flow by the adenylate cyclase receptor complex in the ciliary epithelium. *Am J Ophthalmol 1985; 100:194–198.*
76. Nathanson JA: Human ciliary process adrenergic receptor: pharmacological characterization. *Invest Ophthalmol Vis Sci 1981;21:798–804.*
77. Cepelík J, Cernohorsky M: The effects of adrenergic agonists and antagonists on the adenylate cyclase in albino rabbit ciliary processes. *Exp Eye Res 1981;32:291–299.*
78. Bausher LP, Gregory DS, Sears ML: Interaction between alpha$_2$- and b$_2$-adrenergic receptors in rabbit ciliary processes. *Curr Eye Res 1987; 6:497–505.*
79. Cepelík J, Hynie S: Inhibitory effects of clonidine and dopamine on adenylate cyclase of rabbit ciliary processes. *Curr Eye Res 1990;9: 111–120.*
80. Nilsson SFE: Neuropeptide Y (NPY): A vasoconstrictor in the eye, brain and other tissues in the rabbit. *Acta Physiol Scand 1991; 141:455–467.*
81. Cepelík J, Hynie S: Inhibitory effects of neuropeptide Y on adenylate cyclase of rabbit ciliary processes. *Curr Eye Res 1990;9:121–128.*
82. Bausher LP, Horio B: Neuropeptide Y and somatostatin inhibit stimulated cyclic AMP production in rabbit ciliary processes. *Curr Eye Res, 9:371–378.*
83. Jumblatt JE, Gooch JM: Neuropeptide Y modulates adenylate cyclase in the rabbit iris ciliary body and ciliary epithelium. *Exp Eye Res 51:229–231.*
84. Mittag TW, Tormay A, Podos SM: Vasoactive intestinal peptide and intraocular pressure: Adenylate cyclase activation and binding sites for vasoactive intestinal peptide in membranes of ocular ciliary processes. *J Pharmacol Exp Thera 1987;241:230–235.*
85. Bausher LP, Gregory DS, Sears ML: Alpha$_2$-receptors and VIP receptors in rabbit ciliary processes interact. *Curr Eye Res 1990;8:47–54.*

86. Tobin AB, Osborne NN: Evidence for the presence of cholinergic muscarinic receptors negatively linked to adenylate cyclase in the iris-ciliary body. *Neurochem Int 1988;13:517–523.*
87. Jumblatt JE, North GT, Hackmiller RC: Muscarinic cholinergic inhibition of adenylate cyclase in the rabbit iris-ciliary body and ciliary epithelium. *Invest Ophthalmol Vis Sci 1990;31:1103–1108.*
88. Samuelsson M, Nilsson SFE, Mäepea O, et al: Effects of atrial natriuretic factor (ANF) on intraocular pressure and aqueous humor flow in the cynomolgus monkey. *Exp Eye Res [in press].*
89. Brubaker RF: The effect of intraocular pressure on conventional outflow resistance in the enucleated human eye. *Invest Ophthalmol Vis Sci 1975;14:286–292.*
90. Emi K, Pederson JE, Toris CB: Hydrostatic pressure of the suprachoroidal space. *Invest Ophthalmol Vis Sci 1989;30:233–238.*
91. Kaufman PL: Pressure-dependent outflow, in Ritch E, Shields MB, Krupin T (eds): *The Glaucomas.* St. Louis: CV Mosby, 1989, 199.
92. Casey WJ: Cervical sympathetic stimulation in monkeys and the effects on outflow facility and intraocular volume. A study in the East African vervet (Cercopithecus aethiops). *Invest Ophthalmol Vis Sci 1966;5:33–41.*
93. Neufeld AH: Influences of cyclic nucleotides on outflow facility in the vervet monkey. *Exp Eye Res 1978;27:387–397.*
94. Toris CB, Pederson JE: Effect of intraocular pressure on uveoscleral outflow following cyclodialysis in the monkey eye. *Invest Ophthalmol Vis Sci 1985;26:1745–1749.*
95. Gabelt BT, Kaufman PL: Prostaglandin F_2a increases uveoscleral outflow in the cynomolgus monkey. *Exp Eye Res 1989;49:389–402.*
96. Lütjen–Drecoll E, Tamm E: Morphological study of the anterior segment of cynomolgus monkey eyes following treatment with prostaglandin F_2a. *Exp Eye Res 1988;47:761–769.*
97. Camras CB, Podos SM: The role of endogenous prostaglandins in clinically-used and investigational glaucoma therapy, in Bito LZ, Stjernschantz J (eds): *The Ocular Effects of Prostaglandins and Other Eicosanoids.* New York: Alan R Liss, 1989, 459.
98. Toris CB, Pederson JE: Aqueous humor dynamics in experimental iridocyclitis. *Invest Ophthalmol Vis Sci 1987;28:477–481.*
99. Maren TH: The kinetics of $HC0_3^-$ synthesis related to fluid secretion, pH control, and $C0_2$ elimination. *Annu Rev Physiol 1988;50:695–717.*
100. Maren TH: The development of ideas concerning the role of carbonic anhydrase in the secretion of aqueous humor: Relation to the treatment of glaucoma, in Drance SM, Neufeld AH (eds): *Glaucoma: Applied Pharmacology in Medical Treatment.* Orlando, FL: Grune & Stratton, 1984, 325.
101. Maren TH: Ion secretion into the posterior aqueous humor of dogs and monkeys. *Exp Eye Res 1977;(suppl 25):245–247.*
102. Cantley L, Carilli CT, Farley RA, et al: Location of binding sites on the (Na,K)-ATPase for fluorescein-5-isothiocyanate and ouabain. *Ann NY Acad Sci 1982;402:289–291.*
103. Bartels SP: Aqueous formation: Fluid production by a sodium pump, in Ritch R, Shields MB, Krupin T (eds): *The Glaucomas,* Vol. I. St. Louis: CV Mosby, 1989, 199.
104. Jorgenson PL: Mechanism of the Na^+, K^+ pump: Protein structure and conformations of the pure (N^+ + K^+)-ATPase. *Biochim Biophys Acta 1982;694:27–68.*
105. Katz AI: Role of Na-K-ATPase in kidney function, in Skou J, Norby JG, Maunsbach AB, Esmann M: *The Na^+, K^+ Pump, Part B: Cellular Aspects.* New York: Alan R Liss, 1988, 207.
106. Cole DF: Electrochemical changes associated with the formation of the aqueous humor. *Br J Ophthalmol 1961;45:202–217.*
107. Friedland BR, Maren TH: Carbonic anhydrase: Pharmacology of inhibitors and treatment of glaucoma, in Sears ML (ed): *Handbook of Experimental Pharmacology, Pharmacology of the Eye,* Vol 69. Berlin: Springer-Verlag, 1984, 279.

108. Conroy CW, Maren TH: The permeability of hydrophobic membranes to ^{22}Na salts and $^{14}CO_2$ in low dielectric media. *Biophys Chem 1989;34:177–184.*
109. Wistrand PJ, Schenholm M, Lönnerholm G: Carbonic anhydrase isoenzymes CA I and CA II in the human eye. *Invest Ophthalmol Vis Sci 1986;27:419–428.*
110. Murakami M, Sears M, Mori N, et al: The loci of carbonic anhydrase activity in the ciliary epithelium of the rabbit eye. *Acta Histochem Cytochem 1992;25:1–8.*
111. Lehmann B, Linner E, Wistrand PJ: The pharmacokinetics of acetazolamide in relation to its use in the treatment of glaucoma and its effects as an inhibitor of carbonic anhydrases, in Rospe G (ed): *Schering Workshop in Pharmakokinetics, Advances in the Biosciences 5.* New York: Pergamon, 1969, 197.
112. Higginbotham EJ: Topical carbonic anhydrase inhibitors. *Ophthalmol Clin North Am 1989;2:113–130.*
113. Maren TH, Bar-Ilan A, Conroy CW, et al: Chemical and pharmacological properties of MK-927, a sulfonamide carbonic anhydrase inhibitor that lowers intraocular pressure by the topical route. *Exp Eye Res 1990;50:27–36.*
114. Brechue WF, Maren TH: Correlation of drug accession with IOP reduction following local and intravenous carbonic anhydrase inhibitors (abstract). *Invest Ophthalmol Vis Sci 1991;32:1256.*
115. Sugrue MF, Mallorga P, Schwam H, et al: A comparison of L-671,152 and MK-927, two topically effective ocular hypotensive carbonic anhydrase inhibitors, in experimental animals. *Curr Eye Res 1990; 9:607–615.*
116. Helbig H, Korbmacher C, Erb C, et al: Coupling of ^{22}Na and ^{36}Cl uptake in cultured pigmented ciliary epithelial cells: A proposed role for the isoenzymes of carbonic anhydrase. *Curr Eye Res 1989;8: 1111–1119.*
117. Wiederholt M, Helbig H, Korbmacher C: Ion transport across the ciliary epithelium: Lessons from cultured cells and proposed role of the carbonic anhydrase, in Botrè F, Gross G (eds): *Carbonic Anhydrase.* Cambridge, New York: Verlag-Chemie, 1992, 232–244.
118. Wilcox CS: Diuretics, in Brenner BM, Rector FC (eds): *The Kidney,* Vol. II. Philadelphia: WB Saunders, 1991, 2123.
119. Maren TH, Vogh BP: Timolol appears to dissociate flow and Na^+ entry to the aqueous. *Invest Ophthalmol Vis Sci 1990;(suppl 31):182.*
120. Kishida K, Miwa Y, Iwata C: 2-substituted 1,3,4-thiadiazole-5-sulfonamides as carbonic anhydrase inhibitors: Their effects on the transepithelial potential difference of the isolated rabbit ciliary body and on the intraocular pressure of the living rabbit eye. *Exp Eye Res 1986; 43:981–995.*
121. Alvarado JA, Wood I, Polansky JR: Human trabecular cells II. Growth pattern and ultrastructural characteristics. *Invest Ophthalmol Vis Sci 1982;23:464–478.*
122. Polansky JR, Weinreb R, Alvarado JA: Studies on human trabecular cells propagated in vitro. *Vis Res 1981;21:155–160.*
123. Hernandez MR, Weinstein BI, Schwartz J, et al: Human trabecular meshwork cells in culture: Morphology and extracellular matrix components. *Invest Ophthalmol Vis Sci 1987;28:1655–1660.*
124. Crean EV, Tyson SL, Richardson TM: Factors influencing glycosaminoglycan synthesis by calf trabecular meshwork cell cultures. *Exp Eye Res 1986;43:365–374.*
125. Acott TS, Kingsley PD, Samples JR, Van Buskirk EM: Human trabecular meshwork organ culture: Morphology and glycosaminoglycan synthesis. *Invest Ophthalmol Vis Sci 1988;29:90–100.*
126. Shields MB: *Textbook of Glaucoma,* ed 2. Baltimore: Williams & Wilkins, 1987, 1–44.
127. Kolker AE, Hetherington J Jr (eds): *Becker–Shaffer's Diagnosis and Therapy of the Glaucomas,* ed 5. St. Louis: CV Mosby, 1983, 21–41.

128. Acott TS: Trabecular extracellular matrix regulation, in Drance SM, Van Buskirk EM, Neufeld AH (eds): *Applied Pharmacology of the Glaucomas.* Baltimore: Williams & Wilkins [in press].
129. Bárány EH, Scotchbrook S: Influence of testicular hyaluronidase on the resistance to flow through the angle of the anterior chamber. *Acta Physiol Scand 1954;30:240-248.*
130. Knepper PA, Farbman AI, Telser AG: Exogenous hyaluronidases and degradation of hyaluronic acid in the rabbit eye. *Invest Ophthalmol Vis Sci 1984;25:286-293.*
131. Grant WM: Experimental aqueous perfusion in enucleated human eyes. *Arch Ophthalmol 1963;69:783-801.*
132. Grant WM, Trotter RR: Tonographic measurements in enucleated eyes. *Arch Ophthalmol 1955;53:191–200.*
133. Van Buskirk EM, Grant WM: Influence of temperature and the question of involvement of cellular metabolism in aqueous outflow. *Am J Ophthalmol 1974;77:565–572.*
134. Epstein DL, Hashimoto JM, Anderson PJ, Grant WM: Effect of iodoacetamide perfusion on outflow facility and metabolism of the trabecular meshwork. *Invest Ophthalmol Vis Sci 1981;20:625-631.*
135. Hogan MJ, Alvarado JA, Weddell JE: *Histology of the Human Eye: An Atlas and Textbook.* Philadelphia: WB Saunders, 1971.
136. Eriksson A, Svedbergh B: Transcellular aqueous humor outflow: A theoretical and experimental study. *Graefes Arch Clin Exp Ophthalmol 1980;212:187-197.*
137. Tripathi RC: The functional morphology of the outflow systems of ocular and cerebrospinal fluids. *Exp Eye Res 1977;(suppl):65-116.*
138. Ethier CR, Kamm RD, Palaszwski BA, et al: Calculations of flow resistance in the juxtacanalicular meshwork. *Invest Ophthalmol Vis Sci 1986;27:1741–1750.*
139. McEwen WK: Application of Poiseuille's law to aqueous outflow. *Arch Ophthalmol 1958;60:290-294.*
140. Seiler T, Wollensak J: The resistance of the trabecular meshwork to aqueous humor outflow. *Graefes Arch Clin Exp Ophthalmol 1985; 223:88-91.*
141. Perkins TW, Alvarado JA, Polansky JR, et al: Trabecular meshwork cells grown on filters. *Invest Ophthalmol Vis Sci 1988;29:1836-1846.*
142. Perkins TW, Alvarado JA, Polansky JR, et al: Flow resistance measurements in cultured cells using a filter support system. *Invest Ophthalmol Vis Sci 1987;28(suppl):132.*
143. Nguyen K, Weiss H, Karageuzian LN, et al: Glutathione reductase of calf trabecular meshwork. *Invest Ophthalmol Vis Sci 1985;26:877–890.*
144. de Kater AW, Spurr-Michaud SJ, Gipson IK: Localization of smooth muscle myosin-containing cells in the aqueous outflow pathway. *Invest Ophthalmol Vis Sci 1990;31:347–353.*
145. Weinreb RN, Mitchell MD: Experimental investigation of intraocular eicosanoids: Cultured human trabecular cells and laser photocoagulation of the rabbit iris. *Curr Eye Res 1985;4:281–290.*
146. Richardson TM: Distribution of glycosaminoglycans in the aqueous outflow system of the cat. *Invest Ophthalmol Vis Sci 1982;22:319–329.*
147. Tawara A, Varner HH, Hollyfield JG: Distribution and characterization of sulfated proteoglycans in the human trabecular tissue. *Invest Ophthalmol Vis Sci 1989;30:2215–2231.*
148. Hascall VC, Hascall GK: Proteoglycans, in Hay ED (ed): *Cell Biology of Extracellular Matrix.* New York: Plenum Press, 1981, 39–63.
149. Wight TN, Mecham RP (eds): *Biology of Proteoglycans.* New York: Academic Press, 1987.
150. Heinegard D, Paulsson M: Structure and metabolism of proteoglycans, in Piez KA, Reddi AH (eds): *Extracellular Matrix Biochemistry.* New York: Elsevier, 1984, 277–328.
151. Hascall VC, Kimura JH: Proteoglycans: Isolation and characterization. *Methods Enzymol 1982;82:769-800.*
152. Evered D, Whelan J (eds): *Functions of the Proteoglycans. Ciba Foundation Symposium 124.* New York: John Wiley & Sons, 1986.

153. Arnott S, Rees DA, Morris ER: *Molecular Biophysics of the Extracellular Matrix.* Clifton, NJ: Humana Press, 1984.
154. Ruoslahti E: Proteoglycans in cell regulation. *J Biol Chem 1989; 264:13369–13372.*
155. Jackson RL, Busch SJ, Cardin AD: Glycosaminoglycans: Molecular properties, protein interactions, and role in physiological processes. *Physiol Rev 1991;71:481–539.*
156. Ruoslahti E: Structure and biology of proteoglycans. *Annu Rev Cell Biol 1988;4:229–255.*
157. Acott TS, Westcott M, Passo MS, Van Buskirk EM: Trabecular meshwork glycosaminoglycans in human and cynomolgus monkey eyes. *Invest Ophthalmol Vis Sci 1985;26:1320–1329.*
158. Schachtschabel DO, Bigalke B, Rohen JW: Production of glycosaminoglycans by cell cultures of the trabecular meshwork of the primate eye. *Exp Eye Res 1977;24:71–80.*
159. Schachtschabel DO, Rohen JW, Wever J, Sames K: Synthesis and composition of glycosaminoglycans by cultured human trabecular meshwork cells. *Graefes Arch Clin Exp Ophthalmol 1982;218:113–117.*
160. Breen M, Knepper PA, Weinstein HG, et al: Microanalysis of glycosaminoglycans. *Anal Biochem 1981;113:416–422.*
161. Knepper PA, Farbman AI, Telser AG: Aqueous outflow pathway glycosaminoglycans. *Exp Eye Res 1981;32:265-277.*
162. Grierson I, Lee WR: Acid mucopolysaccharides in the outflow apparatus. *Exp Eye Res 1975;21:417–431.*
163. Gum GC, Goossens W, Knepper PA: Histochemical localization of glycosaminoglycans in the glaucomatous and normal canine eye. *Invest Ophthalmol Vis Sci 1987;28(suppl):131.*
164. Greirson I, Lee WR, Abraham S: A light microscopic study of the effects of testicular hyaluronidase on the outflow system of a baboon (Papio cynocephalus). *Invest Ophthalmol Vis Sci 1979;18:356–360.*
165. Mathews CK, van Holde KE: *Biochemistry.* Redwood City, CA: Benjamin/Cummings, 1990.
166. Acott TS, Truesdale AT, Samples JR, Van Buskirk EM: Trabecular extracellular matrix synthesis in human explant organ culture. *Invest Ophthalmol Vis Sci 1986;26 (suppl):211.*
167. Acott TS, Nobis CA, Van Buskirk EM: Studies of human trabecular extracellular matrix proteoglycans. *Proc Int Soc Eye Res 1986;4:184.*
168. Hassell JR, Newsome DA, Balintine EJ: Synthesis of extracellular matrix components by trabecular meshwork in organ culture. *Invest Ophthalmol Vis Sci 1978;19 (suppl):273.*
169. Murphy CG, Yun AJ, Newsome DA, Alvarado JA: Localization of extracellular proteins of the trabecular meshwork by indirect immunofluorescence. *Am J Ophthalmol 1987;104:33m.*
170. Ogston AG: The biological functions of the glycosaminoglycans, in Balazs EA (ed): *Chemistry and Molecular Biology of the Intercellular Matrix.* Vol 3. New York: Academic Press, 1970, 1231–1240.
171. Bettelheim FA: Physical chemistry of acidic polysaccharides, in Vies A (ed): *Biological Polyelectrolytes.* New York: Marcel Dekker, 1970, 131–209.
172. Maroudas A: Physiochemical properties of cartilage in the light of ion exchange theory. *Biophys J 1968;8:575-595.*
173. Harper GS, Comper WD, Preston GN: Dissipative structures in proteoglycan solutions. *J Biol Chem 1984;259:10582-10589.*
174. Comper WD, Williams RPW: Hydrodynamics of concentrated proteoglycan solutions. *J Biol Chem 1987;262:13464-13471.*
175. Moroudas A, Jizrahi J, Katz EP, et al: Physiochemical properties and functional behavior of normal and osteoarthritic human cartilage, in Kuettner KE, Schleyerbach R, Hascall VC (eds): *Articular Cartilage Biochemistry.* New York: Raven Press, 1986, 311–329.
176. Matalon R: Mucopolysaccharidoses, in Gershwin ME, Robbins DL (eds): *Musculoskeletal Diseases of Children.* New York: Grune & Stratton, 1983, 381–445.
177. Kanwar YS, Linker A, Farquhar MG: Increased permeability of the glomerular basement membrane to ferritin after removal of gly-

cosaminoglycans (heparan sulfate) by enzyme digestion. *J Cell Biol 1980;86:688–693.*
178. Kanwar YS, Hascall VC, Farquhar MG: Partial characterization of newly synthesized proteoglycans isolated from the glomerular basement membrane. *J Cell Biol 1981;90:527–532.*
179. Kanwar YS, Rosenzweig LJ: Clogging of the glomerular basement membrane. *J Cell Biol 1982;93:489–494.*
180. Silvert CK, Kleinman HK: Studies of cultured human fibroblasts in diabetes mellitus: Changes in heparan sulfate. *Diabetes 1979; 28:61–64.*
181. Rohrbach DH, Hassell JR, Kleinman HK, Martin GR: Alterations in the basement membrane (heparan sulfate) proteoglycan in diabetic mice. *Diabetes 1982;31:185–188.*
182. Rohrbach DH, Wagner CW, Star VL, et al: Reduced synthesis of basement membrane heparan sulfate proteoglycan in streptozoticin-induced diabetic mice. *J Biol Chem 1983;258:11672–11677.*
183. Kramer RH, Vogel KG, Nicolson GL: Solubilization and degradation of subendothelial matrix glycoproteins and proteoglycans by metastatic tumor cells. *J Biol Chem 1982;257:2678–2686.*
184. Nakajima M, Irimura T, Di Ferrant N, Nicolson GL: Metastic melanoma cell heparanase. *J Biol Chem 1984;259:2283–2290.*
185. Lark MW, Laterra J, Culp LA: Close and focal contact adhesions of fibroblasts to a fibronectin-containing matrix. *Fed Proc 1985;44: 394–403.*
186. Hook M: Cell-surface glycosaminoglycans. *Annu Rev Biochem 1984; 53:847–869.*
187. Gallagher JT, Lyon M, Steward WP: Structure and function of heparan sulfate proteoglycans. *Biochem J 1986;236:313–325.*
188. Hassell JR: Proteoglycan core protein families. *Annu Rev Biochem 1986; 55:539–567.*
189. Gordon PB, Choi HU, Conn G, et al: Extracellular matrix heparan sulfate proteoglycans modulate the mitogenic capacity of acidic FGF. *J Cell Physiol 1989;140:584–592.*
190. Sommer A, Rifkin DB: Interaction of heparin with human basic FGF: Protection of the angiogenic protein from proteolytic degradation by a glycosaminoglycan. *J Cell Physiol 1989;138:215–220.*
191. Vigny M, Ollier-Hartmann MP, Lavigne M, et al: Specific binding of basic FGF to basement membrane-like structures and to purified heparan sulfate proteoglycan of the EHS tumor. *J Cell Physiol 1988; 137:321–328.*
192. Saksela O, Moscatelli D, Sommer A, Rifkin DB: Endothelial cell-derived heparan sulfate binds basic FGF and protects it from proteolytic degradation. *J Cell Biol 1988;107:743–751.*
193. Globus RK, Plouet J, Gospodarowicz D: Cultured bovine bone cells synthesize basic fibroblast growth factor and store in their extracellular matrix. *Endocrinology 1989;124:1539–1547.*
194. Klein-Soyer C, Beretz A, Cazenave J-P, et al: Sulfated polysaccharides modulate effects of acidic and basic fibroblast growth factors on repair of injured confluent human vascular endothelium. *Arteriosclerosis 1989;9:147-153.*
195. Timpl R: Structure and biological activity of basement membrane proteins. *Eur J Biochem 1989;180:487–502.*
196. Martin GR, Timpl R: Laminin and other basement membrane components. *Ann Rev Cell Biol 1987;3:57–85.*
197. Beck K, Hunter I, Engel J: Structure and function of laminin: anatomy of a multidomain protein. *FASEB J 1990;4:148–160.*
198. Ehrig K, Leivo I, Argraves WS, et al: Merosin, a tissue-specific basement membrane protein, is a laminin-like protein. *Proc Natl Acad Sci USA 1990;87:3264–3268.*
199. Sanes JR, Engvall E, Butkowski R, Hunter DD: Molecular heterogeneity of basal laminae: Isoforms of laminin and collagen IV at the neuromuscular junction and elsewhere. *J Cell Biol 1990;111:1685–1699.*
200. Panayotou G, End P, Aumailley M, et al: Domains of laminin with growth factor activity. *Cell 1989;56:93–101.*

201. Danemoto T, Reich R, Royce L, et al: Identification of an amino acid sequence from the laminin A chain that stimulates metastasis and collagenase IV production. *Proc Natl Acad Sci USA 1990;87:2279–2283.*
202. Yue BYJT, Higginbotham EJ, Chang IL: Ascorbic acid modulates the production of fibronectin and laminin by cells from an eye tissue–trabecular meshwork. *Exp Cell Res 1990;187:65–68.*
203. Kurosawa A, Elner VM, Yue BYJT, et al: Cultured trabecular-meshwork cells: Immunohistochemical and lectin-binding characteristics. *Exp Eye Res 1987;45:239–251.*
204. Polansky JR, Wood IS, Maglio MT, Alvarado JA: Trabecular meshwork cell culture in glaucoma research: Evaluation of biological activity and structural properties of human trabecular cells in vitro. *Ophthalmology 1984;91:580-595.*
205. Worthen DM, Cleveland PH: Fibronectin production by cultured human trabecular meshwork cells. *Invest Ophthalmol Vis Sci 1982; 23:265–269.*
206. Ruoslahti E: Fibronectin and its receptors. *Annu Rev Biochem 1988; 57:375–413.*
207. Hynes R: Molecular biology of fibronectin. *Annu Rev Cell Biol 1985; 1:67–90.*
208. Kornblihtt AR, Gutman A: Molecular biology of the extracellular matrix proteins. *Biol Rev 1988;63:465–507.*
209. Yurchenco PD, Schittny JC: Molecular architecture of basement membranes. *FASEB J 1990;4:1577–1590.*
210. Mayne R, Burgeson RE (eds): *Structure and Function of Collagen Types.* New York: Academic Press, 1987.
211. Rodrigues MM, Katz SI, Foidart J-M, Spaeth GL: Collagen, factor VIII antigen, and immunoglobulins in the human aqueous drainage channels. *Ann Acad Ophthalmol 1980;87:337–344.*
212. Hirano K, Kobayashi M, Kobayashi K, et al: Experimental formation of 100 nm periodic fibrils in the mouse corneal stroma and trabecular meshwork. *Invest Ophthalmol Vis Sci 1989;30:869–874.*
213. Lutjen-Drecoll E, Bittig M, Rauterberg J, et al: Immunomicroscopical study of type VI collagen in the trabecular meshwork of normal and glaucomatous eyes. *Exp Eye Res 1989;48:139–47.*
214. Sandberg LB, Soskel NT, Wolt TB: Structure of the elastic fiber: an overview. *J Invest Dermatol 1982;79:128s–132s* (and following reviews).
215. Sakai LY, Keene DR, Engvall E: Fibrillin, a new 350-kD glycoprotein, is a component of extracellular microfibrils. *J Cell Biol 1986;103: 2499–2509.*
216. Maddox BK, Sakai L, Keene DR, Glanville RW: Connective tissue microfibrils. Isolation and characterization of three large pepsin-resistant domains of fibrillin. *J Biol Chem 1989;264:21381–21385.*
217. Yamashita T, Rosen DA: The elastic tissue of primate trabecular meshwork. *Invest Ophthalmol Vis Sci 1964;3:85–95.*
218. Iwamoto T: Light and electron microscopy of the presumed elastic components on the trabeculae and scleral spur of the human eye. *Invest Ophthalmol Vis Sci 1964;3:144–156.*
219. Rohen JW, Lutjen–Drecoll E: Biology of the trabecular meshwork, in Lutjen-Drecoll E (ed): *Basic Aspects of Glaucoma Research.* Stuttgart: Schattauer Verlag, 1982, 141–166.
220. Rohen JW, Lutjen–Drecoll E: Ageing- and non-ageing processes within the connective tissues of the anterior segment of the eye, in Muller WEG, Rohen JW (eds): *Biochemical and Morphological Aspects of Ageing.* Weisbaden: Steiner Verlag, 1981, 157–174.
221. Lutjen–Drecoll E, Shimizu T, Rohrbach M, Rohen JW: Quantitative analysis of 'plaque material' in the inner- and outer wall of Schlemm's canal in normal- and glaucomatous eyes. *Exp Eye Res 1986;42: 443–455.*
222. Gong H, Trinkaus–Randall V, Freddo TF: Ultrastructural immunocytochemical localization of elastin in normal human trabecular meshwork. *Curr Eye Res 1989;8:1071–1082.*
223. Ruoslahti E, Pierschbacher MD: New perspectives in cell adhesion: RGD and integrins. *Science 1987;238:491–497.*

224. Hynes RO: Integrins: A family of cell surface receptors. *Cell 1987; 48:549–554.*
225. Albelda SM, Buck CA: Integrins and other cell adhesion molecules. *FASEB J 1990;4:2868–2880.*
226. Roden L: Structure and metabolism of connective tissue proteoglycans, in Lennarz WJ (ed): *The Biochemistry of Glycoproteins and Proteoglycans.* New York: Plenum Press, 1980, 267-371.
227. Kusche M, Torri G, Casu B, Lindahl U: Biosynthesis of heparin. *J Biol Chem 1990;265:7292–7300.*
228. Nuwayhic N, Glaser JH, Johnson JC, et al: Xylosylation and glucuronosylation reactions in rat liver Golgi apparatus and endoplasmic reticulum. *J Biol Chem 1986;261:12936–12941.*
229. Ratcliffe A, Fryer PR, Hardingham TE: Proteoglycan biosynthesis in chondrocytes: Protein A-gold localization of proteoglycan protein core and chondroitin sulfate within the Golgi subcompartments. *J Cell Biol 1985;101:2355–2365.*
230. Schwartz NB, Dorfman A: Purification of rat chondrosarcoma xylosyltransferase. *Arch Biochem Biophys 1975;171:136–144.*
231. Stoolmiller AC, Schwartz NB, Dorfman A: Biosynthesis of chondroitin 4-sulfate-proteoglycan by a transplantable rat chondrosarcoma. *Arch Biochem Biophys 1975;171:124–135.*
232. Stoolmiller AC, Horwitz AL, Dorfman A: Biosynthesis of the chondroitin sulfate proteoglycan: Purification and properties of xylosyltransferase. *J Biol Chem 1972;247:3525-3532.*
233. Schwartz NB, Roden L: Biosynthesis of chondroitin sulfate. Purification of UDP-Dxylose:core protein β-D-xylosyltransferase by affinity chromatography. *Carbohydr Res 1974;37:167–180.*
234. Schwartz NB: Biosynthesis of chondroitin sulfate: Role of phospholipids in the activity of UDP-D-galactose:D-xylose galactosyltransferase. *J Biol Chem 1976;252:285–291.*
235. Schwass DE, Pham JT, Acott TS: Human and bovine ocular tissues contain xylosyltransferase, a key enzyme in proteoglycan biosynthesis. *Exp Eye Res [in review].*
236. Pham JT, Acott TS, Schwass DE: Xylosyltransferase occurance and activity in the human and bovine eye. *J Cell Biol 1989;107:158a.*
237. Bourdon MA, Krusius T, Campbell S, et al: Identification and synthesis of a recognition signal for the attachment of glycosaminoglycans to proteins. *Proc Natl Acad Sci USA 1987;84:3194-3198.*
238. Mali M, Jaakkola P, Arvilommi A-M, Jalkanen M: Sequence of human syndecan indicates a novel gene family of integral membrane proteoglycans. *J Biol Chem 1990;265:6884–6889.*
239. Doege K, Sasaki M, Horigan E, et al: Complete primary structure of the rat cartilage proteoglycan core protein deduced from cDNA clones. *J Biol Chem 1987;262:17757–17767.*
240. Krueger RC Jr, Fields JA, Hildreth JIV, Schwartz NB: Chick cartilage chondroitin sulfate proteoglycan core protein. *J Biol Chem 1990; 265:12075–12087.*
241. Sugumaran G, Silbert JE: Biosynthesis of chondroitin sulfate: Organization of sulfation. *J Biol Chem 1989;264:3864–3868.*
242. Shuman MA, Polansky JR, Merkel C, Alvarado JA: Tissue plasminogen activator in cultured human trabecular meshwork cells. *Invest Ophthalmol Vis Sci 1988;29:401–405.*
243. Park JK, Tripathi RC, Tripathi BJ, Barlow GH: Tissue plasminogen activator in the trabecular endothelium. *Invest Ophthalmol Vis Sci 1987; 28:1341–1345.*
244. Alexander JP, Samples JR, Van Buskirk EM, Acott TS: Expression of matrix metalloproteinases and inhibitor by human trabecular meshwork. *Invest Ophthalmol Vis Sci 1991;32:172–180.*
245. Dano K, Andreasen PA, Grondahl-Hansen J, et al: Plasminogen activators, tissue degradation, and cancer. *Adv Cancer Res 1985;44:139–266.*
246. Quigley JP, Gold LI, Schwimmer R, Sullivan LM: Limited cleavage of cellular fibronectin by plasminogen activator purified from transformed cells. *Proc Natl Acad Sci USA 1987;84:2776–2780.*

247. Gold LI, Schwimmer R, Quigley JP: Human plasma fibronectin as a substrate for human urokinase. *Biochem J 1989;262:529–534.*
248. Birkedal–Hansen H: Catabolism and turnover of collagens: Collagenases. *Methods Enzymol 1987;144:140–171.*
249. Emonard H, Grimaud J-A: Matrix metalloproteinases—A review. *Cell Mol Biol 1990;36:131–153.*
250. Liotta LA, Stetler–Stevenson WG: Metalloproteinases and cancer invasion. *Cancer Biol 1990;1:99–106.*
251. Matrisian LM, Hogan BLM: Growth factor-regulated proteases and extracellular matrix remodeling during mammalian development. *Curr Top Dev Biol 1990;24:219–259.*
252. Alexander JP, Bradley JMB, Gabourel JD, Acott TS: Expression of matrix metalloproteinases and inhibitor by retinal pigment epithelium. *Invest Ophthalmol Vis Sci 1990;31:2520–2528.*
253. Van Wart HE, Birkedal–Hansen H: The cysteine switch: A principle of regulation of metalloproteinase activity with potential applicability to the entire matrix metalloproteinase gene family. *Proc Natl Acad Sci USA 1990;87:5578–82.*
254. Springman EB, Angleton EL, Birkedal–Hansen H, Van Wart HE: Multiple modes of activation of latent human fibroblast collagenase: Evidence for the role of a Cys^{73} active-site zinc complex in latency and a "cysteine switch" mechanism for activation. *Proc Natl Acad Sci USA 1990;87:364–368.*
255. Alexander JP, Fisk A, Acott T, Samples JR: Effects of steroids and interleukin-l on metalloproteinase production by the cells of the anterior segment. *Invest Ophthalmol Vis Sci 1991; 32 (suppl):874.*
256. Huang WD, Polansky JR, Wang A, et al: Changes in mRNA for extracellular matrix (ECM) and related proteinases following prolonged glucocorticoid (GC) treatment of cultured human trabecular meshwork. *Invest Ophthalmol Vis Sci 1991; 32(suppl):789.*
257. Stetler–Stevenson WG, Brown PD, Onisto M, et al: Tissue inhibitor of metalloproteinases-2 (TIMP-2) mRNA expression in tumor cell lines and human tumor tissues. *J Biol Chem 1990;265:13933–13938.*
258. Stetler–Stevenson WG, Krutzsch HC, Liotta LA: Tissue inhibitor of metalloproteinase (TIMP-2). A new member of the metalloproteinase inhibitor family. *J Biol Chem 1989;264:17374–17378.*
259. DeClerck YA, Yean T-D, Ratzkin BJ, et al: Purification and characterization of two related but distinct metalloproteinase inhibitors secreted by bovine aortic endothelial cells. *J Biol Chem 1989;264: 17445–17453.*
260. Cawston TE, Curry VA, Clark IM, Hazleman BL: Identification of a new metalloproteinase inhibitor that forms tight-binding complexes with collagenase. *Biochem J 1990;269:183–187.*
261. Higginbotham EJ, Yue BYJT, Crean E, Peace J: Effects of ascorbic acid on trabecular meshwork cells in culture. *Exp Eye Res 1988;46:507–516.*
262. Knepper PA, Breen M, Weinstein HG, Blacik LJ: Intraocular pressure and glycosaminoglycan distribution in the rabbit eye: Effects of age and dexamethasone. *Exp Eye Res 1978;27:567-575.*
263. Knepper PA, Collins JA, Frederick R: Effect of dexamethasone, progesterone and testosterone on IOP and GAGs in the rabbit eye. *Invest Ophthalmol Vis Sci 1985;26:1093-1100.*
264. Nobis CA, Polansky J, Acott TS, et al: Evaluations of proteoglycans and glycoproteins from cultured human trabecular cells. *Invest Ophthalmol Vis Sci 1986; 27(suppl):164.*
265. Johnson DH, Bradley JMB, Acott TS, et al: The effect of steroids on human trabecular meshwork in perfusion organ culture. *Invest Ophthalmol Vis Sci 1989; 30(suppl):223.*
266. Higginbotham EJ, Richardson TM: The effect of vitamin A on glycoconjugate synthesis in the trabecular meshwork. *Exp Eye Res 1987; 44:697–702.*
267. Parshley DL, Alexander JP, Bradley JMB, et al: Trabecular meshwork secretion of matrix metalloproteinases is affected by several growth factors. *Invest Ophthalmol Vis Sci 1990;31(suppl):339.*

268. Lewin B: *Genes*, ed 3. New York: John Wiley & Sons, 1987.
269. Atwater JA, Wisdom R, Verma IM: Regulated mRNA stability. *Annu Rev Genet 1990;24:519–541.*
270. Sawadogo M, Sentenac A: RNA polymerase B (II) and general transcription factors. *Annu Rev Biochem 1990;59:711–754.*
271. Mitchell PJ, Tjian R: Transcriptional regulation in mammalian cells by sequence-specific DNA binding proteins. *Science 1989;245:371–378.*
272. Ransome LJ, Verma IM: Nuclear proto-oncogenes Fos and Jun. *Annu Rev Cell Biol 1990;6:539–557.*
273. Struhl K: Helix-turn-helix, zinc-finger, and leucine-zipper motifs for eukaryotic transcriptional regulatory proteins. *Trends Biochem Sci 1989;14:137–140.*
274. Muller MM, Gerster T, Schaffner W: Enhancer sequences and the regulation of gene transcription. *Eur J Biochem 1988;176:485–495.*
275. Adhya S, Garges S: Positive control. *J Biol Chem 1990;265: 10797–10800.*
276. Jones H: Transcriptional regulation by dimerization: Two sides to an incestuous relationship. *Cell 1990;61:9–11.*
277. Johnson PF, McKnight SL: Eukaryotic transcriptional regulatory proteins. *Annu Rev Biochem 1989;58:799–839.*
278. Angel P, Baumann I, Stein B, et al: 12-0-tetradecanoyl-phorbol-13-acetate induction of the human collagenase gene is mediated by an inducible enhancer element located in the 5′-flanking region. *Mol Cell Biol 1987;7:2256–2266.*
279. Kim S-J, Lafyatis R, Kim KY, et al: Regulation of collagenase gene expression by okadaic acid, an inhibitor of protein phosphatases. *Cell Regul 1990;1:269–278.*
280. Kerr LD, Hold JT, Matrisian LM: Growth factors regulate transin gene expression by c-fos-dependent and c-fos-independent pathways. *Science 1988;242:1424–1427.*
281. Fini ME, Plucinska IM, Mayer AS, et al: A gene for rabbit synovial cell collagenase: Member of a family of metalloproteinases that degrade the connective tissue matrix. *Biochemistry 1987;26:6156-6165.*
282. Auwerx J, Staels B, Sassone–Corsi P: Coupled and uncoupled induction of fos and jun transcription by different second messengers in cells of hematopoietic origin. *Nucleic Acids Res 1990;18:221–228.*
283. Binetruy B, Smeal T, Karin M: Ha-Ras augments c-Jun activity and stimulates phosphorylation of its activation domain. *Nature 1991; 351:122–127.*
284. Montminy MR, Gonzales GA, Yamamoto KK: Regulation of cAMP-inducible genes by CREB. *Rec Prog Horm Res 1990;46:219–229.*
285. Akerblom IE, Slater EP, Beato M, et al: Negative regulation by glucocorticoids through interference with a cAMP responsive enhancer. *Science 1988;241:350–353.*
286. Diamond MI, Milner JN, Yoshinaga SK, Yamamoto KR: Transcription factor interactions: Selectors of positive and negative regulation from a single DNA element. *Science 1990;249:1266–72.*
287. Nicholson RC, Mader S, Nagpal S, et al: Negative regulation of the rat stromelysin gene promoter by retinoic acid is mediated by an API binding site. *EMBO J 1990;9:4443–4454.*
288. Lin Y-S, Carey M, Ptashne M, Green MR: How different eukaryotic transcriptional activators can cooperate promiscuously. *Nature 1990; 345:359–361.*
289. Ptashne M: How eukaryotic transcriptional activators work. *Nature 1988;335:683–689.*
290. Ptashne M, Gann AAF: Activators and targets. *Nature 1990;346: 329–331.*
291. Frisch SM, Morisaki JH: Positive and negative transcriptional elements of the human type IV collagenase gene. *Mol Cell Biol 1990;10: 6524–6532.*
292. Bylsma SS, Samples JR, Acott TS, Van Buskirk EM: Trabecular cell division after argon laser trabeculoplasty. *Arch Ophthalmol 1988; 106:544–547.*

293. Van Buskirk EM, Pond V, Rosenquist RC, Acott TS: Argon laser trabeculoplasty: Studies of mechanism of action. *Ophthalmology 1984; 91:1005-1010.*
294. Dueker DK, Norberg M, Johnson DH, et al: Stimulation of cell division by argon and Nd:YAG laser trabeculoplasty in cynomolgus monkeys. *Invest Ophthalmol Vis Sci 1990;31:115–124.*
295. Acott TS, Samples JR, Bradley JMB, et al: Trabecular repopulation by anterior trabecular meshwork cells after laser trabeculoplasty. *Am J Ophthalmol 1989;107:1–6.*
296. Ruddat MS, Alexander JP, Samples JR, et al: Early changes in trabecular metalloproteinase mRNA levels in response to laser trabeculoplasty are induced by a media-borne factor. *Invest Ophthalmol Vis Sci 1989; 30(suppl):280.*
297. Hadaegh A, Bradley JMB, Gibson S, et al: Analysis of changes in trabecular stromelysin immunolocalization in response to laser trabeculoplasty. *Invest Ophthalmol Vis Sci 1991;32(suppl):875.*
298. Ken J, Wolf P: Presence and distribution of vimentin in cynomolgus monkey trabecular cells. *Anat Rec 1988;222:309–316.*
299. Sherwood ME, Richardson TM: Phagocytosis by trabecular meshwork cells: Sequence of events in cats and monkeys. *Exp Eye Res 1988;46: 881–895.*
300. Rohen JW, van der Zypen E: The phagocytic activity of the trabecular meshwork endothelium: An electron-microscopic study of the vervet (Cercopithecus aethiops). *Graefes Arch Clin Exp Ophthalmol 1968; 175:143–160.*
301. Shirato S, Murphy CG, Bloom E, et al: Alvarado JA: Kinetics of phagocytosis in trabecular meshwork cells. *Invest Ophthalmol Vis Sci 1989; 30:2499–2511.*
302. Grierson I, Lee WR: Erythrocyte phagocytosis in the human trabecular meshwork. *Br J Ophthalmol 1973;57:400–415.*
303. Gipson IK, Anderson RA: Actin filaments in cells of human trabecular meshwork and Schlemm's canal. *Invest Ophthalmol Vis Sci 1979; 18:547–561.*
304. Ryder MI, Weinreb RN, Alvarado J, Polansky J: The cytoskeleton of the cultured human trabecular cell. *Invest Ophthalmol Vis Sci 1988;29:251-260.*
305. Weinreb RN, Ryder MI: In situ localization of cytoskeletal elements in the human trabecular meshwork and cornea. *Invest Ophthalmol Vis Sci 1990;31:1839–1847.*
306. Grierson I, Millar L, De Yong J, et al: *Invest Ophthalmol Vis Sci 1986; 27:1318–1330.*
307. Kaufman PL, Bill A, Barany EH: Effect of cytochalasin B on conventional drainage of aqueous humor in the cynomolgus monkey. *Exp Eye Res 1977; (suppl):411–414.*
308. Kaufman PL, Barany EH: Cytochalasin B reversibly increases outflow facility in the eye of the cynomolgus monkey. *Invest Ophthalmol Vis Sci 1977;16:47–53.*
309. Yue BYJT, Elner VM, Davis HR: Lysosomal enzyme activities in cultured trabecular meshwork cells. *Exp Eye Res 1987;44:891–898.*
310. Jeng S, Weinreb RN, Miller AL: Characterization of lysosomal enzymes from cultured cynomolgus monkey trabecular meshwork cells. *Invest Ophthalmol Vis Sci 1990;31:1560–1566.*
311. Epstein DL, Anderson PJ: The biochemistry of outflow mechanisms, in Drance SM (ed): *Glaucoma: Applied Pharmacology in Medical Treatment.* New York: Grune & Stratton, 1984, 135–150.
312. Anderson PJ, Wang J, Epstein DL: Metabolism of calf trabecular (reticular) meshwork. *Invest Ophthalmol Vis Sci 1980;19:13–20.*
313. Anderson PJ, Karageuzian LN, Cheng H-M, Epstein DL: Hexokinase of calf trabecular meshwork. *Invest Ophthalmol Vis Sci 1984;25: 1258–1261.*
314. Anderson PJ, Karageuzian LN, Epstein DL: Phosphofructokinase of calf trabecular meshwork. *Invest Ophthalmol Vis Sci 1984;25: 1262–1266.*

315. Nguyen K, Lee DA, Anderson PJ, Epstein DL: Glucose 6-phosphate dehydrogenase of calf trabecular meshwork. *Invest Ophthalmol Vis Sci 1986;27:992–997.*
316. Alvarado J, Murphy C, Polansky J, Juster R: Age-related changes in trabecular meshwork cellularity. *Invest Ophthalmol Vis Sci 1981;21: 714–727.*
317. Alvarado J, Murphy C, Juster R: Trabecular meshwork cellularity in primary open-angle glaucoma and nonglaucomatous normals. *Ophthalmology 1984;91:564–579.*
318. Knepper PA, Hvizd MG, Goossens W, et al: GAG profile of human TM in primary open-angle glaucoma. *Invest Ophthalmol Vis Sci 1989; 30(suppl):224.*
319. Knepper PA, Hvizd MG, Higbee RG, et al: Heparitin sulfates and GAG-ase resistant material of normal human and primate trabecular meshwork. *Invest Ophthalmol Vis Sci 1988;29(suppl):128.*
320. Anderson PJ, Karageuzian LN, Suzuki R, et al: Effects of oxidative stress on calf trabecular meshwork and pulmonary aortic endothelial cells in culture. *Invest Ophthalmol Vis Sci 1988;29(suppl):129.*
321. Freedman SF, Anderson PJ, Epstein DL: Superoxide dismutase and catalase of calf trabecular meshwork. *Invest Ophthalmol Vis Sci 1985; 26:16–21.*
322. Scott DR, Karageuzian LN, Anderson PJ, Epstein DL: Glutathione peroxidase of calf trabecular meshwork. *Invest Ophthalmol Vis Sci 1984; 25:599–602.*
323. Epstein DL, De Kater AW, Lou M, Patel J: Influences of glutathione and sulfhydryl containing compounds on aqueous humor outflow function. *Exp Eye Res 1990;50:785–793.*
324. Lindenmayer JM, Kahn MG, Hertzmark E, Epstein DL: Morphology and function of the aqueous outflow system in monkey eyes perfused with sulfhydryl reagents. *Invest Ophthalmol Vis Sci 1983;24:710-717.*
325. Russell P, Garland D, Epstein DL: Analysis of the proteins of calf and cow trabecular meshwork: Development of a model system to study aging effects and glaucoma. *Exp Eye Res 1989;48:251–260.*
326. Polansky JR, Alvarado JA: Isolation and evaluation of target cells in glaucoma research: Hormone receptors and drug responses. *Curr Eye Res 1985;4:267–279.*
327. Kon S-WM, Yue BYJT: Effects of agonists on the intracellular cyclic AMP concentration in monkey trabecular meshwork cells. *Curr Eye Res 1988;7:75–80.*
328. Karnezis TA, Tripathi BJ, Dawson G, et al: Effects of dopamine receptor activation on the level of cyclic AMP in the trabecular meshwork. *Invest Ophthalmol Vis Sci 1989;30:1090–1094.*
329. Neufeld AH, Dueker DK, Vegge T, Sears ML: Adenosine 3′,5′-monophosphate increases the outflow of aqueous humor from the rabbit eye. *Invest Ophthalmol 1975;14:40–42.*
330. Neufeld AH, Sears ML: Cyclic-AMP in ocular tissues of the rabbit, monkey, and human. *Invest Ophthalmol 1974;13:475–477.*
331. Birnbaumer L: Transduction of receptor signals into modulation of effector activity by G proteins: The first 20 years or so. *FASEB J 1990; 4:3068–3078.*
332. Wax MB, Molinoff PB, Alvarado J, Polansky J: Characterization of β-adrenergic receptors in cultured human trabecular cells and in human trabecular meshwork. *Invest Ophthalmol Vis Sci 1989; 30:51–57.*
333. Jampel HD, Lynch MG, Brown RH, et al: β-adrenergic receptors in human trabecular meshwork. *Invest Ophthalmol Vis Sci 1987;28: 772–779.*
334. Weinreb RN, Bloom E, Baxter JD, et al: Detection of glucocorticoid receptors in cultured human trabecular cells. *Invest Ophthalmol Vis Sci 1981;21:403–407.*
335. Weinreb RN, Mitchel MD, Alvarado JA, Polansky JR: Glucocorticoid regulation of eicosanoid biosynthesis in cultured human trabecular cells, in Ticho U, Davis R (eds): *Recent Advances in Glaucoma.* Amsterdam: Elsevier, 1984, 213–218.

336. Yun AJ, Murphy CG, Polansky JR, et al: Proteins secreted by human trabecular cells. *Invest Ophthalmol Vis Sci 1989;30:2012–2022.*
337. Weinstein BI, Munnangi P, Grodon GG, Southern AL: Defects in cortisol-metabolizing enzymes in primary open-angle glaucoma. *Invest Ophthalmol Vis Sci 1985;26:890–893.*
338. Partridge CA, Weinstein BI, Southern AL, Gerritsen ME: Dexamethasone induces specific proteins in human trabecular meshwork cells. *Invest Ophthalmol Vis Sci 1989;30:1843–1847.*
339. Weinreb RN, Mitchell MD, Polansky JR: Prostaglandin production by human trabecular cells: In vitro inhibition by dexamethasone. *Invest Ophthalmol Vis Sci 1983;24:1541–1545.*
340. Tripathi BJ, Tripathi RC, Swift HH: Hydrocortisone-induced DNA endoreplication in human trabecular cells in vitro. *Exp Eye Res 1989; 49:259–270.*
341. Polansky J, Palmberg P, Matulich D, et al: Cellular sensitivity to glucocorticoids in patients with POAG. Steroid receptors and responses in cultured skin fibroblasts. *Invest Ophthalmol Vis Sci 1985; 26:805–809.*
342. Tschumper RC, Johnson DH, Bradley JMB, Acott TS: Glycosaminoglycans of human trabecular meshwork in perfusion organ culture. *Curr Eye Res 1990;9:363–369.*
343. Hanihara H, Ohuchi T, Yoshimura N, et al: Heterogeneous response in calcium signaling by adrenergic and cholinergic stimulation in cultured bovine trabecular cells. *Exp Eye Res 1991;52:393–396.*
344. Kerppola TK, Curran T: DNA bending by Fos and Jun: The flexible hinge model. *Science 1991;254:1210–1214.*

CHAPTER 2
THE NORMAL POSTERIOR SEGMENT

1. Duke–Elder S: *System of Ophthalmology,* Vol III, Part I. *Embryology*. St. Louis: CV Mosby, 1963.
2. Mann I: *Development of the Human Eye*. Cambridge, UK: Cambridge Press, 1949.
3. Barber AN: *Embryology of the Human Eye*. St. Louis: CV Mosby, 1955.
4. Haden H: The development of the ectodermal framework of the optic nerve with special reference to the glial lamina cribrosa. *Am J Ophthalmol 1947;30:1205–1214.*
5. Ikeda H, Wright MJ: How large is the receptive field of a single retinal ganglion cell? *J Physiol (Lond) 1971;217:52–53.*
6. Miller NR: *Walsh and Hoyt's Clinical Neuro-Ophthalmology*. Baltimore: Williams & Wilkins, 1982.
7. Radius RL, Anderson DR: The histology of retinal nerve fiber bundles and bundle defects. *Arch Ophthalmol 1979;97:948–950.*
8. Ogden TE: Nerve fiber layer astrocytes of the primate retina: Morphology, distribution and density. *Invest Ophthalmol Vis Sci 1978; 17:499-510.*
9. Wolter JR: The cells of remak and the astroglia of the normal human retina. *Arch Ophthalmol 1955;53:832–838.*
10. Anderson DR: Ultrastructure of human and monkey lamina cribrosa and optic nerve head. *Arch Ophthalmol 1969;82:800–814.*
11. Anderson DR: Ultrastructure of the optic nerve head. *Arch Ophthalmol 1970;83:63–73.*
12. Anderson DR, Hoyt WF: Ultrastructure ofthe intraorbital portion of human and monkey optic nerve. *Arch Ophthalmol 1969;82:506–530.*
13. Anderson DR, Hoyt WF, Hogan MJ: The fine structure of the astroglia in the human optic nerve and optic nerve head. *Trans Am Ophthalmol Soc 1967;65:275–305.*
14. Hogan MJ, Alvarado JA, Weddell JE *Histology of the Human Eye. An Atlas and Textbook.* Philadelphia: WB Saunders, 1971.
15. Hoyt WF, Schlicke B, Eckelhoff RJ: Fundoscopic appearance of a nerve fiber bundle defect. *Br J Ophthalmol 1972;56:577–583.*
16. Quigley HA, Addicks EM, Green WR: Optic nerve damage in human glaucoma. III. Quantitative correlation of nerve fiber loss and visual field defect in glaucoma, ischemic neuropathy, papilledema, and toxic neuropathy. *Arch Ophthalmol 1982;100:135–146.*

17. Radius RL, Anderson DR: The course of axons through the retina and optic nerve head. *Arch Ophthalmol 1979;97:1154–1158.*
18. Radius RL, DeBruin J: Anatomy of the retinal nerve fiber layer. *Invest Ophthalmol Vis Sci 1981;21:745–749.*
19. Radius RL: Thickness of the retinal nerve fiber layer in primate eyes. *Arch Ophthalmol 1980;98:1625–1629.*
20. Hoyt WF: Anatomic considerations of arcuate scotomas associated with lesions of the optic nerve and chiasm. Nauta axon degeneration study in the monkey. *Bull Johns Hopkins Hosp 1962;111:57–74.*
21. Hoyt WF, Luis OL: Visual fiber anatomy in the infrageniculate pathway of the primate; uncrossed and crossed retinal quadrant fiber projections studied with Nauta silver stain. *Arch Ophthalmol 1962; 68:94–106.*
22. Hoyt WF, Tudor RC: The course of peripapillary temporal retinal axons through the anterior optic nerve: A Nauta degeneration study in the primate. *Arch Ophthalmol 1963;69:503–507.*
23. Ronne H: Der anatomische Projektion der Macula im Corpus geniculatum externa. *Z Gesell Neurol Pschiat 1914;22:469–485.*
24. Minkler DS: The organization of nerve fiber bundles in the primate optic nerve head. *Arch Ophthalmol 1980;98:1630–1636.*
25. Ogden TE: Nerve fiber layer of the macaque retina: Retinotopic organization. *Invest Ophthalmol Vis Sci 1983;24:85–98.*
26. Ogden TE: Nerve fiber layer of the owl monkey retina: Retinotopic organization. *Invest Ophthalmol Vis Sci 1983;24:265–269.*
27. Anderson DR, Braverman S: Reevaluation of the optic disk vasculature. *Am J Ophthalmol 1976;82:165–174.*
28. Francois J, Neetens A: Functional importance of the anterior optic nerve supply. *Ophthalmologica 1974;168:122–127.*
29. Hayreh SS: Blood supply of the optic nerve head and its role in optic atrophy, glaucoma, and oedema of the optic disc. *Br J Ophthalmol 1969;53:721–748.*
30. Henkind P, Levitsky M: Angioarchitecture of the optic nerve head. *Am J Ophthalmol 1969;68:979–986.*
31. Lieberman MF, Maumenee AE, Green WR: Histologic studies of the vasculature of the anterior optic nerve. *Am J Ophthalmol 1976; 82:405–423.*
32. Ben-Sira I, Riva CE: Fluorescein diffusion in the human optic disc. *Invest Ophthalmol Vis Sci 1975;14:205–211.*
33. Grayson MC, Laties AM: Ocular localization of sodium fluorescein: Effects of administration in rabbit and monkey. *Arch Ophthalmol 1971;85:600–609.*
34. Olsson Y, Kristensson K: Permeability of blood vessels and connective tissue sheaths in retina and optic nerve. *Acta Neuropathol 1973; 26:147–156.*
35. Alm A, Bill A: The oxygen supply to the retina. II. Effects of high intraocular pressure and of increased arterial carbon dioxide on uveal and retinal blood flow in cats. A study with radioactively labelled microspheres including flow determinations in brain and other tissues. *Acta Physiol Scand 1972;84:306–319.*
36. Alm A, Bill A: Ocular and optic nerve blood flow at normal and increased intraocular pressures in monkeys (Macaca irus): A study with radioactively labelled microspheres including flow determinations in brain and other tissues. *Exp Eye Res 1973;15:15–29.*
37. Geijer C, Bill A: Effects of raised intraocular pressure on retinal, prelaminar, laminar and retrolaminar optic nerve blood flow in monkeys. *Invest Ophthalmol Vis Sci 1979;18:1030–1042.*
38. Quigley HA, Hohman RM, Sanchez R, Addicks EM: Optic nerve head blood flow in chronic experimental glaucoma. *Arch Ophthalmol 1986;103:956–962.*
39. Sossi N, Anderson DR: Effect of elevated intraocular pressure on blood flow; occurrence in cat optic nerve head studied with iodoantipyrine 1925. *Arch Ophthalmol 1983;101:98–101.*

40. Anderson DR: The optic nerve in glaucoma, in Duane TD, Yaeger ER (eds): *Thomas C. Duane's Clinical Ophthalmology.* Philadelphia: Harper & Row, 1985.
41. Guist G: *Coincident Ophthalmoscopy and Histology of the Optic Nerve.* Vienna: Guist, 1934.
42. Potts AM, Hodges D, Shelman CB, et al: Morphology of the primate optic nerve. Invest. *Ophthalmol Vis Sci 1972;11:980–988.*
43. Teal PK, Morin JD, McCulloch C: Assessment of the normal disc. *Trans Am Ophthalmol Soc 1972;70:164–177.*
44. Minkler DS, McLean IW, Tso MOM: Distribution of axonal and glial elements in the rhesus optic nerve head studied by electron microscopy. *Am J Ophthalmol 1976;82:179–187.*
45. Elschnig A: Das Colobom am Sehnerveneintritte und der Conus nach unten. *Graefes Arch Ophthalmol 1900;51:391–430.*
46. Emery JK, Landis D, Paton D: The lamina cribrosa in normal and glaucomatous eyes. *Trans Am Acad Ophthalmol Otolaryngol 1974;78: OP290–297.*
47. Quigley HA, Addicks EM: Quantitative studies of nerve fiber layer defects in glaucoma. *Arch Ophthalmol 1982;100:807–814.*
48. Radius RL: Regional specificity in anatomy at the lamina cribrosa. *Arch Ophthalmol 1981;99:478–480.*
49. Radius RL, Gonzales M: Anatomy at the lamina cribrosa in human eyes. *Arch Ophthalmol 1981;99:2159–2162.*
50. Kuhnt H: Zur Kenntnis des Sehnerven und der Netzhaut. *Graefes Arch Ophthalmol 1879;25:179–288.*
51. Jacoby E: Über den Neuroglia der Sehnerven. *Klin Mbl Augenheilk 1905; 43:129–137.*
52. Cohen AI: Ultrastructural aspects of the human optic nerve. *Invest Ophthalmol Vis Sci 1967:6:294–308.*
53. Yamamoto T: Electron microscopic observation of the human optic nerve. *Jpn J Ophthalmol 1966;10:40–53.*
54. Konomi K, Hayashi T, Sano J, et al: Immunohistochemical localization of type I, III, and IV collagens in the sclera and choroid of bovine, rat and normal and pathological human eyes. *Biomed Res 1983;4:451–458.*
55. Tengroth B, Ammitzboll T: Changes in the content and composition of collagen in the glaucomatous eye—basis for a new hypothesis for the genesis of chronic open angle glaucoma. *Acta Ophthalmol 1984; 62:999–1008.*
56. Hay ED: *Cell Biology of Extracellular Matrix,* ed 2. New York: Plenum Press, 1983.
57. Hernandez MR, Luo XX, Igoe F, Neufeld AH: Extracellular matrix of the human lamina cribrosa. *Am J Ophthalmol 1987;104:567–576.*
58. Anderson DA: Ultrastructure of human and monkey lamina cribrosa and optic nerve head. *Arch Ophthalmol 1969;82:800–814.*
59. Hernandez MR, Igoe F, Neufeld AH: Extracellular matrix of the human optic nerve head. *Am J Ophthalmol 1986;102:139–148.*
60. Elkington AR, Inman CBE, Steart PV, Weller RO: The structure of the lamina cribrosa of the human eye: An immunocytochemical and electron microscopical study. *Eye 1990;4:42–57.*
61. Hernandez MR, Luo XX, Andrzejewska W, Neufeld AH: Age-related changes in the extracellular matrix of the human optic nerve head. *Am J Ophthalmol 1989;107:476–484.*
62. Goldbaum MH, Jeng S, Logemann R, Weinreb RN: The extracellular matrix of the human optic nerve. *Arch Ophthalmol 1989;107: 1225–1231.*
63. Ogden TE, Duggan J, Danley K, et al: Morphometry of nerve fiber bundle pores in the optic nerve head of the human. *Exp Eye Res 1988; 46:559–568.*
64. Vrabec F: Age changes of the human optic nerve. A neurohistologic study. *Graefe's Arch Clin Exp Ophthalmol 1977;202:231–236.*
65. Repka MX, Quigley HA: The effect of age on normal human optic nerve fiber number and diameter. *Ophthalmology 1989;96:26–32.*

66. Quigley HA, Green WR: The histology of human glaucoma cupping and optic nerve damage: Clinicopathologic correlation in 21 eyes. *Ophthalmology 1979;86:1803–1830.*
67. Kaplan E, Lee BB, Shapley RM: New views of primate retinal function, in Osborne N, Chader J, (eds): *Progress in Retinal Research,* Vol 9. New York: Pergamon Press, 1990, 273–336.
68. Shapley R, Perry VH: Cat and monkey retinal ganglion cells and their visual functional roles. *Trends Neurosci 1986;9:229–235.*
69. Leventhal AG, Rodieck RW, Dreher B: Retinal ganglion cell classes in the old world monkey: Morphology and central projections. *Science 1981;213:1139–1142.*
70. Quigley HA, Dunkelberger GR, Green WR: Chronic human glaucoma causing selectively greater loss of large optic nerve fibers. *Ophthalmology 1988;95:357–363.*
71. Quigley HA, Dunkelberger GR, Green WR: Retinal ganglion cell atrophy correlated with automated perimetry in human eyes with glaucoma. *Am J Ophthalmol 1989;107:453–464.*
72. Glovinsky Y, Quigley HA, Dunkelberger GR: Retinal ganglion cell loss is size dependent in experimental glaucoma. *Invest Ophthalmol Vis Sci 1991;32:484–491.*

CHAPTER 3
DIAGNOSTIC TECHNIQUES OF THE ANTERIOR SEGMENT

1. Stamper RL: *Glaucoma, Lens, and Anterior Segment Trauma.* Section 8. *Basic and Clinical Science Course.* San Francisco: American Academy of Ophthalmology, 1987.
2. Krupin T: *Manual of Glaucoma: Diagnosis and Management.* New York: Churchill Livingstone, 1988, 7–18.
3. Ritch R, Reyes A: Moustache glaucoma. *Arch Ophthalmol 1988; 106:1503.*
4. Minckler DS, Baerveldt G, Heuer D, et al: Clinical evaluation of the Oculab Tono-pen to the Goldmann applanation tonometer. *Am J Ophthalmol 1990;104:168–173.*
5. Lim JI, Blair NP, Higginbotham EJ, et al: Assessment of intraocular pressure in vitrectomized gas-containing eyes. *Arch Ophthalmol 1990;108:684–688.*
6. Kao SF, Lichter PR, Bergstrom TJ, et al: Clinical comparison of the Oculab Tono-pen to the Goldmann applanation tonometer. *Ophthalmologia 1987;94:1541–1544.*
7. Grant WM: Tonography: Past, present, and future. *Ophthalmology 1978;85:252–258.*
8. Grant WM: A tonographic method for measuring the facility and rate of aqueous flow in human eyes. *Arch Ophthalmol 1950;44:204–214.*
9. Grant WM: Clinical measurements of aqueous outflow. *Arch Ophthalmol 1951;46:113–131.*
10. Goldmann H: Abflussdruck, Minutenvolumen und Widerstand der Kammerwasserstromung des Menschen. *Doc Ophthalmol 1951; 5–6:278–356.*
11. Goldmann H: Über Fluorescein in der menschlichen Vorderkammer. Das Kammerwasser-Minutenvolumen des Menschen. *Ophthalmologica 1950;119:65–95.*
12. Grotte D, Mattox V, Brubaker RF: Fluorescent, physiological and pharmacokinetic properties of fluorescein glucuronide. *Exp Eye Res 1985;40:23–33.*
13. Jones RF, Maurice DM: New methods of measuring the rate of aqueous flow in man with fluorescein. *Exp Eye Res 1966;5:208–220.*
14. Maurice DM: A new objective fluorophotometer. *Exp Eye Res 1963;2:33–38.*
15. Coakes RL, Brubaker RF: Method of measuring aqueous humor flow and corneal endothelial permeability using a fluorophotometry nomogram. *Invest Opthalmol Vis Sci 1979;18:288–302.*
16. Yablonski ME, Zimmerman TJ, Waltman SR, Becker B: A fluorophotometric study of the effect of topical timolol on aqueous humor dynamics. *Exp Eye Res 1978;27:135–142.*

17. Araie M, Takase M: Effects of various drugs on aqueous humor dynamics in man. *Jpn J Ophthalmol 1981;25:91–111.*
18. Bloom JN, Levene RZ, Thomas G, et al: Fluorophotometry and the rate of aqueous flow in man: I. Instrumentation and normal values. *Arch Ophthalmol 1976;94:435–443.*
19. Brubaker RF: The flow of aqueous humor in the human eye. *Trans Am Ophthalmol Soc 1982;80:391–474.*
20. Langham M, Wybar KC: Fluorophotometric apparatus for the objective determination of fluorescence in the anterior chamber of the living eye. *Br J Ophthalmol 1954;38:52–57.*
21. Waltman DR, Kaufman HE: A new objective slit lamp fluorophotometer. *Invest Ophthalmol 1970;9:247–249.*
22. McLaren JW, Brubaker RF: A two-dimensional scanning ocular fluorophotometer. *Invest Ophthalmol Vis Sci 1985;26:144–152.*
23. Johnson S, Coakes RL, Brubaker RF: A simple photogrammetric method of measuring anterior chamber volume. *Am J Ophthalmol 1978;85:469–474.*
24. Brubaker RF: Clinical evaluation of the circulation of aqueous humor, in Duane TD (ed): *Clinical Ophthalmology.* Philadelphia: Harper & Row, 1986, 1–11.
25. O'Rourke J, Macri FJ: Studies in uveal physiology. II. Clinical studies of the anterior chamber clearance of isotopic tracers. *Arch Ophthalmol 1970;84:415–420.*
26. O'Rourke J: *Nuclear Ophthalmology, Dynamic Function Studies in Intraocular Disease.* Philadelphia: WB Saunders, 1976, 82–86.
27. Holm O: A photogrammetric method for estimation of the pupillary aqueous flow in the living eye. *Acta Ophthalmol 1968;46:254–277.*
28. Brubaker RF, Penniston JT, Grotte DA, et al: Measurement of fluorescein binding in human plasma fluorescence polarization. *Arch Ophthalmol 1982;100:625–630.*
29. Brubaker RF, Nagataki S, Townsend DJ, et al: The effect of age on aqueous humor formation in man. *Ophthalmology 1981;88:283–287.*
30. Becker B: The decline in aqueous secretion and outflow facility with age. *Am J Ophthalmol 1958;46:731–736.*
31. Ericson LA: Twenty-four hourly variations on the aqueous flow: Examination with periimbal suction cup. *Acta Ophthalmol (Copenh) 1958; (suppl 50):1–95.*
32. Reiss GR, Lee DA, Topper JE, et al: Aqueous humor flow during sleep. *Invest Ophthalmol Vis Sci 1984;25:776–778.*
33. Gharagozloo NZ, Relf SJ, Brubaker RF (1988): Aqueous flow is reduced by the alpha-adrenergic agonist, apraclonidine hydrochloride (ALO 2145). *Ophthalmology 1988;95:1217–1220.*
34. Topper JE, Brubaker RF: Effects of timolol, epinephrine, and acetazolamide on aqueous flow during sleep. *Invest Ophthalmol Vis Sci 1985;26:1315–1319.*
35. Koskela T, Brubaker RF: The nocturnal suppression of aqueous humor flow in humans is not blocked by bright light. Submitted.
36. Heinrich S, Koskela T, Klee GG, et al: The effect of melatonin on aqueous humor flow in humans during the day. *Invest Ophthalmol Vis Sci 1990;(suppl 31):234.*
37. Coakes RL, Brubaker RF: The mechanism of timolol in lowering intraocular pressure. *Arch Ophthalmol 1978;96:2045–2048.*
38. Brubaker RF, Carlson KH, Kullerstrand LJ, et al: Topical forskolin (Colforsin) and aqueous flow in humans. *Arch Ophthalmol 1987;105: 637–641.*
39. McCannel C, Brubaker RF: Acetazolamide but not timolol lowers aqueous humor flow in sleeping humans. Submitted.
40. Anselmi P, Bron AJ, Maurice DM: Action of drugst on the aqueous flow in man measured by fluorophotometry. *Exp Eye Res 1968; 7:487–496.*
41. Lee DA, Brubaker RF: Effect of phenylephrine on aqueous humor flow. *Curr Eye Res 1982;2:89–92.*
42. Nagataki S, Brubaker RF: Effect of pilocarpine on aqueous humor formation in human beings. *Arch Ophthalmol 1982;100:818–821.*

43. Kerstetter JR, Brubaker RF, Wilson SE, et al: Prostaglandin F_2alpha-1-isopropylester lowers intraocular pressure without decreasing aqueous humor flow. *Am J Ophthalmol 1988;105:30–34.*
44. Adams B, Brubaker RF: Caffeine has no clinically significant effect on aqueous humor flow in the normal human eye. *Ophthalmology 1990; 97:1030–1031.*
45. Townsend DJ, Brubaker RF: Immediate effect of epinephrine on aqueous formation in the normal human eye as measured by fluorophotometry. *Invest Ophthalmol Vis Sci 1980;19:256–266.*
46. Coakes RL, Siah PB: Effects of adrenergic drugs on aqueous humor dynamics in the normal human eye. I. Salbutamol. *Br J Ophthalmol 1984;68:393–397.*
47. Larson RS, Brubaker RF: Isoproterenol stimulates aqueous flow in humans with Horner's syndrome. *Invest Ophthalmol Vis Sci 1988; 29:621–625.*
48. Gharagozloo NZ, Larson RS, Kullerstrand LJ, et al: Terbutaline stimulates aqueous humor flow in humans during sleep. *Arch Ophthalmol 1988;106:1218–1220.*
49. Carlson KH, McLaren JW, Topper JE, et al: Effect of body position on intraocular pressure and aqueous flow. *Invest Ophthalmol Vis Sci 1987;28:1346–1352.*
50. Sears M, Mead A: A major pathway for the regulation of intraocular pressure. *Int Ophthalmol 1983;6:201–212.*
51. Caprioli J, Sears M: The adenylate cyclase receptor complex and aqueous humor formation. *Yale J Biol Med 1984;57:283–300.*
52. Nathanson JA: Direct application of a guanylate cyclase activator lowers intraocular pressure. *Eur J Pharmacol 1988;147:155–156.*
53. van Herick W, Shaffer RN, Schwartz A: Estimation of width of angle of anterior chamber. Incidence and significance of the narrow angle. *Am J Ophthalmol 1969;68:626–629.*
54. Palmberg P: Gonioscopy, in Ritch E, Shields MB, Krupin T (eds): *The Glaucomas*. St. Louis: CV Mosby, 1989, 347.
55. Spaeth GL: The normal development of the human anterior chamber angle: A new system of descriptive grading. *Trans Ophthalmol Soc UK 1971;91:709–739.*
56. Lichter PR: Iris processes in 340 eyes. *Am J Ophthalmol 1969;68: 872–878.*
57. Henkind P: Angle vessels in normal eyes. A gonioscopic evaluation and anatomic correlation. *Br J Ophthalmol 1964;48:551–557.*
58. Shihab AM, Lee PF: The significance of normal angle vessels. *Ophthalmic Surg 1985;16:382–385.*
59. Spaeth GL: Gonioscopy: Uses old and new. The inheritance of occludable angles. *Trans Am Acad Ophthalmol Otolaryngol 1978;85:222–232.*
60. Fontana ST, Brubaker RF: Volume and depth of the anterior chamber in the normal aging human eye. *Arch Ophthalmol 1980;98:1803–1808.*
61. Forbes M: Gonioscopy with corneal indentation. A method for distinguishing between appositional closure and synechial closure. *Arch Ophthalmol 1966;76:488–492.*
62. Hoskins HD, Kass MA (eds): *Becker–Shaffer's Diagnosis and Therapy of the Glaucomas,* ed 6. St. Louis: CV Mosby, 1989, 106,107.
63. Shaffer RN: Gonioscopy, ophthalmoscopy and perimetry. *Trans Am Acad Ophthalmol Otolaryngol 1960;64:112–125.*
64. Scheie HG: Width and pigmentation of the angle of the anterior chamber. *Arch Ophthalmol 1957;58:510–512.*

CHAPTER 4
DIAGNOSTIC TECHNIQUES OF THE POSTERIOR SEGMENT

1. Quigley HA, Dunkelberger GR, Green WR: Retinal ganglion cell atrophy correlated with automated perimetery in eyes with glaucoma. *Am J Ophthalmol 1989;107:453–463.*
2. Sommer A, D'Anna SA, Kues HA, et al: High resolution photography of the retinal nerve fiber layer. *Am J Ophthalmol 1983;96:535–539.*
3. Duke-Elder S, Smith RJH: Ophthalmoscopic photography, in Duke-Elder S (ed): *System of Ophthalmology, Vol 7. The Foundation of Ophthalmology*. St. Louis: CV Mosby, 1962, 303–307.

4. Justice T: *Ophthalmic Photography.* Boston: Little, Brown, 1982.
5. Wong D: *Textbook of Ophthalmic Photography.* Amble, PA: Interoptics Publisher, 1982.
6. Coppinger JM, Maio M, Miller R: *Ophthalmic Photography.* Thorofare, NJ: Charles Slack, 1988.
7. Lichter PR: Variability of expert observers in evaluating the optic disc. *Trans Am Ophthalmol Soc 1978;84:532–572.*
8. Leydhecker W, Krieglstein GK, Collani E: Observer variation in applanation tonometry and estimation of the cup disk ratio, in Krieglstein GK, Leydhecker W (eds): *Glaucoma Update.* Berlin: Springer-Verlag, 1979, 101–111.
9. Bengtsson B, Holman C, Krakau CET: Disc haemorrhage and glaucoma. *Acta Ophthalmol 1981;59:1–14.*
10. Gloster J: Incidence of optic disc hemorrhages in chronic simple glaucoma and ocular hypertension. *Br J Ophthalmol 1981;65:452–456.*
11. Heijl A: Frequent disc photography and computerized perimetry in eyes with optic disc hemorrhage. *Acta Ophthalmol 1986;64:274–281.*
12. Frisen L: Photography of the retinal nerve fiber layer: An optimized procedure. *Br J Ophthalmol 1980;64:641–650.*
13. Airaksinen PJ, Nieminen H, Mastonen E: Retinal nerve fiber layer photography with a wide angle fundus camera. *Acta Ophthalmol 1982;60:362–368.*
14. Airaksinen PJ, Nieminen H: Retinal nerve fiber layer photography in glaucoma. *Ophthalmology 1985;92:877–879.*
15. Peli E, Hedges TR, McInnes T, et al: Nerve fiber layer photography. A comparative study. *Acta Ophthalmol 1987;65:71–80.*
16. Schwartz B, Rieser JC, Fishbein SL: Fluorescein angiographic defects of the optic disc in glaucoma. *Arch Ophthalmol 1977;95:1961–1974.*
17. Donaldson DD: A new camera for stereoscopic fundus photography. *Trans Am Ophthalmol Soc 1962;62:429–458.*
18. Donaldson DD, Prescot R, Kennedy S: Simultaneous stereoscopic fundus camera incorporating a single axis. *Invest Ophthalmol Vis Sci 1980;19:289–298.*
19. Falconer DG, Peppers NA, Kottler MS, Rosenthal AR: Twin-prism separator for retinal stereophotography. *Appl Optics 1976;15:29–31.*
20. Rosenthal AR, Kottler MS, Donaldson DD, Falconer DG: Comparative reproducibility of the digital photogrammetric procedure utilizing three methods of stereophotography. *Invest Ophthalmol 1977;16:54–60.*
21. Fraunfelder FT, Scofidi A: Possible adverse effects from topical ocular 10% phenylephrine. *Am J Ophthalmol 1978;85:447–453.*
22. Portney GL, Purcell TW: The influence of tropicamide on intraocular pressure. *Ann Ophthalmol 1975;7:31–34.*
23. Takamoto T, Kennedy S, Schwartz B: Image distortions of the Donaldson stereoscopic fundus camera. *Proc Am Soc Photogrammetry 1981; 326–334.*
24. Schwartz B: Cupping and pallor of the optic disc. *Arch Ophthalmol 1973;89:272–277.*
25. Fishman RS: Optic disc asymmetry. A sign of ocular hypertension. *Arch Ophthalmol 1970;84:590–594.*
26. Kirsch RE, Anderson DR: Clinical recognition of glaucomatous cupping. *Am J Ophthalmol 1973;75:442–454.*
27. Weisman RL, Assef CF, Phelps CD, et al: Vertical elongation of the optic cup in glauocma. *Trans Am Acad Ophthalmol Otolaryngol 1973; 77–OP:157–161.*
28. Drance SM: Disc hemorrhages in the glaucomas. *Surv Ophthalmol 1989;33:331–337.*
29. Iwata K, Nanba K, Abe H: Die beginninde Fundus veränderung infolge rezidivierender kleiner Krisen beim Posner-Schlossman-Syndrom. *Klin Mbl Augenheilkd 1982;180:20–24.*
30. Nagin P, Schwartz B, Reynolds G: Measurement of fluorescein angiograms of the optic disc and retina using computerized image analysis. *Ophthalmology 1985;92:547–552.*

31. Britton RJ, Drance SM, Schulzer M, et al: The areas of the neuroretinal rim of the optic nerve in normal eyes. *Am J Ophthalmol 1987;103:497–504.*
32. Caprioli J, Miller JM: Optic disc rim area is related to disc size in normal subjects. *Arch Ophthalmol 1987;105:1683–1685.*
33. Jonas JB, Gusek GC, Naumann GOH: Optic disc cup and neuroretinal rim size configuration and correlations in normal eyes. *Invest Ophthalmol Vis Sci 1988;29:1151–1158.*
34. Bengtsson B, Krakau CET: Some essential features of the Zeiss fundus camera. *Acta Ophthalmol 1977;55:123–131.*
35. Littmann H: Zur Bestimmüng der wahren Grösse eines objektes auf dem Hintergrund des lebenden Auges. *Klin Mbl Augenheilkd 1982;180:286–289.*
36. Yannuzzi L, Rohrer KT, Tindel LJ, et al: Fluorescein angiography complication survey. *Ophthalmology 1986;93:611–617.*
37. Spaeth G: *The Pathogenesis of Nerve Damage in Glaucoma: Contributions of Fluorescein Angiography.* New York: Grune & Stratton, 1977.
38. Tsukahara J: Hypermeable disc capillaries in glaucoma. *Adv Ophthalmol 1978;35:65–72.*
39. Richard G: Videoangiography: A new technique for the quantification of the retinal circulation, in Lambrou GN, Greve EL (eds): *Ocular Blood Flow in Glaucoma.* Amsterdam: Kugler and Ghedini, 1989, 267–273.
40. Peli E: Electro-optic fundus imaging. *Surv Ophthalmol 1989;34:113–122.*
41. Webb RH, Hughes GW: Scanning laser ophthalmoscope. *IEEE Trans Biomed Eng 1981;BME-28:88–492.*
42. Nagin P, Schwartz B, Nanba K: The reproducibility of computerized boundary analysis for measuring optic disc pallor in the normal optic disc. *Ophthalmology 1985;92:243–251.*
43. Delori FC, Fitch KA, Feke GT, et al: Evaluation of micrometric and microdensitometric methods for measuring the width of retinal vessel images on fundus photographs. *Graefes Arch Clin Exp Ophthalmol 1988;226:393–399.*
44. Takamoto T, Schwartz B: Photogrammetric measurement of nerve fiber layer thickness. *Ophthalmology 1989;96:1315–1319.*
45. Takamoto T, Schwartz B: Reproduciblity of photogrammetric optic disc cup measurements. *Invest Ophthalmol Vis Sci 1985;26:814–817.*
46. Caprioli J, Ortiz-Colberg R, Miller JM, Tressler C: Measurements of peripupillary nerve fiber layer contour in glaucoma. *Am J Ophthalmol 1989;108:404–413.*
47. Radius RL, Anderson DR: The histology of retinal nerve fiber layer bundles and bundle defects. *Arch Ophthalmol 1979;97:948–950.*
48. Minckler DS: The organization of the nerve fiber bundles in the primate optic nerve head. *Arch Ophthalmol 1980;98:1630–1636.*
49. Ogden TE: Nerve fiber layer of the macaque retina: Retinotopic organization. *Invest Ophthalmol Vis Sci 1983;24:85–98.*
50. Radius RL, Anderson DR: The course of axons through the retina and optic nerve head. *Arch Ophthalmol 1979;97:1154–1158*
51. Jonas JB, Nguyen NX, Naumann GOH: The retinal nerve fiber layer in normal eyes. *Ophthalmology 1989;96:627–632.*
52. Quigley HA, Addicks EM: Quantitative studies of retinal nerve fiber layer defects. *Arch Ophthalmol 1982;100:807–814, 1154–1158.*
53. Hoyt WF, Frisen L, Newman NM: Funduscopy of nerve fiber layer defects in glaucoma. *Invest Ophthalmol 1973;12:814–829.*
54. Miller NR, George TW: Monochromatic (red-free) photography and ophthalmoscopy of the peripapillary retinal nerve fiber layer. *Invest Ophthalmol Vis Sci 1978;17:1121–1124.*
55. Airaksinen PJ, Nieminen H: Retinal nerve fiber layer photography in glaucoma. *Ophthalmology 1985;92:877–879.*
56. Peli E, Hedges TR, McInnes T, et al: Nerve fiber layer photography. A comparative study. *Acta Ophthalmol 1987;65:71–80.*

57. Frisen L: Photography of the retinal nerve fiber layer. An optimized procedure. *Br J Ophthalmol 1980;64:641–650.*
58. Sommer A, Miller NR, Pollack I, et al: The nerve fiber layer in the diagnosis of glaucoma. *Arch Ophthalmol 1977;95:2149–2156.*
59. Quigley HA: Examination of the retinal nerve fiber layer in the recognition of early glaucoma damage. *Trans Am Ophthalmol Soc 1986; 84:921–966.*
60. Kottler MS, Rosenthal AR, Falconer DG: Digital photogrammetry of the optic nerve head. *Invest Ophthalmol Vis Sci 1974;13:116–120.*
61. Takamoto T, Schwartz B: Photogrammetric measurement of the optic disc cup in glaucoma. *Int Arch Photogrammetry 1980;23:732–741.*
62. Nagin P, Schwartz B: Reproducibility of computerized boundary analysis for measuring disc pallor in the normal optic disc. *Ophthalmology 1985;92:243–251.*
63. Caprioli J, Miller MM: Videographic measurements of optic nerve topography in glaucoma. *Invest Ophthalmol Vis Sci 1988;29: 1294–1298.*
64. Shields BM, Martone JF, Shelton AR, et al: Reproducibility of topographic measurements with the optic nerve head analyzer. *Am J Ophthalmol 1987;104:581–586.*
65. Mikelberg FS, Airaksinen PJ, Douglas GR, et al: The correlation between optic disk topography measured by the videoophthalmolgraph (Rodenstock Analyzer) and clinical measurement. *Am J Ophthalmol 1985;100:417–419.*
66. Mikelberg FS, Douglas GR, Schulzer M, et al: Reliability of optic disk topographic measurements recorded with a videoopthalmograph. *Am J Ophthalmol 1984;98:98–102.*
67. Katz B, Weinreb RN: Imaging the optic disk and nerve fiber layer in glaucoma and other optic neuropathies. *Pacific Coast Oto-Ophthalmol Soc 1985;66:225–233.*
68. Weinreb RN, Dreher AW, Bille JF: Quantitative assessment of the optic nerve head with the laser tomographic scanner. *Int Ophthalmol 1989;13:25–29.*
69. Caprioli J, Miller JM: Correlation of structure and function in glaucoma. *Ophthalmology 1988;95:723–727.*
70. Weinreb RN, Nelson MR, Goldbaum MH, et al: Digital image analysis of optic disc topography, in Blodi F, Brancats R, Cristin G (eds): *Acts XXV Concilium Ophthalmologicum.* Berkeley, CA: Kugler Publications, 1988, 1509–1512.
71. Weinreb RN: Laser scanning tomography to diagnose and monitor glaucoma. *Curr Opin Ophthalmol 1993;4:3–7.*
72. Bishop KI, Werner EB, Krupin T, et al: Variability and reproducibility of optic disk topographic measurements with the Rodenstock optic nerve head analyser. *Am J Ophthalmol 1988;106:696–702.*
73. Mikelberg FS, Douglas GR, Schulzer M, et al: The correlation between cup-disk ratio, neuroretinal rim area, and optic disk area measured by the video-ophthalmograph (Rodenstock analyser) and clinical measurement. *Am J Ophthalmol 1986;101:7–12.*
74. Weinreb RN, Morsman CD, Bartsch D, Lusky M: Effect of repetitive imaging on optic nerve topograghy. *Arch Ophthalmol 1993;111: 636–638.*
75. Peli E, Hedges TR, Schwartz B: Computerized enhancement of retinal nerve fiber layer. *Acta Ophthalmol 1986;64:113–122.*
76. Cooper RL, Eikelboom RH, Barry C: Computerized densitometry of red-free retinal photographs correlated with automatic perimetry. *Curr Eye Res 1988;7:789–798.*
77. Caprioli J, Miller M: Measurement of relative nerve fiber layer surface height in glaucoma. *Ophthalmology 1989;96:633–639.*
78. Knighton RW, Jacobson SG, Kemp CM: The spectral reflectance of the nerve fiber layer of the macaque retina. *Invest Ophthalmol Vis Sci 1989;30:2393–2402.*
79. Weinreb RN, Dreher AW, Coleman A, et al: Histopathologic validation of Fourier-ellipsometry measurements of retinal nerve fiber layer thickness. *Arch Ophthalmol 1990;108:557–560.*

80. Caprioli J: The contour of the juxtapapillary nerve fiber layer in glaucoma. *Ophthalmology 1990;97:358–365.*
81. Weinreb RN: Discussion of contour of the juxtapapillary nerve fiber layer in glaucoma. *Ophthalmology 1990;97:365–366.*
82. Zeimer RC, Mori MT, Rhoobehi B: Feasibility test of a new method to measure retinal thickness noninvasively. *Invest Ophthalmol Vis Sci 1989;30:2099–2105.*

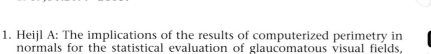

CHAPTER 5
VISUAL FUNCTION

1. Heijl A: The implications of the results of computerized perimetry in normals for the statistical evaluation of glaucomatous visual fields, Krieglstein GK, Leydhecker W (eds): *Glaucoma Update III.* Berlin, Heidelberg: Springer-Verlag, 1987, 115–122.
2. Drance SM, Lakowski R, Schulzer M, Douglas GR: Acquired color vision changes in glaucoma. *Arch Ophthalmol 1981;99:829–831.*
3. Breton ME, Knupin T: Age co-variance between 100-hue color scores and quantitative perimetry in primary open angle glaucoma. *Arch Ophthalmol 1987;105:642–645.*
4. Bengtsson B: Optic disc haemorrhages preceding manifest glaucoma. *Acta Ophthalmol 1990;68:450–454.*
5. Airaksinen PJ, Mustonen E, Alanko H: Optic disc haemorrhages precede retinal nerve fibre layer defect in ocular hypertension. *Acta Ophthalmol 1981;59:627–641.*
6. Drance SM: Disc haemorrhages in glaucomas. *Surv Ophthalmol 1989; 33:331–337.*
7. Airaksinen PJ, Heijl A: Visual field and retinal nerve fibre layer in early glaucoma after optic disc haemorrhage. *Acta Ophthalmol 1983;61: 186–194.*
8. Pedersen JE, Anderson DR: The mode of progressive disc cupping in ocular hypertension and glaucoma. *Arch Ophthalmol 1980;98: 490–495.*
9. Heijl A, Bengtsson Boel: Diagnosis of early glaucoma with flicker comparisons of serial disc photographs. *Invest Ophthalmol Vis Sci 1989; 30:2376–2384.*
10. Ouigley HA: Histology of human glaucoma optic nerve damage compared to clinical findings in the same eye, Krieglstein GK, Leydhecker W (eds): *Glaucoma Update II.* Berlin: Springer-Verlag, 1983; 83–87.
11. Traquair HM: *An Introduction to Clinical Perimetry.* London: Kimpton, 1927.
12. Riddoch G: Dissociation in visual perception due to occipital injuries, with special reference to appreciation of movement. *Brain 1917; 40:15–57.*
13. Heijl A: Automatic perimetry in glaucoma visual field screening. A clinical study. *Graefes Arch Clin Exp Ophthalmol 1976;200:21–37.*
14. Schmied U: Automatic (Octopus) and manual (Goldmann) perimetry in glaucoma. *Graefes Arch Clin Exp Ophthalmol 1980;213:239–244.*
15. Dyster-Aas K, Heijl A, Lundqvist L: Computerized visual field screening in the management of patients with ocular hypertension. *Acta Ophthalmol 1980;58:918–928.*
16. Goldmann H: Ein selbstregistrierendes Projektionskugel perimeter. *Ophthalmologica 1945;109:71–79.*
17. Heijl A: The Humphrey Field Analyzer, in Drance SM, Anderson D (eds): *Automatic Perimetry in Glaucoma.* New York: Grune & Stratton, 1985.
18. Heijl A, Lindgren G, Olsson J: A package for the statistical analysis of computerized visual fields. *Doc Ophthalmol Proc Series 1987; 49:153–168.*
19. Heijl A, Lindgren G, Lindgren A, et al: Extended empirical statistical package for evaluation of single and multiple fields in glaucoma: Statpac 2. Perimetry Update 1990/91, in: *Proceedings of the IXth International Perimetric Society Meeting.* Amsterdam: Kugler, 1991, 303–315.

20. Bodis-Wollner I: Visual acuity and contrast sensitivity in patients with cerebral lesions. *Science 1972;178:769–771.*
21. Francois J, Verriest G: Les dyschromatopsies acquises dans le glaucome primaire. >*Ann Ocul (Paris) 1959;192:191–199.*
22. Fishman GA, Rriss A, Fishman M: Acquired colour defects in patients with open angle glaucoma and ocular hypertension. *Mod Prob Ophthalmol 1974;13:335–338.*
23. Lakowski R, Drance SM: Acquired dyschromatopsias: The earliest functional losses in glaucoma. *Doc Ophthalmol Proc Ser 1979; 19:159–165.*
24. Schade OH: Optical and photoelectric analog of the eye. *J Opt Soc Am 1956;46:721–739.*
25. Campbell FW, Green DC: Optical and retinal factors affecting visual resolution. *J Physiol (Lond) 1965;181:576–595.*
26. Arden GB, Jacobson JJ: A simple grating test for contrast sensitivity: Preliminary results indicate value in screening for glaucoma. *Invest Ophthalmol Vis Sci 1978;17:23–32.*
27. Bodis-Wollner I: Test your eyes in 7 minutes. *Am Health 1982; 1:52–58.*
28. Regan D, Neima D: Low contrast letter charts as a test of visual function. *Ophthalmology 1983;90:1192–1200.*
29. Ginsburg AP: A new contrast sensitivity vision test chart. *Am J Optom Physiol Opt 1984;61:403–407.*
30. Pelli DG, Robson JG, Wilkins AJ: The design of a new letter chart for measuring contrast sensitivity. *Clin Vis Sci 1988;2:187–199.*
31. Wilkins AJ, Della Sala S, Somazzi L, Nimmo-Smith I: Age-related norms for the Cambridge Low Contrast Gratings including details concerning their design and use. *Clin Vis Sci 1988;2:201–212.*
32. Sokol S, Domar A, Moskowitz A: Utility of the Arden grating test in glaucoma screening: High false-positive rate in normals over 50 years of age. *Invest Ophthalmol Vis Sci 1980;19:1529–1533.*
33. Vaegan, Halliday BL: Senile changes in visual acuity. *Trans Ophthalmol Soc UK 1982;95:36–38.*
34. Findlay JM: A spatial integration effect in visual acuity. *Vis Res 1969; 9:157–166.*
35. McCann JJ, Savoy RL, Hall JA Jr: Visibility of low frequency sine wave targets: Dependence on number of cycle and surround parameters. *Vis Res 1978;18:891–894.*
36. Quigley HA, Addicks EM, Green WR: Optic nerve damage in human glaucoma: III. Quantitative correlation of nerve fiber loss and visual field defect in glaucoma, ischemic neuropathy, papilledema, and toxic neuropathy. *Arch Ophthalmol 1982;100:135–146.*
37. Quigley HA, Dunkelberger GR, Green WR: Retinal ganglion cell atrophy correlated with automated perimetry in human eyes with glaucoma. *Am J Ophthalmol 1989;107:453–464.*
38. Quigley HA, Addicks EM, Green WR: Optic nerve damage in human glaucoma: III. Quantitative correlation of nerve fiber loss and visual field defect in glaucoma, ischemic optic neuropathy, papilledema and toxic optic neuropathy. *Arch Ophthalmol 1982;100:136–146.*
39. Pickford R, Lakowski R: The Pickford-Nicholson anomaloscope: For testing and measuring color sensitivity and color blindness, and other tests and experiments. *Br J Physiol Optics 1901;17:131.*
40. Farnsworth D: The Farnsworth-Munsell 100-Hue and dichotomous tests for color vision. *J Opt Soc Am 1943;38:568.*
41. Adams AJ, Rodic R, Husted R, Stamper R: Spectral sensitivity and color discrimination changes in glaucoma and glaucoma-suspect patients. *Invest Ophthalmol Vis Sci, 1982;23:516–524.*
42. Lanthony P: The desaturated panel D-15. *Doc Ophthalmol 1978;46: 1185–1189.*
43. Pinker SA, Nabbe B, Bogaara PVD: Le test 15 hue desaturé de Lanthony. *Ann Oculist 1976;209:731–738.*
44. Drance SM: The early field defects in glaucoma. *Invest Ophthalmol 1969;8:84–91.*

45. Armaly MF: Visual field defects in early open angle glaucoma. *Trans Am Ophthalmol Soc 1971;69:147–62.*
46. Hart WM Jr, Becker B: The onset and evolution of glaucomatous visual field defects. *Ophthalmology 1982;89:268–79.*
47. Feree CE, Rand F, Monroe MM: Studies in perimetry: 2. Preliminary work on a diagnostic scale for the color fields. *Am J Ophthalmol 1929; 12:269–285.*
48. Committee on Vision, Assembly of Behavioural and Social Sciences National Research Council: Report of working group 39. First inter professional standard for visual field testing. *Adv Ophthalmol 1980; 40:173–224.*
49. Verduyn-Lunel HFE, Crone RA: Determination of peripheral spectral sensitivity and saturation discrimination characteristics with a modified Goldmann perimeter. *Mod Probl Ophthalmol 1978;19:181–186.*
50. Drum BA: Chromatic saturation derived from increment thresholds for white and colored targets; a technique for projector color perimetry. *Mod Probl Opthalmol 1976;17:79–85.*
51. Hedin A, Verriest G: Is clinical colour perimetry useful? *Doc Ophthalmol Proc Ser 1981;26:161–184.*
52. Logan N, Anderson DR: Detecting early glaucomatous visual field changes with a blue stimulus. *Am J Ophthalmol 1983;95:432–434.*
53. Mindel JS, Safir A, Schare PW: Visual field testing with red targets. *Arch Ophthalmol 1983;101:927–929.*
54. Carlow JF, Flynn JT, Shipley T: Color perimetry. *Arch Ophthalmol 1976;94:1492–1496.*
55. Heijl A, Drance SM: Changes in differential threshold in patients with glaucoma during prolonged perimetry. *Br J Ophthalmol 1983; 67:512–516.*
56. Lakowski R, Oliver K: Effect of pupil diameter on colour vision test performance. *Mod Probl Ophthalmol 1974;13:307.*
57. Pokorny J, Smith V, Verriest G, et al: *Congenital and Acquired Color Vision Defects.* New York: Grune & Stratton, 1979, 66.
58. Verriest G, Uvijls A: Spectral increment thresholds on a white background in different age groups of normal subjects and in acquired ocular diseases. *Doc Ophthalmol 1977;43:217–248.*
59. Pokorny J, et al: *Procedures for Testing of Color Vision: Report of Working Group 41.* Washington: National Academy Press, 1981, 14–94.
60. Hardy LH, Rand G, Ritter MC: The HRR polychromatic plates. *J Opt Soc Am 1954;44:509–523.*
61. Hardy LH: Standard illuminants in relation to color testing procedures. *Arch Ophthalmol 1945;34:278–282.*
62. Schmidt I: Effect of illumination in testing color vision with pseudoisochromatic plates. *J Opt Soc Am 1952;42:951–955.*
63. Alvis DL: Electroretinographic changes in controlled chronic open-angle glaucoma. *Am J Ophthalmol 1966;61:121–131.*
64. Henkes HE: The electroretinogram in glaucoma. *Ophthalmologica 1951;121:44–46.*
65. Fazio DT, Heckenlively JR, Martin DA, Christensen RE: The electroretinogram in advanced open-angle glaucoma. *Doc Ophthalmol 1986;63:45–54.*
66. Conte MM, Brodie SE: Altered contrast and luminance contributions to the pattern ERG in glaucoma (abstr). *Invest Ophthalmol Vis Sci 1987;(suppl 28):129.*
67. Abe H, Hasegawa S, Itata K: Constant sensitivity and pattern visual evoked potential in patients with glaucoma. *Doc Ophthalmol Proc Ser 1987;65:65–70.*
68. Schmeisser ET, Smith TJ: High-frequency flicker visual-evoked potential losses in glaucoma. *Ophthalmology 1988;96:620–623.*
69. Drance SM, Airaksinen PJ, Price M, et al: The use of psychophysical, structural, and electrodiagnostic parameters to identify glaucomatous damage. *Graefes Arch Clin Exp Ophthalmol 1987;225:365–368.*
70. Gafner F, Goldmann H: Experimentelle Untersuchungen ueber den Zusammenhang von Augendrucksteigerung und Gesichtsfeldschaedigung. *Ophthalmologica 1955;130:357–377.*

71. Hayreh SS: Structure and blood supply of the optic nerve, in Richardson K, Heilmann K (eds): *Glaucoma–Conceptions of Disease.* Stuttgart/New York: Thieme, 1978, 78–96.
72. Duke-Elder WS: The arterial pressure in the eye. *J Physiol 1926; 62:1–12.*
73. Galin MA, Baras I, Cavero R: Ophthalmodynamometry using suction. *Arch Ophthalmol 1969;18:494–500.*
74. Gee W, Oller DW, Homer LD, Bailey CR: Simultaneous bilateral determination of the systolic pressure of the ophthalmic artery by ocular pneumoplethysmography. *Invest Ophthalmol Vis Sci 1977;16:86–92.*
75. Ulrich WD, Ulrich C: Okulooszillodynamographie, ein neues Verfahren zur Bestimmung des Ophthalmikablutdruckes und zur okulaeren Pulskurvenanalyse. *Klin Mbl Augenheilk 1985;186:385–388.*
76. Weigelin E, Lobstein A: *Ophthalmodynamometrie.* Basel: Karger, 1962.
77. Pillunat LE, Stodtmeister R, Marquardt R, Mattern A: Ocular perfusion pressures in different types of glaucoma. *Intern Ophthalmol* [in press].
78. Kirchheim H: Kreislaufregulation, in Busse R (ed): *Kreislaufphysiologie.* Stuttgart: Thieme, 1982, 167–210.
79. Roehler R: *Biologische Kybernetik.* Stuttgart: Teubner, 1973.
80. Stodtmeister R, Wilmanns I, Pillunat L: Methodik okulaerer Kreislaufdiagnostik beim Glaukom, in Stodtmeister R (ed): *Okulaere Durchblutungsstoerungen.* Stuttgart: Enke Verlag, 1987, 95–101.
81. Regan D: Comparison of transient and steady-state methods. *Ann NY Acad Sci 1982;338:45–71.*
82. Mikuni M, Yoneyama J: Ein neues Dynamometer. *Acta Soc Ophthalmol Jpn 1955;59:412–419.*
83. Draeger J, Vogel H: Ophthalmodynamometrie mit einem einfachen Unterdruckgeraet. *Graefes Arch Clin Exp Ophthalmol 1966;170: 209–219.*
84. Boeck J, Bornschein H, Hommer K: Die Erholungslatenz der Helligkeitsempfindung und des Elektroretinogramms nach retinaler Ischaemie. *Graefes Arch Clin Exp Ophthalmol 1964;167:276–282.*

CHAPTER 6

STRUCTURE AND APPEARANCE OF THE OPTIC NERVE HEAD AND RETINAL NERVE FIBER LAYER IN GLAUCOMA

1. Radius RL: Regional specificity in anatomy at the lamina cribrosa. *Arch Ophthalmol 1981;99:478–480.*
2. Quigley HA, Addicks EM: Regional differences in the structure of the lamina cribrosa and their relation to glaucomatous optic nerve damage. *Arch Ophthalmol 1981;99:137–143.*
3. Quigley HA, Addicks EM, Green WR, Maumenee AE: Optic nerve damage in human glaucoma. II. The site of injury and susceptibility to damage. *Arch Ophthalmol 1981;99:635–649.*
4. Quigley HA, Green WR: The histology of human glaucoma cupping and optic nerve damage: Clinicopathologic correlation in 21 eyes. *Ophthalmology 1979;86:1803–1827.*
5. Radius RL, Pederson JE: Laser-induced primate glaucoma. II. Histology. *Arch Ophthalmol 1984;102:1693–1698.*
6. Spaeth GL: Morphologic damage of the optic nerve, in Heilman K, Richardson KT (eds): *Glaucoma: Concepts of Disease Pathogenesis, Diagnosis, Therapy.* Philadelphia: WB Saunders, 1978.
7. Spaeth GL: Appearances of the optic disc in glaucoma: A pathologic classification, in *Symposium on Glaucoma. Transactions of the New Orleans Academy of Ophthalmology* St. Louis: CV Mosby, 1981.
8. Quigley HA, Dunkelberger GR, Green WR: Chronic human glaucoma causing selectively greater loss of large optic nerve fibers. *Ophthalmology 1988;95:357–363.*
9. Quigley HA, Dunkelberger GR, Green WR: Retinal ganglion cell atrophy correlated with automated perimetry in human eyes with glaucoma. *Am J Ophthalmol 1989;107:453–463.*
10. Glovinsky Y, Quigley HA, Dunkelberger GR: Retinal ganglion cell loss is size dependent in experimental glaucoma. *Invest Ophthalmol Vis Sci 1991;32:484–490.*

11. Lalit D, Hendrickson A, Quigley HA: Selective effects of experimental glaucoma on axonal transport by retinal ganglion cells to the dorsal lateral geniculate nucleus. *Invest Ophthalmol Vis Sci 1991;32:1593–1599.*
12. Quigley HA, Addicks EM: Chronic experimental glaucoma in primates. II. Effect of extended intraocular pressure elevation on optic nerve head and axonal transport. *Invest Ophthalmol Vis Sci 1980;19:137–152.*
13. Quigley HA, Hohman RM, Addicks EM: Morphologic changes in the lamina cribrosa correlated with neural loss in open-angle glaucoma. *Am J Ophthalmol 1983;95:673–691.*
14. Quigley HA, Hohman RM, Addicks EM: Blood vessels of the glaucomatous disc in experimental primate and human eyes. *Invest Ophthalmol Vis Sci 1984;25:918–931.*
15. Quigley HA, Hohman RM, Addicks EM: Quantitative study of optic nerve head capillaries in experimental optic disc pallor. *Am J Ophthalmol 1982;93:689–699.*
16. Lampert PW, Vogel MH, Zimmerman LE: Pathology of the optic nerve in acute experimental glaucoma. Electron microscopic studies. *Invest Ophthalmol Vis Sci 1968;7:199–213.*
17. Hernandez MR, Andrzejewska WM, Neufeld AH: Changes in the extracellular matrix of the human optic nerve head in primary open angle glaucoma. *Am J Ophthalmol 1990;109:180–188.*
18. Morrison J, Dorman ME, Dunkelberger GR, Quigley H: Optic nerve head extracellular matrix in primary optic atrophy and experimental glaucoma. *Invest Ophthalmol Vis Sci, 1990;108:1020–1024.*
19. Minckler DS, Spaeth GL: Optic nerve damage in glaucoma. *Surv Ophthalmol 1981;26:128–148.*
20. Zeimer RC, Ogura Y: The relation between glaucomatous damage and optic nerve head mechanical compliance. *Arch Ophthalmol 1989;107:1232–1234.*
21. Keene DR, Engvall E, Glanville RW: Ultrastructure of type VI collagen in human skin and cartilage suggests an anchoring function for this filamentous network. *J Cell Biol 1988;107:1995–2006.*
22. Hernandez MR, Igoe F, Neufeld AH: Cell culture of the human lamina cribrosa. *Invest Ophthalmol Vis Sci 1988;29:78–89.*
23. Richardson WD, Pringle N, Mosley MJ, et al: A role for platelet-derived growth factor in normal gliogenesis in the central nervous system. *Cell 1988;53:309–319.*
24. Hernandez MR, Hanley NM, Neufeld AH: Gene expression for type I collagen and elastin in human lamina cribrosa cells in culture. *Invest Ophthalmol Vis Sci (ARVO Suppl 30) 1989;3:201.*
25. Singer RH, Lawrence JB, Villnave C: Optimization of in situ hybridization using isotopic and non-isotopic detection methods. *BioTechniques 1986;4:230–243.*
26. Hernandez MR, Hanley NM, Neufeld AH: Localization of collagen types I and IV mRNAs in human optic nerve head by in situ hybridization. *Invest Ophthalmol Vis Sci 1991;32:2169–2177.*
27. Armaly MF: Cup/disc ratio in early open-angle glaucoma. *Doc Ophthalmol 1969;26:526–533.*
28. Diehl DL, Quigley HA, Miller NR, et al: Prevalence and significance of optic disc hemorrhage in a longitudinal study of glaucoma. *Arch Ophthalmol 1990;108:545–550.*
29. Betz P, Camps F, Collignon–Brach J, et al: Biometric study of the disc cup in open-angle glaucoma. *Graefes Arch Clin Exp Ophthalmol 1982;218:40–74.*
30. Quigley HA, Addicks EM, Green R: Optic nerve damage in human glaucoma. *Arch Ophthalmol 1982;100:135–146.*
31. Cher I, Robinson VLP: 'Thinning' of the neural rim of the optic nerve-head. *Trans Ophthalmol Soc UK 1973;93:213–242.*
32. Kolker AE, Hetherington J: *Becker–Shaffer's Diagnosis and Therapy of the Glaucomas*, ed 5. St. Louis: CV Mosby, 1983.

33. Buus DR, Anderson DR: Peripapillary crescents and halos in normal-tension glaucoma and ocular hypertension. *Ophthalmology 1989; 96:16–19.*
34. Jonas JB, Fernandez MC, Naumann GOH: Glaucomatous optic nerve atrophy in small discs with low cup-to-disc ratios. *Ophthalmology 1990;97:1211–1215.*
35. Airaksinen PJ, Alanko HI: Effect of retinal nerve fiber loss on the optic nerve head configuration in early glaucoma. *Graefes Arch Clin Exp Ophthalmol 1983;220:193–196.*
36. Sommer A, Katz J, Quigley HA, et al: Clinically detectable nerve fiber atrophy precedes the onset of glaucomatous field loss. *Arch Ophthalmol 1991;109:77–83.*
37. Iwata K, Nanba K, Abe H: Typical slit-like retinal nerve fiber layer defect and corresponding scotoma. *Acta Soc Ophthalmol Jpn 1981; 85:1791–1803.*
38. Airaksinen PJ, Drance SM, Douglas GR, et al: Diffuse and localized nerve fiber loss in glaucoma. *Am J Ophthalmol 1984;98:566–571.*
39. Tuulonen A, Airaksinen PJ: Initial glaucomatous optic disk and retinal nerve fiber layer abnormalities and their progression. *Am J Ophthalmol 1991;111:485–490.*
40. Tuulonen A, Airaksinen PJ, Montagna A, et al: Screening for glaucoma with a non-mydriatic fundus camera. *Acta Ophthalmol 1990;68: 445–449.*
41. Caprioli J, Ortiz–Colberg R, Miller JM, et al: Measurements of peripapillary nerve fiber layer contour in glaucoma. *Am J Ophthalmol 1989;108:404–413.*
42. Takamoto T, Schwartz B: Photogrammetric measurements of nerve fiber layer thickness. *Ophthalmology 1989;96:1315–1319.*
43. Plesch A, Klingbeil U, Bille J: Digital laser scanning fundus camera. *Appl Optics 1987;26:1480–1486.*
44. Weinreb RN, Dreher AW, Bille JF: Quantitative assessment of the optic nerve head with the laser tomographic scanner. *Int Ophthalmol 1989;13:25–29.*
45. Read RM, Spaeth GL: The practical clinical appraisal of the optic disc in glaucoma. The natural history of cup progression and some specific disc-field correlations. *Trans Am Acad Ophthalmol Otolaryngol 1975;78:OP255–274.*
46. Sommer A, Pollack I, Maumenee AE: Optic disc parameters and onset of glaucomatous field loss. I. Methods and progressive changes in disc morphology. *Arch Ophthalmol 1975;97:1444–1448.*
47. Pederson JE, Anderson DR: The mode of progressive disc cupping in ocular hypertension and glaucoma. *Arch Ophthalmol 1980;98: 490–495.*
48. Quigley HA, Addicks EM, Green WR: Optic nerve damage in human glaucoma. II. Quantitative correlation of nerve fiber loss and visual field defect in glaucoma, ischemic neuropathy, papilledema, and toxic neuropathy. *Arch Ophthalmol 1982;100:135–146.*
49. Odberg T, Riise D: Early diagnosis of glaucoma: The value of successive stereophotography of the optic disc. *Acta Ophthalmol 1985; 63:257–263.*
50. Caprioli J, Miller JM, Sears M: Quantitative evaluation of the optic nerve head in patients with unilateral visual field loss from primary open-angle glaucoma. *Ophthalmology 1987;94:1484–1487.*
51. Lichter PR: Variability of expert observers in evaluating the optic disc. *Trans Am Ophthalmol Soc 1976;74:532–572.*
52. Hoyt WF, Frisen L, Newman NM: Funduscopy of nerve fiber layer defects in glaucoma. *Invest Ophthalmol Vis Sci 1973;12:814–829.*
53. Sommer A, Miller NR, Pollsck I, et al: The nerve fiber layer in the diagnosis of glaucoma. *Arch Ophthalmol 1977;95:2149–2156.*
54. Airaksinen PJ, Nieminen H: Retinal nerve fiber layer photography in glaucoma. *Ophthalmology 1985;92:877–879.*
55. Takamoto T, Schwartz B: Reproducibility of photogrammetric optic disc cup measurements. *Invest Ophthalmol Vis Sci 1985;26:814.*

56. Nagin P, Schwartz B, Kinba K: The reproducibility of computerized boundary analysis for measuring disc pallor in the normal optic disc. *Ophthalmology 1985;92:243.*
57. Nagin P, Schwartz B: Detection of increased pallor over time. *Ophthalmology 1984;91:252.*
58. Balazsi AG, Drance SM, Schulzer M, et al: Neuroretinal rim area in suspected glaucoma and early chronic open-angle glaucoma: Correlation with parameters of visual function. *Arch Ophthalmol 1984;102:1011–1014.*
59. Airaksinen PJ, Drance SM, Schulzer M: Neuroretinal rim area in early glaucoma. *Am J Ophthalmol 1985;99:1–4.*
60. Caprioli J, Miller JM: Videographic measurements of optic nerve topography in glaucoma. *Invest Ophthalmol Vis Sci 1988;29:1294–1298.*
61. Airaksinen PJ, Drance SM, Douglas GR, et al: Neuroretinal rim areas and visual field indices in glaucoma. *Am J Ophthalmol 1985;99:107–110.*
62. Caprioli J, Miller JM: Correlation of structure and function in glaucoma: Quantitative measurements of disc and field. *Ophthalmology 1988;95:723–727.*
63. Caprioli J: Quantitative measurements of the optic nerve head, in Ritch R, Krupin T, Shields MD (eds): *The Glaucomas: A Multi-volume Reference.* St. Louis: CV Mosby, 1989, 495.
64. Zeimer RC, Mori MT, Rhoobehi B: Feasibility test of a new method to measure retinal thickness noninvasively. *Invest Ophthalmol Vis Sci 1989;30:2099–2105.*
65. Takamoto T, Schwartz B: Photogrammatic measurement of nerve fiber layer thickness. *Ophthalmology 1989;96:1315–1319.*
66. Weinreb RN, Dreher AW, Coleman A, et al: Histopathologic validation of Fourier-ellipsometry measurements of retinal nerve filter layer thickness. *Arch Ophthalmol 1990;108:557–560.*
67. Caprioli J, Miller JM: Measurement of relative nerve fiber layer surface height in glaucoma. *Ophthalmology 1989;96:633–641.*
68. Caprioli J: The contour of the juxtapapillary nerve fiber layer in glaucoma. *Ophthalmology 1989;97:358–366.*

CHAPTER 7
VISUAL FUNCTION IN GLAUCOMA

1. Sloan LL: Instruments and techniques for the clinical testing of light sense. *Arch Ophthalmol 1939;22:233–251.*
2. Harms H, Aulhorn E: Early visual field defects in glaucoma, in Leydhecker W (ed): *Glaucoma.* Basel: Karger, 1966, 151–175.
3. Goldmann H: Ein Selbstregistrieren des Projektions Kugel Perimeter. *Ophthalmologica 1945;109:71–79.*
4. Drance SM, Berry V, Hughes A: Studies on the effects of age on the central and peripheral isopters of the visual field in normal subjects. *Am J Ophthalmol 1967; 63:1667–1672.*
5. Werner EB, Drance SM: Early visual field disturbances in glaucoma. *Arch Ophthalmol 1977;95:1173–1177.*
6. Quigley HA, Addicks EM, Green WR: Optic nerve damage in human glaucoma: III quantitative correlation of nerve fibre loss and visual field defect in glaucoma, ischemic optic neuropathy, papilledema, and toxic optic neuropathy. *Arch Ophthalmol 1982;100:135–146.*
7. Flammer J, Drance SM, Zulauf M: Differential light threshold: Short and long term fluctuation in patients with glaucoma, normal controls and glaucoma suspects. *Arch Ophthalmol 1984;102:704–706.*
8. Gouras P: Identification of cone mechanisms in monkey ganglion cells. *J Physiol 1968;199:533–547.*
9. Kaplan E, Shapley RM: The primate retina contains two types of ganglion cells with high and low contrast sensitivity. *Proc Natl Acad Sci USA 1986;83:2755–2757.*
10. Perry VH, Cowey A: The ganglion cell and cone distributions in the monkey's retina: Implications for central magnification factors. *Vis Res 1985;25:1795–1810.*

11. D'Zmura M, Lennie P: Shared pathways for rod and cone vision. *Vis Res 1986;26:1273–1280.*
12. Gouras P, Link K: Rod and cone interaction in dark-adapted monkey ganglion cells. *J Physiol 1966;184:499–510.*
13. Polyak SL: *The Retina.* Chicago: University of Chicago Press, 1941.
14. Wiesel TN, Hubel DH: Spatial and chromatic interactions in the lateral geniculate body of the rhesus monkey. *J Neurophysiol 1966;29: 1115–116.*
15. de Monasterio FM: Asymmetry of on- and off-pathways of blue-sensitive cones of the retina of macaques. *Brain Res 1979;166:39–48.*
16. Ingling CR, Drum BA: Retinal receptive fields: correlations between psychophysics and electrophysiology. *Vis Res 1973;13:1151–1163.*
17. Ingling CR, Marlinez–Uriegas E: The spaciotemporal properties of the R-G X-cell channel. *Vis Res 1985;25:33–38.*
18. Quigley HA, Sanchez RM, Dunkelberger GR, et al: Chronic glaucoma selectively damages large optic nerve fibres *Invest Ophthalmol Vis Sci 1987;28:913–920.*
19. Quigley HA, Dunkelberger GR, Green WR: Chronic human glaucoma causing selectively greater loss of large optic nerve fibres. *Ophthalmology 1988;95:357–363.*
20. Maunsell JHR, Newsome WT: Visual processing in the monkey extrastriate cortex. *Annu Rev Neurosci 1987;10:363–401.*
21. Livingston MS, Hubel DH: Segregation of form, color, movement and depth: Anatomy, physiology, and perception. *Science 1988;240: 740–749.*
22. Livingstone MS, Hubel DH: Psychophysical evidence for separate channels for the perception of form, color and depth. *J Neurosci 1987; 7:3416–3468.*
23. Fitzke FW, Poinoosawmy D, Ernst W, Hitchings RA: Peripheral displacement threshold in normal, ocular hypertensives and glaucoma, in Greve EL, Heijl A (eds): *Seventh International Visual Field Symposium.* Dordrecht: Martinus Nijhol/Dr. W. Junk Publishers, 1987, 447–452.
24. Silverman SE, Trick GL, Hart WM: Motion perception is abnormal in primary open-angle glaucoma and ocular hypertension. *Invest Ophthalmol Vis Sci 1990;31:722–728.*
25. Drance SM, Lakowski R, Schulzer M, Douglas GR: Acquired color vision changes in glaucoma. *Arch Ophthalmol 1981;99:829–831.*
26. DuBois–Poulson A, Magis C: Les procédés d'examen de la fonction visuelle dans le glaucome chronique. *Ophthalmologica 1960;139: 155–213.*
27. Francois J, Verriest G: Les dyschormatopsies acquises dans le glaucome primaire. *Ann Ocul (Paris) 1959;192:191–199.*
28. Krill AE, Fishman GA: Acquired color vision defects. *Trans Am Acad Ophthalmol Otolaryngol 1971;75:1095–1112*
29. Lakowski R, Drance SM: Acquired dyschromatopsias: The earliest functional losses in glaucoma. *Doc Ophthalmol Proc Ser 1979; 19:159–165.*
30. Pokorny J, Smith V, Verriest G, Pinkers AJ (eds): *Congenital and Acquired Color Vision Defects.* New York: Grune & Stratton, 1979, 57–70.
31. Fishman GA, Krill A, Fishman M: Acquired color defects in patients with open angle glaucoma and ocular hypertension. *Mod Prob Ophthalmol 1974;13:335–338.*
32. Lakowski R, Bryett J, Drance SM: A study of color vision in ocular hypertension. *Can J Ophthalmol 1972;7:86–95.*
33. Motolko M, Drance SM, Douglas GR: The early psychophysical disturbances in chronic open angle glaucoma: A study of visual functions with asymmetric disc cupping. *Arch Opthalmol 1982;100:1632–1634.*
34. Airaksinen PJ, Lakowski R, Drance SM, Price M: Color vision and retinal nerve fiber layer. *Am J Ophthalmol 1986;102:208–213.*
35. Arden GB, Jacobson J: A simple grating test for contrast sensitivity: Preliminary results indicate value for screening in glaucoma. *Invest Ophthalmol Vis Sci 1978;17:23–32.*

36. Hitchings RA, Powell DJ, Arden GB, Carter RM: Contrast sensitivity gratings in glaucoma family screening. *Br J Ophthalmol 1981; 65:515–517.*
37. Kayazawa F, Nishimur K, Tanabe T, et al: Contrast sensitivity function in primary open-angle glaucoma. *Glaucoma 1984;6:13–16.*
38. Motolko MA, Phelps CD: Contrast sensitivity in asymmetric glaucoma. *Int Ophthalmol 1984;7:45–50.*
39. Sokol S, Domar A, Moskowitz A: Utility of the Arden grating test in glaucoma screening: High false-positive rate in normals over 50 years of age. *Invest Ophthalmol Vis Sci 1980;19:1529–1533.*
40. Drance SM, Airaksinen PJ, Price M, et al: The correlation of functional and structural measurements in glaucoma patients and normal subjects. *Am J Ophthalmol 1986;101:612–615.*
41. Lustgarten JS, Marx MS, Podos SM, et al: Contrast sensitivity and computerized perimetry in early detection of glaucomatous change. *Clin Vis Sci 1990;5:407–413.*
42. Regan D, Neima D: Balance between pattern and flicker sensitivities in the visual fields of ophthalmological patients. *Br J Ophthalmol 1984;68:310–315.*
43. Tyler CW: Specific deficits of flicker sensitivity in glaucoma and ocular hypertension. *Invest Ophthalmol Vis Sci 1981;20:204–212.*
44. Brussel EM, White CW, Faubert J, Dixon M: Multi-flash campimetry as an indicator of visual field loss in glaucoma. *Am J Optom Physiol Opt 1986;63:32–40.*
45. Ross JE, Bron AJ, Reeves BC, Emerson PG: Detection of optic nerve damage in ocular hypertension. *Br J Ophthalmol 1985;698:897–903.*
46. Atkin A, Bodis–Wollner I, Wolkstein M, et al: Abnormalities of central contrast sensitivity in glaucoma. *Am J Ophthalmol 1979;88:205–211.*
47. Stamper RL: The effect of glaucoma on central visual function. *Trans Am Ophthalmol Soc 1984;82:792–826.*
48. Lundh BL: Central and peripheral contrast sensitivity for static and dynamic sinusoidal gratings in glaucoma. *Acta Ophthalmol 1985; 63:487–492.*
49. Lachenmayr B, Rothbacher H, Gleissner M: Automated flicker perimetry confined to quantitative static perimetry in early glaucoma, in Heijl A (ed): *Perimetry Updates.* Amsterdam: Kugler & Ghedini, 1988–1989, 359–368.
50. Mafei L, Fiorentini A: Electroretinographic responses to alternating gratings before and after section of the optic nerve *Science 1981; 211:953–955.*
51. Sherman J: Simultaneous pattern reversal eletroretinograms and visual evoked potentials in diseases of the macula and optic nerve. *Ann NY Acad Sci 1982;388:214.*
52. Van Den Berg TJ, Riemslag FC, deVos GW, Verguyn Lunel HF: Pattern ERG and glaucomatous visual field defects. *Doc Ophthalmol 1986; 61:335–341.*
53. Marx MS, Podos SM, Bodis–Wollner I, et al : Flash and pattern electroretinograms in normal and laser-induced glaucomatous primate eyes. *Invest Ophthalmol Vis Sci 1986;27:378–386.*
54. Berninger TA, Arden GB: The pattern electroretinogram. *Eye 1988; (suppl 2):257–283.*
55. Papst N, Bopp M, Schnaudigel OP: Pattern-ERG in patients with elevated intraocular pressure. *Klin Mbl Augenheilk 1984;1985:390–392.*
56. Trick GL, Bickler–Bluth M, Cooper DG, et al: Pattern reversal electroretinogram abnormalities in ocular hypertension: correlation with glaucoma risk factors. *Curr Eye Res 1988;7:201–206.*
57. von Graefe A: Über die Untersuchung des Gesichtsfeldes bei amblyopischen Affectionen. *Arch Ophthalmol II 1856;2:258–298.*
58. Foerster AI: Sitzungsbericht der Ophthalmologischen Gesellschaft im Jahre 1869. *Klin Mbl Augenheilk 1869;7:411–422.*
59. Bjerrum J: Om en tilføjelse til den sædvanlige synsfeltunersögelse samt om synsfeltet ved glaukom. *Nord Ophthalmol Tidsskrift 1889;II:141–185.*

60. Rønne H: Über das Gesichfeld beim Glaukom. *Klin Mbl Augenheilk 1909;47:12–33.*
61. Drance SM: The glaucoma visual field defect and its progression, in Drance SM, Anderson DR (eds): *Automatic Perimetry in Glaucoma. A Practical Guide.* Orlando: Grune & Stratton, 1985, 43–54.
62. Primrose J: Early signs of the glaucomatous disc. *Ophthalmol 1971; 55:820–825.*
63. Aulhorn E, Harms H: Early visual field defects in glaucoma, in Leydhecker W (ed): *Glaucoma, Symposium Tutzing Castle 1966* Basel, New York: Karger, 1967, 151–186.
64. Aulhorn E, Karmeyer H: Frequency distribution in early glaucomatous field defects. *Doc Ophthalmol Proc Ser 1977;14:75–83.*
65. Werner EB, Drance SM: Early visual field disturbances in glaucoma. *Arch Ophthalmol 1977;95:1173–1175.*
66. Caprioli J, Spaeth GL: Static threshold examination of the peripheral nasal visual field in glaucoma. *Arch Ophthalmol 1985;103:1150–1154.*
67. LeBlanc RP, Lee A, Baxter M: Peripheral nasal field defects. *Doc Ophthalmol Proc Ser 1985;42:377–381.*
68. Werner EB, Drance SM: Increased scatter of responses as a precursor of visual field changes in glaucoma. *Can J Ophthalmol 1977; 12:140–142.*
69. Holmin C, Krakau CET: Variability of glaucomatous field defects in computerized perimetry. *Graefes Arch Clin Ophthalmol 1979;210: 235–250.*
70. Antcil JL, Anderson DR: Early foveal involvement and generalized depression of the visual field in glaucoma. *Arch Ophthalmol 1984; 102:363–370.*
71. Drance SM, Doublas GR, Airaksinen PJ, et al: Diffuse loss in chronic open-angle glaucoma and low-tension glaucoma. *Am J Ophthalmol 1987;104:577–580.*
72. Glowaski A, Flammer J: Is there a difference between glaucoma patients with rather localized field damage and patients with more diffuse visual field damage? *Doc Ophthalmol Proc Ser 1987;49:317–320.*
73. Caprioli J, Sears M: Pattern of early visual field loss in open angle glaucoma. *Doc Ophthalmol Proc Ser 1987;49:307–315.*
74. Heijl A: Lack of diffuse loss of differential light sensitivity in early glaucoma. *Acta Ophthalmol 1989: 67:353–360.*
75. Langerhorst CT: Fluctuation behavior and general and local reduction of sensitivity, *Automated Perimetry in Glaucoma.* Amstelveen: Kugler, 1988, 136.
76. Flammer J, Drance SM, Augustiny L, Funkhouser A: Quantification of glaucomatous field defects with automated perimetry. *Invest Ophthalmol Vis Sci 1985;26:176–181.*
77. Heijl A, Lindgren G, Olsson J: A package for the statistical analysis of visual fields. *Doc Ophthalmol Proc Ser 1987;49:153–168.*
78. Heijl A: Some characteristics of glaucomatous visual field loss, in Krieglstein GK (ed): *Glaucoma Update IV.* Berlin, Heidelberg: Springer, *(in press).*
79. Minckler D: The organization of nerve fiber bundles in the primate optic nerve head. *Arch Ophthalmol 1980;98:1630–1636.*
80. Heijl A: Automatic perimetry in glaucoma visual field screening: A clinical study. *Graefes Arch Clin Ophthalmol 1976;200:21–37.*
81. Schmied U: Automatic (Octopus) and manual (Goldmann) perimetry in glaucoma. *Graefes Arch Clin Ophthalmol 1980;213:239–244.*
82. Johnson CA, Keltner JL: Automated suprathreshold static perimetry. *Am J Ophthalmol 1980;89:731–741.*
83. Dyster–Aas K, Heijl A, Lundquist L: Computerized visual field screening in the management of patients with ocular hypertension. *Acta Ophthalmol 1980;58:918–928.*
84. Anderson DR: *Perimetry: With and Without Automation.* St. Louis: CV Mosby, 1987, 41.
85. Greve EL: *Single and Multiple Stimulus Static Perimetry in Glaucoma: The Two Phases of Visual Field Examination.* The Hague: Junk Publishers, 1973.

86. Armaly MF: Selective perimetry for glaucomatous defects in ocular hypertension. *Arch Ophthalmol 1972;87:518–524.*
87. Rock WJ, Drance Sm, Morgan RW: Visual field screening in glaucoma: An evaluation of the Armaly technique for screening glaucomatous visual fields. *Arch Ophthalmol 1973;89:287–290.*
88. Mikelberg FS, Drance SM: The mode of progression of visual field defects in glaucoma. *Am J Ophthalmol 1984;98:443–445.*
89. Haley MJ: *The Humphrey Field Analyzer Primer,* ed 2. San Leandro, CA: Allergan–Humphrey, 1987.
90. Heijl A, Drance SM: Changes in differential threshold in patients with glaucoma during prolonged perimetry. *Br J Ophthalmol 1983; 67:512–516.*
91. Heijl A, Lindgren G, Olsson J: Reliability parameters in computarized perimetry. *Doc Ophthalmol Proc Ser 1987;49:593–600.*
92. LeBlanc RP: Abnormal values in computerized perimetry, in Whalen WR, Spaeth GL (eds): *Computerized Visual Fields. What They Are and How to Use Them.* Thorofare NJ: Slack, 1985, 167.
93. Heijl A, Lindgren G, Olsson J, Åsman P: Visual field interpretation with empiric probability maps. *Arch Ophthalmol 1989;107:204–208.*
94. Heijl A, Lindgren G, Olsson J: Normal variability of static perimetric threshold values across the central visual field. *Arch Ophthalmol 1987;105:1544–1549.*
95. Lewis RA, Johnson CA, Keltner JL, et al: Variability of quantitative automated perimetry in normal observers. *Ophthalmology 1986; 93:878–881.*
96. Holmin C, Krakau CET: Visual field decay in normal subjects and in cases of chronic glaucoma. *Graefes Arch Clin Ophthalmol 1980; 213:291–298.*
97. Sommer A, Enger C, Witt K: Screening for glaucomatous visual field loss with automated threshold perimetry. *Am J Ophthalmol 1987; 103:681–684.*
98. Åsman P, Heijl A: Glaucoma hemifield test. Automated visual field evaluation. *Arch Ophthalmol 1992; 100:812–819.*
99. Wood JM, Wild JM, Hussey MK, et al: Serial examination of the normal visual field using Octopus automated projection perimetry. *Acta Ophthalmol 1987;65:326–333.*
100. Heijl A, Lindgren G, Olsson J: The effect of perimetric experience in normal subjects. *Arch Ophthalmol 1989;107:81–86.*
101. Chauhan BC, Drance SM, Douglas GR: The use of visual field indices in detecting changes in the visual field in glaucoma. *Invest Ophthalmol Vis Sci 1990;31:512–520.*
102. Heijl A, Lindgren A, Lindgren G: Test-retest variability in glaucomatous visual fields. *Am J Ophthalmol 1989;108:130–135.*
103. Heijl A, Lindgren A, Lindgren G, Patella M: Inter-test threshold variability in glaucoma: Importance of censored observations and general field status, in Mills RP, Heijl A (eds): *Perimetry Update 1990/91* Amsterdam, New York: Kugler & Ghedini, 1991, 189–192.
104. *Statpac 2, Manual:* San Leandro, CA: Allergan–Humphrey, 1989.
105. Holmin C, Krakau CET: Regression analysis of the central visual field in chronic glaucoma cases. *Acta Ophthalmol 1982;60:267–274.1989.*
106. Fankhauser F, Jenni A: Programs Sargon and Delta: two new principles for the automated analysis of the visual field. *Graefes Arch Clin Ophthalmol 1981;216:41–48.*
107. Hills JF, Johnson CA: Evaluation of the t-test as a method of detecting visual field changes. *Ophthalmology 1988;95:261–266.*
108. Krakau CET: Hazards in evaluation of visual field decay. *Doc Ophthalmol 1986;63:239–246.*
109. Arden GB, Jacobson JJ: A simple grating test for contrast sensitivity: Preliminary results indicate value in screening for glaucoma. *Invest Ophthalmol Vis Sci 1978;17:23–32.*
110. Hitchings RA, Powell DJ, Arden GB, Carter RM: Contrast sensitivity gratings in glaucoma family screening. *Br J Ophthalmol 1981;65: 515–517.*

111. Sokol S, Domar A, Moskowitz A: Utility of the Arden grating test in glaucoma screening: High false-positive rate in normals over 50 years of age. *Invest Ophthalmol Vis Sci 1980;19:1529–1533.*
112. Atkin A, Bodis–Wollner I, Wolkstein M, et al: Abnormalities of central contrast sensitivity in glaucoma. *Am J Ophthalmol 1978;88:205–211.*
113. Atkin A, Wolkstein M, Bodis–Wollner I, et al: Interocular comparison of contrast sensitivities in glaucoma patients and suspects. *Br J Ophthalmol 1980;64:858–862.*
114. Wolkstein M, Atkin A, Bodis–Wollner I: Contrast sensitivity in retinal disease. *Ophthalmol 1980;87:1140–1149.*
115. Quigley HA, Addicks EM, Green WR: Optic nerve damage in human glaucoma: III. Quantitative correlation of nerve fiber loss and visual field defect in glaucoma, ischemic neuropathy, papilledema, and toxic neuropathy. *Arch Ophthalmol 1982;100:135–146.*
116. Glovinsky Y, Quigley HA, Dunkelberger GR: Retinal ganglion cell loss is size dependent in experimental glaucoma. *Invest Ophthalmol Vis Sci 1991;32:484–491.*
117. Weinstein GW, Arden GB, Hitchings RA, et al: The pattern electroretinogram (PERG) in ocular hypertension and glaucoma. *Arch Ophthalmol 1988;106:923–928.*
118. Bobak P, Bodis–Wollner I, Harnois C, et al: Pattern electroretinograms and visual evoked potentials in glaucoma and multiple sclerosis. *Am J Ophthalmol 1983;96:72–83.*
119. Trick GL: PRRP abnormalities in glaucoma and ocular hypertension. *Invest Ophthalmol Vis Sci 1986;27:1730–1740.*
120. Trick GL, Bickler–Bluth M, Cooper DG, et al: Pattern reversal electroretinogram abnormalities in ocular hypertension: correlation with risk factors. *Curr Eye Res 1988;7:201–206*
121. Drance SM, Airaksinen PJ, Price M, et al: The use of psychophysical, structural, and electrodiagnostic perameters to identify glaucomatous damage. *Graefes Arch Clin Exp Ophthalmol 1987;225:365–368.*
122. Falcao–Reis F, O'Donoghue E, Buceti R, et al: Peripheral contrast sensitivity in glaucoma and ocular hypertension. *Br J Ophthalmol 1990; 74:712–716.*
123. Lundh BL: Central contrast sensitivity tests in the detection of early glaucoma. *Acta Ophthalmol 1985;63:481–486.*
124. Tyler CW: Specific deficits of flicker sensitivity in glaucoma and ocular hypertension. *Invest Ophthalmol Vis Sci 1981;20:204–212.*
125. Brussell EM, Mucramans M, White CW, et al: Chromatic flicker deficits in glaucoma patients and suspects, in Heijl A (ed): *Perimetry Update.* Amsterdam: Kugler & Ghendini, 1989, 45–52.
126. Regan D, Neima D: Balance between pattern and flicker sensitivities in the visual fields of ophthalmological patients. *Br J Ophthalmol 1984;68:310–315.*
127. Korth M, Horn F, Storck B, Jonas JB: Spatial and spatiotemporal contrast sensitivity of normal and glaucoma eyes. *Graefes Arch Clin Exp Opthalmol 1989;227:428–435.*
128. Ross JE, Bron AJ, Clarke DD: Contrast sensitivity and visual disability in chronic simple glaucoma. *Br J Ophthalmol 1984;68:821–827.*
129. Ross JE: Clinical detection of abnormalities in central vision in chronic simple glaucoma using contrast sensitivity. *Int Ophthalmol 1985;8:167–177.*
130. Ross JE, Bron AJ, Reeves BC, Emmerson PG: Detection of optic nerve damage in ocular hypertension. *Br J Ophthalmol 1985;69:897–903.*
131. Lustgarten JS, Marx MS, Podos SM, et al: Contrast sensitivity and computerized perimetry in early detection of glaucomatous change. *Clin Vis Sci 1990;5:407–413.*
132. Montanaro M, Gandolfo E, Giodano G, Alitta P: Studio comparativo del campo visivo e della sensibilita al contrasto nel glaucoma iniziale. *Boll Oculist 1988;67:89–93.*
133. Motolko M, Drance SM, Douglas GR: The early psychophysical disturbances in chronic open-angle glaucoma. A study of visual functions with asymmetric cupping. *Arch Ophthalmol 1982;100:1632–1634.*

134. Lundh BL: Central and peripheral contrast sensitivity for static and dynamic sinusoidal gratings in glaucoma. *Acta Ophthalmol 1985;63:487–492.*
135. Lundh BL: Eccentric contrast sensitivity loss in glaucoma. *Acta Ophthalmol 1981;59:21–24.*
136. Pokorny J, Smith V, Verriest G, Pinkers AJ (eds): *Congenital and Acquired Colour Vision Defects.* New York: Grune & Stratton, 1979, 57–70.
137. Davson H: *Physiology of the Eye.* New York: Academic Press, 1980, 327–359.
138. Sample PA, Weinreb RN, Boynthon RM: Acquired dyschromatopsia in glaucoma. *Surv Ophthalmol 1986;31:54–64.*
139. Drance SM, Lakowski R, Schulzer M, Douglas GR: Acquired colour vision changes in glaucoma. *Arch Ophthalmol 1981;99:829–831.*
140. Francois J, Verriest G: Les dyschromatopsies dan le glaucome primaire. *Ann Ocul (Paris) 1959;192:191–199.*
141. DuBois–Poulson A, Magis C: Les procédés d'examen de la fonction visuelle dans le glaucome chronique. *Ophthalmologica 1960;139:155–213.*
142. Krill AE, Fishman GA: Acquired colour vision defects. *Trans Am Acad Ophthalmol Otolaryngol 1971;75:1095–1112.*
143. Lakowski R, Drance SM: Acquired dyschromatopsias: The earliest functional losses in glaucoma. *Doc Ophthalmol Proc Ser 1979;19:159–165.*
144. Pokorny J, Smith V, Verriest G, Pinkers AJ (eds): *Congenital and Acquired Colour Vision Defects.* New York: Grune & Stratton, 1979, 57-70.
145. Verriest G, Uvijls A: Spectral increment thresholds on a white background in different age groups of normal subjects and in acquired ocular disease. *Doc Ophthalmol 1977;43:217–248.*
146. Marmion VJ: The color vision deficiency in open angle glaucoma. *Mod Pro Ophthalmol 1979;19:305.*
147. Flammer J, Drance SM: Correlation between colour vision scores and quantitative perimetry in suspected glaucoma. *Arch Ophthalmol 1984;102:38–39.*
148. Heron G, Adams AJ, Husted R: Central fields for short losses wavelength sensitive pathways in glaucoma and hypertension. *Invest Ophthalmol Vis Sci 1988;29:64–70.*
149. Drum B, Armaly MF, Huppert W: Scotopic sensitivity loss in glaucoma. *Arch Ophthalmol 1986;43:712–717.*
150. Lakowski R, Airaksinen PJ, Drance SM, Yamazaki Y: Chromatic functional loss and its relation to the morphology of the retina in the glaucomatous eye, in Drum B, Verriest G (eds): Dordreist, Netherlands: Kluwer Academic Publishers, 1989.
151. Drance SM, Douglas GR, Airaksinen PJ, et al: Diffuse visual field loss in chronic open-angle glaucoma and low-tension glaucoma. *Am J Ophthalmol 1987;104:577–580.*
152. Yamazaki Y, Lakowski R, Drance SM: A comparison of the blue colour mechanism in high and low tension glaucoma. *Ophthalmology 1989;96:12–15.*
153. Fishman GA, Krill A, Fishman M: Acquired colour defects in patients with open angle glaucoma and ocular hypertension. *Mod Prob Ophthalmol 1974;13:335–338.*
154. Lakowski R, Bryett J, Drance SM: A study of colour vision in ocular hypertension. *Can J Ophthalmol 1972;7:86–95.*
155. Motolko M, Drance SM, Douglas GR: The early psychophysical disturbances in chronic open angle glaucoma: A study of visual function with asymmetric disc cupping. *Arch Ophthalmol 1982;100:1632–1634.*
156. Hamill TR, Post RB, Johnson CA, Keltner JL: Correlation of color vision deficits and observable changes in the optic disc in a population of ocular hypertensives. *Arch Ophthalmol 1984;102:1637–1639.*
157. Hart WM, Silverman SE, Trick GL, et al: Glaucoma visual field damage. *Invest Ophthalmol Vis Sci 1990;31:359–367.*

158. Hart WM: Acquired dyschromatopsias. *Surv Ophthalmol 1987;32: 10–31.*
159. Brussell EM, Mucramans M, White CW, et al: Chromatic flicker deficits in glaucoma patients and suspects, in Heijl A (ed): *Perimetry Update.* Amsterdam: Kugler & Ghedini, 1988–1989, 45–52.
160. Adams AJ, Rodic R, Husted R, Stamper R: Spectral sensitivity and color discrimation changes in glaucoma and glaucoma-suspect patients. *Invest Ophthalmol Vis Sci 1982;23:516–524.*
161. Hart WM, Gordon MO: Color perimetry of glaucomatous visual field defects. *Ophthalmology 1984;91:338–346.*
162. Maffei L, Fiorentini A: Electroretinographic responses to alternating gratings before and after section of the optic nerve. *Science 1981; 211:953–955.*
163. Fiorentini A, Maffei L, Pirchio M, Spinelli D, Porciatti V: The ERG in reponse to alternating gratings in patients with diseases of the peripheral visual pathway. *Invest Ophthalmol Vis Sci 1981;21:490–493.*
164. Maffei L, Fiorentini A, Bisti S, Hollander H: Pattern ERG in the monkey after section of the optic nerve. *Exp Brain Res 1985;59:423–425.*
165. Marx MS, Podos SM, Bodis–Wollner I, et al: Flash and pattern eletroretinograms in normal and laser-induced glaucomatous primate eyes. *Invest Ophthalmol Vis Sci 1986;27:378–386.*
166. Berninger TA, Arden GB: The pattern electroretinogram. *Eye 1988; (suppl 2): 257–283.*
167. Trick GI, Bickler–Bluth M, Cooper DG, et al: Pattern reversal electroretinogram (PRERG) abnormalities in ocular hypertension: Correlation with glaucoma risk factors. *Curr Eye Res 1988;7:201–206.*
168. Weinstein GW, Arden GB, Hitchings RA, et al: The pattern electroretinogram (PERG) in ocular hypertension and glaucoma. *Arch Ophthalmol 1988;106:923–928.*
169. Conte MM, Brodie SE: Altered contrast and luminance contributions to the pattern ERG in glaucoma (abstr). *Invest Ophthalmol Vis Sci 1987;(suppl 28):129.*
170. Papst N, Bopp M, Schnaudigel OP: Pattern-ERG in patients with elevated intraocular pressure. *Klin Mbl Augenheilk 1984;185:390–392.*
171. O'Sullivan F, Arden GB, Hitchings R, et al: Longitudinal changes in a cohort of patients with ocular hypertension and glaucoma, tested with the pattern ERG (abstr). *Invest Ophthalmol Vis Sci 1991;(suppl 32):1192.*
172. Trick GL: Visual impairments in glaucoma and ocular hypertension (OHT): Results of a 4-year prospective study (abstr). *Invest Ophthalmol Vis Sci 1991;(suppl 32):1192.*
173. Bresnick GH, Palta M: Oscillatory potential amplitudes. Relation to severity of diabetic retinopathy. *Arch Ophthalmol 1987;105:929–933.*
174. Gur M, Zeevi YY, Bielik M, Neumann E: Changes in the oscillatory potentials of the electroretinogram in glaucoma. *Curr Eye Res 1987; 6:457–466.*
175. Brodie SE, Frisch S, Siebold E, et al: Fourier analysis of the oscillatory potentials in glaucoma and ocular hypertension (abstr). *Invest Ophthalmol Vis Sci 1988;(suppl 29): 239.*
176. Abe H, Hasegawa S, Itaka K: Contrast sensitivity and pattern visual evoked potential in patients with glaucoma. *Doc Ophthalmol Proc Ser 1987;65:65–70.*
177. Schmeisser ET, Smith TJ: High-frequency flicker visual-evoked potential losses in glaucoma. *Ophthalmology 1988;96:620–623.*
178. Drance SM, Airaksinen PJ, Price M, et al: The use of psychophysical, structural, and electrodiagnostic parameters to identify glaucomatous damage. *Graefes Arch Clin Exp Ophthalmol 1987;225:365–368.*
179. Bartl G: Das Elektroretinogramm und das evozierte Sehrindenpotential bei normalen und an Glaukom erkrankten Augen. *Graefes Arch Clin Exp Ophthalmol 1978;207:243–269.*

CHAPTER 8
SPECIFIC TYPES OF GLAUCOMA

1. Shields MB: Primary angle-closure glaucoma, in Shields MB (ed): *Textbook of Glaucoma*, ed 3. Baltimore: Williams & Wilkins, 1992, 198–219.
2. Hoskins HD Jr, Kass MA: Angle-closure glaucoma with pupillary block, in Hoskins HD Jr, Kass MA (eds): *Becker–Shaffer's Diagnosis and Therapy of the Glaucomas*, ed 6. St. Louis: CV Mosby, 1989, 208–237.
3. Tornquist R: Chamber depth in primary acute glaucoma. *Br J Ophthalmol 1956;40:421–429.*
4. Fontana ST, Brubaker RF: Volume and depth of the anterior chamber in the normal aging human eye. *Arch Ophthalmol 1980;98:1803–1808.*
5. Wilensky J: Racial influences in glaucoma. *Ann Ophthalmol 1977; 9:1545.*
6. Drance SM: Angle closure glaucoma among Canadian Eskimos. *Can J Ophthalmol 1973;8:252–254.*
7. Hagan JC III, Lederer CM Jr: Primary angle closure glaucoma in a myopic kinship. *Arch Ophthalmol 1985;103:363–365.*
8. Lowe RF: Anterior lens displacement with age. *Br J Ophthalmol 1970; 54:117–121.*
9. Appleby RS Jr, Kinder RSL: Bilateral angle-closure glaucoma in a 14–year-old boy. *Arch Ophthalmol 1971;86:449–450.*
10. Mandelkorn RM, Zimmerman TJ: Effects of nonsteroidal drugs on glaucoma, in Ritch R, Shields MB, Krupin T (eds): *The Glaucomas*. St. Louis: CV Mosby, 1989, 1169–1184.
11. Mapstone R: Mechanics of pupil block. *Br J Ophthalmol 1968; 52:19–25.*
12. Anderson DR, Davis EB: Sensitivities of ocular tissues to acute pressure-induced ischemia. *Arch Ophthalmol 1975;93:267–274.*
13. Anderson DR: Pathology of the glaucomas. *Br J Ophthalmol 1972; 56:146–157.*
14. Zimmerman LE, de Venecia G, Hamasaki DI: Pathology of the optic nerve in experimental acute glaucoma. *Invest Ophthalmol 1967; 6:109–125.*
15. Douglas GR, Drance SM, Schulzer M: The visual field and nerve head in angle-closure glaucoma. A comparison of the effects of acute and chronic angle closure. *Arch Ophthalmol 1975;93:409–411.*
16. McNaught EI, Rennie A, McClure E, Chisholm IA: Pattern of visual damage after acute angle-closure glaucoma. *Trans Ophthalmol Soc UK 1974;94:406–415.*
17. Airaksinen PJ, Saari KM, Tiainen TJ, Jaanio E-AT: Management of acute closed-angle glaucoma with miotics and timolol. *Br J Ophthalmol 1979;63:822–825.*
18. Wand M, Grant WM: Thymoxamine hydrochloride: An alpha-adrenergic blocker. *Surv Ophthalmol 1980;25:75–84.*
19. Allinson RW, Gerber DS, Bieber S, Hodes BL: Reversal of mydriasis by dapiprazole. *Ann Ophthalmol 1990;22:131–138.*
20. Anderson DR: Corneal indentation to relieve acute angle-closure glaucoma. *Am J Ophthalmol 1979;88:1091–1093.*
21. Ritch R: Argon laser treatment for medically unresponsive attacks of angle-closure glaucoma. *Am J Ophthalmol 1982;94:197–204.*
22. Campbell DG, Vela A: Modern goniosynechialysis for the treatment of synechial angle-closure glaucoma. *Ophthalmology 1984;91: 1052–1060.*
23. Lowe RF: Acute angle-closure glaucoma: An analysis of 200 cases. *Br J Ophthalmol 1962;46:641–645.*
24. Chandler PA, Trotter RR: Angle-closure glaucoma. Subacute types. *Arch Ophthalmol 1955;53:305–317.*
25. Lowe RF: Primary creeping angle-closure glaucoma. *Br J Ophthalmol 1964;48:544–550.*
26. Tielsch JM, Sommer A, Katz J, et al: Racial variations in the prevalence of glaucoma: the Baltimore Eye Survey, *Invest Ophthalmol Vis Sci 1990;31(suppl 4):431.*

27. Forbes M: Gonioscopy with corneal indentation: A method for distinguishing between appositional closure and synechial closure. *Arch Ophthalmol 1966;76:488–492.*
28. Wand M, Grant WM, Simmons RJ, Hutchinson BT: Plateau iris syndrome. *Trans Am Acad Ophthalmol Otolaryngol 1977;83:122–130.*
29. Friedman Z, Neumann E: Comparison of prone-position, dark-room, and mydriatic tests for angle-closure glaucoma before and after peripheral iridectomy. *Am J Ophthalmol 1972;74:24–27.*
29A. Wilensky JT, Kaufman PL, Frolichstein D, et al: Follow-up of angle-closure glaucoma suspects. *Am J Ophthalmol 1993;115:338–346.*
30. Hoskins HD Jr, Kass MA: Angle-closure glaucoma without pupillary block, in Hoskins HD Jr, Kass MA (eds): *Becker-Shaffer's Diagnosis and Therapy of the Glaucomas*, ed 6. St. Louis: CV Mosby, 1989, 238–276.
31. Shields MB: Glaucoma associated with disorders of the retina, vitreous, and choroid, in Shields MB (ed): *Textbook of Glaucoma*, ed 3. Baltimore: Williams & Wilkins, 1992, 307–328.
32. Wand M: Neovascular glaucoma, in Ritch R, Shields MB, Krupin T (eds): *The Glaucomas*. St. Louis: CV Mosby, 1989, 1063–1110.
33. Ohrt V: The frequency of rubeosis iridis in diabetic patients. *Acta Ophthalmol (Copenh) 1971;49:301–307.*
34. Blankenship G, Cortez R, Machemer R: The lens and pars plana vitrectomy for diabetic retinopathy complications. *Arch Ophthalmol 1979;97:1263–1267.*
35. Machemer R, Blankenship G: Vitrectomy for proliferative diabetic retinopathy associated with vitreous hemorrhage. *Ophthalmology 1981;88:643–646.*
36. Hayreh SS, Rojas P, Podhajsky P, et al: Ocular neovascularization with retinal vascular occlusion. III. Incidence of ocular neovascularization with retinal vein occlusion. *Ophthalmology 1983;90:488–506.*
37. Servais GE, Thompson HS, Hayreh SS: Relative afferent pupillary defect in central retinal vein occlusion. *Ophthalmology 1986; 93:301–303.*
38. Magargal LE, Donoso LA, Sanborn GE: Retinal ischemia and risk of neovascularization following central retinal vein obstruction. *Ophthalmology 1982;89:1241–1245.*
39. Hayreh SS, Podhajsky P: Ocular neovascularization with retinal vascular occlusion. II. Occurrence in central and branch retinal artery occlusion. *Arch Ophthalmol 1982;100:1585–1596.*
40. Magargal LE, Brown GC, Augsburger JJ, Parrish RK: Neovascular glaucoma following branch retinal vein obstruction. *Glaucoma 1981; 3:333–337.*
41. Brown GC, Magargal LE, Schachat A, Shah H: Neovasclar glaucoma: Etiologic considerations. *Ophthalmology 1984;91:315–320.*
42. Weiss DI, Shaffer RN, Nehrenberg TR: Neovascular glaucoma complicating carotid-cavernous fistula. *Arch Ophthalmol 1963;69:304–307.*
43. Glaser BM, D'Amore PA, Michaels RG, et al: The demonstration of angiogenic activity from ocular tissues. Preliminary report. *Ophthalmology 1980;87:440–446.*
44. Thompson JT, Glaser BM: Role of lensectomy and posterior capsule in movement of tracers from vitreous to aqueous. *Arch Ophthalmol 1985;103:420–421.*
45. Pries I, Langer R, Brem S, Folkman J: Inhibition of neovascularization by an extract derived from vitreous. *Am J Ophthalmol 1977;84: 323–328.*
46. Williams GA, Eisenstein R, Schumacher B, et al: Inhibitor of vascular endothelial cell growth in the lens. *Am J Ophthalmol 1984;97: 366–371.*
47. Poliner LS, Christianson DJ, Escoffery RF, et al: Neovascular glaucoma after intracapsular and extracapsular cataract extraction in diabetic patients. *Am J Ophthalmol 1985;100:637–643.*
48. Weinreb RN, Wasserstrom JP, Parker W: Neovascular glaucoma following neodymium:YAG laser posterior capsulotomy. *Arch Ophthalmol 1986;104:730–731.*

49. Ehrenberg M, McKuen BW II, Schindler RH, Machemer R: Rubeosis iridis: Preoperative iris fluorescein angiography and periocular steroids. *Ophthalmology 1984;91:321–325.*
50. John T, Sassani JW, Eagle RC Jr: The myofibroblastic component of rubeosis iridis. *Ophthalmology 1983;90:721–728.*
51. Grant WM: Management of neovascular glaucoma, in Leopold IH (ed): *Symposium on Ocular Therapy*, Vol 7. St. Louis: CV Mosby, 1974, 36–61.
52. Wand M: Neovascular glaucoma, in Ritch R, Shields MB (eds): *The Secondary Glaucomas*. St. Louis: CV Mosby, 1982, 162–193.
53. Tano Y, Chandler D, Machemer R: Treatment of intraocular proliferation with intravitreal injection of triamcinolone acetonide. *Am J Ophthalmol 1980;90:810–816.*
54. Murphy RP, Egbert PR: Regression of iris neovascularization following panretinal photocoagulation. *Arch Ophthalmol 1979;97:700–702.*
55. Magargal LE, Brown GC, Augsburger JJ, Donoso LA: Efficacy of panretinal photocoagulation in preventing neovascular glaucoma following ischemic central retinal vein obstruction. *Ophthalmology 1982; 89:780–783.*
56. May DR, Bergstrom TJ, Parmet AJ, Schwartz JG: Treatment of neovascular glaucoma with transscleral panretinal cryotherapy. *Ophthalmology 1980;87:1106–1111.*
57. Simmons RJ, Depperman SR, Dueker DK: The role of gonio-photocoagulation in neovascularization of the anterior chamber angle. *Ophthalmology 1980;87:79–82.*
58. Allen RC, Bellows AR, Hutchinson BT, Murphy SD: Filtration surgery in the treatment of neovascular glaucoma. *Ophthalmology 1982;89: 1181–1187.*
59. Rockwood EJ, Parrish RK II, Heuer DK, et al: Glaucoma filtering surgery with 5-fluorouracil. *Ophthalmology 1987;94:1071–1078.*
60. Skuta GL, Beeson CC, Higginbotham EJ, et al: Intraoperative mitomycin versus postoperative 5-fluorouracil in high-risk glaucoma filtering surgery. *Ophthalmology 1992;99:438–444.*
61. Minckler DS, Heuer DK, Hasty B, et al: Clinical experience with the single-plate Molteno implant in complicated glaucomas. *Ophthalmology 1988;95:1181–1188.*
62. Shields MB: Glaucomas following ocular surgery, in Shields MB (ed): *Textbook of Glaucoma*, ed 3. Baltimore: Williams & Wilkins, 1992, 400–428.
63. Luntz MH, Rosenblatt M: Malignant glaucoma. *Surv Ophthalmol 1987;32:73–93.*
64. Shaffer RN, Hoskins HD Jr: Ciliary block (malignant) glaucoma. *Ophthalmology 1978;85:215–221.*
65. Chandler PA, Grant WM: Mydriatic-cycloplegic treatment in malignant glaucoma. *Arch Ophthalmol 1962;68:353–359.*
66. Levene R: A new concept of malignant glaucoma. *Arch Ophthalmol 1972;87:497–506.*
67. Shaffer RN: The role of vitreous detachment in aphakic and malignant glaucoma. *Trans Am Acad Ophthalmol Otolaryngol 1954; 58:217–231.*
68. Simmons RJ, Thomas JV, Yaqub MK: Malignant glaucoma, in Ritch R, Shields MB, Krupin T (eds): *The Glaucomas*. St. Louis: CV Mosby, 1989, 1251–1263.
69. Simmons RJ: Malignant glaucoma, in Ritch R, Shields MB (eds): *The Secondary Glaucomas*. St. Louis: CV Mosby, 1982, 331–344.
70. Hanish SJ, Lamberg RL, Gordon JM: Malignant glaucoma following cataract extraction and intraocular lens implant. *Ophthal Surg 1982; 13:713–714.*
71. Rieser JC, Schwartz B: Miotic-induced malignant glaucoma. *Arch Ophthalmol 1972;87:706–712.*
72. Schwartz AL, Anderson DR: "Malignant glaucoma" in an eye with no antecedent operation or miotics. *Arch Ophthalmol 1975;93:379–381.*

73. Kushner BJ: Ciliary block glaucoma in retinopathy of prematurity. *Arch Ophthalmol 1982;100:1078–1079.*
74. Herschler J: Laser shrinkage of the ciliary processes. A treatment for malignant (ciliary block) glaucoma. *Ophthalmology 1980;87: 1155–1159.*
75. Momeda S, Hayashi H, Oshima K: Anterior pars plana vitrectomy for phakic malignant glaucoma. *Jpn J Ophthalmol 1983;27:73–76.*
76. Epstein DL, Steinert RF, Puliafito CA: Neodymium:YAG laser therapy to the anterior hyaloid in aphakic malignant (ciliovitreal block) glaucoma. *Am J Ophthalmol 1984;98:137–143.*
77. Cashwell LF, Martin TJ: Malignant glaucoma after laser iridectomy. *Ophthalmology 1992;99:651–658.*
78. Alward WLM: Uveitic glaucoma, in Tasman W, Jaeger EA (eds): *Duane's Clinical Ophthalmology,* Vol 3. Philadelphia: JB Lippincott, 1989, chap 54D,1–11.
79. Gressel MG: Lens-induced glaucoma, in Tasman W, Jaeger EA (eds): *Duane's Clinical Ophthalmology,* Vol 3. Philadelphia: JB Lippincott, 1989, chap 54A,1–9.
80. Van Buskirk EM: Pupillary block after intraocular lens implantation. *Am J Ophthalmol 1983;95:55–59.*
81. Weinreb RN, Wasserstrom JP, Forman JS, Ritch R: Pseudophakic pupillary block with angle-closure glaucoma in diabetic patients. *Am J Ophthalmol 1986;102:325–328.*
82. Shields MB: Progressive essential iris atrophy, Chandler's syndrome, and iris-nevus (Cogan-Reese) syndrome: A spectrum of disease. *Surv Ophthalmol 1979;24:3–20.*
83. Phelps CD: Glaucoma associated with diseases of the retina, in Ritch R, Shields MB (eds): *The Secondary Glaucomas.* St. Louis: CV Mosby, 1982, 150–161.
84. Burton TC, Folk JC: Laser iris retraction for angle-closure glaucoma after retinal detachment surgery. *Ophthalmology 1988;95:742–748.*
85. Grant WM: Shallowing of the anterior chamber following occlusion of the central retinal vein. *Am J Ophthalmol 1973;75:384–389.*
86. Vela A, Rieser JC, Campbell DG: The heredity and treatment of angle-closure glaucoma secondary to iris and ciliary body cysts. *Ophthalmology 1983;91:332–337.*
87. Singh OS, Simmons RJ, Brockhurst RJ, Trempe CL: Nanophthalmos: A perspective on identification and therapy. *Ophthalmology 1982;89: 1006–1012.*
88. Kimbrough RL, Trempe CS, Brockhurst RJ, Simmons RJ: Angle-closure glaucoma in nanophthalmos. *Am J Ophthalmol 1979;88:572–579.*
89. Brockhurst RJ: Nanophthalmos with uveal effusion. A new clinical entity. *Arch Ophthalmol 1975;93:1289–1299.*
90. Trelstad RL, Silbermann NN, Brockhurst RJ: Nanophthalmic sclera: Ultrastructural, histochemical, and biochemical observations. *Arch Ophthalmol 1982;100:1935–1938.*
91. Sommer A: Intraocular pressure and glaucoma. *Am J Ophthalmol 1989;107:186–188.*
92. Anderson DR: Glaucoma: The damage caused by pressure. XLVI Edward Jackson Memorial Lecture. *Am J Ophthalmol 1989; 108:485–495.*
93. Hollows FC, Graham PA: The Ferndale glaucoma survey, in Hunt LB (ed): *Glaucoma: Epidemiology, Early Diagnosis, and Some Aspects of Treatment.* London: E & S Livingstone, 1966.
94. Bankes JLK, Perkins ES, Tsolakis S, Wright JE: The Bedford glaucoma survey. *Br Med J 1968;1:791–796..*
95. Armaly MF: Ocular pressure and visual fields. A ten-year follow-up study. *Arch Ophthalmol 1969;81:25–40.*
96. Zeimer RC: Circadian variations in intraocular pressure, in Ritch R, Shields MB, Krupin T (eds): *The Glaucomas.* St Louis: CV Mosby, 1989, 319–336.
97. Drance SM: The significance of the diurnal tension variation in normal and glaucomatous eyes. *Arch Ophthalmol 1960;64:494–501.*

98. Grant WM, Burke JF: Why do some people go blind from glaucoma? *Ophthalmology 1982;89:991–998.*
99. Sponsel WE: Tonometry in question: Can visual screening tests play a more decisive role in glaucoma diagnosis and management? *Surv Ophthalmol 1989;(suppl)33:291–300.*
100. Beck RW, Messner DK, Musch DC, et al: Is there a racial difference in physiologic cup size? *Ophthalmology 1985;92:873–876.*
101. Wilensky JT, Gandhi N, Pan T: Racial influences in open-angle glaucoma. *Ann Ophthalmol 1978;10:1398–1402.*
102. Martin MJ, Sommer A, Gold EB: Race and primary open-angle glaucoma. *Am J Ophthalmol 1985;99:383–387.*
103. Mason RP, Kosoko O, Wilson R, et al: National Survey of the prevalence and risk factors of glaucoma in St. Lucia, West Indies. Part I: Prevalence findings. *Ophthalmology 1989;96:1363–1368.*
104. Leske MC, Troutman HT, Brook S, Connell A: Glaucoma in Barbados. *Arch Ophthalmol 1989;107:169.*
105. Hiller R, Kahn HA: Blindness from glaucoma. *Am J Ophthalmol 1975;80:62–69.*
106. Kahn HA, Roy CM: Alternative definitions of open-angle glaucoma: Effect on prevalence and associations in the Framingham Eye Study. *Arch Ophthalmol 1980;98:2172–2711.*
107. Kolker AE: Glaucoma family study: ten-year follow-up (preliminary report). *Israel J Med Sci 1972;8:1357–1361.*
108. Paterson G: A nine-year follow-up of studies on first-degree relatives of patients with glaucoma simplex. *Trans Ophthalmol Soc UK 1971;90:515.*
109. Becker B: Diabetes mellitus and primary open-angle glaucoma. *Am J Ophthalmol 1971;70:1–16.*
110. Wilson MR, Hertzmark E, Walker AM, et al: A case-control study of risk factors in open-angle glaucoma. *Arch Ophthalmol 1987;105:1066–1071.*
111. Henry JC, Krupin T, Schmitt M, et al: Long-term follow-up of pseudoexfoliation and the development of elevated intraocular pressure. *Ophthalmology 1987;94:545–552.*
112. Farrar SM, Shields MB, Miller KN, Storep CM: Risk factors for the development and severity of glaucoma in pigment dispersion syndrome. *Am J Ophthalmol 1989;108:223–239.*
113. Perkins ES, Phelps CD: Open-angle glaucoma, ocular hypertension, low-tension glaucoma, and refraction. *Arch Ophthalmol 1982;100:1464–1467.*
114. Podos SM, Becker B, Morton WR: High myopia and primary open-angle glaucoma. *Am J Ophthalmol 1966;62:1039–1043.*
115. Armaly MF, Kreuger DE, Maunder L, et al: Biostatistical analysis of the collaborative glaucoma study I. Summary report of the risk factors for glaucomatous visual field defects. *Arch Ophthalmol 1980;98:2163–2172.*
116. Kolker AE, Hetherington J: *Becker–Shaffer's Diagnosis and Therapy of the Glaucomas*, ed 5. St. Louis: CV Mosby, 1983.
117. Trobe JD, Glaser JS, Cassady J, et al: Nonglaucomatous excavation of the optic disc. *Arch Ophthalmol 1980;98:1046–1050.*
118. Rohen JW, Witmer R: Electron microscope studies on the trabecular meshwork in glaucoma simplex. *Graefes Arch Clin Exp Ophthalmol 1972;83:251–266.*
119. Rodrigues MM, Spaeth GL, Livalingam E, Weinreb S: Histopathology of 150 trabeculectomy specimens in glaucoma. *Trans Ophthalmol Soc UK 1976;96: 245–255.*
120. Lütjen–Drecoll E, Shimizu T, Rohrbach M, Rohen JW: Quantitative analysis of "plaque material" in the inner and outer wall of Schlemm's canal in normal and glaucomatous eyes. *Exp Eye Res 1986;42:443–455.*
121. Lütjen–Drecoll E, Shimizu T, Rohrbach M, Rohen JW: Quantitative analysis of "plaque material" between ciliary muscle tips in normal and glaucomatous eyes. *Exp Eye Res 1986;42:457–465.*

122. Alvarado J, Murphy C, Juster R: Trabecular meshwork cellularity in primary open-angle glaucoma and nonglaucomatous normals. *Ophthalmology 1984;91:564–579.*
123. Grierson I, Wang Q, McMenamin PG, Lee WR: The effects of age and antiglaucoma drugs on the meshwork cell population. *Res Clin Forums 1982;4:69–92.*
124. Scheie HG, Cameron JD: Pigment dispersion syndrome: A clinical study. *Br J Ophthalmol 1981;65:264–269.*
125. Mandelkorn RM, Hoffman ME, Olander KW, Zimmerman T, Harsha D: Inheritance and the pigment dispersion syndrome. *Ann Ophthalmol 1983;15:577–582.*
126. McDermott JA, Ritch R, Berger A, Wang RF: Inheritance of pigment dispersion syndrome. *Invest Ophthalmol Vis Sci 1987;(suppl)28:153.*
127. Sugar HS: Pigmentary glaucoma: A 25–year review. *Am J Ophthalmol 1966;62:499–507.*
128. Migliazzo CV, Shaffer RN, Nykin R, Magee S: Long-term analysis of pigment dispersion syndrome and pigmentary glaucoma. *Ophthalmology 1986;93:1528–1536.*
129. Berger A, Ritch R, McDermott JA, Wang RF: Pigmentary dispersion, refraction and glaucoma. *Invest Ophthalmol Vis Sci 1987;(suppl)28:134.*
130. Lotufo D, Ritch R, Sperling M, et al: Pigmentary and POAG in young patients. *Invest Ophthalmol Vis Sci 1986;(suppl)27:166.*
131. Farrar SM, Shields MB, Miller KN, Stoup CM: Risk factors for the development and severity of glaucoma in the pigment dispersion syndrome. *Am J Ophthalmol 1989;108:223–229.*
132. Bellows AR, Jocson VL, Sears ML: Iris pigment granule obstruction of the aqueous outflow channels in enucleated monkey eyes. *Invest Ophthalmol Vis Sci 1974;13(suppl):38.*
133. Grant WM: Experimental aqueous perfusion in enucleated human eyes. *Arch Ophthalmol 1963;69:783–801.*
134. Kristensen P: Mydriasis-induced pigment liberation in the anterior chamber associated with acute rise in intraocular pressure in open-angle glaucoma. *Acta Ophthalmol 1965;43:714–724.*
135. Schenker HI, Luntz M, Kels B, Podos SM: Exercise-induced increase of IOP in the pigmentary dispersion syndrome. *Am J Ophthalmol 1980; 89:598–600.*
136. Smith DL, Kau SF, Rabbani R, Musch DC: The effects of exercise on IOP in pigmentary glaucoma patients. *Ophthal Surg 1989;20:561–567.*
137. Epstein DL, Boger WP III, Grant WM: Phenylephrine provocative testing in the pigment dispersion syndrome. *Am J Ophthalmol 1978;85:43.*
138. Campbell DG: Pigmentary dispersion and glaucoma: A new theory. *Arch Ophthalmol 1979;97:1667.*
139. Kampik A, Green WR, Quigley HA, Pierce LH: Scanning and transmission electron microscopic studies of two cases of pigment dispersion syndrome. *Am J Ophthalmol 1981;91:573.*
140. Richardson TM: Pigmentary glaucoma, in Ritch R, Shields MB, Krupin T (eds): *The Glaucomas*. St. Louis: CV Mosby, 1982, 981–995.
141. Fine BS, Yanoff M, Scheie HG: Pigmentary "glaucoma": A histologic study. *Trans Am Acad Ophthalmol Otolaryngol 1974;78:314–325.*
142. Kupfer C, Kuwabara T, Kaiser–Kupfer M: The histopathology of pigment dispersion syndrome with glaucoma. *Am J Ophthalmol 1975; 80:857–862.*
143. Richardson TM, Hutchinson BT, Grant WM: The outflow tract in pigmentary glaucoma: A light and electron microscopic study. *Arch Ophthalmol 1977;95:115–125.*
144. Lichter PR, Shaffer RM: Diagnostic and prognostic signs in pigmentary glaucoma. *Trans Am Acad Ophthalmol Otolaryngol 1970;74: 984–998.*
145. Speakman JS: Pigmentary dispersion. *Br J Ophthalmol 1981;65: 249–251.*
146. Ritch R: Nonprogressive low-tension glaucoma. *Am J Ophthalmol 1982;94:190–196.*

147. Ritch R, Manusow D, Podos SM: Remission of pigmentary glaucoma in a patient with subluxed lenses. *Am J Ophthalmol 1982;94:812–813.*
148. Lunde MW: Argon laser trabeculoplasty in pigment dispersion syndrome with glaucoma. *Am J Ophthalmol 1983;96:721–725.*
149. Hagadus J, Ritch R, Pollack I, et al: Argon laser trabeculoplasty in pigmentary glaucoma. *Invest Ophthalmol Vis Sci 1984;25(suppl):94.*
150. Liebmann J, Ritch R, Pollack I, et al: Argon laser trabeculoplasty in pigmentary glaucoma: Long-term follow-up. *Invest Ophthalmol Vis Sci 1990;31(suppl):18.*
151. Streeten BW, Bookman L, Ritch R, et al: Pseudoexfoliative fibrillopathy in the conjunctiva. A relation to elastic fibers and elastosis. *Ophthalmology 1987;94:1439–1449.*
152. Aasved H: Mass screening for fibrillopathia epitheliocapsularis. *Acta Ophthalmol 1971;49:334–343.*
153. Krause U, Alanko HI, Karna J, et al: Prevalence of exfoliation syndrome in Finland. *Acta Ophthalmol 1988;66(suppl 184):120–122.*
154. Hiller R, Sperduto RD, Krueger DE: Pseudoexfoliation, intraocular pressure, and senile lens changes in a population based survey. *Arch Ophthalmol 1982;100:1080–1082.*
155. Cashwell LF, Shields MB: Exfoliation syndrome. Prevalence in a southeastern United States population. *Arch Ophthalmol 1988; 106:335–336.*
156. Aasved H: The geographical distribution of fibrillopathia epitheliocapsularis. *Acta Ophthalmol 1969;47:792–810.*
157. Forsius H: Prevalence of pseudoexfoliation of the lens in Finns, Lapps, Icelanders, Eskimos, and Russians. *Trans Ophthalmol Soc UK 1979; 99:296–298.*
158. Henry JC, Krupin T, Schmitt M, et al: Long-term follow-up of pseudoexfoliation and the development of elevated intraocular pressure. *Ophthalmology 1987;94:545–549.*
158A. Schlotzer-Schrehardt UM, Koca MR, Naumann GOH, Volkholz H: Pseudoexfoliation syndrome. Ocular manifestation of a systemic disorder? *Arch Ophthalmol 1992;110:1752–1756.*
158B. Streeten BW, Li ZI, Wallace RN, Eagle RC, Keshgegian AA: Pseudoexfoliative fibrillopathy in visceral organs of a patient with pseudoexfoliation syndrome. *Arch Ophthalmol 1992;110:1757–1762.*
159. Forsius M: Exfoliation syndrome in various ethnic populations. *Acta Ophthalmol 1988;66(suppl 184):71–85.*
160. Kozart DM, Yanoff M: Intraocular pressure status in 100 consecutive patients with exfoliation syndrome. *Ophthalmology 1982;89:214–218.*
161. Aasved H: Incidence of defects in the pigmented pupillary ruff in eyes with and without fibrillopathia epitheliocapsularis. *Acta Ophthalmol 1973;5l:7l0–715.*
162. Norn MS: Iris pigment defects in normals. *Acta Ophthalmol 1971; 49:887–894.*
163. Prince AM, Ritch R: Clinical signs of the pseudoexfoliation syndrome. *Ophthalmology 1986;93:803–807.*
164. Vannas A: Fluorescein angiography of the vessels of the iris in pseudoXF of the lens capsule, capsular glaucoma and other forms of glaucoma. *Acta Ophthalmologica 1969;l05(suppl):37.*
165. Brooks AMV, Gillies WE: The development of microneovascular changes in the iris in pseudoXF of the lens capsule. *Ophthalmology 1987;94:1090–1097.*
166. Vannas A, Setala K, Rurisuraara P: Endothelial cells in capsular glaucoma. *Acta Ophthalmol 1977;55:951–958.*
167. Brooks AMV, Grant G, Gillies WE: Differentiation and assessment of corneal endothelial changes associated with diseases of the anterior segment of the eye. *Aust NZ J Ophthalmol 1987;15:65–70.*
168. Miyake K, Matsuda M, Inaba M: Corneal endothelial changes in pseudoexfoliation syndrome. *Am J Ophthalmol 1989;108:49–52.*
169. Prince AM, Streeten BW, Ritch R, et al: Preclinical diagnosis of pseudoexfoliation syndrome. *Arch Ophthalmol 1987;105:1076–1082.*
170. Layden WE, Shaffer RN: Exfoliation syndrome. *Am J Ophthalmol 1974;78:835–841.*

171. Wishart PK, Spaeth GL, Poryzees EM: Anterior chamber angle in the exfoliation syndrome. *Br J Ophthalmol 1985;69:103–107.*
172. Morrison JC, Green WR: Light microscopy of the exfoliation syndrome. *Acta Ophthalmol 1988;66(suppl 184):5–27.*
173. Speakman JS, Ghosh M: The conjunctiva in senile lens exfoliation. *Arch Ophthalmol 1976;94:l757–1759.*
174. Ringvold A, Vegge T: Electron microscopy of the trabecular meshwork in eyes with exfoliation syndrome (pseudoexfoliation of the lens capsule). *Virchows Arch [A] 1971;353:ll0–127.*
175. Richardson M, Epstein DL: Exfoliation glaucoma. A quantitative perfusion and ultrastructural study. *Ophthalmology 1981;88:968–980.*
176. Ito N, Inomata H: Histopathological study of the trabecular meshwork and iris in exfoliation syndrome with glaucoma. *Acta Soc Ophthalmol Jpn 1985;29:838–849.*
177. Benedikt O, Roll P: The trabecular meshwork of a non-glaucomatous eye with the exfoliation syndrome. *Virchows Arch [A] 1979;384: 347–355.*
178. Eagle RC Jr, Font RL, Fine BS: The basement membrane exfoliation syndrome. *Arch Ophthalmol 1979;97:510–515.*
179. Davanger M: Studies on the pseudoexfoliation material. *Graefes Arch Clin Exp Ophthalmol 1978;208:65–68.*
180. Baba H: Histochemical and polarization optical investigation for glycosaminoglycans in XF syndrome. *Graefes Arch Clin Exp Ophthalmol 1983;221:106–109.*
181. Harnisch JP, Barrach JH, Hassell JR, Sinha PK: Identification of a basement membrane proteoglycan in exfoliation material. *Graefes Arch Clin Exp Ophthalmol 1981;215:273–278.*
182. Streeten BW, Gibson SA, Li Z-Y: Lectin binding to pseudoexfoliative material and the ocular zonules. *Invest Ophthalmol Vis Sci 1986; 27:1516–1521.*
183. Garner A, Alexander RA: Pseudoexfoliative disease: Histochemical evidence of an affinity with zonular fibers. *Br J Ophthalmol 1984;68: 574–580.*
184. Streeten BW, Licari PA, Marucci AA, Dougherty M: Immunohistochemical comparison of ocular zonules and the microfibrils of elastic tissue. *Invest Ophthalmol 1981;21:130–135.*
185. Streeten BW, Gibson SA, Dark AJ: Pseudoexfoliative material contains an elastic microfibrillar-associated glycoprotein. *Trans Am Ophthalmol Soc 1986;84:304–320.*
186. Li Z-Y, Streeten BW, Wallace RN: Association of elastin with pseudoexfoliative material: an immunoEMic study. *Curr Eye Res 1988;7: 1163–1172.*
187. Li Z-Y, Streeten BW, Yohai N: Amyloid P protein in pseudoexfoliative fibrillopathy. *Curr Eye Res 1989;8:217–227.*
188. Airaksinen PJ: The long-term hypotensive effect of timolol maleate compared with the effect of pilocarpine in simple and capsular glaucoma. *Acta Ophthalmol 1979;57:425–434.*
189. Ritch R, Podos SM: Laser trabeculoplasty in the exfoliation syndrome. *Bull NY Acad Med 1983;59:339–344.*
190. Pohjanpelto P: Late results of laser trabeculoplasty for increased intraocular pressure. *Acta Ophthalmol 1983;61:998–1008.*
191. Raitta C, Setala K: Intraocular lens implantation in exfoliation syndrome and capsular glaucoma. *Acta Ophthalmol 1986;64:130–133.*
192. Guzek JP, Holm M, Cotter JB, et al: Risk factors for intraoperative complications in 1000 extracapsular cataract cases. *Ophthalmology 1987; 94:461–466.*
193. Skuta GL, Parrish RK II, Hodapp E, et al: Zonular dialysis during extracapsular cataract extraction in pseudoexfoliation syndrome. *Arch Ophthalmol 1987;105:632–634.*
194. Savage JA, Thomas JV, Belcher CD III, Simmons RJ: Extracapsular cataract extraction and posterior chamber intraocular lens implantation in glaucomatous eyes. *Ophthalmology 1985;92:1506–1516.*

195. Delori F, Pomerantzeff O, Cox MS: Deformation of the globe under high-speed impact. Its relation to contusion injuries. *Invest Ophthalmol 1969;8:290–301.*
196. Canavan YM, Archer DB: Anterior segment consequences of blunt ocular injury. *Br J Ophthalmol 1982;66:549–555.*
197. Collins ET: On the pathological examination of three eyes lost from concussion. *Trans Ophthalmol Soc UK 1892;12:180–186.*
198. Kaufman JH, Tolpin DW: Glaucoma after traumatic angle recession. *Am J Ophthalmol 1974;78:648–654.*
199. Green K, Paterson CA, Siddiqui A: Ocular blood flow after experimental alkali burns and prostaglandin administration. *Arch Ophthalmol 1985;103:569–571.*
200. Paterson CA, Pfister RR: Intraocular pressure changes after alkali burns. *Arch Ophthalmol 1974;91:211–218.*
201. Toris CB, Pederson JE: Aqueous humor dynamics in experimental iridocyclitis. *Invest Ophthalmol Vis Sci 1987;28:477–481.*
202. Epstein DL, Hasimoto JM, Grant WM: Serum obstruction of aqueous outflow in enucleated eyes. *Am J Ophthalmol 1978;86:101–105.*
203. Herschler J, Davis EB: Modified goniotomy for inflammatory glaucoma. Histologic evidence for the mechanism of pressure reduction. *Arch Ophthalmol 1980;98:684–687.*
204. Roth M, Simmons RJ: Glaucoma associated with precipitates on the trabecular meshwork. *Ophthalmology 1976;86:16131618.*
205. Smith RE, Godfrey WA, Kimura SJ: Complications of chronic cyclitis. *Am J Ophthalmol 1976;82:277–282.*
206. Womack LW, Liesgang TJ: Complications of Herpes zoster ophthalmicus. *Arch Ophthalmol 1983;101:42–45.*
207. Krupin T: Glaucoma associated with uveitis, in Ritch R, Shields MB (eds): *The Secondary Glaucomas*. St. Louis: CV Mosby, 1982, 290–306.
208. Posner A, Schlossman A: Syndrome of unilateral recurrent attacks of glaucoma with cyclitic symptoms. *Arch Ophthalmol 1948;39:517–535.*
209. Hollwich F: Clinical aspects and therapy of the Posner-Schlossman-syndrome. *Klin Mbl Augenheilk 1978;172:736–744.*
210. Hung PT, Chang JM: Treatment of glaucomatocyclitic crises. *Am J Ophthalmol 1974;77:169–172.*
211. Fuchs E: Uber Komplikationen der Heterochromie. *Zeitschr Augenheil 1906;15:191–212.*
212. Loewenfeld IE, Thompson HS: Fuchs' heterochromic iridocyclitis: A critical review of the literature. *Surv Ophthalmol 1973;17:394–457.*
213. Franceschetti A: Heterochromic cyclitis (Fuchs' syndrome). *Am J Ophthalmol 1955;39:50–58.*
214. Kimura SJ, Hogan MJ, Thygeson P: Fuchs' syndrome of heterochromic cyclitis. *Arch Ophthalmol 1955;54:179–186.*
215. Perry HD, Yanoff M, Scheie HG: Rubeosis in Fuchs heterochromic iridocyclitis. *Arch Ophthalmol 1975;93:337–339.*
216. Sugar HS: Late glaucoma associated with inactive syphilitic interstitial keratitis. *Am J Ophthalmol 1962;53:602–605.*
217. Grant WM: Late glaucoma after interstitial keratitis. *Am J Ophthalmol 1975;79:87–91.*
218. Watson PG, Hayreh SS: Scleritis and episcleritis. *Br J Ophthalmol 1976;60:163–191.*
219. Richter CU, Epstein DL: Lens induced open angle glaucoma, in Ritch R, Shields MB, Krupin T (eds): *The Glaucomas*, Vol 2. St. Louis: CV Mosby, 1989, 1017–1026.
220. Chandler PA: Narrow-angle glaucoma. *Arch Ophthalmol 1952;47: 695–716.*
221. Hyams SW, Neumann E: Transient angle closure glaucoma after retinal vein occlusion. Report of two cases. *Br J Ophthalmol 1972;56: 353–355.*
222. Grant WM: Shallowing of the anterior chamber following occlusion of the central retinal vein. *Am J Ophthalmol 1973;75:384–389.*
223. Chandler PA: Choice of treatment in dislocation of the lens. *Arch Ophthalmol 1964;71:765–786.*

224. Jarrett WH: Dislocation of the lens. A study of 166 hospitalized cases. *Arch Ophthalmol 1967;78:289–296.*
225. Ritch R, Wand M: Treatment of the Weill-Marchesani syndrome. *Ann Ophthalmol 1981;13:665–667.*
226. Epstein DL: Diagnosis and management of lens-induced glaucoma. *Ophthalmology 1982;89:227–230.*
227. Bartholomew RS, Rebello PF: Calcium oxalate crystals in the aqueous. *Am J Ophthalmol 1979;88:1026–1028.*
228. Yanoff M: In discussion of Shields MB, McCracken JS, Klintworth GK, Campbell DG: Corneal edema in essential iris atrophy. *Ophthalmology 1979;86:1549–1550.*
229. Harms C: Eiseitige spontane Luckenbildung der Iris durch Atrophie ohne mechanische Zerrung. *Klin Mbl Augenheilk 1903;41:522–528.*
230. Chandler PA: Atrophy of the stroma of the iris. Endothelial dystrophy, corneal edema, and glaucoma. *Am J Ophthalmol 1956;41:607–615.*
231. Cogan DG, Reese AB: A syndrome of iris nodules, ectopic Descemet's membrane, and unilateral glaucoma. *Doc Ophthalmol 1969;26:424–433.*
232. Shields MB: Progressive essential iris atrophy, Chandler's syndrome, and the iris nevus (Cogan-Reese) syndrome: A spectrum of disease. *Surv Ophthalmol 1979;24:3–20.*
233. Campbell DG, Shields NB, Smith TR: The corneal endothelium and the spectrum of essential iris atrophy. *Am J Ophthalmol 1978;86:317–324.*
234. Waring GO III, Rodrigues MM, Laibson PR: Corneal dystrophies. II. Endothelial dystrophies. *Surv Ophthalmol 1978;23:147–168.*
235. Crouch ER Jr, Frenkel, M: Aminocaproic acid in the treatment of traumatic hyphema. *Am J Ophthalmol 1976;81:355–360.*
236. Coles WH: Traumatic hyphema: An analysis of 235 cases. *South Med J 1968;61:813–816.*
237. Spaeth GL, Levy PM: Traumatic hyphema: Its clinical characteristics and failure of estrogens to alter its course. A double-blind study. *Am J Ophthalmol 1966;62:1098–1106.*
238. Edwards WC, Layden WE: Traumatic hyphema. A report of 184 consecutive cases. *Am J Ophthalmol 1973;75:110–116.*
239. Rakusin W: Traumatic hyphema. *Am J Ophthalmol 1972;74:284–292.*
240. Goldberg MF: The diagnosis and treatment of secondary glaucoma after hyphema in sickle cell patients. *Am J Ophthalmol 1979;87:43–49.*
241. Goldberg, MF: Sickled erythrocytes, hyphema and secondary glaucoma: 1. The diagnosis and treatment of sickled erythrocytes in human hyphemas. *Ophthalmic Surg 1979;10:17–31.*
242. Goldberg MF, Tso MOM: Sickled erythrocytes, hyphema, and secondary glaucoma: VII. The passage of sickled erythrocytes out of the anterior chamber of the human and monkey eye: Light and electron microscopic studies. *Ophthalmic Surg 1979;10:89–123.*
243. Campbell DG, Simmons RJ, Grant WM: Ghost cells as a cause of glaucoma. *Am J Ophthalmol 1976;81:441–450.*
244. Cobb B: Vascular tufts at the pupillary margin: A preliminary report on 44 patients. *Trans Ophthalmol Soc UK 1968;88:211–221.*
245. Fenton RH, Zimmerman LE: Hemolytic glaucoma. An unusual cause of acute open-angle secondary glaucoma. *Arch Ophthalmol 1963;70:236–239.*
246. Brubaker RF: Determination of episcleral venous pressure in the eye. A comparison of three methods. *Arch Ophthalmol 1967;77:110–114.*
247. Phelps CD, Thompson HS, Ossoining KC: The diagnosis and prognosis of atypical carotid-cavernous fistula (red-eyed shunt syndrome). *Am J Ophthalmol 1982;93:423–436.*
248. Weiss DI, Shaffer RN, Nehrenberg TR: Neovascular glaucoma complicating carotid-cavernous fistula. *Arch Ophthalmol 1963;69:304–307.*
249. Grove AS Jr: The dural shunt syndrome. Pathophysiology and clinical course. *Ophthalmology 1983;91:31–44.*
250. Radius RL, Maumenee AE: Dilated episcleral vessels and open-angle glaucoma. *Am J Ophthalmol 1978;86:31–35.*

251. Talusan ED, Fishbein SL, Schwartz B: Increased pressure of dilated episcleral veins with open-angle glaucoma without exophthalmos. *Ophthalmology 1983;90:257–265.*
252. Phelps CD: The pathogenesis of glaucoma in Sturge-Weber syndrome. *Ophthalmology 1978;85:276–286.*
253. Bellows RA, Chylack LT, Epstein DL, Hutchinson BT: Choroidal effusion during glaucoma surgery in patients with prominent episcleral vessels. *Arch Ophthalmol 1979;97:493–497.*
254. Yanoff M: Glaucoma mechanisms in ocular malignant melanomas. *Am J Ophthalmol 1970;70:898–904.*
255. Shields MB, Klintworth GK: Anterior uveal melanomas and intraocular pressure. *Ophthalmology 1980;87:503–517.*
256. Jakobiec FA, Silbert G: Are most iris "melanomas" really nevi? A clinicopathologic study of 189 lesions. *Arch Ophthalmol 1981;99:2117–2132.*
257. Yanoff M, Scheie HG: Melanomalytic glaucoma. Report of a case. *Arch Ophthalmol 1970;84:471–473.*
258. Van Buskirk EM, Leure–duPree AE: Pathophysiology and electron microscopy of melanomalytic glaucoma. *Am J Ophthalmol 1978;85:160–166.*
259. Chandler PA: Glaucoma in aphakia. *Trans Am Acad Ophthalmol Otolaryngol 1963;67:483–487.*
260. Van Buskirk EM: Pseudophakic glaucoma, in Weinstein GW (ed): *Contemporary Issues in Ophthalmology: Open Angle Glaucoma,* Vol 3. 1986, 133–154.
261. Passo MS, Ernest JT, Goldstick TK: Hyaluronate increases intraocular pressure when used in cataract extraction. *Br J Ophthalmol 1985;69:572–575.*
262. Cherfan GM, Rich WJ, Wright G: Raised intraocular pressure and other problems with sodium hyaluronate and cataract surgery. *Trans Ophthalmol Soc UK 1983;103:277–279.*
263. Berson FG, et al: Obstruction of aqueous outflow by sodium hyaluronate in enucleated eyes. *Am J Ophthalmol 1983;95:668–672.*
264. Pape LG: Intraocular and extracapsular technique of lens implantation with Healon. *Am Intraocul Implant Soc J 1980;6:342–343.*
265. Chandler PA, Simmons RJ, Grant WM: Malignant glaucoma. Medical and surgical treatment. *Am J Ophthalmol 1968;66:495–502.*
266. Simmons RJ: Malignant glaucoma. *Br J Ophthalmol 1972;56:263–272.*
267. Weiss DI, Shaffer RN: Ciliary block (malignant) glaucoma. *Trans Am Acad Ophthamol Otolaryngol 1972;76:450–461.*
268. Epstein DL, Steinert RF, Puliafito CA: Neodymium-YAG laser therapy to the anterior hyaloid in aphakic malignant (ciliovitreal block) glaucoma. *Am J Ophthalmol 1984;98:137–143.*
269. Becker B, Shaffer RN: in Hoskins HD, Kass M (eds): *Diagnosis and Therapy of the Glaucomas,* ed 6. St. Louis: CV Mosby, 1989.
270. Hoskins HD: Evaluation technique for congenital glaucomas. *J Ped Ophthalmol 1971;8:81–87.*
271. Radtke ND, Cohen BE: Intraocular pressure measurement in the newborn. *Am J Ophthalmol 1974;78:501–504.*
272. Dominguez A, Banos MS, Alvarez MG: Intraocular pressure measurement in infants under general anesthesia. *Am J Ophthalmol 1974;78:110–116.*
273. Hoskins HD Jr, Hetherington J Jr, Shaffer RN, Welling AM: Developmental glaucomas: Diagnosis and classification, in *New Orleans Academy of Ophthalmology. Symposium on Glaucoma.* St. Louis: CV Mosby, 1981, 172–190.
274. Shaffer RN: Pathogenesis of congenital glaucoma: Gonioscopic and microscopic anatomy. *Trans Am Acad Ophthalmol Otolaryngol 1955;59:297–308.*
275. Anderson DR: The development of trabecular meshwork and its abnormality in primary infantile glaucoma. *Trans Am Ophthalmol Soc 1981;79:458–485.*
276. Richardson KT, Shaffer RN: Optic nerve cupping in congenital glaucoma. *Am J Ophthalmol 1966;62:507–509.*

277. Quigley HA: Childhood glaucoma: Results with trabeculectomy and study of reverse cupping. *Ophthalmology 1982;89:219–225.*
278. deLuise VP, Anderson D: Primary infantile glaucoma. *Surv Ophthalmol 1983;28:1–19.*
279. Nelson LB, Spaeth GL, Nowinski TS, et al: Aniridia: A review. *Surv Ophthalmol 1984;28:621–642.*
280. Phelps CD: The pathogenesis of glaucoma in Sturge-Weber syndrome. *Ophthalmology 1978;85:276–286.*
281. Cibis GW, Tripathi RC and Tripathi BJ: Glaucoma in Sturge-Weber syndrome. *Ophthalmology 1984;91:1061–1071.*
282. Grant WM, Walton DS: Distinctive gonioscopic findings in glaucoma due to neurofibromatosis. *Arch Ophthalmol 1968;79:127–134.*
283. Waring GO III, Rodriguez MM, Laibson PR: Anterior chamber cleavage syndrome: A stepladder classification. *Surv Ophthalmol 1975; 20:3–27.*
284. Wolff SM: The ocular manifestation of congenital rubella: A prospective study of 328 cases of congenital rubella. *Trans Am Ophthalmol Soc 1972;70:577–614.*
285. Zimmerman TJ, Kooner KS, Morgan KS: Safety and efficacy of timolol in pediatric glaucoma. *Surv Ophthalmol 1983;28:262–292.*
286. McMahon CD, Hetherington J, Hoskins HD, Shaffer RN: Timolol and pediatric glaucoma. *Ophthalmology 1981;88:249–252.*
287. Barkan O: Technique of goniotomy. *Arch Ophthalmol 1938;19: 217–221.*
288. Barkan O: Operation for congenital glaucoma. *Am J Ophthalmol 1942;25:552–568.*
289. Barkan O: Surgery of congenital glaucoma: Review of 196 eyes operated by goniotomy, *Am J Ophthalmol 1953;36(2):1523–1534.*
290. Broughton WL, Parks MM: An analysis of treatment of congenital glaucoma by goniotomy. *Am J Ophthalmol 1981;91:566–572.*
291. Hoskins HD, Shaffer RN, Hetherington J: Goniotomy vs trabeculotomy. *J Pedriatr Ophthalmol Strabismus 1984;21:153–158.*
292. Anderson DR: Trabeculotomy compared to goniotomy for glaucoma in children. *Ophthalmology 1983;90:805–86.*
293. Allen L, Burian HM: Trabeculectomy ab externo. A new glaucoma operation. Technique and results of experimental surgery. *Am J Ophthalmol 1962;53:19–26.*
294. Gressel MG, Heuer DK, Parrish RK II: Trabeculectomy in young patients. *Ophthalmology 1984;91:1242–1246.*
295. Heuer DK, Parrish RK II, Gressel MG, et al: 5–Fluorouracil and glaucoma filtering surgery—a pilot study. *Ophthalmology 1984;91: 384–394.*
296. Molteno ACB, Ancker E, VanBiljon G: Surgical technique for advanced juvenile glaucoma. *Arch Ophthalmol 1984;102:51–57.*
297. Aminlar A: Cyclocryotherapy in congenital glaucoma. *Glaucoma 1981;1:331–332.*
298. Morin JD, Bryars JH: Causes of loss of vision in congenital glaucoma. *Arch Ophthalmol 1980;98:1575–1576.*

CHAPTER 9
THERAPY OF GLAUCOMA

1. Garratt S (ed): *Primary Open-Angle Glaucoma, Preferred Practice Plan.* San Francisco: American Academy of Ophthalmology, 1989.
2. Leydhecker W: Is glaucoma therapy useless? in Kriegelstein GK, Leydhecker W (eds): *Glaucoma Update II.* Berlin: Springer-Verlag, 1983, 95–102.
3. Mao LK, Steward WC, Shields MB: Correlation between intraocular pressure control and progressive glaucomatous damage in primary open-angle glaucoma. *Am J Ophthalmol 1991;111:51–55.*
4. O'Brien C, Schwartz B, Takamoto T, Wu DC: Intraocular pressure and the rate of visual field loss in chronic open-angle glaucoma. *Am J Ophthalmol 1991;11 1:491–500.*
5. Sommer A: Intraocular pressure and glaucoma. *Am J Ophthalmol 1989;107:186–188.*

6. Sommer A, Tielsch JM, Katz J, et al: Baltimore Eye Survey Research Group: Relationship between intraocular pressure and primary open angle glaucoma among white and black Americans. *Arch Ophthalmol 1991;109:109 1095.*
7. Cartwright MJ, Anderson DR: Correlation of asymmetric damage with asymmetric intraocular pressure in normal-tension glaucoma (low tension glaucoma). *Arch Ophthalmol 1988:106:898–900.*
8. Crichton A, Drance SM, Douglas GR, Schulzer M: Unequal intraocular pressure and its relation to asymmetric visual field defects in low-tension glaucoma. *Ophthalmology 1989;96:1312–1314.*
9. Quigley HA, Addicks EM: Chronic experimental glaucoma in primates. II. Effect of extended intraocular pressure elevation on optic nerve head and axonal transport. *Invest Ophthalmol Vis Sci 1980; 19:137–152.*
10. Eddy DM, Billings J: *The Quality of Medical Evidence and Medical Practice.* National Leadership Commission on Health Care, 1987.
11. Spaeth GL: The effect of change in intraocular pressure on the natural history of glaucoma: Lowering intraocular pressure in glaucoma can result in improvement of visual fields. *Trans Ophthalmol Soc UK 1985;104:256–64.*
12. Spaeth GL: Control of glaucoma: A new definition. *Ophthal Surg 1983; 14:303–304.*
13. Epstein DL, Krug JH, Hertzmark E, et al: A long-term clinical trial of timolol therapy versus no treatment in the management of glaucoma suspects. *Ophthalmology 1989;96:1460–1467.*
14. Kass MA, Gordon MO, Hoff MR, et al: Topical timolol administration reduces the incidence of glaucomatous damage in ocular hypertensive individuals. *Arch Ophthalmol 1989;l07:1590–l598.*
15. Shin DH, Kolker AE, Kass MA, et al: Long-term epinephrine therapy of ocular hypertension. *Arch Ophthalmol 1976;94:2059–2060.*
16. David R, Livingston DG, Luntz MH: Ocular hypertension—A long-term follow-up of treated and untreated patients. *Br J Ophthalmol 1977;61:668–674.*
17. Schulzer M, Drance SM, Douglas GR: A comparison of treated and untreated glaucoma suspects. *Ophthalmology 1991;98:301–307.*
18. deJong N, Greve EL, Hoyng PFI, Geilssen HC: Results of a filtering procedure in low tension glaucoma. *Int Ophthalmol 1989;l3:131–138.*
19. Hart WM, Becker B: The onset and evolution of glaucomatous visual field defects. *Ophthalmology 1982;89:268–279.*
20. Mikelberg FS, Schulzer M, Drance SM, Lau W: The rate of progression of scotomas in glaucoma. *Am J Ophthalmol 1986;101:1–6.*
21. Kolker AE: Visual prognosis in advanced glaucoma: A comparison of medical and surgical therapy for retention of vision in 101 eyes with advanced glaucoma. *Trans Am Ophthalmol Soc 1977;75:539–554.*
22. Leydhecker W, Gramer E: Long-term studies of visual field changer by means of computerized perimetry (Octopus 201) in eyes with glaucomatous field defects after normalization of the intra-ocular pressure. *Int Ophthalmol 1989;13:113–117.*
23. Vogel R, Crick RP, Newson RB, et al: Association between intraocular pressure and loss of visual field in chronic simple glaucoma. *Br J Ophthalmol 1990;74:3:6.*
24. Niesel P, Flammer J: Correlations between intraocular pressure, visual field and visual acuity, based on 11 years of observations of treated chronic glaucomas. *Int Ophthalmol 1980;3:31–35.*
25. Zeimer RC, WilenskyJT, Gieser DK, Viana MAG: Association between intraocular pressure peaks and progression of visual field loss. *Ophthalmology 1991;98:64–69.*
26. Holmin C, Storr-Paulsen A: The visual field after trabeculectomy. A followup study using computerized perimetry. *Acta Ophthalmol 1984;62:230234.*
27. Grant WM, Burke JF: Why do some people go blind from glaucoma? *Ophthalmology 1982;89:991–998.*

28. Odberg T: Visual field prognosis in advanced glaucoma. *Acta Ophthalmologica 1987;65(suppl 182):27–29.*
29. Quigley HA, Maumenee AE: Long-term follow-up of treated open-angle glaucoma. *Am J Ophthalmol 1979;87:519–525.*
30. Roth SM, Spaeth GL, Starita RJ, et al: The effects of postoperative corticosteroids on trabeculectomy and the clinical course of glaucoma: Five year follow-up study. *Ophthalmic Surg 1991;22:724–729.*
31. Kidd M, O'Connor: Progression of field loss after trabeculectomy: A five-year follow-up. *Br J Ophthalmol 1985;69:827–831.*
32. Werner EB, Drance SM, Schulzer M: Trabeculectomy and the progression of glaucomatous visual field loss.*Arch Ophthalmol 1977;95: 1374–1377.*
33. Greve EL, Dake CL: Four-year follow-up of a glaucoma operation. Prospective study of the double flap Scheie. *Int Ophthalmol 1979;1: 139–145.*
34. Rollins DF, Drance SM: *Five-Year Follow-Up of Trabeculectomy in the Management of Chronic Open Angle Glaucoma. Symposium on Glaucoma. New Orleans Academy of Ophthalmology.* St. Louis: CV Mosby, 1981, 295–30.
35. Anderson DR: Glaucoma: The damage caused by pressure. XLVI Edward Jackson Memorial Lecture. *Am J Ophthalmol 1989;108: 485–495.*
36. Migdal C, Hitchings R: Control of chronic simple glaucoma with primary medical, surgical and laser treatment. *Trans Ophthalmol Soc UK 1986;105:653–656.*
37. Glaucoma Laser Trial Research Group. The glaucoma laser trial (GLT). 2. Results of argon laser trabeculoplasty versus topical medicines. *Ophthalmology 1990;97:1403–13.*
38. Molteno ACB: Use of Molteno implants to treat secondary glaucoma, in Caims JE (ed): *Glaucoma.* Vol 1. New York: Grune & Stratton, 1986, 211–238.
39. Kaufman PL: Aqueous humor dynamics, in Duane TD (ed): *Clinical Ophthalmology.* Vol 3. Philadelphia: Harper & Row, 1985, 1–24.
40. Ly AM, Michaelis EK: Solubilization, partial purification and reconstitution of glutamate and N-methyl-D aspartate-activated cation channels from brain synaptic membranes. *Biochemistry 1991; 30:4307–4316.*
41. Paul AK, Marala RB, Jaiswal RK, Sharma RK: Coexistence of guanylate cydase and atrial natriuretic factor in a 180 kDa protein. *Science 1987;235:1224–1226.*
42. Bremner HM, Ballerman BJ, Gunning ME, Zeidel ML: Diverse biological actions of atrial natriuretic protein. *Physiol Rev 1990;70:665–687.*
43. Stone RA, Glembotski CC: Immunoreactive atrial natriuretic peptide in the rat eye; molecular forms in anterior uvea and retina. *Biochem Biophys Res Commun 1986;134:102–1028.*
44. Bianchi C, Anand-Srivastava MB, DeLeon A, et al: Localization and characterization of specific receptors for atrial natriuretic factor in the ciliary process of the eye. *Curr Eye Res 1986;5:283–293.*
45. Mittag TW, Tormay A, Ortega M, Severin C: Atrial natriuretic peptide (ANP), guanylate cyclase, and intraocular pressure in the rabbit eye. *Curr Eye Res 1987;6:1189–1196.*
46. Kaupp UB, Niidome T, Tanabe T, et al: Primary structure and functional expression from a complimentary DNA of the rod photoreceptor cGMP-gated channel. *Nature 1989;42:762–766.*
47. Ahmad I, Redmond LJ, Barnstable CJ: Developmental and tissue specific expression of the rod photoreceptor cGMP-gated ion channel gene. *Biochem Biophys Res Commun 1990;173:463–470.*
48. Bredt DS, Snyder SH: Isolation of nitric oxide synthetase, a calmodulin requiring enzyme. *Proc Natl Acad Sci USA 1990;87:682–685.*
49. Ignaro LJ: Endothelium derived nitrous oxide: Actions and properties. *FASEBJ 1989;3:31–36.*
50. Bausher LP, Gregory DS, Sears ML: Interaction between α_2 and $\mathbf{b}_2$ adrenergic receptors in rabbit ciliary processes. *Curr Eye Res 1987; 6:497–505.*

51. Brown AM, Birmbaumer L: Direct G-protein gating of ion channels. *Am J Physiol 1988;254:H40 1–H410.*
52. DeFrancesco D, Tortora P: Direct activation of cardiac pace-maker channels by intracellular cyclic AMP. *Nature 1991;351:145–147.*
53. Hartzel H-C, Mery P-F, Fischmeister R, Zabo G: Sympathetic regulation of cardiac calcium current is due exdusively to cAMP-dependent phosphorylation. *Nature 1991;351:573–576.*
54. Ehara T, Ishihara K: Anion channels activated by adrenaline in cardiac myocytes. *Nature 1990;347:284–286.*
55. Dhallan RS, Yau K-W, Schrader KA, Reed RR: Primary structure and functional expression of a cydic nucleotide activated channel from olfactory neurons. *Nature 1990;347:184-187.*
56. Welsh MJ: Abnormal regulation of ion channels in cystic fibrosis epithelia. *FASEBJ 1990;2716–2725.*
57. Kurachi Y, Ito H, Sugimoto T, et al: Arachidonic acid metabolites as intracellular modulators of the G-protein-gated cardiac K+ channel. *Nature 1989;337:555–557.*
58. Kaufman PL, Gabelt BT: Cholinergic mechanisms and aqueous humor dynamics. Circa 1990, in Drance SM, Neufeld AH, Van Buskirk EM (eds): *Applied Pharmacology of the Glaucomas.* Baltimore: Williams & Wilkins [in press.]
59. Suzuki R, Oso T, Kobayashi S: Cholinergic inhibitory response in the bovine iris dilator muscle. *Invest Ophthalmol Vis Sci 1983;24:760–765.*
60. Kaufman PL, Wiedman T, Robinson JR: Cholinergics, in Sears ML (ed): *Pharmacology of the Eye. Handbook of Experimental Pharmacology Series.* Vol 69. Berlin: Springer-Verlag, 1984, 149–191.
61. Gharagozloo NZ, Relf SJ, Brubaker RF: Aqueous flow is reduced by the alphaadrenergic agonist, apraclonidine hydrochloride (ALO 2145). *Ophthalmology 1988;95:1217–1220.*
62. Robin AL: Short-term effects of unilateral 1% apraclonidine therapy. *Arch Ophthalmol 1988;106:912–915.*
63. Mittag TW, Tormay A, Severin C, Podos SM: Alpha-adrenergic antagonists: Correlation of the effect on intraocular pressure and on α_2-adrenergic receptor binding specificity in the rabbit eye. *Exp Eye Res 1985;40:59 1–598.*
64. DeVries GW, Mobasser A, Wheeler LA: Stimulation of endogenous cAMP levels in ciliary body by SKF A2526, a novel dopamine receptor agonist. *Curr Eye Res 1986;5:449–55.*
65. Mittag TW, Tormay A: Drug responses of adenylate cyclase in iris-ciliary body determined by adenine labelling. *Invest Ophthalmol Vis Sci 1985;26:39–40.*
66. Mittag TW: Adrenergic and dopaminergic drugs in glaucoma, in Ritch R, Shields MB, Krupin T (eds): *The Glaucomas.* St. Louis: CV Mosby, 1989, 523–537.
67. Rorsman T, Bokvist K, Ammala C, et al: Activation by adrenaline of a low conductance G-protein-dependent K^+ channel in mouse pancre atic Bcells. *Nature 1991;349:77–79.*
68. Jumblatt JE, Liu JGH, North GT: Alpha-2 adrenergic modulation of norepinephrine secretion in perfused rabbit iris-ciliary body. *Curr Eye Res 1987;6: 767–773.*
69. Potter DE, Burke JA: An in vivo model for dissociating α_2 or DA_2 adrenoreceptor activity in ocular adnexa: Utility of the cat nictitating membrane preparation. *Curr Eye Res 1984;3:1289–1296.*
70. Liu JHK, Dacus AC: Endogenous hormonal changes and circadian elevation of intraocular pressure. *Invest Ophthalmol Vis Sci 1991; 32:496–503.*
71. Polansky JR: Beta-adrenergic therapy for glaucoma. *Int Ophthalmol Clin 1990;30:219–229.*
72. Van Alphen GWHM, Kern R, Robinette SL: Adrenergic receptors of the intraocular muscles: Comparison to cat, rabbit and monkey. *Arch Ophthalmol 1965;74:253–259.*
73. Jampel HP, Lynch MG, Brown RH, et al: Beta-adrenergic receptors in human trabecular meshwork. *Invest Ophthalmol Vis Sci 1987; 28:772–779.*

74. Kaufman PL: Pressure-dependent outflow, in Ritch R, Shields M, Bruce, Krupin T (eds): *The Glaucomas,* Vol 1. St. Louis: CV Mosby, 1989, 219–240.
75. Robinson IC, Kaufman PL: Cytochalasin B potentiates epinephrine's facility increasing effect. *Invest Ophthalmol Vis Sci 1991;32:1614–1618.*
76. Bill A: Early effects of epinephrine on aqueous humor dynamics in vervet monkeys *(Cercopithecus ethiops). Exp Eye Res 1969;8:35–43.*
77. Townsend DI, Brubaker RF: Immediate effects of epinephrine on aqueous formation in the normal human eye as measured by fluorophotometry. *Invest Ophthalmol Vis Sci 1980;19:256–266.*
78. Bhattacherjee P, Hammond BR: Effect of indomethacin on the ocular hypotensive action of adrenaline in the rabbit. *Exp Eye Res 1977; 24:307–313.*
79. Camras CB, Feldman SG, Podos SM, et al: Inhibition of the epinephrine induced reduction of intraocular pressure by systemic indomethacin in humans. *Am I Ophthalmol 1985; 100:169–175.*
80. Nilsson SFE, Samuelsson M, Bill A, Stjernschantz J: Increased uveosderal outflow as a possible mechanism of ocular hypotension caused by prostaglandin $F_{2\alpha}$-1-isopropylester in the cynomolgus monkey. *Exp Eye Res 1989;48:707–716.*
81. Gabelt BT, Kaufman PL: Prostaglandin $F_{2\alpha}$ increases uveoscleral outflow in the cynomolgus monkey. *Exp Eye Res 1989;49:389402.*
82. Lütjen-Drecoll E, Tamm E: Morphological study of the anterior segment of cynomolgus monkey eyes following treatment with prostaglandin F2α. *Exp Eye Res 1988;47:761–769.*
83. Schneider TL, Brubaker RF: The effect of chronic epinephrine on aqueous humor flow during the day and during sleep in heaithy volunteers. *Invest Ophthalmol Vis Sci 1990;31(ARVO suppl):148.*
84. Topper JE, Brubaker RF: Effects of timolol, epinephrine, and acetazolamide on aqueous flow during sleep. *Invest Ophthalmol Vis Sci 1985;26:1315–1319.*
85. Boas RS, Messenger M, Mittag TW, Podos SM: The effects of topically applied epinephrine on intraocular pressure and aqueous humor camp in the rabbit. *Exp Eye Res 1981;32:681–689.*
86. Wax MB, Molinoff PB: Distribution and properties of β-adrenergic receptors in human iris-ciliary body. *Invest Ophthalmol Vis Sci 28:420–430.*
87. Gregory BS, Bausher LP, Bromberg BB, Sears ML: The β-adrenergic receptors and adenylyl cyclase of rabbit ciliary processes, in Sears ML (ed): *New Directions in Ophthalmic Research.* New Haven, London: Yale University Press, 1981, 127–148.
88. Vareilles P, Silverstone D, Plazonnet B, et al: Comparison of the effects of timolol and other adrenergic agents on intraocular pressure in the rabbit. *Invest Ophthalmol Vis Sci 1977;16:987–996.*
89. Wentworth WO, Brubaker RF: Aqueous humor dynamics in a series of patients with third neuron Horner's syndrome. *Am J Ophthalmol 1981;92:407–415.*
90. Robinson JC, Kaufman PL: Effects and interactions of epinephrine, norepinephrine, timolol, and betaxolol on outflow facility in the cynomolgus monkey. *Am J Ophthalmol 1990;109:189–194.*
91. Gilmartin B, Hogan RE, Thompson SM: The effect of timolol maleate on tonic accommodation, tonic vergence, and pupil diameter. *Invest Ophthalmol Vis Sci 1984;25:763–770.*
92. Wiederholt M, Helbig H, Korbmacher C: lon transport across the ciliary epithelium: Lessons from cultured cells and proposed role of the carbonic anhydrase, in Botre F, Gross G, Storey BT (eds): *Carbonic Anhydrase.* Weinheim, New York, Basel, Cambridge: VCH, 1991, 232–244.
93. Chu TC, Candia OA, Podos SM: Electrical parameters of the isolated monkey ciliary epithelium and effects of pharmacological agents. *Invest Ophthalmol Vis Sci 1987;28:1644–1648.*
94. Hoskins HD Jr, Kass MA: Betaxolol, in Dunbar Hoskins H Jr, Kass MA (eds): Becker-Shaffer's Diagnosis and Therapy of the Glaucomas. St. Louis: CV Mosby, 1989, 457–458.

95. Schenker HI, Yablonski ME, Podos SM, Linder L: Fluorophotometric study of epinephrine and timolol in human subjects. *Arch Ophthalmol 1981;99:1212–1216.*
96. Gaul GR, Will Nl, Brubaker RF: Comparison of a noncardioselective betaadrenergic blocker and a cardioselective blocker in reducing aqueous flow in humans. *Arch Ophthalmol 1989;107:1308–1311.*
97. Daily RA, Brubaker RF, Bourne WB: The effects of timolol maleate and acetazolamide on the rate of aqueous formation in normal human subjects. *Am J Ophthalmol 1982;93:232–23 7.*
98. Podos SM, Serle JB: Topically active carbonic anhydrase inhibitors for glaucoma. *Arch Ophthalmol 1982;109:38–40.*
99. Kolker AE: Hyperosmotic agents in glaucoma. *Invest Ophthalmol Vis Sci 1970;9:418–423.*
100. Crawford KS, Kaufman PL: Dose-related effects of prostaglandin F2α isopropylester on intraocular pressure, refraction and pupil diameter in monkeys. *Invest Ophthalmol Vis Sci 1991;32:510–519.*
101. Crawford KS, Kaufman PL, Gabelt BT: Effects of topical PGF2α on aqueous humor dynamics in cynomolgus monkeys. *Curr Eye Res 1987;6:1035–1044.*
102. Gabelt BT, Kaufman PL: The effect of PGF2α on trabecular outflow facility in cynomolgus monkeys. *Exp Eye Res 1990;51:879 1 .*
103. Hayashi M, Yablonski ME, Bito LZ: Eicosanoids as a new class of ocular hypotensive agents. 2. Comparison of the apparent mechanism of the ocular hypotensive effects of A and F type prostaglandins. *Invest Ophthalmol Vis Sci 1987;28: 1639–1643.*
104. Kaufman PL, Crawford KS: Aqueous humor dynamics: How PGF2α lowers intraocular pressure, in Bito LZ, Stjernschantz I (eds): *The Ocular Effects of Prostaglandins and Other Eicosanoids.* New York: Alan R Liss, 1989, 387–416.
105. Tamm E, Rittig M, Lutjen-Drecoll E: Elektronenmikroskopische und immunhistochemische Untersuchungen zur augendrucksenkenden Wirkung von Prostaglandin $F_{2\alpha}$. *Fortschr Ophthalmol 1990; 87:623–629.*
106. Toris CB, Pederson JE: Aqueous humor dynamics in experimental iridocyclitis. *Invest Ophthalmol Vis Sci 1987;28;477–481.*
107. McGetrick JJ, Wilson DG, Dortzbach RK, et al: A search for lymphatic drainage of the monkey orbit. *Arch Ophthalmol 1989;l07:255–260.*
108. Bill A: Blood circulation and fluid dynamics in the eye. *Physiol Rev 1975;55:383–417.*
109. Camras CB, Siebold EC, Lustgarten JS, et al: Maintained reduction of intraocular pressure by prostaglandin $F_{2\alpha}$-l-isopropylester applied in multiple doses in ocular hypertensive and glaucoma patients. *Ophthalmology 1989;96:1329–1335.*
110. Crawford KS, Kaufman PL: Pilocarpine antagonizes $PGF_{2\alpha}$-induced ocular hypotension: Evidence for enhancement of uveoscleral outflow by $PGF_{2\alpha}$. *Arch Ophthalmol 1987;105:1112–1116.*
111. Anderson DR: Glaucoma: The damage caused by pressure. XLVI Edward Jackson Memorial Lecture. *Am J Ophthalmol 1989;108: 485–495.*
112. Sommer A, Tielsch JM, Katz J, et al: Intraocular pressure and open angle glaucoma: The Baltimore Eye Survey. *Invest Ophthalmol Vis Sci 1990;31(ARVO suppl):502.*
113. Jay JL, Murray SB: Early trabeculectomy versus conventional management in primary open angle glaucoma. *Br J Ophthalmol 1988; 72:881–889.*
114. Kass MA, Gordon ML, Hoff M, et al: Topical-timolol administration reduces the incidence of glaucomatous damage in ocular hypertensive individuals. *Arch Ophthalmol 1989;107:1590–1598.*
115. Schulzer M, Drance SM, Douglas GR: A comparison of treated and untreated glaucoma suspects. *Ophthalmology 1991;98:301–307.*
116. Grunwald JE: Effect of timolol maleate on the retinal circulation of human eyes with ocular hypertension. *Invest Ophthalmol Vis Sci 1990;31:521–526.*

117. Kass MA, Gordon M, Morley RE Jr, et al: Compliance with topical timolol treatment. *Am J Ophthalmol 1987;103:188–193.*
118. Krasnov MM: Laseropuncture of the anterior chamber angle in glaucoma. *Am J Ophthalmol 1973;75:674–678.*
119. Worthen DM, Wickham MG: Laser trabeculotomy in monkeys. *Invest Ophthalmic Vis Sci 1973;12:707–711.*
120. Gaasterland DE, Kupfer C: Experimental glaucoma in the rhesus monkey. *Invest Ophthalmol Vis Sci 1974;13:455–457.*
121. Wise JB, Witter SL: Argon laser therapy for open-angle glaucoma; a pilot study. *Arch Ophthalmol 1979;97:319–322.*
122. Wilensky JT, Jampol LM: Laser therapy for open-angle glaucoma. *Ophthalmology 1981;88:213–217.*
123. Schwartz AL, Whitten ME, Bleiman B, Martin D: Argon laser trabeculoplasty in uncontrolled phakic open-angle glaucoma. *Ophthalmology 1981;88:203–212.*
124. Van Buskirk EM: Pathophysiology of laser trabeculoplasty. *Surv Ophthalmol 1989;33:264–272.*
125. Byslma SB, Samples JR, Acott TS, Van Buskirk EM: Trabecular cell division after argon laser trabeculoplasty. *Am I Ophthalmol 1988; 106:544–547.*
126. Wilensky JT, Weinreb RN: Low dose trabeculoplasty. *Am J Ophthalmol 1983;95:423–426.*
127. Reiss G, Wilensky JT, Higginbotham EJ: Laser trabeculoplasty. *Surv Ophthalmol 1991;35:407–428.*
128. Rouhiainen HJ, Terasvirta ME, Tuovinen EJ: The effect of some treatment variables on the results of trabeculoplasty. *Arch Ophthalmol 1988;106:611:614.*
129. Thomas JV, Simmons RJ, Belcher CD: Argon laser trabeculoplasty in the presurgical glaucoma patient. *Ophthalmology 1982;89:187–197.*
130. Higginbotham EJ, Richardson TM: Response of exfoliation glaucoma to laser trabeculoplasty. *Br J Ophthalmol 1986;709:837–839.*
131. Brown SLV, Thomas JV, Budenz DL, et al: Effect of cataract surgery on intraocular pressure reduction obtained with laser trabeculoplasty. *Am J Ophthalmol 1985;100:3 73–376.*
132. Traverso CE, Greenidge KC, Spaeth GL: Formation of peripheral anterior synechiae following argon laser trabeculoplasty. *Arch Ophthalmol 1984; 102:861–863.*
133. Wilensky JT, Weinreb RN: Early and late failures of argon laser trabeculoplasty. *Arch Ophthalmol 1983;101:895–897.*
134. Safran MJ, Robin AL, Pollack IP: Argon laser trabeculoplasty in younger patients with primary open-angle glaucoma. *Am J Ophthalmol 1984;97:292–295.*
135. Traverso CE, Spaeth GL, Starita RJ, et al: Factors affecting the results of argon laser trabeculoplasty in open-angle glaucoma. *Ophthal Surg 1986;17:554–559.*
136. Schwartz AL, Love DC, Schwartz MH: Long-term follow-up of argon laser trabeculoplasty for uncontrolled glaucoma. *Arch Ophthalmol 1985; 103: 1482–1484.*
137. Glaucoma Laser Trial Research Group: The Glaucoma Laser Trial. 1. Acute effects of argon laser trabeculoplasty on intraocular pressure. *Arch Ophthalmol 1989;107:1135–1142.*
138. Weinreb RN, Ruderman I, Justin R, Zweig K: Immediate intraocular pressure response to argon laser trabeculoplasty. *Am J Ophthalmol 1983;95:279–281.*
139. Ofner S, Samples JR, Van Buskirk EM: Pilocarpine and the increase in intraocular pressure after trabeculoplasty. *Am J Ophthalmol 1984; 97:647–649.*
140. Robin AL, Pollack IP, Hause B, Enger C: Effect of ALO-2145 on intraocular pressure following argon laser trabeculoplasty. *Arch Ophthalmol 1987; 105:646–650.*
141. Pappas HR, Berry DP, Partamian L, et al: Topical indomethacin therapy before argon laser trabeculoplasty. *Am J Ophthalmol 1985; 99:571–575.*

142. Hoskins HD, Hetherington J, Minckler DS, et al: Complications of laser trabeculoplasty. *Ophthalmology 1983;90:796–799.*
143. Shingleton BJ, Richter CU, Bellows AR, et al: Long-term efficacy of argon laser trabeculoplasty. *Ophthalmology 94:1513–1518.*
144. Starita RJ, Fellman RL, Spaeth GL, Poryzees E: The effect of repeating full-circumference argon laser trabeculoplasty. *Ophthal Surg 1984 ;15:41–43.*
145. Brown SVL, Thomas JV, Simmons RJ: Laser trabeculoplasty retreatment. *Am J Ophthalmol 1985;99:8–10.*
146. Grayson DK, Camras CB, Podos SM, Lustgarten JS: Long-term reduction of intraocular pressure after repeat argon laser trabeculoplasty. *Am J Ophthalmol 1988;106:312–321.*
147. Tuulonen A, Niva AK, Alanko HI: A controlled five-year follow-up study of laser trabeculoplasty as primary therapy for open-angle glaucoma. *Am I Ophthalmol 1987;104:334–338.*
148. Migdal C, Hitchings R: Control of chronic simple glaucoma with primary medical surgical and laser treatment. *Trans Ophthalmol Soc UK 1986; 105:653–656.*
149. Glaucoma Laser Trial Research Group: The Glaucoma Laser Trial. 1. Acute effects of argon laser trabeculoplasty versus topical medication. *Ophthalmology 1990;97:1403–1413.*
150. Hoskins HD Jr, Kass MA: Laser treatment for internal flow block, in Hoskins HD Jr, Kass MA (eds): *Becker-Shaffer's Diagnosis and Therapy of the Glaucomas,* ed 6. St. Louis: CV Mosby, 1989, 499–510.
151. Shields MB: Surgery of the iris, in Shields MB (ed): *Textbook of Glaucoma,* ed 3. Baltimore: Williams & Wilkins, 1992, 561–576.
152. Higginbotham EJ, Shahbazi MF: Laser therapy in glaucoma: An overview and update. *Int Ophthalmol Clin 1990;30:187–197.*
153. Schwartz AL, Martin NF, Weber PA: Corneal decompensation after argon laser iridotomy. *Arch Ophthalmic 1988;106:1572–1574.*
154. Moster MR, Schwartz LW, Spaeth GL, et al: Laser iridectomy: A controlled study comparing argon and neodymium:YAG. *Ophthalmology 1986;93:20–24.*
155. Robin AL, Pollack IP, deFaller JM: Effects of ALO 2145 (p-aminoclonidine hydrochloride) on the intraocular pressure rise after argon laser iridotomy. *Arch Ophthalmol 1987;105:1208–1211.*
156. Robin AL, Pollack IP: A comparison of neodymium:YAG and argon laser iridectomies. *Ophthalmology 1984;91:1011–1016.*
157. Goins K, Schmeisser E, Smith T: Argon laser pretreatment in Nd:YAG iridotomy. *Ophthal Surg 1990;21:497–500.*
158. Kimbrough RL, Trempe CS, Brockhurst RJ, Simmons RJ: Angle-closure glaucoma in nanophthalmos. *Am J Ophthalmol 1979;88:572–579.*
159. Burton TC, Folk JC: Laser iris retraction for angle-closure glaucoma after retinal detachment surgery. *Ophthalmology 1988;95:742–748.*
160. Benedikt O: Die darstellung des kammer wasserabflusses normalen und glaucomlkranker menschlicher augen durch fullung der vorderkammer mit fluorescein. *Graefes Arch Clin Exp Ophthalmol 1976;199:45–67.*
161. Kronfeld PC: Chemical demonstration of transconjunctival passage after antiglaucomatous operations. *Am J Ophthalmol 1952;35(#5,part 2;ARVO Proceedings):38–45.*
162. Scheie H: Retraction of scleral wound edges as a fistulizing procedure for glaucoma. *Am J Ophthalmol 1958;45:20–228.*
163. Hoskins Jr HD, Kass M: *Becker-Shaffer's Diagnosis and Therapy of the Glaucomas,* ed. 6. St Louis: CV Mosby, 1989, 554–560, 564–565.
164. Holth S: Iridenclesis cum iridotomia meridionali. *Arch Ophthalmol 1930;4:803–816.*
165. Melamed S, Fiore PM: Molteno implant surgery in refractory glaucoma. *Surv Ophthalmol 1990;34:441–448.*
166. Cairns JE: Trabeculectomy. Preliminary report of a new method. *Am J Ophthalmol 1968;66:673–679.*
167. Grant M: Further studies on facility of flow through the trabecular meshwork. *Arch Ophthalmol 1958;60:523–533.*

168. Starita RJ, Fellman RL, Spaeth GL, Poryzees E: Effect of varying size of scleral flap and corneal block on trabeculectomy. *Ophthalmic Surg 1984;15:484–487.*
169. Lamping K, Bellows R, Hutchinson T, Afran S: Long-term evaluation of initial filtration surgery. *Ophthalmology 1986;93:91–101.*
170. Skuta G, Parrish R: Wound healing in glaucoma filtering surgery. *Surv Ophthalmol 1987;32:149–170.*
171. Radius RL, Herschler J, Claflin A, Fiorentino G: Aqueous humor changes after experimental filtering surgery. *Am J Ophthalmol 1980;89:250–254.*
172. Joseph JP, Miller MH, Hitchings RA: Wound healing as a barrier to successful filtration surgery. *Eye 1988;2:5113–5123.*
173. The Fluorouracil Filtering Surgery Study Group: Fluorouracil filtering surgery study one-year follow-up. *Am J Ophthalmol 1989;108: 625–635.*
174. Grehn F, Mauthe S, Pfeiffer N: Limbus-based versus fornix-based conjunctival flap in filtering surgery. *Int Ophthalmol 1989;13:139–143.*
175. Alpar JJ: Sodium hyaluronate (Healon) in glaucoma filtering procedures. *Ophthalmic Surg 1986;17:724–730.*
176. Kolker AE, Hetherington J: *Becker-Shaffer's Diagnosis and Therapy of the Glaucomas,* ed 5. St. Louis: CV Mosby, 1983, 453–454, 509.
177. Watson PG, Grierson I: The place of trabeculectomy in the treatment of glaucoma. *Ophthalmology 1981;88:175–196.*
178. Heuer DK, Gressel MG, Parrish RK, et al: Trabeculectomy in aphakic eyes. *Ophthalmology 1984;91:1045–1051.*
179. Bellows AR, Johnstone MA: Surgical management of chronic glaucoma in aphakia. *Ophthalmology 1983;90:807–813.*
180. Schwartz AL, Anderson DR: Trabecular surgery. *Arch Ophthalmol 1974;92:134–138.*
181. Parrish RK, Hershler J: Eyes with endstage neovascular glaucoma; natural history following successful modified filtering operation. *Arch Ophthalmol 1983;101:745–746.*
182. Herschler J, Agness D: A modified filtering operation for neovascular glaucoma. *Arch Ophthalmol 1979;97:2339–2341.*
183. Madsen PH: Experiences in the surgical treatment of haemorrhagic glaucoma: A follow-up study. *Acta Ophthalmol 1973;120(suppl):88–91.*
184. Gressel MG, Heuer DK, Parrish RK: Trabeculectomy in young patients. *Ophthalmology 1984;91:1242–1246.*
185. Beauchamp GR, Parks MM: Filtering surgery in children: Barriers to success. *Ophthalmology 1979;86:170–180.*
186. Miller RD, Barber IC: Trabeculectomy in black patients. *Ophthal Surg 1981;12:46–50.*
187. Maumenee AE: External filtering operations for glaucoma: The mechanism of function and failure. *Trans Am Ophthalmol Soc 1960;58:319–325.*
188. Skuta GL, Parrish RK: Wound healing in glaucoma filtering surgery. *Surv Ophthalmol 1987;32:149–170.*
189. Tahery MM, Lee DA: Review: Pharmacologic control of wound healing in glaucoma filtration surgery. *Ocul Pharmacol 1989;5:155–178.*
190. Cameron IL: Perspectives on drugs and the cell cycle, in Zimmerman AM, Padilla GM, Cameron IL (eds): *Drugs and the Cell Cycle.* New York: Academic Press, 1973, 6.
191. The Fluorouracil Filtering Surgery Study Group: Fluorouracil filtering surgery study one-year follow-up. *Am J Ophthalmol 1989;108:625–635.*
192. Weinreb RN: Adjusting the dose of 5-fluorouracil after filtration surgery to minimize side effects. *Ophthalmology 1987;94:564–570.*
193. Heuer DK, Parrish RK, Gressel MG, et al: 5-Fluorouracil and glaucoma filtering surgery: III. Intermediate follow-up of a pilot study. *Ophthalmology 1986;93:1537–1546.*
194. Rockwood EJ, Parrish RK, Heuer DK, et al: Glaucoma filtering surgery with 5–fluorouracil. *Ophthalmology 1987;94:1071–1078.*

195. Knapp A, Heuer DK, Stern GA, Driebe WT: Serious corneal complications of glaucoma filtering surgery with postoperative 5-fluorouracil. *Am Ophthalmol 1987;103:183–187.*
196. Nakano Y, Araie M, Shirato S: Effect of postoperative subconjunctival 5-fluorouracil injections on the surgical outcome of trabeculectomy in the Japanese. *Graefes Arch Clin Exp Ophthalmol 1989;227:569–574.*
197. Loftfleld K, Ball SF: 5-Fluorouracil (5-FU) in primary trabeculectomy: A randomized trial. *Invest Ophthalmol Vis Sci 1991;32(suppl):745.*
198. Mills KB: Trabeculectomy: A retrospective long-term follow-up of 444 cases. *Br J Ophthalmol 1981;65:790–795.*
199. Beeson CC, Skuta GS, Higginbotham EJ, et al: Randomized clinical trial of intraoperative subconjunctival mitomycin-C versus postoperative 5-fluorouracil. *Invest Ophthalmol Vis Sci 1991;32(suppl):1122.*
200. Chen C-W, Huang H-T, Sheu M-M: Enhancement of IOP control effect of trabeculectomy by local application of anticancer drug. *Acta XXV Concilium Ophthalmologicum, Rome, 1986;2:1487-1491.*
201. Palmer SS: Mitomycin as adjunct chemotherapy with trabeculectomy. *Ophthalmology 1991;98:317–321.*
202. Hayasaka S, Noda S, Yamamoto Y, et al: Postoperative instillation of lowdose mitomycin C in the treatment of primary pterygium. *Am J Ophthalmol 1988;106:715–718.*
203. Herbert H: Subconjunctival fistula formation. *Trans Ophthalmol Soc UK 1903;23:324–346.*
204. Holth S: Iridencleisis antiglaucoma. *Ann Ocul 1907;37:345–350.*
205. Elliot RH: A preliminary note on a new operative procedure for the establishment of a filtering cicatrix in the treatment of glaucoma. *Ophthalmoscope 1912;10:258–261.*
206. Rollett M, Moreau M: Traitement de phypopyon par le drainage capillaire de la chambre anterieure. *Rev Gen Ophthalmol 1906;25:481–489.*
207. Zorab A: The reduction of tension in chronic glaucoma. *Ophthalmoscope 1912;10:258–261.*
208. Mayou MS: A note on Zorab's operation of aqueoplasty. *Ophthalmoscope 1912;10:254–257.*
209. Wood CA: The sclerocomeal seton in the treatment of glaucoma. *Ophthamol Rec Chicago 1915;24:235–240.*
210. MacDonald RK, Pierce HF: Silicone setons. *Am I Ophthalmol 1965;59(4):635–646.*
211. Vail DT: Retained silk thread or 'seaton' drainage from vitreous chamber to Tenon's lymph channel for the relief of glaucoma. *Ophthamol Rec Chicago 1915;24:184–186.*
212. Row H: Operation to control glaucoma: preliminary report. *Arch Ophthalmol 1934;12:325–329.*
213. Troncosco MU: Cyclodialysis with insertion of a metal implant in the treatment of glaucoma: A preliminary report. *Arch Ophthalmol 1940;23:270–300.*
214. Troncosco MU: Use of tantalum implants for inducing a permanent hypotony in rabbits' eyes. *Am J Ophthalmol 1949;32:499–508.*
215. Stefansson J: An operation for glaucoma. *Am J Ophthalmol 1925; 8:681693.*
216. Pinnas G, Boniuk M: Cyclodialysis with teflon tube implants. *Am J Ophthalmol 1969;68:879–883.*
217. Ellis RA: Reduction of intraocular pressure using plastics in surgery. *Am J Ophthalmol 1960;50:733–743.*
218. Lehman RN, McCaslin MF: Gelatin film used as a seton in glaucoma. *Am J Ophthalmol 1959;47:690–691.*
219. Stone W: Alloplasty in surgery of the eye, I. *N Engl J Med 1958;258:48 490.*
220. Stone W: Alloplasty in surgery of the eye, II. *N Engl J Med 1958; 258:533–540.*
221. Richards RD, Van Bijsterveld OP: Artificial drainage tubes for glaucoma. *Am J Ophthalmol 1965;60:405–408.*
222. Mascati NT: A new surgical approach for the control of a class of glaucomas. *Int Surg 1967;47:10–15.*

223. Rajah-Sivayoham IS-S: Camero-venous shunt for secondary glaucoma following orbital venous obstruction. *Br J Ophthalmol 1968;52:843–845.*
224. Lee P-F, Wong W-T: Aqueous-venous shunt for glaucoma: Report on 15 cases. *Ann Ophthalmol 1974;6:1083–1088.*
225. Honrubia FM, Grijalbo MP, Gomez ML, Lopez A: Surgical treatment of neovascular glaucoma. *Trans Ophthalmol Soc UK 1979;99:89–91.*
226. Krupin T, Podos SM, Becker B, Newkirk JB: Valve implants in filtering surgery. A preliminary report. *Am J Ophthalmol 1976;81:232–235.*
227. Krupin T, Kaufman P, Mandell A, et al: Filtering valve implant for eyes with neovascular glaucoma. *Am J Ophthalmol 1980;89:338–343.*
228. Krupin T, Kaufman P, Mandell AI, et al: Long-term results of valve implants in filtering surgery for eyes with neovascular glaucoma. *Am I Ophthalmol 1983;95:775–782.*
229. Molteno ACB: New implant for glaucoma clinical trial. *Br J Ophthalmol 1969;53:606–615.*
230. Molteno ACB: Mechanisms of intraocular inflammation. *Trans Ophthalmol Soc NZ 1980;32:69–72.*
231. Schocket SS, Lakhanpal V, Richards RD: Anterior chamber tube shunt to an encircling band in the treatment of neovascular glaucoma. *Ophthalmology 1982;89:1188–1194.*
232. Kupin T, Ritch R, Camras CB, et al: A long Klupin-Denver valve implant attached to a 180 scleral explant for glaucoma surgery. *Ophthalmology 1988;95:1174–1180.*
233. Joseph NJ, Sherwood MB, Trantas G, Hitchings RA: A one piece drainage system for glaucoma surgery. *Trans Ophthalmol Soc UK 1986;105:657664.*
234. Molteno ACB: Use of Molteno implants to treat secondary glaucoma, in Cairns (ed): *Glaucoma.* London: Grune & Stratton, 1986 211–238.
235. Minckler DS, Shammas A, Wilcox M, Ogden T: Experimental studies of aqueous filtration using the Molteno implant. *Trans Am Ophthalmol Soc 1987;84:368–392.*
236. Schocket SS: Investigations of the reasons for success and failure in the anterior shunt-to-the-encircling-band procedure in the treatment of refractory glaucoma. *Trans Am Ophthalmol Soc 1986;84:743–798.*
237. Minckler DS, Krupin T: *Oral Presentation at the 1990 Meeting of the American Glaucoma Society,* MacKinaw Island, MI, 1990.
238. Molteno ACB, Strachan J, Ancker E: Long tube implants in the management of glaucoma. *S Afr Med 1976;50:1062–1066.*
239. Minckler DS, Heuer DK, Hasty B, et al: Clinical experience with the singleplate Molteno implant in complicated glaucomas. *Ophthalmology 1988;95:1181–1188.*
240. Heuer DK: *Single Versus Two-Plate Molteno Implant. Presentation at the American Academy of Ophthalmology Meeting.* Atlanta, GA: AAO, 1990.
241. Cohen JS, Osher RH: Releasable scleral flap suture, in Krupin T, Wax MB (eds): *New Techniques in Glaucoma Surgery.* Philadelphia: WB Saunders, 1988, 187-197.
242. Price FW, Whitson WE: Polypropylene ligatures as a means of controlling intraocular pressure with Molteno implants. *Ophthalmic Surg 1989;20:781–783 .*
243. Lieberman MF, Egbert PR: Internal suture occlusion of the Molteno glaucoma implant for the prevention of postoperative hypotony. *Ophthalmic Surg 1989;20:53–56.*
244. Ball SF, Loftfield K, Scharfenberg J: Molteno rip-cord suture hypopyon. *Ophthalmic Surg 1990;21:407–410.*
245. Baerveldt G, Smith RE, Heuer D, et al: Molteno implant for control of glaucoma in eyes after penetrating keratoplasty. *Ophthalmology 1988;95:364–369.*
246. Traverso CE, Tomey KF, al-Kaff A: The long-tube single plate Molteno implant for the treatment of recalcitrant glaucoma. *Int Ophthalmol 1989; 13: 159–162.*
247. Schocket SS, Nirankari VS, Lakhanpal V, et al: Anterior chamber tube shunt to an encirding band in the treatment of neovascular glau-

coma and other refractory glaucomas: A long term study. *Ophthalmology 1985;92:553–562.*

248. Wilson RP: The Schocket shunt, in Krupin T, Wax MB (eds): *New Techniques in Glaucoma Surgery.* Philadelphia: WB Saunders, 1988, 225–232.
249. Sherwood MB, Joseph NH, Hitchings RA: Surgery for refractory glaucoma: Results and complications with a modified Schocket technique. *Arch Ophthalmol 1987;l05:562–569.*
250. Hitchings RA, Joseph NH, Sherwood MB, et al: Use of one-piece valved tube and variable surface area explant for glaucoma drainage surgery. *Ophthalmology 1987;94:1079–1084.*
251. Krupin T: Setons in glaucoma surgery, in Waltman SR, Keates RH, Hoyt CS, et al (eds): *Surgery of the Eye.* New York: Churchill Livingstone, 1988,377–385.
252. Dewecker L: La sclerotomie interne. *Ann Ocul 1895;114:95–101.*
253. LaGrange F: De l'Iridectomie et de la sclerectomie combinées dans le traitement du glaucoma chronique. Procédé nouveau pour l'establissement de la cicatrice filtrante. *Bull Mem Soc Fr Ophthalmol 1906; 23:477–511.*
254. Elliot RH:*Sclero-Corneal Trephining in the Operative Treatment of Glaucoma,* ed 2. London George Pulman & Sons, 1914, 78.
255. Brown RH, Bruner WE, Denhan DB, et al: Trabeculectomy ab interno. *Invest Ophthalmol Vis Sci 1982;22(suppl):256.*
256. Brown RH, Lynch MG, et al: Ab interno filtering surgery. *Ophthalmol Clin North Am 1988;12:199–207.*
257. March WF, Gherezghiher T, Koss MC, et al: Experimental YAG laser sclerostomy. *Arch Ophtalmol 1984;102:1834–1836.*
258. L'Esperance F: *Ocular Photocoagulation.* St. Louis: CV Mosby, 1983.
259. March WF, Gherezghiher T, Koss MC, et al: Histologic study of a neodymium:YAG laser sclerostomy. *Arch Ophthalmol 1985;l03 860–863.*
260. Hoskins DH, Iwach AG, Vassiliadis A, et al: Subconjunctival THC:YAG laser thermal sclerostomy. *Ophthalmology 1991;98:1394–1400.*
261. Latina MA, March WF, Dobrogowski M, Birngruber R: Laser sclerostomy by pulsed dye laser and goniolens. *Arch Ophthalmol 1990;108: 1745–1750.*
262. Gaasterland DE, Hennings DR, Boutacoff TA, et al: Ab interno and ab extemo filtering operations by laser contact surgery. *Ophthal Surg 1987;18:254–257.*
263. Jaffe GJ, Williams GA, Mieler WF, et al: Ab interno sclerostomy with a high-powered argon endolaser. *Am J Ophthalmol 1988;106:391–396.*
264. Wilson RP, Javitt JC, Federman JL, et al: Contact Nd:YAG laser thermal sclerostomy ab interno in primates. *Ophthalmology 1988; 95(suppl):168.*
265. Federman IL, Wilson RP, Ando F, et al: Contact laser: Thermal sclerostomy ab interno. *Ophthal Surg 1987;18:726–727.*
266. Bietti G: Surgical intervention on the ciliary body. New trends for the relief of glaucoma. *JAMA 1950;142:889–897.*
267. Wilkes TDI, Fraunfelder FT: Principles of cryosurgery. *Ophthal Surg 1979; 10:21–30.*
268. Prost M: Cyclocryotherapy for glaucoma. Evaluation of techniques. *Surv Ophthalmol 1983;28:93–100.*
269. Caprioli J, Sears N: Regulation of intraocular pressure during cydocryotherapy for advanced glaucoma. *Am J Ophthalmol 1986; 101:542–545.*
270. Weekers R, Lavergne G, Watillon M, et al: Effects of photocoagulation of ciliary body upon ocular tension. *Am J Ophthalmol 1961; 52:156–163.*
271. Vucicevic ZM, Tsou KC, Nazarian IH, et al: A cytochemical approach to the laser coagulation of the ciliary body. *Mod Probl Ophthalmol 1969;8:467–478.*
272. Beckman H, Waeltermann J: Transscleral ruby laser cyclocoagulation. *Am J Ophthalmol 1984;98:788–795.*

273. Hampton C, Shields MB: Transscleral neodymium:YAG cyclophotocoagulation. A histologic study of human autopsy eyes. *Arch Ophthalmol 1988;106:1121–1123.*
274. Blasini M, Simmons R, Shields MB: Early tissue response to transscleral neodymium:YAG cyclophotocoagulation. *Invest Ophthalmol Vis Sci 1990;31:1114–1118.*
275. Allingham RR, de Kater AW, Bellows AR, Hsu J: Probe placement and power levels in contact transscleral neodymium:YAG cyclophotocoagulation. *Arch Ophthalmol 1990;108: 738–742.*
276. Schubert HD, Federman JL: The role of inflammation on CW Nd:YAG contact transsderal photocoagulation and cryopexy. *Invest Ophthalmol Vis Sci 1989;30:543–549.*
277. Shields MB, Blasini M, Simmons R, Erickson PJ: A contact lens for transscleral Nd:YAG cyclophotocoagulation. *Am J Ophthalmol 1989;108:457–458.*
278. Schuman JS, Puliafito CA, Allingham RR, et al: Contact transscleral continuous wave Nd:YAG laser cyclophotocoagulation. *Ophthalmology 1990;97:571–580.*
279. Hampton C, Shields MB, Miller KM, Blasini M: Evaluation of a protocol for transscleral neodymium:YAG cyclophotocoagulation in one hundred patients. *Ophthalmology 1990;97:910–917.*
280. Lee P-F, Pomerantzeff O: Transpupillary cyclophotocoagulation of rabbit eyes. An experimental approach to glaucoma surgery. *Am J Ophthalmol 1971;71:911–920.*
281. Shields S, Stewart WC, Shields MB: Transpupillary argon laser cyclophotocoagulation in the treatment of glaucoma. *Ophthal Surg 1988;l9:171–175.*
282. Shields MB: Cyclodestructive surgery for glaucoma: Past, present, and future. *Trans Am Ophthalmol Soc 1985;83:285–303.*
283. Zarbin MA, Michels RG, de Bustros S, et al: Endolaser treatment of the ciliary body for severe glaucoma. *Ophthalmology 1988;95:1639–1648.*
284. Shields MB, Chandler DB, Hickingbotham D, Klintworth GK: Intraocular cyclophotocoagulation. Histopathologic evaluation in primates. *Arch Ophthalmol 1985;103:1731–1735.*
285. Purnell EW, Sokollu A, Torchia R, Taner N: Focal chorioretinitis produced by ultrasound. *Invest Ophthalmol 1964;3:657–664.*
286. Coleman DJ, Lizzi FL, Driller J, et al: Therapeutic ultrasound in the treatment of glaucoma. II. Clinical applications. *Ophthalmology 1985; 92:347–353.*

INDEX

NUMBERS IN BOLD REFER TO FIGURES

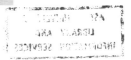